W9-BIZ-551

CANADIAN ESSENTIALS OF
NURSING
RESEARCH

Carmen G. Loiselle, PhD, RN
Assistant Professor
McGill University School of Nursing

Senior Researcher
Centre for Nursing Research, SMBD Jewish General Hospital
Montreal, Quebec
Canada

Joanne Profetto-McGrath, PhD, RN
Associate Professor
University of Alberta Faculty of Nursing
Edmonton, Alberta
Canada

Denise F. Polit, PhD
President
Humanalysis, Inc.
Saratoga Springs, New York

Cheryl Tatano Beck, DNSc,
   CNM, FAAN
Professor
University of Connecticut
   School of Nursing
Storrs, Connecticut

SECOND EDITION

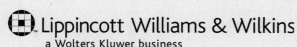
Lippincott Williams & Wilkins
a Wolters Kluwer business
Philadelphia · Baltimore · New York · London
Buenos Aires · Hong Kong · Sydney · Tokyo

Senior Acquisitions Editor: Margaret Zuccarini
Managing Editor: Helen Kogut
Editorial Assistant: Delema Caldwell-Jordan
Senior Production Manager: Helen Ewan
Senior Managing Editor/Production: Erika Kors
Art Director: Doug Smock
Design Coordinator: Joan Wendt
Manufacturing Manager: William Alberti
Indexer: Gaye Tarallo
Compositor: TechBooks
Printer: R. R. Donnelley/Crawfordsville

2nd Edition

Copyright © 2007 by Lippincott Williams & Wilkins.
Copyright © 2004 by Lippincott Williams & Wilkins. All rights reserved. This book is protected by copyright. No part of it may be reproduced, stored in a retrieval system, or transmitted, in any form or by any means—electronic, mechanical, photocopy, recording, or otherwise—without prior written permission of the publisher, except for brief quotations embodied in critical articles and reviews and testing and evaluation materials provided by publisher to instructors whose schools have adopted its accompanying textbook. Printed in the United States of America. For information write Lippincott Williams & Wilkins, 530 Walnut Street, Philadelphia PA 19106.

Materials appearing in this book prepared by individuals as part of their official duties as U.S. Government employees are not covered by the above-mentioned copyright.

9   8   7   6   5   4   3

Library of Congress Cataloging-in-Publication Data

ISBN: 13 978-0-7817-8416-0
ISBN: 0-7817-8416-6

Canadian essentials of nursing research / Carmen G. Loiselle . . . [et al.].—2nd ed.
    p. ; cm.
  Includes bibliographical references and index.
  ISBN 0-7817-8416-6 (alk. paper)
  I. Nursing—Research—Methodology.   2. Nursing—Research—Canada.   I. Loiselle, Carmen G.
  [DNLM: I. Nursing Research—methods—Canada. WY 20.5 C2115 2006]
  RT81.5.C355 2006
  610.73072—dc22

                                                                        2005028084

Care has been taken to confirm the accuracy of the information presented and to describe generally accepted practices. However, the authors, editors, and publisher are not responsible for errors or omissions or for any consequences from application of the information in this book and make no warranty, express or implied, with respect to the content of the publication.

The authors, editors, and publisher have exerted every effort to ensure that drug selection and dosage set forth in this text are in accordance with the current recommendations and practice at the time of publication. However, in view of ongoing research, changes in government regulations, and the constant flow of information relating to drug therapy and drug reactions, the reader is urged to check the package insert for each drug for any change in indications and dosage and for added warnings and precautions. This is particularly important when the recommended agent is a new or infrequently employed drug.

Some drugs and medical devices presented in this publication have Food and Drug Administration (FDA) clearance for limited use in restricted research settings. It is the responsibility of the health care provider to ascertain the FDA status of each drug or device planned for use in his or her clinical practice.

CANADIAN ESSENTIALS OF
NURSING
RESEARCH

Canadian Reviewers

Patricia Grainger, RN, BN, MN
Nurse Educator
Centre for Nursing Studies
St. John's, Newfoundland and Labrador

Anne Kearney, PhD, RN
Coordinator of Research Office; Faculty Member
Centre for Nursing Studies
St. John's, Newfoundland and Labrador

P. Jane Milliken, BSc (Nu), MA, PhD, RN
Associate Professor
School of Nursing, University of Victoria
Victoria, British Columbia

Beth Perry RN, BScN, PhD
Associate Professor
Athabasca University
Athabasca, Alberta

Pammla Petrucka, BScN, MN, PhD (C)
Assistant Professor
University of Saskatchewan
Regina, Saskatchewan

Jan Seeley, RN, HBScN, MEd, MScN(c)
Professor of Nursing
Confederation College
Thunder Bay, Ontario

Katherine M. Cox Stevenson, RN, BSN, MSN, PhD(c)
Nursing Faculty
Camosun College
Victoria, British Columbia

Gail Blair Storr, RN, MEd, MN, PhD
Professor
University of New Brunswick, Faculty of Nursing
Fredericton, New Brunswick

Preface

This second edition of *Canadian Essentials of Nursing Research* features state-of-the-art research undertaken by Canadian nurse researchers, as well as Canadian content relating to the history of nursing research, ethical considerations, models of nursing, and models of research utilization. At the same time, this edition contains all the innovative features that made the original award-winning text so popular. *Essentials of Nursing Research: Methods, Appraisal, and Utilization* is hailed worldwide by faculty, clinicians, and students alike for its up-to-date, clear, concise, and "user-friendly" presentation.

Nursing research is the conduct of systematic studies to generate new knowledge pertaining to health and illness-related experiences. Nurse researchers are scientists who seek answers to pressing questions through systematic observation and recording of phenomena relating to nursing practice. There is a growing expectation that nurses—especially those in clinical practice—will increasingly utilize the results of scientific studies as a basis for their practice. The need to apply new knowledge from research requires that we overcome the challenges related to accessing, reading, understanding, and translating research findings into practice. One main purpose of this book is to assist consumers of nursing research in evaluating the adequacy of research findings in terms of their scientific merit and potential for utilization.

The twenty-first century is a very exciting era for nursing research in Canada. The information age is revolutionizing the way we as nurses teach, practice, and conduct research. Current nursing research agendas are more dynamic, more responsive to social and health care delivery developments, and more accessible to nurse researchers, other health researchers, research users, funding agencies, and the public. The explosion of information technology has enabled clinicians and researchers to readily transcend geographical distances and disciplinary boundaries so that they may work together to answer important nursing questions. In addition, an ever increasing critical mass of well-funded nurse researchers makes for a more visible, productive, and collaborative health-related research enterprise. The unprecedented availability of funding for nursing research originates from new and innovative partnerships among federal and provincial governments, professional nursing associations, and private industry. We are also witnessing more concerted efforts on the part of nurse researchers to involve key stakeholders (e.g., lay individuals, nurses involved in direct care, clinical nurse specialists) in the design, conduct, evaluation, and dissemination of nursing research. One challenge for the future of Canadian nursing research, however, will be to augment the means through which research findings are more broadly disseminated—both academic and professional nursing journals in Canada remain scant.

Growing evidence indicates that the presentation of knowledge that is personally relevant to students contributes to optimal learning. The first Canadian adaptation of this textbook has clearly shown that students' timely exposure to research activities conducted by Canadian nurse researchers has enhanced their understanding and appreciation of nursing research.

The material gathered for this second Canadian edition is a testimony to the breadth and high quality of research conducted by these nurse researchers across the country. This second edition will continue to stimulate students to become well-informed consumers of research and to become more actively involved in the discovery of nursing knowledge. Research now plays a pivotal role in shaping the profession and the discipline of nursing and continues its contribution to better care and optimal health-related outcomes for Canadians. We are honored to have the opportunity to update *Canadian Essentials of Nursing Research* at a most promising moment in the history of nursing research in Canada.

New to This Edition

Enhanced Assistance in Critiquing Studies

This edition is more focused on the art—and science—of research critiques than ever before. Each chapter offers specific opportunities for critiquing aspects of a study or research report that was discussed in the chapter. In most chapters, students are invited to answer critiquing questions for up to four studies (usually two quantitative and two qualitative). Some exercises are based on studies that are included in their entirety in the appendices of the book (four full studies are included in this edition), while others are based on studies that are summarized at the end of the chapters. Students can then consult the accompanying CD-ROM to find our thoughts about each critiquing exercise, so that students can get immediate feedback about their grasp of material in the chapter. This edition also includes full critiques of two studies that are in the appendices, which students can use as models for a comprehensive research critique. Many more critiquing opportunities are available in the *Study Guide to Accompany Essentials of Nursing Research, Sixth Edition*, which includes seven studies in their entirety in the appendices.

More Emphasis on Evidence-Based Practice Implications

We have made several changes to ensure that this textbook will better help prepare students for evidence-based practice (EBP). We remind readers to think about the implications of research for EBP throughout the book, and emphasize that EBP relies on strong evidence from high-quality research. Some examples of how research evidence has affected nursing practice are introduced in the first chapter. We have also substantially revised the concluding chapter on research utilization and EBP. One particularly important addition is a discussion about how to critique integrative reviews (including meta-analyses and metasyntheses), which have become a cornerstone of EBP. Two integrative reviews are presented in their entirety in appendices of the *Study Guide to Accompany Essentials of Nursing Research, Sixth Edition*.

Better Coverage of Qualitative Research

Every new edition of *Essentials of Nursing Research: Methods, Appraisal, and Utilization* has improved on the quality and quantity of information provided to students about qualitative research. This Canadian edition is no exception. We describe the three main qualitative research traditions (ethnography, phenomenology, grounded theory) early in this book (Chapter 3) and then point out differences and similarities among them in subsequent chapters.

Greater Facilitation in Learning the Basics

Essentials of Nursing Research: Methods, Appraisal and Utilization has been widely hailed for its clear, concise, and "user-friendly" presentation. In this Canadian edition, we have gone to great lengths to write in an even simpler, more straightforward fashion—it is designed to help consumers progress fairly slowly into the complexities of disciplined research. In addition to our consumer "tips" we have added new "How-to-Tell" tips in many chapters that specifically help students learn how to identify fundamental features—for example, how to tell if a study is experimental or nonexperimental—or how to tell if a journal article is a study or something else.

Organization of the Text

The content of this edition is organized into six main parts.

Part 1—*Overview of Nursing Research* serves as the overall introduction to fundamental concepts in nursing research. Chapter 1 introduces and summarizes the history and future of nursing research both in Canada and elsewhere, discusses the philosophical underpinnings of qualitative research versus quantitative research, and describes the major purposes of nursing research. Chapter 2 introduces readers to key terms, with new emphasis on terms related to the quality of research evidence. Chapter 3 presents an overview of the steps in the research process for both qualitative and quantitative studies. Chapter 4 provides an introduction to research reports—what they are and how to read them. Chapter 5 is devoted to a discussion of ethics in research studies.

Part 2—*Preliminary Steps in the Research Process* includes three chapters and focuses on the steps that are taken in getting started on a research project. Chapter 6 focuses on the development of research questions and the formulation of research hypotheses. Chapter 7 discusses how to prepare and critique literature reviews. Chapter 8 presents information about theoretical and conceptual frameworks.

Part 3—*Designs for Nursing Research* presents material relating to the design of qualitative and quantitative nursing studies. Chapter 9 describes some fundamental design principles and discusses many specific aspects of quantitative research design. Chapter 10 addresses the various research traditions that have contributed to the growth of naturalistic inquiry and qualitative research. Chapter 11 provides an introduction to some specific types of research (e.g., evaluations, surveys, secondary analyses, case studies), and also describes integrated qualitative/quantitative designs. Chapter 12 presents various designs for sampling of study participants.

Part 4—*Data Collection* deals with the collection of research data. Chapter 13 discusses the full range of data collection options available to researchers, including both qualitative and quantitative approaches. Chapter 14, an especially important chapter for critiquing qualitative studies, explains methods of assessing data quality.

Part 5—*Data Analysis* is devoted to the organization and analysis of research data. Chapter 15 reviews methods of quantitative analysis. The chapter assumes no prior instruction in statistics and focuses primarily on helping readers to understand why statistics are needed, what tests might be appropriate in a given research situation, and what statistical information in a research report means. Chapter 16 presents a discussion of qualitative analysis, greatly expanded and improved in this edition.

Part 6—*Critical Appraisal and Utilization of Nursing Research* is intended to sharpen the critical awareness of consumers with respect to several key issues. Chapter 17 discusses the interpretation and appraisal of research reports. Chapter 18, the final chapter, offers guidance for research utilization and EBP.

Key Features

Research Examples: Each chapter includes critical thinking exercises that contain summaries of two or more actual research examples. (In this edition, we summarize the studies in an "abstract style" that we think will be more compelling.) Students are asked to evaluate features of these studies using the chapter's critiquing guidelines, with some supplementary questions targeted specifically to the selected study. Our suggested "answers" have been made available to students on the accompanying Student Resource CD-ROM. In addition, we used many actual recent nursing studies to illustrate key concepts in the text. The use of relevant examples is crucial to the development of both an understanding of and interest in the research process.

Consumer Tips: Each chapter contains numerous tips on what to expect in research reports vis-à-vis the topics that have been discussed in the chapter. In these tips, we have paid special attention to helping students read research reports, which are often daunting to those without specialized research training. This feature will enable students to translate the material presented in the textbook into meaningful concepts as they approach the research literature.

Guidelines for Critiquing Research Reports: Each chapter has a section devoted to guidelines for conducting a critique. These sections provide a list of questions that walk students through a study, drawing attention to aspects of the study that are amenable to appraisal by research consumers.

Features for Student Learning

To enhance and reinforce learning, we have used several features to guide students' attention:

Chapter Objectives: Learning objectives are identified on the chapter opener to focus students' attention on critical content.

Chapter Summary Points: A succinct list of summary points that focus on salient chapter content is included in each chapter.

Full-Length Research Examples: This edition includes four recent full-length examples of Canadian studies—two quantitative and two qualitative—that students can read, analyze, and critique. They appear in the appendices of the text.

Critical Thinking Activities: Each chapter of the textbook includes activities designed to reinforce student learning and provide opportunities to practice critiquing skills.

Suggested Readings: A list of methodologic references are provided in each chapter to direct the student's further inquiry.

Teaching-Learning Package

Essentials of Nursing Research: Methods, Appraisal, and Utilization, Sixth Edition has an ancillary package designed with both students and instructors in mind. These materials are available for students and instructors using *Canadian Essentials of Nursing Research.*

The *Study Guide to Accompany Essentials of Nursing Research, Sixth Edition* augments the text and provides students with application exercises for each text chapter. Critiquing skills are emphasized, but there are also activities to support the learning of fundamental research terms. This edition offers exercises designed to reinforce learning while at the same time being "fun"—specifically, crossword puzzles with new terms have been developed for each chapter. Seven recent studies are included in the appendices, and many chapter exercises are based on these studies.

Free CD-ROM: The *Study Guide to Accompany Essentials of Nursing Research, Sixth Edition* also includes a CD-ROM providing 290 review questions to assist students in self-testing. This review program provides the rationale for both correct and incorrect answers, helping students to identify areas of strength and areas needing further study.

The Instructor's Resource CD-ROM for Essentials of Nursing Research, Sixth Edition includes a chapter for every chapter in the textbook. Each chapter of the instructor's manual contains the following: Statement of Intent, Special Class Projects, Answers to Selected Study Guide Exercises, and Test Questions and Answers. In the special class projects, we offer opportunities (new in this edition) for students to develop quantitative and (or) qualitative data sets. With regard to test questions to evaluate student learning, we offer in this edition multiple choice and true/false questions (as in previous editions), but we have added questions specifically designed to test students' comprehension of research reports.

Carmen G. Loiselle, PhD, RN
Joanne Profetto-McGrath, PhD, RN
Denise F. Polit, PhD
Cheryl Tatano Beck, DNSc, CNM, FAAN

In Appreciation

Because of the great success of the first edition of *Canadian Essentials of Nursing Research*, we were excited to undertake the write-up of this second edition. The preparation of the first edition led to such stimulating exchanges with Canadian nurse researchers across the country that when recontacted, their enthusiasm for the project was as keen as ever. We are most thankful to all our nursing colleagues for sharing their research findings with us and for providing "behind the scenes" insights that were incorporated into this revised edition.

We are indebted to the Lippincott team, Carol McGimpsey, Corey Wolfe, Barry Wight, Margaret Zuccarini, and Helen Kogut, who were great believers in the "Canadianization" of *Essentials of Nursing Research* and wonderful promoters of the book. Given its great success, they felt the need to undertake as soon as possible the preparation of this second edition.

Two institutions deserve special mention. McGill University and the University of Alberta provided the authors a wonderfully supportive and stimulating intellectual environment that fostered interesting discussions about nursing research in Canada. We also thank our colleagues Margaret Purden, Nancy Feeley, Susan French, Dorothy Forbes, Laurie Gottlieb, Joan Bottorff, Lesley Degner, Carole Estabrooks, Greta Cummings, Wendy Austin, Connie Winther, and Barbara Dussault for their contagious passion for nursing research, sense of humor, and unwavering support. We wish to acknowledge the precious assistance of medical librarian Robin Canuel, MLIS, from the Centre for Nursing Research at the SMBD Jewish General Hospital in Montreal for his enthusiastic assistance, timely literature searches, and for most efficiently forwarding requested papers to us.

As was true for the first edition of *Canadian Essentials of Nursing Research*, most credit goes to the original authors of *Essentials of Nursing Research: Methods, Appraisal, and Utilization*. Denise Polit, a rigorous, efficient, and dedicated colleague and friend who took the lead in the revised and updated second edition and made sure that all coauthors shared in the decisions to include particular studies and revise, delete, or develop new sections of the book. Our warmest thanks also go to coauthor Cheryl Tatano Beck for her timely feedback, suggestions for improvement, and keen eye for methodologic details.

To each of the above individuals we are indebted. Collectively, they made the production of the second edition a most pleasant, stimulating, and gratifying experience.

Last, we wish to acknowledge our families and friends to whom this book is dedicated. They remained most supportive and understanding throughout its preparation—from beginning to end.

Contents

Overview of Nursing Research

Introducing Research and Its Use in Nursing Practice

STUDENT OBJECTIVES

On completing this chapter, you will be able to:

▶ Describe why research is important in the nursing profession and why evidence-based practice is needed
▶ Describe historical trends and future directions in nursing research
▶ Describe alternative sources of evidence for nursing practice
▶ Describe major characteristics of the positivist and naturalistic paradigms, and discuss similarities and differences between the traditional scientific method (quantitative research) and naturalistic methods (qualitative research)
▶ Identify several purposes of qualitative and quantitative research
▶ Define new terms in the chapter

AN INTRODUCTION TO NURSING RESEARCH

It is an exciting—and challenging—time to be a nurse. Nurses are managing their clinical responsibilities at a time when the nursing profession and the larger health care system require an extraordinary range of skills and talents of them. Nurses are expected to deliver the highest possible quality care in a compassionate manner, while also being mindful of costs. To accomplish these diverse (and sometimes conflicting) goals, nurses continually need to access and evaluate new information, and incorporate it into their clinical decision making. In today's world, *nurses must become lifelong learners,* capable of reflecting on, evaluating, and modifying their clinical practice based on emerging knowledge from nursing and health care research.

What Is Nursing Research?

Research is systematic inquiry that uses disciplined methods to answer questions or solve problems. The ultimate goal of research is to develop and expand a base of knowledge.

Nurses are increasingly engaged in disciplined studies that benefit the profession and its patients. **Nursing research** is designed to develop evidence about issues of importance to nurses, including nursing practice, nursing education, and nursing administration.

In this book, we emphasize clinical nursing research, that is, research designed to generate evidence to guide nursing practice and to improve the care and quality of life of patients. Clinical nursing research typically begins with questions stemming from practice-related problems—problems such as ones you may have already encountered.

Examples of nursing research questions

▶ What is the effect of *waiting,* among patients preparing for first-time elective coronary angiography, on the patients' anxiety and health-related quality of life (DeJong-Watt & Arthur, 2004)?
▶ What are the factors that facilitate or constrain individual efforts to implement changes in health behaviours (Angus, Evans, Lapum, Rukholm, St. Onge, Nolan, & Michel, 2005)?

The Importance of Research in Nursing

Nurses increasingly are expected to adopt an **evidence-based practice** (EBP), which is broadly defined as the use of the best clinical evidence in making patient care decisions. Evidence can come from various sources, but there is general agreement that research findings from rigorous studies constitute the best type of evidence for informing nurses' decisions and actions. Nurses are coming to recognize the need to base specific nursing actions and decisions on evidence indicating that the actions are appropriate, cost-effective, and result in positive client outcomes. Nurses who incorporate high-quality research evidence into their clinical practice are being professionally accountable to their clients. Evidence for clinical nursing decisions comes from both nursing studies and studies in a broad array of other disciplines.

Another reason for nurses to engage in research involves the cost-containment practices being instituted in health care facilities. Now, more than ever, nurses need to document the effectiveness of their practice not only to the profession but also to nursing care consumers, health care administrators, insurance companies, and government agencies. Some research findings will help eliminate nursing actions that do not achieve desired outcomes. Other findings will help nurses identify the practices that improve health care outcomes and contain costs as well.

Example of evidence-based practice

Numerous clinical practice changes over the past two decades reflect the impact of research. For example, "kangaroo care" (the holding of diaper-clad preterm infants skin-to-skin, chest-to-chest by parents) is now practiced in many neonatal intensive care units (NICUs), but this is a new trend. As recently as the early 1990s, only a few NICUs offered kangaroo care options. The adoption of this practice reflects the accumulating evidence that early skin-to-skin contact has clinical benefits to infants and families without any apparent negative side effects (Dodd, 2005). Some of that evidence was developed in rigorous studies by nurse researchers in Canada, the United States, Australia, Taiwan, and other countries. For example, Celeste Johnston and her colleagues at McGill University (2003) found that kangaroo care was effective in diminishing the pain response of preterm neonates (Johnston, Stevens, Pinelli, Gibbins, Fillion, Jack, Stele, Boyer, & Veilleux, 2003).

Nursing research can help in a broad array of problem-solving situations. Research enables nurses to assess the need for an intervention, identify factors that must be considered in planning nursing care, predict the probable outcomes of nursing decisions, control the occurrence of undesired outcomes, provide advice to enhance client health, and initiate activities to promote appropriate client behaviour. These are all activities that nurses already undertake; research findings can enhance the likelihood that the activities will have the desired results.

CONSUMER TIP

Every time you make a clinical decision or undertake a procedure, your action is based on something—perhaps what you learned in school, what you read in a book or journal, what you were told to do by a supervisor, or what your "intuition" tells you is appropriate. It is a professional responsibility to ask: How do I *know* this is really the most effective decision or action? Some practices that are based on tradition rather than on research are simply *not* the best way to do things. ▬

Roles of Nurses in Research

With the current emphasis on EBP, it has become *every* nurse's responsibility to engage in one or more research activities along a continuum of research participation. At one end of the continuum are nurses whose involvement in research is indirect. Users (consumers) of nursing research read research reports to develop new skills and to keep up-to-date on findings that may affect their practice. Nurses are expected to maintain this level of involvement with research, at a minimum. **Research utilization**—the use of findings from research in a practice setting—depends on competent nursing research consumers.

At the other end of the continuum are nurses who design and undertake research. At one time, most nurse researchers were academics who taught in nursing schools, but research is increasingly being conducted by practicing nurses who want to find what works best for their patients.

Example of research by hospital-based nurses

Tranmer, Minard, Fox, and Rebelo (2003), who worked at the Kingston General Hospital in Ontario, undertook a study to better understand the sleep experience of medical and surgical patients during a hospital stay. They found that a number of personal and environmental factors in the unit, many of which were amenable to change, significantly influenced patients' sleep.

Between these two end points lie a rich variety of research-related activities in which nurses engage to improve their effectiveness and enhance their professional lives. Even if you never conduct a study, you may well do one or more of the following:

▶ Participate in a **journal club** in a practice setting, which involves regular meetings among nurses to discuss and critique research articles
▶ Attend research presentations at professional conferences
▶ Evaluate completed research for its possible use in practice
▶ Help to develop an idea for a clinical study
▶ Review a proposed research plan and offer clinical expertise to improve the plan
▶ Assist researchers in collecting information for a study (e.g., distributing questionnaires to clients)
▶ Provide information and advice to clients who are participating in studies
▶ Discuss the implications and relevance of research findings with clients

CONSUMER TIP

Here is a headline about a health study of more than 16,000 nurses that appeared in newspapers throughout Canada and the United States in September 2004: "Walking Might Ward Off Alzheimer's." According to the study, which included nurses aged 70 to 81, even those who walked as little as 1½ hours per week did better on tests of mental function than those who were less active. What would you say if clients asked you about this study? Would you be able to comment on the believability of the findings, based on your assessment of how rigorously the study was conducted? You should be able to do this after completing this course. ■

In all these possible research-related activities, nurses who have some research skills are better able to make a contribution to nursing and to EBP than those who do not. A knowledge of nursing research can improve the depth and breadth of every nurse's practice. Learning about research methods allows you to evaluate and synthesize new information (i.e., become an informed research consumer), acquire knowledge that can be used in practice, and engage meaningfully in various research-related roles.

NURSING RESEARCH: PAST, PRESENT, AND FUTURE

Although nursing research has not always had the prominence and importance it enjoys today, its long and interesting history portends a distinguished future. Table 1.1 summarizes some of the key events in the historical evolution of nursing research.

TABLE 1.1   Historical Landmarks Affecting Nursing Research

YEAR	EVENT
1859	Florence Nightingale's *Notes on Nursing* published
1923	Columbia University in New York establishes first doctoral program for nurses
1932	Weir report, jointly sponsored by the Canadian Nurses Association and the Canadian Medical Association, is published
1930s	*American Journal of Nursing* publishes clinical case studies
1952	The journal *Nursing Research* begins publication
1955	Inception of the American Nurses Foundation to sponsor nursing research
1957	Establishment of nursing research center in the United States at Walter Reed Army Institute of Research
1959	First master's degree is nursing program established at the University of Western Ontario
1963	*International Journal of Nursing Studies* begins publication
1965	American Nurses Association (ANA) begins sponsoring nursing research conferences
1969	*Canadian Journal of Nursing Research* begins publication under the leadership of Dr. Moyra Allen
1971	ANA establishes a Commission on Research
1972	ANA establishes its Council of Nurse Researchers
	Canadian Helen Shore publishes first study on research–practice gap in nursing
1976	Stetler and Marram publish guidelines on assessing research for use in practice
1978	The journals *Research in Nursing & Health* and *Advances in Nursing Science* begin publication
1979	*Western Journal of Nursing Research* begins publication
1982	Alberta Heritage Foundation for Nursing Research is established and becomes first granting agency in Canada to exclusively fund nursing research
	The Conduct and Utilization of Research in Nursing (CURN) project publishes report
1983	*Annual Review of Nursing Research* begins publication
1986	National Center for Nursing Research (NCNR) is established within U.S. National Institutes of Health
1988	The journals *Applied Nursing Research* and *Nursing Science Quarterly* begin publication
1989	U.S. Agency for Health Care Policy and Research is established (renamed Agency for Healthcare Research and Quality, or AHRQ, in 1999)
1991	First fully funded nursing doctoral program established at the University of Alberta; second program established at University of British Columbia later in the year
1992	The journal *Clinical Nursing Research* begins publication
1993	NCNR becomes a full NIH institute, the National Institute of Nursing Research (NINR)
	Cochrane Collaboration is established
1994	The journal *Qualitative Health Research* begins publication under the leadership of renowned Canadian nurse researcher Dr. Janice Morse
1997	Canadian Health Services Research Foundation is established with federal funding
1998	Sigma Theta Tau International, in cooperation with faculty at the University of Toronto, sponsors the first international conference on research utilization
1999	Canadian Government established $25 million Nursing Research Fund to be administered by the Canadian Health Services Research over a period of 10 years
2000	NINR issues funding priorities for 2000–2004; annual funding exceeds $100 million
	Canadian Institutes of Health Research (CIHR) is launched
2004	Sigma Theta Tau International begins publishing the journal *Worldviews on Evidence-Based Nursing*

The Early Years: From Nightingale to the 1960s

Most people would agree that nursing research began with Florence Nightingale. Based on her skilful analyses of factors affecting soldier mortality and morbidity during the Crimean War, she was successful in effecting some changes in nursing care—and, more generally, in public health. Her landmark publication, *Notes on Nursing* (1859), describes her early research interest in environmental factors that promote physical and emotional well-being—an interest of nurses that continues nearly 150 years later.

For many years after Nightingale's work, the nursing literature contained little research. Some attribute this absence to the apprenticeship nature of nursing. The pattern of nursing research that eventually emerged at the turn of the century was closely aligned with the problems confronting nurses. For example, most studies in the early 1900s concerned nursing education. As more nurses received university-based education, studies about nursing students became more numerous. When hospital staffing patterns changed, researchers focused not only on the supply and demand of nurses but also on the amount of time required to perform certain nursing activities. During these years, nursing struggled with its professional identity, and nursing research took a twist toward studying nurses: what they did, how other groups perceived them, and who entered the profession.

In the 1950s, a number of forces combined to put nursing research on the rapidly accelerating upswing it is on today. More nurses with advanced academic preparation, government funding and the establishment of the journal *Nursing Research* in the United States, and upgraded research skills among nursing faculty are some of the forces propelling nursing research. In the late 1950s, the need for studies addressing clinical nursing problems was recognized.

During the 1960s, clinical nursing research began in earnest as practice-oriented research on various clinical topics emerged in the literature. Nursing research advanced worldwide: the *International Journal of Nursing Studies* began publication in 1963, and the *Canadian Journal of Nursing Research* appeared in 1969. Also, the seeds for EBP were planted by the U.K.-based Royal College of Nursing Study of Nursing Care, which began assessing clinical effectiveness.

Nursing Research Since 1970

By the 1970s, the growing number of nursing studies and the increased discussion of theoretical and contextual issues created the need for additional communication outlets. Several other journals that focus on nursing research were established in the 1970s, including *Advances in Nursing Science, Research in Nursing & Health*, the *Western Journal of Nursing Research,* and the *Journal of Advanced Nursing.* During that decade, there was a notable shift in emphasis from areas such as teaching and administration to the improvement of patient care. Nurses also began to pay more attention to the utilization of research findings in nursing practice. A seminal article by Stetler and Marram (1976) offered guidance on assessing research for application in practice settings.

Several events in the 1980s provided impetus for nursing research. For example, the first volume of the *Annual Review of Nursing Research* was published in 1983. These annual reviews include summaries of current research knowledge on selected areas of nursing practice and encourage the use of research findings. In Canada, as elsewhere, the production and dissemination of nursing knowledge have been linked to the availability of government funding. Federal funding for nursing research became available in Canada in the late 1980s through the National Health Research Development Program (NHRDP) and the Medical Research Council of Canada (MRC). Similarly, in the United States, the National Center for Nursing Research (NCNR) within the National Institutes of Health (NIH) was established in 1986. Also in the 1980s, nurses began to conduct formal research utilization projects, and an important new journal was established: *Applied Nursing Research*. This journal includes research reports on studies of special relevance to practicing nurses. And in Australia, the *Australian Journal of Nursing Research* was launched in the 1980s.

Forces outside of nursing in the late 1980s helped to shape today's nursing research landscape. A group from the McMaster Medical School designed a clinical learning strategy that was called evidence-based medicine (EBM). EBM, which promulgated the view that research findings were far superior to the opinions of authorities as a basis for clinical decisions, constituted a profound shift for medical practice and has had a major effect on all health care professions. In 1989, the U.S. government established an agency that is now known as the Agency for Healthcare Research and Quality (AHRQ). AHRQ is the U.S. agency that has been charged with supporting research specifically designed to improve the quality of health care, reduce health costs, and enhance patient safety; it plays a pivotal role in the promulgation of EBP in the United States and also in Canada. International cooperation around the issue of EBP in nursing also began to develop in the 1990s. For example, the Honor Society of Nursing, Sigma Theta Tau International, began to focus attention on research utilization and sponsored the first international research utilization conference, in cooperation with the faculty of the University of Toronto, in 1998.

After a long crusade by nursing organizations in the United States, nursing research was given more visibility and clout in 1993 when NCNR was promoted to full institute status within NIH. The birth of the **National Institute of Nursing Research** (NINR) helped to put nursing research into the mainstream of research activities enjoyed by other health disciplines in the United States. Funding for nursing research has also grown. In 1986, the NCNR had a budget of $16.2 million, whereas in fiscal year 2005, the budget for NINR was more than $130 million.

Funding opportunities for nursing research expanded in Canada as well during the 1990s. The **Canadian Health Services Research Foundation** (CHSRF) was established in 1997 with an endowment from federal funds, and plans for the **Canadian Institutes of Health Research** (CIHR) were underway. Beginning in 1999, the CHSRF earmarked $25 million for nursing research conducted in the health services research domain. Likewise, CIHR, Canada's major federal funding agency for health research, is now becoming an important source of funding for nursing research. However, unlike the United States, the various institutes in the CIHR (13 to date) do not include a separate institute for nursing research. Although this means that Canadian nurse investigators must compete for funding with scientists from all disciplines within the CIHR-designated fields of science, some have argued that this has strengthened nursing science and honed nurse scientists' competitive edge (Estabrooks, 2004). Several CHSRF/CIHR Chair Awards were recently granted to key investigators within the Canadian nursing research community. These 10-year awards are designed to promote knowledge generation and knowledge transfer in various nursing specialties (e.g., oncology nursing, community health, nursing human resources). In addition to federal funding, most provincial governments increasingly have been providing funding to stimulate the development of specific programs of nursing research. For example, in 2002, the Ontario Ministry of Health and Long Term Care awarded nearly $6 million to nurse researchers.

Example of a CHSRF/CIHR Chair Award recipient

Dr. Lesley Degner is a prominent nurse researcher who has focused considerable research on ways to reduce the burden of cancer for individuals and families. She is a professor of nursing at the University of Manitoba and senior investigator of the cancer nursing research group. She and her colleagues have completed numerous studies, including an investigation of the meaning of breast cancer to women at various points after diagnosis (Degner, Hack, O'Neil, & Kristjanson, 2003), a study of participation in medical decision making among women with breast cancer (Hack, Degner, Watson, & Sinha, 2005), and families' and children's experiences of a childhood cancer symptom trajectory (Woodgate & Degner, 2004). Her program as a CHSRF/CIHR Chair is called *Development of Evidence-Based Nursing Practice in Cancer Care, Palliative Care, and Cancer Prevention.*

In addition to growth in funding opportunities for nursing research internationally, the 1990s witnessed the birth of several more journals for nurse researchers, including *Qualitative Health Research*, *Clinical Nursing Research*, and *Clinical Effectiveness*. Another major contribution to EBP was inaugurated in 1993: the Cochrane Collaboration, an international network of institutions and individuals that maintains and updates systematic reviews of hundreds of clinical interventions to facilitate EBP.

In a seminal article that reviewed "breakthroughs" in nursing research over four decades, Donaldson (2000) noted that many of the nurse scientists who were "pathfinders"—who played a strategic role in helping to shape nursing—completed studies during the 1990s. Donaldson's review featured path-breaking research in diverse areas, such as personal and family health, dementia care, pain management, child development, health and violence, site transitional care, women's health, and biobehavioural health. By the turn of the century, nursing research had come of age.

Directions for Nursing Research in the New Millennium

Nursing research continues to develop at a rapid pace and will undoubtedly flourish in the years ahead. Certain trends for the beginning of the 21st century are evident from developments that were taking shape at the turn of the millennium:

▶ *Heightened focus on EBP.* Efforts to translate research findings into practice are sure to continue, and nurses at all levels will be encouraged to engage in evidence-based patient care. In turn, improvements will be needed both in the quality of nursing studies and in nurses' skills in understanding, critiquing, and utilizing study results.

▶ *Stronger knowledge base through multiple confirmatory strategies.* Practicing nurses cannot be expected to change procedures or adopt innovations based on single, isolated studies. Confirmation is needed through **replications**, that is, the repeating of studies with different clients, in different clinical settings, and at different times to ensure that findings are robust.

▶ *Greater emphasis on integrative reviews.* **Integrative reviews** of nursing knowledge, which are considered a cornerstone of EBP, will take on increased importance. The purposes of integrative reviews are to amass comprehensive research information on a topic, weigh pieces of evidence, and use integrated information to draw conclusions about the state of knowledge.

▶ *Increased involvement in transdisciplinary research.* Interdisciplinary collaboration of nurses with researchers in related fields is likely to continue to expand in the 21st century as researchers address fundamental health care problems. Collaborative efforts could result in nurse researchers playing a more prominent role in national and international health care policies. CIHR is supporting such a trend through its recent strategic training initiative programs that seek to support the training of transdisciplinary health researchers. To date, CIHR and other funding partners have provided a total of $3.6 million over 6 years to finance two nursing-led training initiatives, one in cardiovascular nursing called FUTURE—Facilitating Unique Training Using Research and Education—and the other in psychosocial oncology, PORT—Psychosocial Oncology Research Training (Loiselle, Bottorff, Butler, & Degner, 2004).

▶ *Expanded dissemination of research findings.* The Internet and other modes of electronic communication have a big impact on the dissemination of research information, which in turn may help to promote EBP. Through online publishing (e.g., the *Online Journal of Knowledge Synthesis for Nursing*); online resources such as Lippincott's NursingCenter.com; electronic document retrieval and delivery; e-mail; and electronic mailing lists, information about innovations can be communicated more widely and more quickly than ever before.

▶ *Increased interest in outcomes research.* **Outcomes research** is designed to assess and document the effectiveness of health care services. The growing number of studies that can be characterized as outcomes research has been stimulated by the need for cost-effective care that achieves positive outcomes without compromising quality. Nurses are increasingly engaging in outcomes research that is focused both on patients and on the overall health care delivery system.

▶ *Emphasis on the visibility of nursing research.* Efforts to increase the visibility of nursing research will likely expand. Most people are unaware that many nurses are scholars and researchers. Nurse researchers must market themselves to professional and consumer organizations and to the corporate world to increase support for their research. As Baldwin and Nail (2000) have noted, nurse researchers constitute one of the best qualified groups to meet the need in today's world for clinical outcomes research, but they are not recognized for their expertise.

In terms of substantive areas, research priorities and goals for the future are also under discussion. The Think Tank on Nursing Science in Canada, a group of nurse researchers that sets the agenda for research goals and priorities, has identified two main goals: (1) minimizing barriers to the conduct of nursing research through more collaborative efforts between universities and teaching hospitals, and (2) increasing designated funding for nursing research through formal research training programs at the master's and doctoral levels. In terms of research priorities, along with the Academy of Canadian

Executive Nurses (ACEN), they have identified three main areas: (1) patient safety and quality-of-life issues; (2) nursing work environments and workload; and (3) evidence-based decision making. In the United States, groups of experts convened by NINR helped to formulate five research themes that are part of NINR planning for the future. In a statement issued in 2003, NINR announced the following themes: (1) changing lifestyle behaviours for better health; (2) managing the effects of chronic illness to improve quality of life; (3) identifying effective strategies to reduce health disparities; (4) harnessing advanced technologies to serve human needs; and (5) enhancing the end-of-life experience for patients and their families.

SOURCES OF EVIDENCE FOR NURSING PRACTICE

As a nursing student, you are being taught how to practice nursing, but it is important to recognize that learning about best-practice nursing will continue throughout your career. Some of what you have learned thus far is based on systematic research, but much of it is not. Nursing practice relies on a collage of information sources that vary in dependability. Increasingly there are discussions of **evidence hierarchies** that acknowledge that certain types of evidence are superior to others. A brief review of alternative sources of evidence shows how research-based information is different.

Tradition and Authority

Within Western culture and within nursing, certain beliefs are accepted as truths—and certain practices are accepted as effective—simply based on custom. However, tradition may undermine effective problem solving. Traditions may be so entrenched that their validity or usefulness is not questioned. There is growing concern that many nursing interventions are based on tradition and "unit culture" rather than on sound evidence.

Another common source of knowledge is an authority, a person recognized for specialized expertise. Reliance on nursing authorities (such as nursing faculty) is to some degree unavoidable; however, like tradition, authorities as a knowledge source have limitations. Authorities are not infallible (particularly if their expertise is based mainly on personal experience), yet their knowledge often goes unchallenged.

Clinical Experience and Intuition

Our own clinical experience is a functional source of knowledge. The ability to recognize regularities and to make predictions based on observations is a hallmark of the human mind. Nevertheless, personal experience has limitations as a source of evidence for practice because each person's experience is too narrow to be useful in general terms, and personal experiences are often coloured by biases.

Nurses sometimes rely on "intuition" in their practice. Intuition is a type of knowledge that cannot be explained on the basis of reasoning or prior instruction. Although intuition undoubtedly plays a role in nursing practice—as it does in the conduct of research—it cannot serve as the basis for policies and practices for nurses.

Trial and Error

Sometimes we tackle problems by successively trying out alternative solutions. This approach may in some cases be practical, but it is often fallible and inefficient. The method tends to be haphazard, and the solutions are, in many instances, idiosyncratic.

Assembled Information

In making clinical decisions, health care professionals use information that has been assembled for various purposes. For example, local, national, and international *benchmarking data* provide information on such issues as the rates of using various procedures (e.g., rates of caesarean deliveries) or rates of infection (e.g., nosocomial pneumonia rates), and can help in evaluating clinical practices. *Quality improvement and risk data*, such as medication error reports, can be used to assess practices and determine the need for practice changes. Such sources, while offering information that can be used in practice, provide no mechanism for determining whether improvements in patient outcomes result from their use.

Disciplined Research

Research conducted within a disciplined format is the most sophisticated method of acquiring evidence that humans have developed. Nursing research combines aspects of logical reasoning with other features to create systems of problem solving that, although fallible, tend to be more reliable than other methods of acquiring knowledge.

The current emphasis on evidence-based health care requires nurses to base their clinical practice to the greatest extent possible on research-based findings rather than on tradition, intuition, or personal experience—although nursing will always remain a rich blend of art and science.

PARADIGMS AND METHODS FOR NURSING RESEARCH

A **paradigm** is a world view, a general perspective on the complexities of reality. Disciplined inquiry in the field of nursing is being conducted mainly (although not exclusively, as we discuss in Chapter 10) within two broad paradigms. This section describes the two paradigms and broadly outlines the research methods associated with them.

The Positivist/Postpositivist Paradigm

A paradigm that dominated thinking about disciplined inquiry for decades is known as *positivism*. Positivism is rooted in 19th-century thought, guided by such philosophers as Newton and Locke. Positivism is a reflection of a broader cultural phenomenon (*modernism*) that emphasizes the rational and scientific.

As shown in Table 1.2, a fundamental assumption of positivists is that there is a reality *out there* that can be studied and known. Adherents of positivism assume that nature

TABLE 1.2	Major Assumptions of the Positivist and Naturalistic Paradigms	
TYPE OF ASSUMPTION	POSITIVIST PARADIGM	NATURALISTIC PARADIGM
The nature of reality	Reality exists; there is a real world driven by real natural causes	Reality is multiple, subjective, and mentally constructed by individuals
The relationship between the researcher and those being studied	The researcher is independent from those being researched	The researcher interacts with those being researched, and findings are the creation of the interaction
The role of values in the inquiry	Values are to be held in check; objectivity is sought	Subjectivity and values are inevitable and desirable
Best methods for obtaining evidence/ knowledge	▶ Seeks generalizations ▶ Emphasis on discrete concepts ▶ Fixed design ▶ Focus on the objective and quantifiable ▶ Measured, quantitative information; statistical analysis ▶ Control over context; decontextualized ▶ Outsider knowledge—researcher as external ▶ Verification of researcher's hunches ▶ Focus on the product	▶ Seeks patterns ▶ Emphasis on the whole ▶ Flexible design ▶ Focus on the subjective and nonquantifiable ▶ Narrative information; qualitative analysis ▶ Context-bound; contextualized ▶ Insider knowledge—researcher as internal ▶ Emerging interpretations grounded in participants' experiences ▶ Focus on product and process

is basically ordered and regular and that an objective reality exists independent of human observation, awaiting discovery. In other words, the world is assumed not to be merely a creation of the human mind. The related assumption of **determinism** refers to the positivists' belief that *phenomena* (observable facts and events) are not haphazard or random, but rather have antecedent causes. If a person develops lung cancer, the scientist in a positivist tradition assumes that there must be one or more reasons that can be potentially identified. Within the **positivist paradigm**, much research is aimed at understanding the underlying causes of natural phenomena.

Because of their belief in an objective reality, positivists seek to be objective in their search for knowledge. Their approach calls for disciplined procedures with tight controls over the research situation to test researchers' hunches about the nature of the phenomena being studied and relationships among them.

Strict positivist thinking has been challenged and undermined, and few researchers adhere to the tenets of pure positivism. In the *postpositivist paradigm*, there is still a belief in reality and a desire to understand it, but postpositivists recognize the impossibility of total objectivity. They do, however, see objectivity as a goal and strive to be as neutral as possible. Postpositivists also appreciate the impediments to knowing reality with certainty and therefore seek *probabilistic* evidence—that is, what the true state of a phenomenon *probably* is, with a high and ascertainable degree of likelihood. This modified positivist position remains a dominant force in scientific research. For the sake of simplicity, we refer to it as positivism.

The Naturalistic Paradigm

The **naturalistic paradigm** (also referred to as the *constructivist paradigm*) began as a countermovement to positivism with writers such as Weber and Kant. The naturalistic paradigm represents a major alternative system for conducting disciplined inquiry. Table 1.2 compares four major assumptions of the positivist and naturalistic paradigms.

For the naturalistic inquirer, reality is not a fixed entity but rather a construction of the individuals participating in the research; reality exists within a context, and many constructions are possible. Naturalists thus take the position of relativism: if there are always multiple interpretations of reality that exist in people's minds, then there is no process by which the ultimate truth or falsity of the constructions can be determined.

The naturalistic paradigm assumes that knowledge is maximized when the distance between the inquirer and the participants in the study is minimized. The voices and interpretations of those under study are keys to understanding the phenomenon of interest, and subjective interactions are the primary way to access them. The findings from a naturalistic inquiry are the product of the interaction between the inquirer and the participants.

Paradigms and Methods: Quantitative and Qualitative Research

Research methods are the techniques researchers use to structure a study and to gather and analyze information relevant to a research question. The two alternative paradigms have strong implications for the research methods to be used to develop evidence. The methodologic distinction typically focuses on differences between **quantitative research,** which is most closely allied with the positivist tradition, and **qualitative research,** which is most often associated with naturalistic inquiry—although positivists sometimes undertake qualitative studies, and naturalistic researchers sometimes collect quantitative information. The use of different approaches does not exclusively reflect philosophical disagreements about the nature of reality—different approaches are used to answer different types of questions about that reality, as we discuss later in this chapter.

THE SCIENTIFIC METHOD AND QUANTITATIVE RESEARCH

The traditional, positivist **scientific method** is a general set of orderly, disciplined procedures used to acquire information. Quantitative researchers typically move in a systematic fashion from the definition of a problem and the selection of concepts on which to focus, to the solution of the problem. By *systematic* we mean that the investigator progresses logically through a series of steps, according to a prespecified plan of action. The researcher uses mechanisms designed to control the study, which involves imposing conditions on the research situation so that biases are minimized and precision and validity are maximized.

Quantitative researchers gather **empirical evidence**—evidence rooted in objective reality and gathered directly or indirectly through the senses rather than through personal hunches. In the positivist paradigm, information is gathered systematically, using formal instruments. Usually the information gathered is quantitative—that is, numeric information that results from formal measurement and that is analyzed with statistical procedures. Scientists strive to go beyond the specifics of a research situation; the degree to which research findings can be generalized is a widely used criterion for assessing the quality and importance of quantitative studies.

Example of internationally renowned Canadian quantitative nurse researchers

A team of researchers at the University of British Columbia—notably Joan Bottorff, Joy Johnson, and Pamela Ratner—have worked together for more than a decade and have established a strong program of research. Their early collaboration focused on health promotion—for example, they conducted a sophisticated study of a model to explain health promotion behaviour (Johnson, Ratner, Bottorff, & Hayduk, 1993), and they examined the relationship between gender and health promotion (Ratner, Bottorff, Johnson, & Hayduk, 1994). More recently, however, much of their joint work has focused on smoking. For example, they designed and tested an intervention to prevent smoking relapse in postpartum women (Johnson, Ratner, Bottorff, Hall, & Dahinten, 2000), examined the social-demographic factors associated with smoking in high school students (Johnson, Tucker, Ratner, Bottorff, Prkachin, Shoveller, & Zumbo, 2004), and developed a tool to measure tobacco dependence in adolescence (Johnson, Ratner, Tucker, Bottorff, Zumbo, Prkachin, & Shoveller, 2005). They also designed and tested an intervention to help smokers abstain from smoking before surgery (Ratner, Johnson, Richardson, Bottorff, Moffat, Mackay, Fofonoff, Kingsbury, Miller, & Budz, 2004). Much (although not all) of their collaborative research has used quantitative methods.

The traditional scientific method used by quantitative researchers has enjoyed considerable stature, and it has been used productively by nurse researchers studying a wide range of nursing problems. This is not to say, however, that this approach can solve all nursing problems. One important limitation—common to both quantitative and qualitative research—is that research methods usually cannot be used to answer moral or ethical questions. Many intriguing questions fall into this area (e.g., Should euthanasia be practiced? Should abortion be legal?). Given the many moral issues that are linked to health care, it is inevitable that the nursing process will never rely exclusively on scientific information.

The scientific method also must contend with problems of *measurement*. In studying a phenomenon, scientists attempt to measure it—that is, to attach numeric values that express quantity. For example, if the phenomenon of interest were patient morale, a researcher might want to know whether a patient's morale were high or low, or higher under some conditions than under others. Although physiologic phenomena such as blood pressure can be measured with accuracy and precision, the same cannot be said of psychological phenomena, such as hope or self-esteem.

A final issue is that most nursing research focuses on human beings, who are inherently complex and diverse. Within any given study, the scientific method typically focuses on a relatively small portion of the human experience (e.g., weight gain, chemical dependency). Complexities are controlled and, insofar as possible, eliminated in scientific studies rather than studied directly. Sometimes this narrow focus obscures insights. Finally and relatedly, quantitative research in the positivist paradigm has sometimes been accused of a narrowness and inflexibility of vision, a "sedimented view" of the world that does not fully capture the reality of experiences.

NATURALISTIC METHODS AND QUALITATIVE RESEARCH

Naturalistic methods of inquiry deal with human complexity by exploring it directly. Researchers in the naturalistic tradition stress the inherent depth of humans, the ability of humans to shape and create their own experiences, and the idea that "truth" is a composite of realities. Consequently, naturalistic investigations emphasize *understanding* the human experience as it is lived, usually through the collection and analysis of qualitative materials that are narrative and subjective.

Researchers who reject the traditional scientific method believe that a major limitation of the classical model is that it is *reductionist*—that it reduces human experience to a few concepts under investigation, and that the concepts are defined in advance by researchers rather than emerging from the experiences of those under study. Naturalistic researchers tend to focus on the dynamic, holistic, and individual aspects of phenomena and attempt to capture those aspects in their entirety, within the context of those who are experiencing them.

Flexible, evolving procedures are used to capitalize on findings that emerge in the course of the study. Naturalistic inquiry takes place in naturalistic settings (in the *field*), frequently over an extended period of time. The collection of information and its analysis typically progress concurrently. As the researcher sifts through the existing information and gains insight, new questions emerge, calling for additional evidence to amplify the insights. Through an inductive process, the researcher integrates the evidence to develop a framework that helps explain the processes under observation.

Example of an internationally renowned Canadian qualitative nurse researcher

Dr. Janice Morse is one of the leading qualitative nurse researchers not only in Canada but also in the world. She holds doctoral degrees in Nursing and Anthropology. She is Director of the International Institute for Qualitative Methodology and Professor of Nursing at the University of Alberta. Dr. Morse is also the editor of a prestigious qualitative journal, *Qualitative Health Research*. Dr. Morse's prolific program of research has focused on exploring comfort and comforting, enduring and suffering. She has explored such topics as the experience of comfort (Morse, Bottorff, & Hutchinson, 1994), the experience of agony (Morse & Mitcham, 1998), the experience of nurses comforting patients in extreme distress (Morse & Mitcham, 1997), and the identification of signals of suffering (Morse, Beres, Spiers, Mayan, & Olson, 2003).

Naturalistic studies yield rich, in-depth information that can potentially clarify the multiple dimensions of a complicated phenomenon (e.g., the process by which patients with cancer cope with their illness). The findings from in-depth qualitative research are typically grounded in the real-life experiences of people with first-hand knowledge of a phenomenon. However, the approach has several limitations. Human beings are the direct instruments through which qualitative information is gathered, and humans are intelligent and sensitive—but fallible—tools. The highly personal approach that enriches the analytic insights of skilful researchers can sometimes result in petty and trivial "findings" by less competent ones.

Another potential limitation involves the subjective nature of the inquiry, which can raise questions about the idiosyncratic nature of the conclusions. Would two naturalistic researchers studying the same phenomenon in the same setting arrive at the same findings? Moreover, most naturalistic studies involve a relatively small group of participants. Thus, the utility of the findings from naturalistic inquiries for other settings can sometimes be called into question.

CONSUMER TIP

Researchers usually do not discuss the underlying paradigm of their studies in their reports, so don't expect to find this stated explicitly. Qualitative researchers are more likely to mention the naturalistic paradigm (or to say they have undertaken a naturalistic inquiry) than are quantitative researchers to mention positivism. ■

Multiple Paradigms and Nursing Research

Paradigms are lenses that help us to sharpen our focus on a phenomenon; they are not blinders that limit our intellectual curiosity. The emergence of alternative paradigms for studying nursing problems is a healthy and desirable trend in the pursuit of new evidence for practice. Nursing knowledge would be meagre, indeed, without a rich array of approaches and methods available within the two paradigms—methods that are often complementary in their strengths and limitations.

We have emphasized the differences between the positivist and naturalistic paradigms and their associated methods so that their distinctions would be easy to understand. Despite their differences, however, the alternative paradigms have many features in common:

▶ *Ultimate goals.* The ultimate aim of disciplined inquiry, regardless of the paradigm, is to gain understanding. Both quantitative and qualitative researchers seek "the truth" about an aspect of the world in which they are interested, and both can make significant—and mutually beneficial—contributions.
▶ *External evidence.* Although the word *empiricism* has come to be allied with the scientific method, researchers in both traditions gather and analyze evidence empirically, that is, through their senses. Neither qualitative nor quantitative researchers are "armchair" analysts, relying on their own beliefs to generate information.
▶ *Reliance on human cooperation.* Evidence for nursing research comes primarily from humans, so the need for human cooperation is essential. To understand people's

experiences, researchers must persuade them to participate in the investigation *and* to act and speak candidly. The need for candour and cooperation can be a challenging requirement—for researchers in either tradition.

▶ *Ethical constraints.* Research with human beings is guided by ethical principles that may interfere with the researcher's ultimate goal. As discussed in Chapter 5, ethical dilemmas often confront researchers, regardless of paradigms or methods.

▶ *Fallibility of disciplined research.* Virtually all studies—in either paradigm—have limitations. Every research question can be addressed in many different ways, and inevitably there are tradeoffs. Financial constraints are one issue, but limitations may exist even with abundant resources. This does not mean that small, simple studies intrinsically have no value. It means that no single study can ever definitively answer a research question. Completed studies add to a body of accumulated evidence. The fallibility of any single study makes it important for you as a research consumer to understand and critique researchers' decisions when evaluating the quality of their evidence.

Thus, despite philosophical and methodologic differences, researchers using the traditional scientific method or naturalistic methods share overall goals and face many similar challenges. The selection of an appropriate method depends to some degree on the researcher's personal philosophy but largely on the nature of the research question. If a researcher asks, "What are the effects of surgery on circadian rhythms (biologic cycles)?" the researcher needs to express the effects through the careful quantitative measurement of bodily processes subject to rhythmic variation. On the other hand, if a researcher asks, "What is the process by which parents learn to cope with the death of a child?" the researcher would be hard pressed to quantify the process. Researchers' personal world views help to shape the types of question they ask.

In reading about the alternative paradigms for nursing research, you were probably more attracted to one of the two paradigms—the paradigm that corresponds most closely to your view of the world and of reality. Learning about and respecting both approaches to disciplined inquiry, however, and recognizing the strengths and limitations of each are important. In this textbook, we provide an overview of the methods associated with both qualitative and quantitative research and offer guidance on how to understand, critique, and use findings from both.

 HOW-TO-TELL TIP

How can you tell whether a study is qualitative or quantitative? As you progress through this book, you should be able to identify most studies as qualitative or quantitative based simply on the title, or based on terms appearing in the abstract at the beginning of the report. At this point, though, it may be easiest to distinguish the two types of studies based on how many *numbers* appear in the report, especially in tables. Qualitative studies may have no tables with numeric information, or only a single table with numbers describing participants' characteristics (e.g., how many were male or female). Quantitative studies typically have several tables with numbers and statistical information. Qualitative studies, by contrast, may have "word tables" or diagrams illustrating processes inferred from the narrative information gathered. ▬

PURPOSES OF NURSING RESEARCH

The general purpose of nursing research is to answer questions or solve problems of relevance to the nursing profession. Sometimes a distinction is made between basic and applied nursing research. *Basic research* is undertaken to extend the base of knowledge in a discipline. For example, a researcher may do a study to better understand grieving processes, without having *explicit* nursing applications in mind. *Applied research* focuses on finding solutions to problems. For example, a study to test the effectiveness of a nursing intervention to ease grieving would be applied. Basic research is appropriate for discovering general principles of human behaviour and biophysiology; applied research is designed to show how these principles can be used to solve problems in nursing practice. In nursing, the findings from applied research may pose questions for basic research, and the results of basic research often suggest clinical applications.

CONSUMER TIP

Researchers rarely specify whether their intent is to address a pragmatic problem or to generate basic knowledge. The study's intent generally has to be inferred and, in some cases, may be ambiguous. ■

The specific purposes of nursing research include identification, description, exploration, explanation, prediction, and control. Within each purpose, nurse researchers address various types of questions; certain questions are more amenable to qualitative than to quantitative inquiry, and vice versa.

Identification and Description

Many qualitative studies focus on phenomena about which little is known. In some cases, so little is known that the phenomenon has yet to be clearly identified—or has been inadequately defined or conceptualized. The in-depth, probing nature of qualitative research is well suited to answering such questions as, "What is this phenomenon?" and "What is its name?" (Table 1.3). In quantitative research, by contrast, researchers begin with a phenomenon that has been defined previously, sometimes in a qualitative study. Thus, in quantitative research, identification typically precedes the inquiry.

Qualitative example of identification

Dewar (2003) conducted an in-depth study to determine how individuals are able to live with catastrophic illnesses and injuries. She called one of the strategies they used *boosting*—people's efforts to improve their self-esteem—which helped them to endure their circumstances.

TABLE 1.3	Research Purposes and Research Questions	
PURPOSE	**TYPES OF QUESTIONS: QUANTITATIVE RESEARCH**	**TYPES OF QUESTIONS: QUALITATIVE RESEARCH**
Identification		What is this phenomenon? What is its name?
Description	How prevalent is the phenomenon? How often does the phenomenon occur? What are the characteristics of the phenomenon?	What are the dimensions of the phenomenon? What variations exist? What is important about the phenomenon?
Exploration	What factors are related to the phenomenon? What are the antecedents of the phenomenon?	What is the full nature of the phenomenon? What is really going on here? What is the process by which the phenomenon evolves or is experienced?
Explanation	What are the measurable associations between phenomena? What factors cause the phenomenon? Does the theory explain the phenomenon?	How does the phenomenon work? Why does the phenomenon exist? What is the meaning of the phenomenon? How did the phenomenon occur?
Prediction and control	What will happen if we alter a phenomenon or introduce an intervention? If phenomenon X occurs, will phenomenon Y follow? How can we make the phenomenon happen, or alter its nature or prevalence? Can the occurrence of the phenomenon be controlled?	

Description of phenomena is another important purpose of research. In a descriptive study, researchers observe, count, delineate, elucidate, and classify. Nurse researchers have described a wide variety of phenomena. Examples include patients' stress and coping, health beliefs, and time patterns of temperature readings. Description can be a major purpose for both qualitative and quantitative researchers. Quantitative description focuses on the prevalence, size, and measurable attributes of phenomena. Qualitative researchers, on the other hand, use in-depth methods to describe the dimensions, variations, and importance of phenomena. Table 1.3 compares descriptive questions posed by quantitative and qualitative researchers.

Exploration

Like descriptive research, exploratory research begins with a phenomenon of interest, but exploratory research goes beyond description and investigates the full nature of the

Quantitative example of description

Stewart, D'Arcy, Pitblado, Morgan, Forbes, Remus, Smith, Andrews, Kosteniuk, Kulig, and MacLeod (2005) undertook a study designed to provide a profile of the characteristics of nurses in rural and remote Canada and to describe the nature and scope of their nursing practice.

Qualitative example of description

Lam and Beaulieu (2004) undertook an in-depth study to describe the experiences of family members of patients admitted into a neurologic intensive care unit.

phenomenon and factors to which it is related. For example, a descriptive quantitative study of preoperative stress might document the degree of stress patients experience and the percentage of patients who experience it. An exploratory study might ask: What factors are related to a patient's stress level? Do a patient's clinical outcomes change in relation to the level of stress experienced?

Exploratory studies are undertaken when a new area or topic is being investigated, and qualitative methods are especially useful for exploring little-understood phenomena. Exploratory qualitative research is designed to shed light on the various ways in which a phenomenon is manifested and on underlying processes.

Quantitative example of exploration

Secco and Moffatt (2003) explored differences in the psychosocial, situational, and home environment characteristics of adolescent mothers from three cultural groups (Metis, First Nation, and Caucasian) at 4 weeks and 12 to 18 months postpartum.

Qualitative example of exploration

Through interviews with postpartum women, Mackinnon, McIntyre, and Quance (2005) explored what it means to women in labour to have a nurse present during childbirth.

Explanation

The goals of explanatory research are to understand the underpinnings of natural phenomena and to explain systematic relationships among phenomena. Explanatory research is often linked to a *theory*, which represents a method of organizing and integrating ideas about the manner in which phenomena are manifested or interrelated. Whereas descriptive research provides new information, and exploratory research provides promising insights, explanatory research focuses on understanding the causes or full nature of a phenomenon.

In quantitative research, theories or prior findings are used deductively as the basis for generating explanations that are then tested empirically. That is, based on existing theory or a body of evidence, researchers make specific predictions that, if upheld by the findings, lend credibility to the explanation. In qualitative studies, researchers may search for explanations about how or why a phenomenon exists or what a phenomenon means as a basis for developing a theory that is grounded in rich, in-depth, experiential evidence.

Quantitative example of explanation

Cummings, Hayduk, and Estabrooks (2005) tested a model to explain nurses' physical and emotional health during hospital restructuring, with particular emphasis on the explanatory power of nursing leadership.

Qualitative example of explanation

Milliken and Northcott (2003) undertook a study that sought to explain how parents with adult schizophrenic children redefined their identity and caregiving during the erratic course of their child's mental illness. (This study is included in its entirety in Appendix D.)

Prediction and Control

Many research problems defy absolute explanation. Yet it is possible to predict and control phenomena based on research findings, even without complete understanding. For example, research has shown that the incidence of Down syndrome in infants increases with the age of the mother. Therefore, we can predict that a woman aged 40 years is at higher risk for bearing a child with Down syndrome than a woman in her twenties. The incidence of Down syndrome may be partially controlled by educating women about the risks and offering amniocentesis to women older than 35 years of age. Note, however, that the ability to predict and control in this example does not depend on an explanation of *why* older women are at higher risk. There are many examples of nursing studies—typically, quantitative ones—in which prediction and control are key objectives. For example, studies designed to test health care effectiveness are typically concerned with controlling patient outcomes or the costs of care.

Quantitative example of prediction

Lang, Goulet, and Amsel (2004) studied the extent to which a person's internal resources (hardiness) and external resources (social support) predicted the health of couples following foetal or infant death.

CONSUMER TIP

It is the researchers' responsibility to explain the purpose of the study, and this usually happens fairly early in a research report. Most nursing studies have multiple aims. Almost all studies have some descriptive intent. Some exploratory studies are undertaken with the expectation that the results will serve a predictive or control function. Truly explanatory studies are the least common in the nursing literature. ■

ASSISTANCE TO CONSUMERS OF NURSING RESEARCH

This book is designed to help you develop skills that will allow you to read, evaluate, and use nursing studies (i.e., to become skilful consumers and users of nursing research). In each chapter of this book, we present information relating to the methods used by nurse researchers and provide specific guidance to consumers in several ways. First, interspersed throughout the chapters, we offer tips on what you can expect to find in actual research reports with regard to the content in the chapter. These include special "how-to-tell" tips that help you find concepts discussed in this book in research reports. These tips are identified with this icon: 🗒.

Second, we include guidelines for critiquing the aspects of a study covered in each chapter. The questions in Box 1.1 are designed to assist you in using the information in this chapter in an overall preliminary assessment of a research report.

BOX 1.1   Questions for a Preliminary Overview of a Research Report

1. How relevant is the research problem to the actual practice of nursing? Does the study focus on a topic that is considered a priority area for nursing research?
2. Is the research quantitative or qualitative?
3. What is the underlying purpose (or purposes) of the study—identification, description, exploration, explanation, or prediction and control?
4. What might be some clinical implications of this research? To what type of people and settings is the research most relevant? If the findings are accurate, how might the results of this study be used by *me*?

And third, we offer opportunities to apply your newly acquired skills. The critical activities at the end of each chapter guide you through appraisals of real research examples of both qualitative and quantitative studies (some of which are presented in their entirety in the appendices to this book or to the *Study Guide to Accompany Essentials of Nursing Research,* 6th édition). These activities also challenge you to think about how the findings from these studies could be used in nursing practice. A discussion of these critical thinking activities with suggested answers to the questions can be found on the Student Resource CD-ROM.

CONSUMER TIP

The following websites are useful starting points for further information about nursing research and EBP:

▶ *Canadian Association for Nursing Research: http://www.canr.ca*
▶ *Canadian Association of Schools of Nursing: http://www.casn.ca*
▶ *Canadian Health Services Research Foundation (CHSRF): http://www/chsrf.ca*
▶ *Canadian-International Nurse Researcher Database: http://nurseresearcher.com*
▶ *Canadian Institutes of Health Research (CIHR): http://www.cihr-irsc.gc.ca*
▶ *Canadian Nurses Association: http://www.cna-nurses.ca*
▶ *Canadian Nurses Foundation: http://canadiannursesfoundation.ca*
▶ *Cochrane Collaboration: http:www.cochrane.org*
▶ *Lippincott's Nursing Center: http:www.nursingcenter.com*
▶ *National Centre for Knowledge Transfer: http://ckt-ctc.ca*
▶ *National Institute of Nursing Research: http://ninr.nih.gov/ninr*
▶ *Agency for Healthcare Research and Quality: http:www.ahrq.gov*
▶ *Sigma Theta Tau International: http:www.nursingsociety.org*

RESEARCH EXAMPLES   Critical Thinking Activities

 EXAMPLE 1: Quantitative Research

Aspects of a quantitative nursing study, featuring terms and concepts discussed in this chapter, are presented below, followed by some questions to guide critical thinking.

Study
"A randomized trial of a cognitive coping intervention for acutely ill HIV-positive men" (Côté & Pepler, 2002); "Cognitive coping intervention for acutely ill HIV-positive men (Côté & Pepler, 2005)

Study Purpose
Côté and Pepler noted that people who are HIV positive now live longer when they contract AIDS, and consequently may face prolonged periods of stress and depression. They devised and tested a nursing intervention that was specifically focused

(Research Examples continue on page 26)

Critical Thinking Activities (continued)

on strengthening the cognitive coping skills of patients hospitalized for an exacerbation of HIV-related symptoms. The effect of this intervention on psychological well-being was compared with the effect of a more common nursing intervention that focuses on the expression of emotions.

Research Method
A sample of 90 HIV-positive adult men were recruited at two Canadian tertiary care hospitals and were put into one of three groups, at random: (1) a cognitive coping skills (CCS) intervention group; (2) an expression of emotions (EE) intervention group; and (3) a group getting no special intervention. Both the CCS and EE interventions were administered on 3 consecutive days, in 20- to 30-minute daily sessions.

Patient Outcomes
The three groups of men were assessed for mood, psychological distress, and anxiety both before and after the intervention, using formal assessment instruments.

Key Findings
▶ The researchers found that both the CCS and EE interventions produced a beneficial effect on negative mood over time, but no change in positive mood was observed for either group.
▶ The CCS group also experienced a reduction in both distress and anxiety from immediately before to immediately after each session, whereas those in the EE group showed an increase in anxiety during the same period.

Conclusions
Côté and Pepler concluded that the cognitive coping skills nursing intervention was effective in helping regulate emotional responses among HIV-positive patients and is feasible for use by skilled practitioners providing daily care.

Critical Thinking Suggestions*
*See the Student Resource CD-ROM for a discussion of these questions.
1. Answer the questions from Box 1.1 regarding this study.
2. Also consider the following targeted questions, which may assist you in assessing aspects of the study's merit:
   a. Why do you think Côté and Pepler decided to have a group of patients who got an alternative intervention and another group who received no special intervention?
   b. If you wanted to replicate this study to see whether the findings could be confirmed, what might you want to change to maximize the utility of the replication? For example, what type of people would you recruit to participate?
   c. Could this study have been undertaken as a qualitative study? Why or why not?

Critical Thinking Activities (continued)

 ### EXAMPLE 2: Qualitative Research

Aspects of a qualitative nursing study, featuring key terms and concepts discussed in this chapter, are presented below, followed by some questions to guide critical thinking.

Study
"The dyspnea-anxiety-dyspnea cycle—COPD patients' stories of breathlessness: 'It's scary/when you can't breathe' " (Bailey, 2004)

Study Purpose
Bailey did an in-depth study to explore the affective component of dyspnea/anxiety as described by patients living with chronic obstructive pulmonary disease (COPD) characterized by acute illness events.

Research Method
Bailey conducted her study in two general hospitals in a northeastern Ontario mining community. Over a 4-month period, admission clerks in the hospitals' emergency departments notified her about individuals admitted with acute exacerbation events of COPD. Bailey recruited participants by explaining the study and asking them to identify two family members who had been involved in an acute exacerbation event and who had an ongoing commitment to their well-being. Bailey then conducted in-depth interviews with 10 patient-nurse-family units during the hospitalization. The interviews were audiotaped and transcribed for analysis.

Key Findings
A total of 503 "stories" were identified across the interviews. The most frequently told stories were about the patient's emotional functioning—stories in which the patient or family member experienced overwhelming anxiety. Through their accounts, they illustrated their emotional vulnerability as they lived with chronic lung disease. As one study participant explained, "It's very hard to . . . not get into a panic. . . . You've gotta be able to control that" (p. 768).

Conclusions
The researchers concluded that health care providers need to recognize anxiety as an important and potentially measurable sign of invisible dyspnea for end-stage patients with COPD.

Critical Thinking Suggestions
1. Answer the questions in Box 1.1 regarding this study.
2. Also consider the following targeted questions, which may assist you in assessing aspects of the study's merit:
  a. Why do you think Bailey collected data from patients, nurses, *and* family members?

(Research Examples continue on page 28)

Critical Thinking Activities (continued)

b. Why do you think that the researcher audiotaped and transcribed her in-depth interviews with study participants?

c. Do you think it would have been appropriate for Bailey to conduct this study using quantitative research methods? Why or why not?

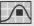 **EXAMPLE 3: Quantitative Research**

1. Read the abstract and the introduction from the study by Feeley and colleagues ("Mother–VLBW Infant Interaction") in Appendix A of this book, and then answer the questions in Box 1.1.

2. Also consider the following targeted questions, which may further sharpen your critical thinking skills and assist you in assessing aspects of the study's merit:

a. What gap in the existing body of research was the study designed to fill?

b. Would you describe this study as applied or basic, based on information provided in the abstract?

c. Could this study have been undertaken as a qualitative study? Why or why not?

d. Who helped to pay for this research? (This information appears in a footnote at the end of the report).

 EXAMPLE 4: Qualitative Research

1. Read the abstract and the introduction from Beck's study ("Birth Trauma") in Appendix B of this book, and then answer the questions in Box 1.1.

2. Also consider the following targeted questions, which may further sharpen your critical thinking skills and assist you in assessing aspects of the study's merit:

a. What gap in the existing research was the study designed to fill?

b. Was Beck's study conducted within the positivist paradigm or the naturalistic paradigm? Provide a rationale for your choice.

CHAPTER REVIEW
Summary Points

❱ **Nursing research** is a systematic inquiry to develop knowledge about issues of importance to nurses and serves to establish a base of knowledge for nursing practice.

❱ Nurses in various settings are pursuing an **evidence-based practice** (EBP) that incorporates research findings into their decisions and their interactions with clients.

❱ Knowledge of nursing research methods enhances the professional practice of all nurses, including both consumers of research (who read, evaluate, and use studies) and producers of research (who design and undertake studies).

❱ Nursing research began with Florence Nightingale but developed slowly until its rapid acceleration in the 1950s. Since the 1970s, nursing research has focused on problems related to clinical practice.

▶ The **Canadian Health Services Research Foundation** (CHSRF) has been funding a series of research chairs and related programs specific to nursing since 1999.

▶ Future emphases of nursing research are likely to include EBP and research utilization projects, **replications** of research, **integrative reviews**, transdisciplinary studies, expanded dissemination efforts, and **outcomes research**.

▶ Disciplined research is widely considered superior to other sources of evidence for nursing practice, such as tradition, authority, clinical experience, trial and error, and intuition.

▶ Disciplined inquiry in nursing is conducted mainly within two broad **paradigms,** or world views with underlying assumptions about the complexities of reality: the positivist paradigm and the naturalistic paradigm.

▶ Researchers in the **positivist paradigm** assume that there is an objective reality and that natural *phenomena* (observable facts and events) are regular and orderly. The related assumption of **determinism** refers to the belief that events are not haphazard but rather the result of prior causes. Pure positivism has been replaced with a *postpositivist* perspective that acknowledges the difficulty of making totally objective observations and knowing reality with certainty.

▶ Researchers in the **naturalistic paradigm** assume that reality is not a fixed entity but is rather a construction of human minds, and thus "truth" is a composite of multiple constructions of reality.

▶ The positivist paradigm is associated with **quantitative research**—the collection and analysis of numeric information. Quantitative research is typically conducted within the traditional **scientific method**, which is a systematic and controlled process. Quantitative researchers base their findings on **empirical evidence** (evidence collected by way of the human senses) and strive for generalizability of their findings beyond a single setting or situation.

▶ Researchers within the naturalistic paradigm emphasize understanding the human experience as it is lived through the collection and analysis of subjective, narrative materials using flexible procedures that evolve in the field; this paradigm is associated with **qualitative research**.

▶ Nursing research can be either *basic* (designed to provide information for the sake of knowledge) or *applied* (designed to solve specific problems). Research purposes include identification, description, exploration, explanation, prediction, and control.

Additional Resources for Review

Chapter 1 of the *Study Guide to Accompany Essentials of Nursing Research,* 6th edition offers various exercises and study suggestions for reinforcing the concepts presented in this chapter. For additional review, see the Student Self-Study Review Questions section of the Student Resource CD-ROM provided with this book.

SUGGESTED READINGS

References for studies cited in the chapter appear at the end of the book.

Methodologic and Theoretical References

Baldwin, K. M., & Nail, L. M. (2000). Opportunities and challenges in clinical nursing research. *Journal of Nursing Scholarship, 32*, 163–166.

Degner, L. F. (2002). Pathfinding for nursing science in the 21st century. Paper presented at the Think Tank Meeting of Canadian Nurse Scientists, sponsored by the Nursing Policy Division of Health Canada, October 2, Toronto, Canada.

Donaldson, S. K. (2000). Breakthroughs in scientific research: The discipline of nursing, 1960–1999. *Annual Review of Nursing Research, 18,* 247–311.

Estabrooks, C. A. (2004). Thoughts on evidence-based nursing and its science: A Canadian perspective. *Worldviews on Evidence-Based Nursing, 1,* 88–91.

Guba, E. G. (Ed.). (1990). *The paradigm dialog.* Newbury Park, CA: Sage Publications.

Lincoln, Y. S., & Guba, E. G. (1985). *Naturalistic inquiry.* Beverly Hills: Sage Publications.

Loiselle, C. G., Bottorff, J. L., Butler, L., & Degner, L. F. (2004). PORT—Psychosocial Oncology Research Training: A newly funded strategic initiative in health research. *CJNR, 36*(1), 159–164.

Nightingale, F. (1859). *Notes on nursing: What it is and what it is not.* Philadelphia: J. B. Lippincott.

Stetler, C. B., & Marram, G. (1976). Evaluating research findings for applicability in practice. *Nursing Outlook, 24,* 559–563.

Comprehending Key Concepts in Qualitative and Quantitative Research

STUDENT OBJECTIVES

On completing this chapter, you will be able to:

▶ Define new terms presented in the chapter
▶ Distinguish terms associated with quantitative and qualitative research
▶ Discuss some of the major challenges faced by researchers in doing rigorous qualitative or quantitative research

THE BUILDING BLOCKS OF RESEARCH

Research, like any other discipline, has its own language and terminology—its own *jargon*. Some terms are used by both qualitative and quantitative researchers, but other terms are used mainly with one or the other research approach.

The Places and Faces of Research

When researchers address a problem or answer a question through disciplined research—regardless of whether it is qualitative or quantitative—they are doing a **study** (or an *investigation*). **Clinical studies** are specifically designed to generate knowledge to guide clinical practice. **Collaborative studies**, involving a team with a mixture of clinical, theoretical, and methodologic skills, are increasingly common in health care research.

Example of a collaborative study

Steven, Fitch, Dhaliwal, Kirk-Gardner, Sevean, Jamieson, and Woodbeck, an interdisciplinary team of colleagues (2004)—including nurses, a physician, a psychologist, and a health care administrator—undertook a collaborative study focusing on the knowledge, attitudes, and practices regarding breast and cervical cancer screening among various ethnocultural groups in northwestern Ontario.

HOW-TO-TELL TIP

How can you tell whether an article appearing in a nursing journal is a *study*? In journals that specialize in research (e.g., *CJNR*), most articles are original research reports, but in specialty journals, there is usually a mix of research and nonresearch articles. Sometimes you can tell by the title, but sometimes you cannot. For example, Duchscher and Cowin (2004) from the Nursing Education Program of Saskatchewan published an article entitled "The Experience of Marginalization in New Nursing Graduates" in *Nursing Outlook*. The title suggests a possible qualitative study, but it is not a research report. Look at the major headings of an article, and if there is no heading called "Method" or "Methodology" (the section that describes what a researcher *did*) and no heading called "Findings" or "Results" (the section that describes what a researcher *learned*), then it is probably not an original study. ◼

Studies with humans involve two sets of people: those who conduct the study and those who provide the information. In a quantitative study, the people being studied are called **subjects** or **study participants,** as shown in Table 2.1. (When participants provide information by answering questions, as in an interview, they may be called **respondents**.) In a qualitative study, the individuals cooperating in the study play an active rather than a passive role and are called **informants, key informants**, or study participants. The person who conducts a study is the **researcher** or *investigator* (or sometimes—more often in quantitative studies—the *scientist*). Studies are sometimes undertaken by a single researcher, but more often involve a research team.

Research can be undertaken in various *settings* (the specific places where information is gathered) and in one or more *sites*. Some studies take place in **naturalistic settings**—in the **field**—(e.g., in people's homes); others are done in highly controlled **laboratory settings**. Qualitative researchers, especially, are likely to engage in **fieldwork** in natural settings because they are interested in the contexts of people's lives and experiences. A site is the overall location for the research—it could be an entire community (e.g., an Italian neighbourhood in Toronto) or an institution in a community (e.g.,

TABLE 2.1	Key Terms Used in Quantitative and Qualitative Research	
CONCEPT	**QUANTITATIVE TERM**	**QUALITATIVE TERM**
Person contributing information	Subject Study participant Respondent	Study participant Informant, key informant
Person undertaking the study	Researcher, investigator	Researcher, investigator
That which is being studied	Concepts Constructs Variables	Phenomena Concepts Constructs
Information gathered	Data (numeric values)	Data (narrative descriptions)
Links between concepts	Relationships (causal, functional)	Patterns of association
Logical reasoning processes	Deductive reasoning	Inductive reasoning
Quality of evidence	Reliability, validity, generalizability	Trustworthiness

a clinic in Edmonton). Researchers sometimes engage in **multisite studies** because the use of multiple sites offers a larger or more diverse group of participants.

Phenomena, Concepts, and Constructs

Research focuses on abstract rather than tangible phenomena. For example, the terms *pain, resilience,* and *grief* are all abstractions of particular aspects of human behaviour and characteristics. These abstractions are referred to as **concepts** (or, in qualitative research, **phenomena**).

Researchers also use the term construct. Kerlinger and Lee (2000) distinguish concepts from constructs by noting that **constructs** are abstractions that are deliberately and systematically invented (or constructed) by researchers for a specific purpose. For example, *self-care* in Orem's model of health maintenance is a construct. The terms *construct* and *concept* may be used interchangeably, although by convention, a construct often refers to a slightly more complex abstraction than a concept.

Theories, Models, and Frameworks

A **theory** is a systematic, abstract explanation of some aspect of reality. In a theory, concepts are knitted together into a system to explain some aspect of the world. Theories play a role in both qualitative and quantitative research.

In a quantitative study, researchers may start with a theory or a **conceptual model** or **framework** (the distinction is discussed in Chapter 8) and, using deductive reasoning, make predictions about how phenomena will behave *if the theory were "true."*

The specific predictions are then tested through research, and the results are used to reject, modify, or lend credence to the theory.

In qualitative research, theories may be used in various ways. Sometimes frameworks derived from various disciplines or qualitative research traditions (which we describe in the next chapter) offer an orienting view with clear conceptual underpinnings. In some qualitative studies, however, theory is the *product* of the research. Information from participants is the starting point for the researcher's conceptualization that seeks to explain patterns and commonalities emerging from researcher–participant interactions. The goal is to develop a theory that explains phenomena as they exist, not as they are preconceived. Theories generated in a qualitative study are sometimes subjected to more controlled confirmation through quantitative research.

Variables

In a quantitative study, concepts are referred to as **variables.** A variable, as the name implies, is something that varies. Weight, anxiety level, and body temperature are all variables (i.e., each of these properties varies from one person to another). In fact, nearly all aspects of human beings and their environment are variables. For example, if everyone weighed 150 pounds, weight would not be a variable; it would be a *constant*. But it is precisely because people and conditions *do* vary that research is conducted. Most quantitative researchers seek to understand how or why things vary and to learn how differences in one variable are related to differences in another. For example, lung cancer research is concerned with the variable of lung cancer. It is a variable because not everybody has the disease. Researchers have studied variables that might be linked to lung cancer and have identified cigarette smoking. Smoking is also a variable because not everyone smokes. A variable, then, is any quality of a person, group, or situation that varies or takes on different values—typically, numeric values.

 CONSUMER TIP

Every study focuses on one or more phenomena, concepts, or variables, but these terms *per se* are not necessarily used in research reports. For example, a report might say: "The purpose of this study is to examine the effect of primary nursing on patient satisfaction." Although the researcher has not explicitly used the term *concept*, the concepts (variables) under study are *type of nursing* and *patient satisfaction.* Key concepts or variables are often indicated in the study title.   ■

Variables are often inherent characteristics of people, such as age, blood type, or height. Sometimes, however, researchers *create* a variable. For example, if a researcher is testing the effectiveness of patient-controlled analgesia compared with intramuscular analgesia in relieving pain after surgery, some patients would be given patient-controlled analgesia and others would receive intramuscular analgesia. In the context of this study, method of pain management is a variable because different patients are given different analgesic methods.

Sometimes a variable can take on a range of different values that can be represented on a continuum (e.g., height or weight). Other variables take on only a few values; sometimes such variables convey quantitative information (e.g., number of children), but others simply involve placing people into categories (e.g., male, female).

DEPENDENT VARIABLES AND INDEPENDENT VARIABLES

Many quantitative studies seek to determine the causes of phenomena. Does a nursing intervention *cause* improved patient outcomes? Does a certain procedure *cause* stress? The presumed cause is called the **independent variable**, and the presumed effect is called the **dependent variable**.

Variation in the dependent variable is presumed to *depend on* variation in the independent variable. For example, researchers investigate the extent to which lung cancer (the dependent variable) depends on or is caused by smoking (the independent variable). Or, researchers might examine the effect of tactile stimulation (the independent variable) on weight gain (the dependent variable) in premature infants. The dependent variable (sometimes called the **outcome variable**) is the variable researchers want to understand, explain, or predict. In lung cancer/smoking research, it is the cancer that researchers are trying to explain and predict, not smoking.

Frequently, the terms *independent variable* and *dependent variable* are used to designate the *direction of influence* between variables rather than cause and effect. For example, suppose a researcher studied the mental health of caretakers caring for spouses with Alzheimer's disease and found better mental health outcomes for wives than for husbands. The researcher might be unwilling to take the position that the spouse's mental health was *caused* by gender. Yet the direction of influence clearly runs from gender to mental health: it makes *no* sense to suggest that mental health status influenced the spouse's gender! Although in this example the researcher does not infer a cause-and-effect connection, it is appropriate to conceptualize mental health as the dependent variable and gender as the independent variable.

Many dependent variables have multiple causes or antecedents. If we were interested in studying influences on people's weight, for example, age, height, physical activity, and eating habits might be the independent variables. Two or more *dependent* variables also may be of interest to researchers. For example, suppose we wanted to compare the effectiveness of two methods of nursing care for children with cystic fibrosis. Several dependent variables could be designated as measures of treatment effectiveness, such as length of hospital stay, recurrence of respiratory infections, presence of cough, and so on. It is common to design studies with multiple independent and dependent variables.

Variables are not *inherently* dependent or independent. A dependent variable in one study may be an independent variable in another study. For example, a study might examine the effect of nurses' contraceptive counselling (the independent variable) on unwanted births (the dependent variable). Another study might investigate the effect of unwanted births (the independent variable) on episodes of child abuse (the dependent variable). The role that a variable plays in a particular study determines whether it is an independent or a dependent variable.

The distinction between dependent and independent variables is often difficult for students. Don't be discouraged—it is something that will become a lot easier with practice.

CONSUMER TIP

Few research reports *explicitly* label variables as dependent and independent, despite the importance of this distinction. Moreover, variables (especially independent variables) are sometimes not fully spelled out. Take the following research question: What is the effect of exercise on heart rate? In this example, heart rate is the dependent variable. Exercise, however, is not in itself a variable. Rather, exercise versus something else (e.g., no exercise) is a variable; "something else" is implied rather than stated in the research question. If exercise were not compared with something else, such as no exercise or different amounts of exercise, then exercise would not be a variable. ■

Example of independent and dependent variables

Research question: Does a special intervention for nursing home residents with dementia help them to find their way in a new environment? (McGilton, Riviera & Dawson, 2003)
Independent variable: Receipt versus nonreceipt of a special way-finding intervention (use of a location map and behavioural training)
Dependent variable: Residents' ability to find their way to specific destinations (e.g., the dining room)

Conceptual and Operational Definitions

Concepts in a study need to be defined and explicated, and dictionary definitions are almost never adequate. Two types of definitions are of particular relevance in a study—conceptual and operational.

The concepts in which researchers are interested are abstractions of "observable" phenomena, and researchers' world views shape how concepts are defined. A **conceptual definition** is the abstract, theoretical meaning of a concept being studied. Even seemingly straightforward terms need to be conceptually defined by researchers. Take as an example the concept of *spirituality*. Chiu, Emblen, Van Hofwegen, Sawatzky, and Meyerhoff (2004) did a comprehensive review of how spirituality was conceptually defined in the research literature and found that current definitions revolve around four distinct themes: existential reality, transcendence, connectedness, and power/force/energy. Researchers undertaking studies of spirituality need to make clear which conceptual definition of spirituality they have adopted. In qualitative studies, conceptual definitions of key phenomena may be a major end product, reflecting an intent to have the meaning of concepts defined by those being studied.

In quantitative studies, however, researchers clarify and define research concepts at the outset because they must indicate how variables will be observed and measured. An **operational definition** of a variable specifies the operations that researchers must perform to collect the required information. Operational definitions should correspond to conceptual definitions.

Variables differ in the ease with which they can be operationalized. The variable weight, for example, is easy to define and measure. We might operationally define weight as follows: the amount that an object weighs in kilograms, to the nearest full kilogram. Note that this definition designates that weight will be determined with one measuring system (kilograms) rather than another (pounds). The operational definition might also specify that subjects' weight will be measured to the nearest kilogram using a spring scale with subjects fully undressed after 10 hours of fasting. This operational definition clearly indicates what is meant by the variable *weight.*

Unfortunately, few variables of interest to nurses are operationalized as easily as weight. There are multiple methods of measuring most variables, and researchers must choose the method that best captures the variables as they conceptualize them. Take, for example, *anxiety*, which can be defined in terms of either physiologic or psychological functioning. For researchers choosing to emphasize physiologic aspects of anxiety, the operational definition might involve a measure such as the Palmar Sweat Index. If, on the other hand, researchers conceptualize anxiety as primarily a psychological state, the operational definition might involve a paper-and-pencil measure such as the State Anxiety Scale. Readers of research reports may not agree with how investigators conceptualized and operationalized variables, but precise definitions have a strong communication value.

Example of conceptual and operational definitions

Beck and Gable (2001) conceptually defined various aspects of *postpartum depression* and then described how the definitions were linked operationally to Beck's Postpartum Depression Screening Scale (PDSS). For example, one aspect of postpartum depression is *cognitive impairment*, conceptually defined as "a mother's loss of control over her thought processes (that) leaves her frightened she may be losing her mind." Operationally, the PDSS captured this dimension by having women indicate their level of agreement with such statements as "I could not stop the thoughts that kept racing in my mind."

CONSUMER TIP

Most research reports never use the term *operational definition* explicitly. Quantitative research reports do, however, provide information on how key variables were measured (i.e., they specify the operational definitions even if they do not use this label). This information is usually included in a section called "Research Measures" or "Instruments." ■

Data

Research **data** (singular, datum) are the pieces of information obtained in a study. All the pieces of data that researchers gather for a study make up their **data set.**

BOX 2.1 **Example of Quantitative Data**

Question

Thinking about the past week, how depressed would you say you have been on a scale from 0 to 10, where 0 means "not at all" and 10 means "the most possible"?

Data

Subject 1: 9
Subject 2: 0
Subject 3: 4

In quantitative studies, researchers identify the variables of interest, develop operational definitions, and then collect relevant data from subjects. The actual values of the variables constitute the study data. In quantitative studies, researchers collect primarily **quantitative data** (i.e., numeric information). For example, suppose we were conducting a quantitative study in which a key variable was *depression*. In such a study, we would try to measure how depressed different participants were. We might ask, "Thinking about the past week, how depressed would you say you have been on a scale from 0 to 10, where 0 means 'not at all' and 10 means 'the most possible'?" Box 2.1 presents some data from three fictitious respondents. The subjects have provided a number corresponding to their degree of depression: 9 for subject 1 (a high level of depression), 0 for subject 2 (no depression), and 4 for subject 3 (very mild depression). The numeric values for all subjects in the study, collectively, would constitute the data on the variable depression.

In qualitative studies, researchers collect primarily **qualitative data,** which are narrative descriptions. Narrative information can be obtained by having conversations with participants, by making notes about how participants behave in naturalistic settings, or by obtaining narrative records (e.g., diaries). Suppose we were studying depression qualitatively. Box 2.2 presents some qualitative data from three participants responding conversationally to the question, "Tell me about how you've been feeling lately. Have you felt sad or depressed at all, or have you generally been in good spirits?" Here, the data consist of rich narrative descriptions of participants' emotional state. The analysis of such qualitative data is a particularly labour-intensive process.

Relationships

Researchers usually study phenomena in relation to other phenomena—they examine relationships. A **relationship** is a bond or connection between two or more phenomena; for example, researchers repeatedly have found that there is a *relationship* between cigarette smoking and lung cancer. Both qualitative and quantitative studies examine relationships, but in different ways.

In quantitative studies, researchers are primarily interested in the relationship between independent variables and dependent variables. Variation in the dependent variable is presumed to be systematically related to variation in the independent variable. Relationships are often explicitly expressed in quantitative terms, such as *more than, less*

BOX 2.2   Example of Qualitative Data

Question

Tell me about how you've been feeling lately—have you felt sad or depressed at all, or have you generally been in good spirits?

Data

Participant 1: "I've been pretty depressed lately, to tell you the truth. I wake up each morning and I can't seem to think of anything to look forward to. I mope around the house all day, kind of in despair. I just can't seem to shake the blues, and I've begun to think I need to go see a shrink."

Participant 2: "I can't remember ever feeling better in my life. I just got promoted to a new job that makes me feel like I can really get ahead in my company. And I've just gotten engaged to a really great guy who is very special."

Participant 3: "I've had a few ups and downs the past week, but basically things are on a pretty even keel. I don't have too many complaints."

than, and so on. For example, let us consider as a possible dependent variable a person's weight. What variables are related to a person's weight? Some possibilities include height, caloric intake, and exercise. For each of these three independent variables, we can make a prediction about its relationship to the dependent variable:

Height: Taller people weigh more than shorter people.

Caloric intake: People with higher caloric intake are heavier than those with lower caloric intake.

Exercise: The lower the amount of exercise, the greater the person's weight.

Each of these statements expresses a presumed relationship between weight (the dependent variable) and a measurable independent variable. Most quantitative research is conducted to determine whether relationships do or do not exist among variables, and often to quantify how strong the relationship is.

CONSUMER TIP

Relationships are expressed in two basic forms, depending on what the variables are like. First, relationships can be expressed as "if more of variable X, then more of (or less of) variable Y." For example, there is a relationship between height and weight: with more height, there tends to be more weight; that is, taller people tend to weigh more than shorter people. The second form is sometimes confusing to students because there is no explicit relational statement. The second form involves relationships expressed as group differences. For example, there is a *relationship* between gender and height: men tend to be taller than women. ■

Variables can be related to one another in different ways. One type of relationship is a **cause-and-effect** (or **causal**) **relationship.** Within the positivist paradigm, natural phenomena are assumed not to be haphazard; they have antecedent causes that are presumably discoverable. In our example about a person's weight, we might speculate that there is a causal relationship between caloric intake and weight: all else being equal, eating more calories causes weight gain.

Example of a study focusing on a causal relationship

Gagnon and her colleagues (Gagnon, Legendre-Parent, Vigneault, Marquis, Paquet, Michaud, & Gauyin, 2004) studied whether a case management approach for total hip and knee arthroplasty patients would result in improvements in terms of length of stay, readmissions, and number of complications.

Not all relationships between variables can be interpreted causally. There is a relationship, for example, between a person's pulmonary artery and tympanic temperatures: people with high readings on one have high readings on the other. We cannot say, however, that pulmonary artery temperature caused tympanic temperature, nor that tympanic temperature caused pulmonary artery temperature, despite the relationship between the two variables. This type of relationship is sometimes referred to as a *functional* (or *associative*) *relationship* rather than a causal one.

Example of a study focusing on a functional/associative relationship

Reutter, Sword, Meagher-Stewart, and Rideout (2004) studied nursing students' beliefs about poverty and health in relation to several background characteristics of students, such as their age and program level.

HOW-TO-TELL TIP

How can you tell if a researcher is testing a causal relationship? The researcher is likely to ask whether the outcome variable is *caused by, affected by, resulted from,* or *influenced by* the independent variable. If the researcher is not seeking to establish a causal relationship, he or she is more likely to ask whether the outcome variable is *related to, linked to,* or *associated with* the independent variable. ■

Qualitative researchers are not concerned with quantifying relationships, nor in testing and confirming causal relationships. Rather, qualitative researchers seek patterns of association as a way of illuminating the underlying meaning and dimensionality of phenomena of interest. Patterns of interconnected themes and processes are identified as a means of understanding the whole.

Example of a qualitative study of patterns

Montbriand (2004) studied the life experiences of seniors with a chronic illness living independently in a Canadian prairie city. She found that seniors with optimistic perceptions did not connect their life experiences with illnesses, but seniors with pessimistic perceptions did connect life experiences (including experiences of abuse) with their present illnesses.

Logical Reasoning

Logical reasoning plays an important role in both qualitative and quantitative research. Two intellectual mechanisms are used in reasoning. **Inductive reasoning** is the process of developing conclusions from specific observations. For example, a nurse may observe various anxious behaviours of (specific) hospitalized children and conclude that (in general) children's separation from their parents is stressful. Inductive reasoning is an important tool in disciplined research and plays an especially important role in qualitative research, in which the emphasis is on weaving together pieces of information into a cohesive pattern.

Deductive reasoning is the process of developing specific predictions from general principles. For example, if we assume that separation anxiety affects hospitalized children (in general), we might predict that (specific) children in Memorial Hospital whose parents do not room-in will manifest symptoms of stress. Quantitative studies would examine the validity of the prediction—that is, test **hypotheses** about how variables are related. In our example, the hypothesized relationship would be between *rooming-in* (versus not rooming-in) and *stress levels* in hospitalized children.

Logical reasoning can be used to solve problems even in the absence of systematic research. However, reasoning in and of itself is limited because the validity of reasoning depends on the accuracy of the information (or premises) with which one starts. Systematic research can be structured to provide maximally useful information, the accuracy of which can be evaluated.

CRITICAL CHALLENGE OF CONDUCTING RESEARCH

Researchers face numerous challenges in conducting research. For example, there are conceptual challenges (e.g., How should key concepts be defined?); financial challenges (How will the study be paid for?); ethical challenges (Can the study achieve its goals without infringing on human rights?); and methodologic challenges (Will the adopted method yield results that can be trusted?). Most of this book provides guidance relating to the last question, and this section highlights key methodologic challenges as a way of introducing important terms and concepts, and illustrating key differences between qualitative and quantitative research. In reading this section, it is important for you to remember that the worth of a study's evidence for evidence-based practice (EBP) is based on how well researchers deal with these challenges.

Reliability, Validity, and Trustworthiness

Researchers want their findings to reflect the *truth*. Research cannot contribute evidence to guide clinical practice if the findings are inaccurate or fail to adequately represent the experiences of the target group. Research users need to assess the quality of evidence in a study by evaluating the conceptual and methodologic decisions researchers made, and researchers need to strive to make good decisions to produce evidence of the highest possible quality.

Quantitative researchers use several criteria to assess the quality of a study, sometimes referred to as its **scientific merit.** Two important criteria are reliability and validity. **Reliability** is the accuracy and consistency of information obtained in a study. The term is most often associated with the methods used to measure research variables. For example, if a thermometer measured Bob's temperature as 98.1°F one minute and as 102.5°F the next minute, the reliability of the thermometer would be highly suspect. The concept of reliability is also important in interpreting statistical analyses. Statistical reliability refers to the probability that the same results would be obtained with a completely new sample of participants—that is, that the results accurately reflect the outcomes of a wider group than just the particular people who participated in the study.

Validity is a more complex concept that concerns the *soundness* of the study's evidence—that is, whether the findings are cogent and well grounded. Like reliability, validity is an important criterion for assessing the method of measuring variables. In this context, the validity question is whether there is evidence to support the assertion that the methods are really measuring the abstract concepts that they purport to measure. Is a paper-and-pencil measure of depression *really* measuring depression? Or is it measuring something else, such as loneliness or low self-esteem? The validity criterion underscores the importance of having solid conceptual definitions of research variables—as well as high-quality methods to operationalize them.

Another aspect of validity concerns the quality of the researcher's evidence regarding the link between the independent variable and the dependent variable. Did a nursing intervention *really* bring about improvements in patients' outcomes—or were other factors responsible for patients' progress? Researchers make numerous methodologic decisions that can influence this type of study validity.

Qualitative researchers use somewhat different criteria (and different terminology) in evaluating a study's quality. Generally, qualitative researchers discuss methods of enhancing the **trustworthiness** of the study's results (Lincoln and Guba, 1985). Trustworthiness encompasses several different dimensions, one of which is credibility.

Credibility, an especially important aspect of trustworthiness, is achieved to the extent that the research methods engender confidence in the "truth" of the data and in the researchers' interpretations of the data. Credibility can be enhanced through various strategies (see Chapter 14), but one in particular merits early discussion because it has implications for the design of all studies, including quantitative ones. **Triangulation** is the use of multiple sources or referents to draw conclusions about what constitutes the "truth." In a quantitative study, this might mean having two different operational definitions of the dependent variable to determine whether results are consistent across the two. In a qualitative study, triangulation might involve trying to understand the full complexity of a poorly understood phenomenon by using multiple means of data collection to converge on the "truth" (e.g., having in-depth conversations with study participants, as well as observing them in natural settings). Nurse researchers are also beginning to triangulate across paradigms—that is, to integrate both qualitative and quantitative data in a single study to offset the limitations of each approach.

Example of triangulation

Leipert and Reutter (2005) studied how women maintain their health in northern geographically isolated settings. Their study involved three in-depth interviews with 25 women in two of the four northern health regions in British Columbia. Observational data about the geographical terrain and distances were also recorded. Written documents (newspapers, local histories) were also used as data sources.

Nurse researchers need to design their studies in such a way that threats to the reliability, validity, and trustworthiness of their studies are minimized, and that users of research must evaluate the extent to which they were successful.

CONSUMER TIP

In reading and evaluating research reports, it is appropriate to assume a "show me" attitude—that is, to expect researchers to build and present a solid case for the merit of their findings. They do this by presenting evidence that the findings are reliable and valid or trustworthy. ■

Bias

Bias is a major concern in research because it can threaten the study's validity and trustworthiness. In general, a **bias** is an influence that produces a distortion in the study results. Biases can affect the quality of evidence in both qualitative and quantitative studies. Bias can result from various factors, including study participants' lack of candour or desire to please, researchers' preconceptions, or faulty methods of collecting data.

To some extent, bias can never be avoided totally because the potential for its occurrence is so pervasive. Some bias is haphazard and affects only small segments of the data. As an example of such random bias, a handful of study participants might fail to provide accurate information because they were tired at the time of data collection. Systematic bias results when the bias is consistent or uniform. For example, if a spring scale consistently measured people's weights as being 2 pounds heavier than their true weight, there would be systematic bias in the data on weight. Rigorous research method aims to eliminate or minimize bias—or, at least, to detect its presence so it can be taken into account in interpreting the data.

Researchers adopt a variety of strategies to address bias. Triangulation is one such approach, the idea being that multiple sources of information or points of view help to counterbalance biases and offer avenues to identify them. In quantitative research, methods to combat bias often entail research control.

Research Control

Quantitative studies typically involve efforts to control various aspects of the research. **Research control** involves holding constant other influences on the dependent variable so that the true relationship between the independent and dependent variables can be understood. In other words, research control attempts to eliminate contaminating factors that might cloud the relationship between the variables that are of central interest.

The issue of confounding factors—**extraneous variables**—can best be illustrated with an example. Suppose we were interested in the question, Does young maternal age affect infant birth weight? Existing studies have shown that teenagers more often have low-birth-weight babies than women in their 20s or 30s; the question here is whether maternal age itself (the independent variable) causes differences in birth weight (the dependent variable) or whether there are other mechanisms that account for or mediate the relationship between age and birth weight. We need to design a study that controls other influences on the dependent variable to clarify the effect of the independent variable.

Two possible extraneous variables are women's nutritional habits and their prenatal care. Teenagers tend to be less careful than older women about their eating patterns during pregnancy, and are also less likely to obtain adequate prenatal care. Both nutrition and the amount of care could, in turn, affect birth weight. Thus, if these two factors are not controlled, then any observed relationship between mother's age and her baby's weight at birth could be caused by the mother's age itself, her diet, or her prenatal care. It would be impossible to know what the underlying cause really is.

These three possible explanations might be portrayed schematically as follows:

1. Mother's age → infant birth weight
2. Mother's age → adequacy of prenatal care → infant birth weight
3. Mother's age → nutritional adequacy → infant birth weight

The arrows here symbolize a causal mechanism or an influence. In examples 2 and 3, the effect of maternal age on infant birth weight is mediated by prenatal care and nutrition, respectively; these are **mediating variables** in these last two models. Some research is specifically designed to test paths of mediation, but in the present example, these variables are extraneous to the research question. Our task is to design a study so that the first explanation can be tested. Both nutrition and prenatal care must be controlled to learn whether explanation 1 is valid. If they are not controlled, they will confound the results.

How can we impose such control? There are a number of ways, as discussed in Chapter 9, but the general principle underlying each alternative is the same: *the extraneous variables of the study must be held constant*. The extraneous variables must be handled so that, *in the context of the study*, they are not related to the independent or dependent variable.

Research control is a fundamental feature of quantitative studies. The world is complex, and variables are interrelated in complicated ways. In quantitative studies, it is difficult to examine this complexity directly. Researchers analyze a few relationships at a time and put the pieces together like a jigsaw puzzle. That is why even modest quantitative studies can make contributions to knowledge. The extent of the contribution, however, is often related to how well a researcher controls confounding influences. In reading reports of quantitative studies, you will need to consider whether the researcher has, in fact, appropriately controlled extraneous variables.

Although research control in quantitative studies is viewed as a critical tool for managing bias and enhancing validity, there are situations in which too much control can introduce bias. For example, if researchers tightly control the ways in which key study variables can manifest themselves, it is possible that the true nature of those variables will be obscured. When key concepts are phenomena that are poorly understood or whose dimensions have not been clarified, then an approach that allows some flexibility (as in a qualitative study) is better suited to the study aims. Research rooted in the naturalistic paradigm does not impose controls. With their emphasis on holism and the individuality of human experience, qualitative researchers typically adhere to the view that to impose controls on a research setting is to remove irrevocably some of the meaning of reality.

Randomness and Reflexivity

For quantitative researchers, a powerful tool for eliminating bias involves the concept of **randomness**—having certain features of the study established by chance rather than by design or personal preference. When people in a community are selected at random to participate in a study, for example, each person in the community has an equal chance of being selected. This in turn means that there are no systematic biases in the make-up of the study group. Men are as likely to be selected as women, for example.

Qualitative researchers do not consider randomness a useful tool for understanding phenomena. Qualitative researchers tend to use information obtained early in the study in a purposeful (nonrandom) fashion to guide their inquiry and to pursue information-rich sources that can help them refine their conceptualizations. Researchers' judgments are viewed as indispensable vehicles for uncovering the complexities of the phenomena of interest. However, qualitative researchers often rely on reflexivity to guard against personal bias in making judgments. **Reflexivity** is the process of reflecting critically on the self, and of analyzing and making note of personal values that could affect data collection and interpretation.

Example of reflexivity

Myrick and Yonge (2004) studied the process used in the preceptorship experience to enhance critical thinking in graduate nursing education. Their study involved interviews with graduate students and preceptors. During the study, both researchers maintained a journal of personal reflections.

Generalizability and Transferability

Nurses increasingly rely on evidence from disciplined research as a guide in their clinical practice. If study findings are totally unique to the people or circumstances of the original research, can they be used as a basis for changes in practice? The answer, clearly, is no.

As noted in Chapter 1, **generalizability** is the criterion used in a quantitative study to assess the extent to which study findings can be applied to other groups and settings. How do researchers enhance the generalizability of a study? First, they must design studies strong in reliability and validity. There is little point in wondering whether results are generalizable if they are not accurate or valid. In selecting participants, researchers must also give thought to the types of people to whom the results might be generalized—and then select them in such a way that an appropriate sample is obtained. If a study is intended to have implications for male and female patients, then men and women should be included as participants. If an intervention is intended to benefit patients in urban and rural hospitals, then perhaps a multisite study is needed.

Qualitative researchers do not specifically seek to make their findings generalizable. Nevertheless, qualitative researchers often seek understandings that might prove useful in other situations. Lincoln and Guba (1985), in their influential book on naturalistic inquiry, discuss the concept of **transferability**, the extent to which qualitative findings can be transferred to other settings, as an aspect of a study's trustworthiness. An important mechanism for promoting transferability is the amount of information qualitative researchers provide about the contexts of their studies. **Thick description**, a widely used term among qualitative researchers, refers to a rich and thorough description of the research setting and of observed processes. Quantitative researchers, like qualitative researchers, need to thoroughly describe their study participants and their research settings so that the utility of the evidence for nursing practice can be assessed.

GENERAL QUESTIONS IN REVIEWING A STUDY

Most of the remaining chapters of this book contain guidelines to help you evaluate different aspects of a research report critically, focusing primarily on the methodologic decisions that the researcher made in conducting the study. Box 2.3 presents some further suggestions for performing a preliminary overview of a research report, drawing on concepts explained in this chapter. These guidelines supplement those presented in Box 1.1, Chapter 1.

 BOX 2.3   **Additional Questions for a Preliminary Overview of a Study**

1. What is the study all about? What are the main phenomena, concepts, or constructs under investigation?
2. If the study is quantitative, what are the independent and dependent variables?
3. Do the researchers examine relationships or patterns of association among variables or concepts? Does the report imply the possibility of a causal relationship?
4. Are key concepts clearly defined, both conceptually and operationally?
5. Are you able to discern any steps the researcher took to enhance the study's reliability, validity, and generalizability (quantitative research) or trustworthiness (qualitative research)?

RESEARCH EXAMPLES   **Critical Thinking Activities**

 EXAMPLE 1: Quantitative Research

Aspects of a quantitative nursing study, featuring key terms and concepts discussed in this chapter, are presented below, followed by some questions to guide critical thinking.

Study
"Impact of preoperative education on pain outcomes after coronary artery bypass graft surgery" (Watt-Watson, Stevens, Katz, Costello, Reid, & David, 2004)

Study Purpose
The study tested the effectiveness of preoperative education regarding postsurgical pain on pain-related outcomes among patients undergoing coronary artery bypass graft (CABG) surgery. The intervention involved giving patients a special booklet, *Pain Relief After Surgery*, that reflects current research evidence on pain and the Canadian Pain Society's position on pain relief. The booklet focuses on communicating pain and the use of analgesics in pain relief.

Research Method
A total of 406 elective patients who were attending a standard education session 2 to 7 days before their CABG surgery were recruited into the study. Half the participants, at random, were put in a group that received standard cardiovascular education plus the special booklet, whereas the other half were put in a group that received standard education only. Outcome data were gathered postoperatively in a cardiovascular surgical unit of a large Toronto hospital.

Outcome Variables
The primary outcome variable was pain-related interference in activities (e.g., sleeping, walking) on days 3 and 5 after surgery, as reported by patients on a 6-question scale. Additionally, the researchers gathered information about the patients' self-reported level of pain, analgesics prescribed and administered (from patients' charts), patients' concerns about reporting pain and taking analgesics, length of hospital stay, and patients' level of satisfaction with pain treatment.

Key Findings
- The two groups were comparable with regard to pain-related interference with activities on day 3, but the intervention group had some reduction in pain-related interference on day 5, especially with regard to deep breathing and coughing.
- The two groups did not differ with regard to pain levels, analgesics administered or prescribed, length of hospital stay, or patient satisfaction.
- Despite moderate pain intensity scores across 5 days, patients in both groups received inadequate analgesics (33% of the prescribed dose).

(Research Examples continue on page 48)

Critical Thinking Activities (continued)

Critical Thinking Suggestions*
*See the Student Resource CD-ROM for a discussion of these questions.

1. Answer questions 1, 2, 3, and 5 from Box 2.3 regarding this study.
2. Also consider the following targeted questions, which may assist you in assessing aspects of the study's merit:
   a. What are some of the extraneous variables the researchers would have wanted to control—what factors other than the treatment could have affected the outcomes?
   b. What is your perception of the validity of the outcome measures?
   c. How did the researchers reduce bias in forming the two groups that were compared?
   d. Would it have been appropriate to address the research question using qualitative research methods? Why or why not?
3. If the results of this study are valid and generalizable, what are some of the uses to which the research evidence might be put in clinical practice?

 EXAMPLE 2: Qualitative Research

Aspects of a qualitative nursing study, featuring key terms and concepts discussed in this chapter, are presented below, followed by some questions to guide critical thinking.

Study
"The experience of waiting and life during breast cancer follow-up" (Gaudine, Sturge-Jacobs, & Kennedy, 2003)

Study Purpose
Gaudine and her colleagues sought to understand and thoroughly describe the experience of waiting and of life in the years following women's diagnosis and treatment for breast cancer.

Research Method
The researchers gathered the stories about women's experiences with waiting— waiting for the next medical intervention, for the next check-up, for the next battery of tests—during follow-up for breast cancer. They interviewed nine women who were breast cancer survivors who had been undergoing follow-up treatment for at least 1 year. The in-depth interviews, lasting 60 to 90 minutes, were audiotaped and transcribed. Six of the interviews were conducted in person, but three interviews (with women living in remote rural areas) were conducted by telephone. Transcriptions were read and re-read by each researcher separately. Data analysis was ongoing, and additional women were interviewed until no new themes emerged. To establish trustworthiness, the three researchers analyzed data separately, then cross-checked each other's categories, themes, and interpretations.

Critical Thinking Activities (continued)

Key Findings

The women's experiences were captured in four themes:

▸ The diagnosis of breast cancer and follow-up care was a *life-changing experience*.

▸ There was a *sense of belonging* by receiving follow-up care through cancer clinics.

▸ *Uncertainty* about life was pervasive—mortality for these women became real and personal, as illustrated by the following quote: "I think what I find most difficult is the uncertainty of it all. What I find most difficult . . . I find waiting extremely difficult. Many times I would prefer just to have that test done and over with, but it is the waiting for the test and what is even worse is the waiting for the results." (p. 160)

▸ *Needing to know*—there was a strong need for knowledge about the disease, treatment options, and ramifications.

Critical Thinking Suggestions

1. Answer questions 1, 3, and 5 from Box 2.3 regarding this study.

2. Also consider the following targeted questions, which may assist you in assessing aspects of the study's merit:

   a. Gaudine and her colleagues did not control extraneous variables, nor did they use randomness in this study. Would these decisions affect the quality of the study?

   b. Some actual data are presented in the summary—indicate what the data are.

   c. Would it have been appropriate to address the research question using quantitative research methods? Why or why not?

3. If the results of this study are trustworthy, what are some of the uses to which the findings might be put in clinical practice?

 EXAMPLE 3: Quantitative Research

1. Read the abstract and the introduction from the study by Feeley and colleagues ("Mother–VLBW Infant Interaction") in Appendix A of this book and then answer questions 1 through 3 in Box 2.3.

2. Also consider the following targeted questions, which may further sharpen your critical thinking skills and assist you in assessing aspects of the study's merit:

   a. Did the researchers randomly assign subjects to groups in this study?

   b. What are some of the extraneous variables that the researchers would have wanted to control in this study?

 EXAMPLE 4: Qualitative Research

1. Read the abstract, introduction, and literature review section of Beck's study ("Birth Trauma") in Appendix B of this book (and skim the remainder of the report) and then answer the relevant questions in Box 2.3.

(Research Examples continue on page 50)

Critical Thinking Activities (continued)

2. Also consider the following targeted questions, which may further sharpen your critical thinking skills and assist you in assessing aspects of the study's merit:
  a. Find an example of actual *data* in this study. (You will need to look at the first few paragraphs of the "Results" section of the report.)
  b. Does Beck's report discuss reflexivity?
  c. Would it have been appropriate for Beck to conduct her study of birth trauma using quantitative research methods? Why or why not?

CHAPTER REVIEW
Summary Points

▶ A research **study** (or *investigation*) is undertaken by one or more **researchers** (or **investigators**). The people who provide information in a study are the **subjects** or **study participants** (in quantitative research) or study participants or **informants** (in qualitative research).

▶ **Collaborative research** involving a research team with both clinical and methodologic expertise is increasingly common in addressing problems of clinical relevance.

▶ The *site* is the overall location for the research; researchers sometimes engage in **multisite studies**. *Settings*—the more specific places where data collection occurs—range from **naturalistic (field) settings** to formal laboratories.

▶ Researchers investigate phenomena or **concepts** (or **constructs**), which are abstractions or mental representations inferred from behaviour or events.

▶ Concepts are the building blocks of **theories,** which are systematic explanations of some aspect of the world.

▶ In quantitative studies, concepts are called variables. A **variable** is a characteristic or quality that takes on different values (i.e., varies from one person to another).

▶ The **dependent** (or **outcome**) **variable** is the behaviour, characteristic, or outcome the researcher is interested in explaining, predicting, or affecting. The **independent variable** is the presumed cause of, antecedent to, or influence on the dependent variable.

▶ A **conceptual** definition clarifies the abstract or theoretical meaning of a concept being studied. An **operational definition** specifies the procedures and tools required to measure a variable.

▶ **Data**—the information collected during the course of a study—may take the form of narrative information (**qualitative data**) or numeric values (**quantitative data**).

▶ Researchers often focus on the relationship between two concepts. A **relationship** is a bond (or pattern of association) between two phenomena; when the independent variable causes or determines the dependent variable, it is a **causal** (or **cause-and-effect**) **relationship**.

▶ **Inductive reasoning** is the process of developing conclusions from specific observations, whereas **deductive reasoning** is the process of developing specific predictions from general principles.

▶ Researchers face numerous conceptual, practical, ethical, and methodologic challenges. The major methodologic challenge is designing studies that are reliable and valid (quantitative studies) or trustworthy (qualitative studies).

▶ **Reliability** refers to the accuracy and consistency of information obtained in a study. **Validity** is a more complex concept that concerns the *soundness* of the study's evidence—that is, whether the findings are cogent and well-grounded.

▶ **Trustworthiness** in qualitative research encompasses several dimensions, including credibility. **Credibility** is achieved to the extent that the research methods engender confidence in the truth of the data and in the researchers' interpretations. **Triangulation**, the use of multiple sources or referents to draw conclusions about what constitutes the truth, is one approach to establishing credibility.

▶ A **bias** is an influence that distorts study results. In quantitative research, a powerful tool to eliminate bias concerns **randomness**—having features of the study established by chance rather than by design or preference.

▶ Qualitative researchers often keep personal biases in check through **reflexivity,** the process of reflecting critically on the self and noting personal values that could affect data collection and interpretation.

▶ Quantitative researchers use various methods of **research control** to hold constant confounding influences on the dependent variable so that its relationship to the independent variable can be better understood. The confounding influences are **extraneous variables**—extraneous to the purpose of the study.

▶ **Generalizability** is the criterion used in a quantitative study to assess the extent to which the findings can be applied to other groups and settings.

▶ A similar concept in qualitative studies is **transferability**, the extent to which qualitative findings can be transferred to other settings. A mechanism for promoting transferability is **thick description**, the rich, thorough description of the research context so that others can make inferences about contextual similarities.

Additional Resources for Review

Chapter 2 of the *Study Guide to Accompany Essentials of Nursing Research,* 6th edition offers various exercises and study suggestions for reinforcing the concepts presented in this chapter. For additional review, see the Student Self-Study Review Questions section of the Student Resource CD-ROM provided with this book.

SUGGESTED READINGS

References for studies cited in the chapter appear at the end of the book.

Methodologic References

Kerlinger, F. N., & Lee, H. B. (2000). *Foundations of behavioral research* (4th ed.). Orlando, FL: Harcourt College Publishers.

Lincoln, Y. S., & Guba, E. G. (1985). *Naturalistic inquiry.* Newbury Park, CA: Sage Publications.

Morse, J. M., & Field, P. A. (1995). *Qualitative research methods for health professionals* (2nd ed.). Thousand Oaks, CA: Sage Publications.

Understanding the Research Process in Qualitative and Quantitative Studies

STUDENT OBJECTIVES

On completing this chapter, you will be able to:

▶ Distinguish experimental and nonexperimental research
▶ Identify the three main disciplinary traditions for qualitative nursing research
▶ Describe the flow and sequence of activities in quantitative and qualitative research, and discuss why they differ
▶ Define new terms presented in the chapter

Researchers usually decide early on whether to conduct a quantitative or qualitative study; they typically work within a paradigm that is consistent with their world view and that gives rise to the types of question that excite their curiosity. After selecting a paradigm, researchers proceed to design and implement their study, but the progression of activities differs in qualitative and quantitative research. In this chapter, we discuss the flow of both types of study.

CONSUMER TIP

The flow of a research project is not transparent to those reading a research report. Researchers rarely articulate the progression of steps they took in initiating and completing a study. This chapter is not, therefore, designed to help you to critique a report (i.e., you will not have to evaluate whether researchers followed an appropriate sequence of steps), but will help you better understand the research process. It is also intended to heighten your awareness of the many decisions that researchers make—decisions that have a strong bearing on study quality. ◼

MAJOR CLASSES OF QUANTITATIVE AND QUALITATIVE RESEARCH

Before describing the evolution of a research project, we briefly describe broad categories of quantitative and qualitative research.

Quantitative Research: Experimental and Nonexperimental Studies

A basic distinction in quantitative studies is between experimental and nonexperimental research. In **experimental research**, researchers actively introduce an intervention or treatment. In **nonexperimental research**, on the other hand, researchers collect data without making changes or introducing treatments. For example, if a researcher gave bran flakes to one group of participants and prune juice to another to evaluate which method facilitated elimination more effectively, the study would be experimental because the researcher intervened in the normal course of things. If, on the other hand, a researcher compared elimination patterns of two groups of people whose regular eating patterns differed—for example, some normally took foods that stimulated bowel elimination and others did not—there is no intervention. Such a study, which focuses on existing attributes, is nonexperimental.

Experimental studies are explicitly designed to test causal relationships. Sometimes nonexperimental studies also seek to elucidate or detect causal relationships, but doing so is tricky and less conclusive. Experimental studies offer the possibility of greater control over extraneous variables than nonexperimental studies.

Example of experimental research

Taylor, Oberle, Crutcher, and Norton (2005) tested the effectiveness of a special nurse–physician collaborative intervention on diabetes-related outcomes among patients with type 2 diabetes. Patients were randomly assigned either to an intervention group that received home visits from a nurse, or to a group that received standard care.

In this example, the researchers intervened by designating that some patients would receive the special support intervention and others would not. In other words, the researchers had control over the independent variable, which in this case was receipt or nonreceipt of the intervention.

Example of nonexperimental research

Voyer, Verreault, Mengue, Laurin, Rochette, Martin, and Baillargeon (2005) searched for factors that are associated with the use of neuroleptic (antipsychotic) drugs among more than 2000 elderly people in nursing homes.

In this nonexperimental study, the researchers did not intervene in any way. They merely measured the participants' characteristics. The independent variables were a range of predictive factors such as the elders' age, cognitive impairment, and insomnia—variables over which the researchers did not have control (i.e., they could not *assign* some elders to having sleeping problems and others to not have such problems— their sleeping patterns were a "given"). Yet the researchers *were* interested in the possibility that the elders' insomnia affected the administration of neuroleptic drugs. We will see in Chapter 9 why making causal inferences in nonexperimental studies is a thorny issue.

Qualitative Research: Disciplinary Traditions

Qualitative studies (which are almost invariably nonexperimental) are often rooted in research traditions that originate in the disciplines of anthropology, sociology, and psychology. Three such traditions have had especially strong influences on qualitative nursing research and are briefly described here so that we can better explain their similarities and differences throughout the book. Chapter 10 provides a fuller discussion of alternative research traditions and the methods associated with them.

The **grounded theory** tradition, which was developed in the 1960s by two sociologists, Glaser and Strauss (1967), seeks to describe and understand the key social-psychological and structural processes that occur in a social setting. Most grounded theory studies focus on an evolving social experience—the social and

Example of a grounded theory study

Woodgate and Degner (2004) conducted a grounded theory study to develop a description, grounded in children's and families' experiences, of the symptom trajectory in childhood cancer. Their core variable was "passage through the transition periods" and included six transition periods starting with "It is just the flu . . . anything but cancer" and ending with "it is dragsville."

psychological stages and phases that characterize a particular event or episode. A major component of grounded theory is the discovery of a *core variable* (or *core category*) that is central in explaining what is going on in that social scene. Grounded theory researchers strive to generate comprehensive explanations of phenomena that are grounded in reality.

Phenomenology, which has its disciplinary roots in both philosophy and psychology, is concerned with the lived experiences of humans. Phenomenology is an approach to thinking about what life experiences of people are like and what they mean. The phenomenologic researcher asks: What is the *essence* of this phenomenon as experienced by these people? Or, What is the meaning of the phenomena to those who experience it?

Example of a phenomenological study

Hayne (2003) conducted a phenomenological study to describe the experience of being given a psychiatric diagnosis—specifically, the experience of being labelled as having a "severe and enduring mental illness"—from the clients' perspectives.

Ethnography is the primary research tradition within anthropology, and provides a framework for studying the patterns and experiences of a defined cultural group in a holistic fashion. Ethnographers typically engage in extensive fieldwork, often participating to the extent possible in the life of the culture of interest. The aim of ethnographers is to learn from (rather than to "study") members of a cultural group, to understand their world view as they perceive and live it.

Example of an ethnographic study

Johnson, Bottorff, Browne, Grewal, Hilton, and Clarke (2004) used ethnographic methods to study *othering* (the process that identifies those who are thought to be different from oneself or the mainstream) within the context of health care services. Women from South Asia described discriminatory experiences within Canadian health care settings.

MAJOR STEPS IN A QUANTITATIVE STUDY

In quantitative studies, researchers move from a start point (posing a question) to an end point (getting an answer) in a fairly linear sequence of steps. This section describes the progression of activities that is typical in a quantitative study; the next section describes how qualitative studies differ.

Phase 1: The Conceptual Phase

The early steps in a quantitative study typically involve activities with a strong conceptual element. During this phase, researchers call on such skills as creativity, deductive reasoning, and a firm grounding in previous research on the topic of interest.

STEP 1: FORMULATING AND DELIMITING THE PROBLEM

The first step is to identify an interesting, significant research problem and to develop research questions. In developing research questions, nurse researchers need to consider substantive issues (Is the question significant?); clinical issues (Could the findings be useful in practice?); methodologic issues (Can a study be designed to yield high-quality evidence?); practical issues (Are adequate resources available to do the study?); and ethical issues (Can this question be rigorously addressed without committing ethical transgressions?).

STEP 2: REVIEWING THE RELATED RESEARCH LITERATURE

Quantitative research is typically conducted within the context of previous knowledge. Quantitative researchers typically strive to understand what is already known about a topic by conducting a thorough **literature review** before any data are collected.

STEP 3: UNDERTAKING CLINICAL FIELDWORK

Researchers embarking on a clinical nursing study often benefit from spending time in clinical settings, discussing the topic with clinicians and administrators, and observing current practices. Such clinical fieldwork can provide perspectives on recent clinical trends and healthcare delivery models; it can also help researchers better understand affected clients and the settings in which care is provided.

STEP 4: DEFINING THE FRAMEWORK AND DEVELOPING CONCEPTUAL DEFINITIONS

When quantitative research is performed within the context of a theoretical framework (i.e., when a theory is used as a basis for predictions that can be tested), the findings may have broader significance. Even when the research question is not embedded in a theory, researchers must have a clear sense of the concepts under study. Thus, an important early task is the development of conceptual definitions.

STEP 5: FORMULATING HYPOTHESES

As noted in Chapter 2, hypotheses state researchers' expectations about relationships among study variables. The research question identifies the variables and asks how they might be related; a hypothesis is the predicted answer. For example, the research question might be: Is preeclamptic toxaemia in pregnant women related to stress experienced during pregnancy? This might lead to the following hypothesis: Pregnant women who report high levels of stress during pregnancy are more likely than women with lower levels of stress to develop preeclamptic toxaemia. Most quantitative studies test hypotheses.

Phase 2: The Design and Planning Phase

In the second major phase of a quantitative study, researchers make decisions about the methods to use to address the research question, and plan for the actual collection of data.

As a consumer, you should be aware that the methodologic decisions that researchers make during this phase affect the integrity, interpretability, and clinical utility of the results. Thus, you must be able to evaluate the decisions so that you can determine how much faith to put in the evidence. A major objective of this book is to help you evaluate methodologic decisions.

STEP 6: SELECTING A RESEARCH DESIGN

The **research design** is the overall plan for obtaining answers to the research questions and for addressing the challenges we described in Chapter 2. In quantitative studies, research designs tend to be highly structured and to include controls to reduce the effects of extraneous variables. There are a wide variety of experimental and nonexperimental research designs.

STEP 7: DEVELOPING PROTOCOLS FOR THE INTERVENTION

In experimental research, researchers create the independent variable, which means that participants are exposed to two or more different treatments or conditions. An **intervention protocol** must be developed, specifying exactly what the intervention will entail (e.g., what it is, who will administer it, how frequently and over how long a period it will last, and so on) *and* what the alternative condition will be. The goal of well-articulated protocols is to have all participants in each group treated the same way. In nonexperimental research, of course, this step would not be necessary.

STEP 8: IDENTIFYING THE POPULATION TO BE STUDIED

Quantitative researchers need to specify a population, indicating what attributes participants should possess, and thereby clarifying the group to which study results can be generalized. A **population** is *all* the individuals or objects with common, defining characteristics. For example, a researcher might specify that the study population consists of all licensed nurses residing in Canada.

STEP 9: DESIGNING THE SAMPLING PLAN

Researchers typically collect data from a **sample,** which is a subset of the population. Using samples is practical, but the risk is that the sample will not adequately reflect the population's traits. In a quantitative study, a sample's adequacy is assessed by the criterion of *representativeness*; that is, how typical, or representative, the sample is of the population. The **sampling plan** specifies in advance *how* the sample will be selected and *how many* study participants there will be.

STEP 10: SPECIFYING METHODS TO MEASURE VARIABLES

Quantitative researchers must develop or borrow methods to measure study variables as accurately as possible. Based on the conceptual definitions, researchers select methods to operationalize the variables (i.e., to collect the data). A variety of quantitative data collection approaches exist; the most common methods are self-reports (e.g., interviews), observations, and biophysiologic measurements.

STEP 11: DEVELOPING METHODS TO PROTECT HUMAN/ANIMAL RIGHTS

Most nursing studies involve human subjects, although some involve animals. In either case, procedures need to be developed to ensure that the study adheres to ethical principles.

Each aspect of the study plan needs to be reviewed to determine whether participants' rights have been adequately protected.

STEP 12: FINALIZING AND REVIEWING THE RESEARCH PLAN

Before collecting data, researchers often seek feedback from colleagues or advisers and perform "tests" to ensure that plans will work smoothly. For example, they may assess the *readability* of written materials to determine whether participants with low reading skills can comprehend them, or they may *pretest* their measuring instruments to assess their adequacy. If researchers have concerns about their study plans, they may undertake a **pilot study**, which is a small-scale version or trial run of the major study.

Example of a pilot study

Nemeth, Harrison, Graham, and Burke (2004) conducted a pilot study focusing on venous leg ulcer pain over a 5-week period in one Canadian community, to determine the feasibility of a larger study that would be conducted over a longer time period.

Phase 3: The Empirical Phase

The empirical phase of a quantitative study involves collecting data and preparing data for analysis. The empirical phase is often the most time-consuming part of the study.

STEP 13: COLLECTING THE DATA

Data collection in a quantitative study normally proceeds according to a preestablished plan. The *data collection plan* specifies procedures for actually collecting the data (e.g., where, when, and how the data will be gathered), for recruiting the sample, and for training those who will collect the data.

STEP 14: PREPARING DATA FOR ANALYSIS

The data collected in a quantitative study are rarely amenable to direct analysis. One preliminary step is **coding,** which is the process of translating data into numeric form. For example, responses to a question about gender might be coded (1) for females and (2) for males. Another typical step involves transferring data from written forms to computer files for analysis.

Phase 4: The Analytic Phase

The quantitative data gathered in the empirical phase are not reported in *raw* form (i.e., as a mass of numbers). They are subjected to analysis and interpretation, which occurs in the fourth major phase of the project.

STEP 15: ANALYZING THE DATA

Research data must be processed and analyzed in an orderly fashion so that relationships can be discerned and hypotheses can be tested. Quantitative data are analyzed through **statistical analyses**, which include some simple procedures as well as complex methods.

STEP 16: INTERPRETING THE RESULTS

Interpretation is the process of making sense of the results and examining their implications. In quantitative studies, researchers attempt to interpret study results in light of prior evidence and theory and in light of the rigor of the research methods. Interpretation also involves determining how the findings can best be used in clinical practice, or what further research is needed before utilization can be recommended.

Phase 5: The Dissemination Phase

In the analytic phase, the researcher comes full circle: the questions posed at the outset are answered. The researcher's job is not completed, however, until the study results are disseminated.

STEP 17: COMMUNICATING THE FINDINGS

A study cannot contribute evidence to practice if the results are not communicated. Another—and often final—task of a research project is the preparation of a *research report* that can be shared with others. We discuss research reports in the next chapter.

STEP 18: UTILIZING RESEARCH EVIDENCE IN PRACTICE

Ideally, the concluding step of a good study is to plan for its use in practice settings. Although nurse researchers may not always be able to undertake a plan for utilizing research findings, they can contribute to the process by developing suggestions for how study findings could be incorporated into nursing practice and by vigorously pursuing opportunities to disseminate their findings to practicing nurses.

ACTIVITIES IN A QUALITATIVE STUDY

Quantitative research involves a fairly linear progression of tasks (i.e., researchers lay out in advance the steps to be taken to maximize the integrity of the study and then follow them as faithfully as possible). In a qualitative study, by contrast, the progression is closer to a circle than to a straight line—qualitative researchers are continually examining and interpreting data and making decisions about how to proceed based on what has already been discovered.

Because qualitative researchers have a flexible approach to collecting and analyzing data, it is impossible to define the flow of activities precisely—the flow varies from one study to another, and researchers themselves do not know ahead of time exactly how the study will unfold. We try to provide a sense of how a qualitative study is conducted, however, by describing some major activities and indicating how and when they might be performed.

Conceptualizing and Planning a Qualitative Study

IDENTIFYING A RESEARCH PROBLEM

Qualitative researchers generally begin with a general topic area, often focusing on an aspect of a topic that is poorly understood and about which little is known. They therefore do not develop hypotheses or pose refined research questions at the outset. Qualitative researchers often proceed with a fairly broad question that allows the focus to be sharpened once they are in the field.

DOING A LITERATURE REVIEW

Qualitative researchers do not all agree about the value of doing an upfront literature review. Some believe that the literature should not be consulted before collecting data. Their concern is that prior studies might unduly influence their conceptualization of the phenomenon under study. According to this view, the phenomenon should be elucidated based on participants' viewpoints rather than on prior information. Others believe that researchers should conduct at least a cursory literature review at the outset. In any event, qualitative researchers typically find a relatively small body of relevant literature because of the types of questions they ask.

SELECTING AND GAINING ENTRÉE INTO RESEARCH SITES

Before going into the field, qualitative researchers must identify an appropriate site. For example, if the topic is the health care beliefs of the urban poor, a low-income inner-city neighbourhood must be identified. In many cases, researchers need to make preliminary contacts with key actors in the site to ensure cooperation and access to informants (i.e., researchers need to **gain entrée** into the site). Gaining entrée typically involves negotiations with *gatekeepers* (or *stakeholders*) who have the authority to permit entry into their world.

DESIGNING QUALITATIVE STUDIES

Quantitative researchers do not collect data before finalizing the research design. Qualitative researchers, by contrast, use an **emergent design**—a design that emerges during the course of data collection. Certain design features are guided by the study's qualitative tradition, but qualitative studies do not have a rigid structure that prohibits changes in the field.

ADDRESSING ETHICAL ISSUES

Qualitative researchers, like quantitative researchers, must also develop plans for addressing ethical issues—and, indeed, there are special concerns in qualitative studies because of the more intimate nature of the relationship that typically develops between researchers and study participants.

Conducting a Qualitative Study

In qualitative studies, the activities of sampling, data collection, data analysis, and interpretation typically take place iteratively. Qualitative researchers begin by talking with or observing people who have first-hand experience with the phenomenon under study. The discussions and observations are loosely structured, allowing participants to express a full range of beliefs and behaviours. Analysis and interpretation are ongoing, concurrent activities, used to guide decisions about whom to sample next and what questions to ask or observations to make. The process of data analysis involves clustering together related types of narrative information into a coherent scheme.

As analysis and interpretation progress, the researcher begins to identify *themes* and categories, which are used to build a descriptive theory of the phenomenon. The kinds of data obtained become increasingly focused and purposeful as a theory emerges. Theory development and verification shape the sampling and data gathering process—as the theory develops, the researcher seeks participants who can confirm and enrich the theoretical understandings as well as participants who can potentially challenge them and lead to further theoretical development.

Quantitative researchers decide in advance how many participants to include in the study, but qualitative researchers' sampling decisions are guided by the data themselves. Many qualitative researchers use the principle of **saturation**, which occurs when themes and categories in the data become repetitive and redundant, such that no new information can be gleaned by further data collection.

Quantitative researchers seek to collect high-quality data by using measuring instruments with demonstrated reliability and validity. Qualitative researchers, by contrast, *are* the main data collection instrument and must take steps to ensure the trustworthiness of the data. The central feature of these efforts is to confirm that the findings accurately reflect participants' experiences and viewpoints, rather than the researchers' perceptions. For example, one confirmatory activity involves going back to participants and sharing preliminary interpretations with them so that they can evaluate whether the researcher's thematic analysis is consistent with their experiences.

Disseminating Qualitative Findings

Quantitative reports almost never contain any **raw data**—data exactly in the form they were collected, which are numeric values. Qualitative reports, by contrast, are usually filled with rich verbatim passages directly from study participants. The excerpts are used in an evidential fashion to support or illustrate researchers' interpretations and thematic construction.

Example of raw data in a qualitative report

Regehr, Kjerulf, Popova, and Baker (2004) studied the experiences and attitudes of operating room nurses participating in the procurement of organs for transplantation. In-depth interviews with 14 operating room nurses revealed that the organ procurement process is highly stressful, as illustrated by the following quote: "During the procedure I have to sort of split my mind up and say I'm removing the kidneys or the liver or whatever, and looking at what I'm doing rather than looking at the whole picture.... Because to me, it's like, oh my God, why are you doing this?" (p. 434)

Like quantitative researchers, qualitative nurse researchers want to see their findings used by others. Qualitative findings can serve as the basis for formulating hypotheses that are tested by quantitative researchers, and for developing measuring instruments used for both research and clinical purposes. Qualitative findings can also provide a foundation for designing effective nursing interventions. Qualitative studies help to shape nurses' perceptions of a problem or situation, their conceptualization of potential solutions, and their understanding of patients' concerns and experiences.

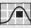

RESEARCH EXAMPLES   Critical Thinking Activities

EXAMPLE 1: Quantitative Research

The progression of activities in a quantitative study by one of this book's authors (Beck) is summarized below, followed by some questions to guide critical thinking.

Study
"Further validation of the Postpartum Depression Screening Scale" (Beck & Gable, 2001)

Study Purpose
Beck and Gable undertook a study to evaluate the Postpartum Depression Screening Scale (PDSS), an instrument designed for use by clinicians and researchers to screen mothers for postpartum depression (PPD).

Phase 1. Conceptual Phase, 1 Month: This phase was the shortest because most of the conceptual work had been done earlier in developing the instrument (Beck & Gable, 2000). The literature had already been reviewed, so the review only needed to be updated. The same framework and conceptual definitions that had been used in the first study were used in the new study.

Phase 2. Design and Planning Phase, 6 Months: The second phase involved fine-tuning the research design, gaining entrée into the hospital where participants were recruited, and obtaining approval of the hospital's ethics review committee. During this period, Beck met with statistical consultants and an instrument development consultant to finalize the design.

Phase 3. Empirical Phase, 11 Months: The design called for administering the PDSS to 150 mothers who were 6 weeks postpartum, and then scheduling a psychiatric diagnostic interview for them to determine whether they were suffering from PPD. Recruitment of participants and data collection took nearly a year.

Phase 4. Analytic Phase, 3 Months: Statistical tests were performed to determine a cut-off score on the PDSS above which mothers would be identified as having screened positive for PPD. Data analysis also was undertaken to determine the accuracy of the PDSS in predicting diagnosed PPD.

Phase 5. Dissemination Phase, 18 Months: The researchers prepared a research report and submitted it to the journal *Nursing Research* for possible publication. It was accepted for publication within 4 months, but it was "in press" (awaiting publication) for 14 months. During this period, the authors presented their findings at conferences, and prepared a report for the agency that funded the research.

Key Findings
Beck and Gable found that the PDSS was a reliable and valid tool for screening mothers and considered that the scale was ready for routine use.

*Critical Thinking Suggestions**
*See the Student Resource CD-ROM for a discussion of these questions.

Critical Thinking Activities (continued)

1. Answers questions 1 and 3 from Box 1.1 (Chapter 1) regarding this study.

2. Also consider the following targeted questions, which may further sharpen your critical thinking skills and assist you in understanding this study:

a. Was the study experimental or nonexperimental? What do you think the *population* for this study was?

b. How would you evaluate Beck and Gable's dissemination plan?

c. What are your thoughts about how time was allocated in this study; that is, how much time was spent in each phase?

d. Would it have been appropriate for the researchers to address the research question using qualitative research methods? Why or why not?

3. If the results of this study are valid and generalizable, what are some of the uses to which the findings might be put in clinical practice?

 EXAMPLE 2: Qualitative Research

The progression of activities in a qualitative study by one of this book's authors (Beck) is summarized below, followed by some questions to guide critical thinking.

Study

"Releasing the pause button: Mothering twins during the first year of life" (Beck, 2002)

Study Purpose

Beck undertook a grounded theory study to explore the phenomenon of mothering twins during the first year after delivery.

Phase 1. Conceptual Phase, 3 Months: Beck became interested in mothers of multiples as a result of her studies on postpartum depression (PPD). These studies had revealed a much higher prevalence of PPD among mothers of multiples than among those of singletons. Beck had not studied multiple births before, and so she carefully reviewed that literature. She easily gained entrée into the research site (a hospital) because she had previously conducted a study there and was known to the hospital's gatekeepers.

Phase 2. Design and Planning Phase, 4 Months: Beck chose a grounded theory design because she wanted to (1) discover the basic problem mothers with twins experience and (2) describe the process these mothers used to cope during the first year of their twins' life. Beck met with the nurse who headed a support group to plan the best approach for recruiting mothers into the study. Plans were also made for Beck to attend the support group's monthly meetings. Once the design was finalized, the research proposal was submitted to ethics review committees.

Phase 3. Empirical/Analytic Phases, 10 Months: Data collection and data analysis occurred simultaneously in this study. Beck attended the "parents of

(Research Examples continue on page 64)

Critical Thinking Activities (continued)

multiples" support group for 10 months. She also conducted in-depth interviews with 16 mothers of twins in their homes, and analyzed her rich and extensive data. Some steps Beck used to enhance the trustworthiness of her findings included (1) audiotaping all the interviews so that she would have verbatim transcripts for data analysis and (2) validating her developing grounded theory with mothers of twins who attended one of the multiple-birth parent meetings at the hospital.

Phase 4. Dissemination Phase, 23 Months: A manuscript describing the study was submitted for publication to *Qualitative Health Research*, which published the report in 2002. Beck also presented the findings at a regional nursing research conference and a neonatal/perinatal symposium.

Key Findings

Beck's analysis indicated that "life on hold" was the basic problem mothers of twins experienced during the first year. As mothers attempted to resume their own lives, they progressed through a four-stage process that Beck called "releasing the pause button."

Critical Thinking Suggestions

1. Answers questions 1 and 3 from Box 1.1 (Chapter 1) regarding this study.

2. Also consider the following targeted questions, which may further sharpen your critical thinking skills and assist you in understanding this study:

   a. What are your thoughts about how time was allocated in this study; that is, how much time was spent in each phase?

   b. Given the focus of the study, do you think that grounded theory was the appropriate research approach?

   c. Who was one of the gatekeepers in the hospital who helped Beck recruit her sample?

   d. Would it have been appropriate for Beck to address the research question using quantitative research methods? Why or why not?

3. If the results of this study are valid and generalizable, what are some of the uses to which the findings might be put in clinical practice?

 EXAMPLE 3: Quantitative Research

The progression of activities in the study by Feeley and colleagues ("Mother–VLBW Infant Interaction") in Appendix A is not spelled out in detail in the report (this is normal), but there are a few clues that provide some insights about scheduling. Answer the following questions regarding the timeframes of the study:

1. When was the study submitted to the journal for publication? (See the footnote at the end of the report.) How long did it take between submission and acceptance, and between acceptance and publication?

2. What is your estimate of how long the study took, from the time it was conceptualized (and an application was submitted for financial support) until the time when the report was published?

Critical Thinking Activities (continued)

EXAMPLE 4: Qualitative Research

The progression of activities in Beck's study ("Birth Trauma") in Appendix B is not spelled out in detail in the report, but there are a few clues that provide some insights about scheduling. Answer the following questions regarding the time-frames of the study:

1. Over how long a period were the data for this study collected? (See the subsection labelled "Procedure.") Why do you think it took this long to collect the data?

2. Did Beck receive funding to complete her study? (Information regarding funding is usually found at the end of a report, just before references, or in a footnote on the first page of a report.)

3. When was the study accepted for publication? (See the end of the report, before the References.) What does this suggest about when the data were analyzed and the report was written?

4. How long did it take between when the report was accepted for publication and when it was published?

5. What is your estimate of how long the study took, from the time it was conceptualized until the time when the report was published?

CHAPTER REVIEW

Summary Points

▶ Quantitative studies are either experimental or nonexperimental. In **experimental research,** researchers actively introduce a treatment or intervention; in **nonexperimental research,** researchers make observations of existing characteristics and behaviour without intervening.

▶ Qualitative nursing research often is rooted in research traditions from the disciplines of anthropology, sociology, and psychology. Three such traditions are ethnography, grounded theory, and phenomenology.

▶ **Grounded theory** seeks to describe and understand key social–psychological processes that occur in social settings.

▶ **Phenomenology** is concerned with lived experiences and is an approach to learning about what people's life experiences are like and what they mean.

▶ **Ethnography** provides a framework for studying the meanings, patterns, and experiences of a defined cultural group in a holistic fashion.

▶ In a quantitative study, researchers progress in a linear fashion from posing a research question to answering it in fairly standard steps.

▶ The main phases in a quantitative study are the conceptual, planning, empirical, analytic, and dissemination phases.

▶ The conceptual phase involves defining the problem to be studied, doing a **literature review**, engaging in clinical fieldwork for clinical studies, developing a framework and conceptual definitions, and formulating hypotheses to be tested.

▶ The design and planning phase entails selecting a **research design**, formulating the **intervention protocol** (in experimental research), specifying the **population**, developing a **sampling plan**, specifying methods to measure the research variables, designing procedures to protect subjects' rights, and finalizing the research plan (and, in some cases, conducting a **pilot study**).

▶ The empirical phase involves collecting the data and preparing the data for analysis (e.g., **coding** the data).

▶ The analytic phase involves analyzing the data through **statistical analysis** and interpreting the results.

▶ The dissemination phase entails communicating the findings and promoting their utilization.

▶ The flow of activities in a qualitative study is more flexible and less linear than in a quantitative study.

▶ Qualitative researchers begin with a broad question that is narrowed through the actual process of data collection and analysis.

▶ In the early phase of a qualitative study, researchers select a site and then take steps to **gain entrée** into it; gaining entrée typically involves enlisting the cooperation of *gatekeepers* or *stakeholders* within the site.

▶ Qualitative studies typically involve an **emergent design**: researchers select informants, collect data, and then analyze and interpret them in an ongoing fashion. Field experiences help to shape the design of the study.

▶ Early analysis leads to refinements in sampling and data collection, until **saturation** (redundancy of information) is achieved.

▶ Qualitative researchers conclude by disseminating findings that can subsequently be used to guide further studies, to develop structured measuring tools, and to influence nurses' perceptions of a problem and their conceptualizations of potential solutions.

Additional Resources for Review

Chapter 3 of the *Study Guide to Accompany Essentials of Nursing Research*, 6th edition offers various exercises and study suggestions for reinforcing the concepts presented in this chapter. For additional review, see the Student Self-Study Review Questions section of the Student Resource CD-ROM provided with this book.

SUGGESTED READINGS

References for studies cited in the chapter appear at the end of the book.

Methodologic References

Creswell, J. W. (1998). *Qualitative inquiry and research design: Choosing among five traditions*. Thousand Oaks, CA: Sage Publications.

Glaser, B. G., & Strauss, A. L. (1967). *The discovery of grounded theory: Strategies for qualitative research*. Chicago: Aldine.

Kerlinger, F. N., & Lee, H. B. (2000). *Foundations of behavioral research* (4th ed.). Orlando, FL: Harcourt College.

4

Reading Research Reports

STUDENT OBJECTIVES

On completing this chapter, you will be able to:

▶ Name types of research reports
▶ Describe the major sections in a research journal article
▶ Characterize the style used in quantitative and qualitative research reports
▶ Distinguish research summaries and research critiques
▶ Define new terms in the chapter

TYPES OF RESEARCH REPORTS

Evidence from nursing studies is communicated through *research reports* that describe what was studied, how it was studied, and what was found. Research reports—especially reports for quantitative studies—are often daunting to readers without research training. This chapter is designed to help make research reports more accessible.

Researchers communicate information about their studies in various ways. The most common types of research reports are theses and dissertations, books, presentations at conferences, and journal articles. You are most likely to be exposed to research results at professional conferences or in journals.

Presentations at Professional Conferences

Research findings are presented at conferences as oral presentations or poster sessions.

▶ *Oral presentations* follow a format similar to that used in journal articles, which we discuss later in this chapter. The presenter of an oral report is typically allotted 10 to 20 minutes to describe the most important aspects of the study.

▶ In **poster sessions,** many researchers simultaneously present visual displays summarizing their studies, and conference attendees circulate around the room perusing these displays.

One attractive feature of conference presentations is that there may be less time elapsed between the completion of a study and the dissemination of findings than is the case with journal articles. Conferences also offer an opportunity for dialogue among researchers and conference attendees. The listeners at oral presentations and viewers of poster displays can ask questions to help them better understand how the study was done or what the findings mean; moreover, they can offer the researchers suggestions about the clinical implications of the study. Thus, professional conferences offer a particularly valuable forum for a clinical audience.

Example of conference presentations

Dr. Cheryl Forchuk, a prominent nurse researcher who teaches at the University of Western Ontario, has made hundreds of presentations at professional conferences. One of her collaborative studies has involved an evaluation of the effectiveness of postoperative pain massage from a significant other for women who have had lymph node dissection surgery. Her findings were published in 2004 (Forchuk, Baruth, Prendergast, Holliday, Bareham, Brimmer, Schulz, Chan, & Yammine, 2004), but preliminary results were presented in a poster session in Toronto in May 2001 and in an oral presentation in Copenhagen in June 2001. (The published study appears in its entirety in Appendix C of this book.)

Research Journal Articles

Research **journal articles** are reports that summarize studies in professional journals. Because competition for journal space is keen, the typical research article is brief—generally only 10 to 25 double-spaced manuscript pages. This means that researchers must condense a lot of information about the study purpose, research methods, findings, interpretation, and clinical significance into a short report.

Publication in journals is competitive. Usually, research articles are reviewed by two or more **peer reviewers** (other researchers doing work in the field) who make recommendations about whether the article should be accepted, rejected, or revised and re-reviewed. These are usually **"blind" reviews**—reviewers are not told researchers' names, and researchers are not told reviewers' names.

In major nursing research journals, the rate of acceptance is low—it can be as low as 5% of submitted manuscripts. Thus, consumers of research articles have some assurance that the reports have already been evaluated by other nurse researchers. Nevertheless, the publication of an article does not mean that the findings can be uncritically accepted. The validity of the findings and their utility for clinical practice depend on how the study was conducted. Research methods courses help consumers to evaluate the quality of research evidence reported in journal articles.

THE CONTENT OF RESEARCH JOURNAL ARTICLES

Research reports in journals tend to follow a certain format and to be written in a particular style. Research reports begin with a title that succinctly conveys (typically in 15 or fewer words) the nature of the study. In qualitative studies, the title includes the central phenomenon and group under investigation; in quantitative studies, the title usually indicates the independent and dependent variables and the population.

Quantitative reports—and many qualitative ones—typically follow a conventional format for organizing content: the **IMRAD format**. This format involves organizing material into four sections—the **I**ntroduction, **M**ethod, **R**esults, **and D**iscussion. The main text of the report is usually preceded by an abstract and followed by references.

The Abstract

The **abstract** is a brief description of the study placed at the beginning of the article. The abstract answers, in about 100 to 200 words, the following questions: What were the research questions? What methods were used to address those questions? What were the findings? and What are the implications for nursing practice? Readers can review an abstract to assess whether the entire report should be read.

Some journals have moved from having traditional abstracts—single paragraphs summarizing the main features of the study—to slightly longer and more informative abstracts with specific headings. For example, abstracts in *Nursing Research* after 1997 present information about the study organized under the following headings: Background, Objectives, Method, Results, Conclusions, and Key Words.

Box 4.1 presents abstracts from two actual studies. The first is a "new style" abstract for a quantitative study entitled "Functional and Self-efficacy Changes of Patients Admitted to a Geriatric Rehabilitation Unit" (McCloskey, 2004). The second is a more traditional abstract for a qualitative study entitled "Daughters Giving Care to Mothers Who Have Dementia: Mastering the 3 Rs of (Re)Calling, (Re)Learning, and (Re)Adjusting" (Perry, 2004). These two studies are used as illustrations throughout this chapter.

The Introduction

The introduction acquaints readers with the research problem and its context. The introduction usually describes the following:

▶ *The central phenomena, concepts, or variables under study.* The problem area under investigation is identified.
▶ *The statement of purpose, research questions, and/or hypotheses to be tested.* Researchers explain what they set out to accomplish by conducting the study.

> **BOX 4.1** **Examples of Abstracts from Journal Articles**

Quantitative Study

Background: Geriatric rehabilitation units (GRUs) have been established to restore functional abilities of older hospitalized patients. Although considerable health care resources have been allocated to these units, few outcome-based research studies have been reported on Canadian GRUs. *Aim:* The aim of this paper is to report a study examining the effect of admission to a GRU on patients' functional ability and self-efficacy in performing everyday activities at home.

Methods: Following Institutional Review Board approval, data were collected from 40 patients aged 65–101 years (mean, 83.8; SD, 6.57) admitted to a 21-bed interdisciplinary GRU over a 7-month period. All were living independently before hospital admission. Data were collected on admission to the unit and on discharge using two instruments: the Functional Independence Measure and the Falls Efficacy Scale.

Results: Statistically significant improvements were found in functional ability and self-efficacy following admission to the GRU.

Conclusions: Although functional level and feelings of self-efficacy on admission to the unit were at levels that may have prevented participants from returning home, most participants were discharged to the community. Results suggest that admission to a GRU helps prepare patients to return to community living (McCloskey, 2004).

Qualitative Study

Using the process of constant comparative analysis to examine interview data, the current study explored the process of taking and continuing to give care to mothers with dementia. The sample consisted of 19 daughters and 1 daughter-in-law; all but one were living with the mother. The core phenomenon of mastery captured the processes of (re)calling, through (re)learning how to be with the mother to (re)adjusting as the daughters try to take care of themselves and consider placing their mother in a nursing home. Through these processes, the daughters essentially deconstruct their images of their mother and rebuild the image to include the impact of the disease process. The inclusion of the cognitive work adds an additional focus for potential intervention with daughters who, in providing care for their mothers, form such a vital part of current health care systems (Perry, 2004).

▶ *A review of the related literature.* Current knowledge relating to the study problem is briefly described so that readers can understand how the study fits in with previous findings and can assess the contribution of the new study.

▶ *The theoretical framework.* In theoretically driven studies, the framework is usually presented in the introduction.

▶ *The significance of and need for the study.* Most research reports include an explanation of why the study is important to nursing.

Thus, the introduction sets the stage for a description of what the researcher did and what was learned. The information in the introduction corresponds roughly to the activities undertaken in the conceptual phase of the project, as described in Chapter 3.

In this paragraph, the researcher described the background of the problem, the population of primary interest (older hospitalized patients), and the need for the study (the paucity of studies outside the United States).

Example from an introductory paragraph

"Acute hospitalization of older adults often results in functional decline and decreased self-care abilities. Research has suggested that up to 50% of older hospitalized patients experience functional decline (Bergman et al. 1997, Herbert 1997, Rosenberg & Moore 1997). In fact, functional decline on admission to hospital has previously been shown to be a predictor of adverse hospital outcomes (Inouye et al. 2000, Fleury 2002, Huckstadt 2002). Geriatric Rehabilitation Units (GRUs) have been recognized as an effective strategy to restore older, hospitalized patients' functional abilities (Rubenstein et al 1984, Batzan et al 2003). However, studies reporting this have been mainly conducted in the United States" (McCloskey, 2004, p. 186).

CONSUMER TIP

The introduction sections of many reports are not specifically labelled "Introduction." The report's introduction immediately follows the abstract. ▪

The Method Section

The method section describes the methods the researcher used to answer the research questions. The method section tells readers about major methodologic decisions and may offer rationales for those decisions. For example, a report for a qualitative study may explain why a qualitative approach was considered to be appropriate and fruitful.

In a report for a quantitative study, the method section usually describes the following, which may be in specifically labelled subsections:

▶ *The research design.* A description of the research design focuses on the overall plan for structuring the study, often including the steps the researcher took to minimize biases and control extraneous variables.
▶ *The sample.* Quantitative research reports describe the population under study, specifying the criteria by which the researcher decided whether a person would be eligible for the study. The method section also describes the actual sample, indicating how people were selected and the number of subjects in the sample.
▶ *Measures and data collection.* Researchers describe the methods and procedures used to collect the data, including how the critical research variables were operationalized; they also present information about the quality of the measuring tools.
▶ *Study procedures.* The method section contains a description of the procedures used to conduct the study, including a description of any intervention. The researcher's efforts to protect participants' rights may also be documented in this section.

Table 4.1 presents excerpts from the method section of the quantitative study by McCloskey (2004), describing aspects of the research design, sample (i.e., participants), data collection strategies (i.e., instruments), and procedures (data collection).

TABLE 4.1	Excerpts From Method Section, Quantitative Report
METHODOLOGIC ELEMENT	**EXCERPT FROM McCLOSKEY, 2004**
Research design	We used an exploratory, one-group, longitudinal design that involved no experimental manipulation of the independent variable (care provided on the geriatric rehabilitation unit [GRU]). (p. 187)
Participants	The setting was a 21-bed GRU located in an urban centre in Canada that services a population of 150 000. Patients were transferred to the unit after resolution of an acute medical or surgical condition that necessitated hospital admission. Those admitted to the unit who met the study criteria from 1 July 1999 to 20 January 2000 were invited to participate. Recruitment criteria were that potential participants must be over 64 years of age, English speaking, having their first admission to the unit, and able to provide informed consent. (pp. 187–188)
Instruments	The FIM (Functional Independence Measure) is a widely used instrument to assess functional status. The tool has 16 items and each is rated on a 7-point scale ranging from completely dependent (1) to completely independent (7). . . . The FES (Falls Efficacy Scale) measures self-efficacy. Confidence in completing 10 activities in the home is rated on a 10-point scale ranging from 1 for "not confident at all" to 10 for "completely confident." (p. 188)
Data collection	Within 72 hours of admission to the GRU, the researcher: (i) met all patients who had agreed to be approached to participate, (ii) obtained informed consent for participation, and (iii) completed the FES in collaboration with the patient. Within 72 hours of the patient's admission to the GRU, the nurse in charge of the study unit from Monday to Friday during the day shift completed the FIM in collaboration with the patient's primary nurse. (p. 188)

Qualitative researchers discuss many of the same issues, but with different emphases. For example, reports for a qualitative study often provide more information about the research setting and the study context and less information on sampling. Also, because formal instruments are not used to collect qualitative data, there is little discussion about data collection methods, but there may be more information on data collection procedures. Qualitative reports increasingly are including descriptions of the researchers' efforts to ensure the trustworthiness of the data. Some qualitative reports also have a subsection on data analysis. There are fairly standard ways of analyzing quantitative data, but such standardization does not exist for qualitative data, so qualitative researchers may describe their analytic approach. Table 4.2 presents excerpts from the method section of the qualitative study by Perry (2004), describing aspects of her sample, data collection, and data analysis.

In quantitative studies, the method section describes decisions made during the design and planning phase of the study and implemented during the empirical phase (see Chapter 3). In qualitative studies, the methodologic decisions are made during the planning stage and also during the course of data collection and fieldwork.

TABLE 4.2	Excerpts From Method Section, Qualitative Report
METHODOLOGIC ELEMENT	**EXCERPT FROM PERRY, 2004**
Recruitment	Staff from support groups and day centers in the Pacific Northwest offered daughters a letter of information. The researcher called all daughters who gave their permission to provide the details of the study and make arrangements for the interviews. . . . (p. 54)
Participants	Participants whose mothers were in early, middle, and advanced stages of dementia were sought to ensure the inclusion of the full range of experiences. . . . Of the participants, 18 daughters who lived at home with their mothers at the time of the first interview, one daughter-in-law who claimed to be very close and who lived with her mother-in-law, and one daughter who recently placed her mother constituted the sample. The daughters' ages ranged between 43 and 60 years with a mean of 49 years. (p. 55)
Data collection	In-depth interviews included questions that addressed how the daughters had assumed the caregiver role, their views and feelings, and how their caregiving went on a day-to-day basis. Questions were open ended and broad based, such as "Tell me about what you saw happening with your mom?" (p. 54)
Data analysis	Verbatim transcripts of the audiotaped interviews and field notes were analyzed throughout the study. Line-by-line coding was undertaken to extract codes and preliminary categories. Categories were continually emerging and were examined for links and connections so that they could be reorganized to a higher level of abstraction. (p. 55)

The Results Section

The results section presents the research **findings** (i.e., the results obtained in the analyses of the data). The text presents a narrative summary of the findings, often accompanied by tables or figures that highlight the most noteworthy results.

Results sections typically contain basic descriptive information, including a description of the participants (e.g., their average age). In quantitative studies, researchers also provide descriptive information about key variables. For example, in a study of the effect of prenatal drug exposure on birth outcomes, the results section might begin by describing the average birth weights and Apgar scores of the infants, or the percentage who were of low birth weight (less than 2500 g).

In quantitative studies, the results section also reports the following information relating to the statistical analyses performed:

▶ *The name of statistical tests used.* A **statistical test** is a procedure for testing hypotheses and evaluating the believability of the findings. For example, if the percentage of low-birth-weight infants in the sample of drug-exposed infants is computed, how probable is it that the percentage is accurate? If the researcher finds that the average birth weight of drug-exposed infants in the sample is lower than the birth weight of infants who were not exposed to drugs, how probable is it that the same would be true for other infants not in the sample? That is, is the relationship between prenatal drug exposure and infant birth weight *real* and likely to be replicated with a new sample of infants? Statistical tests answer such questions. Statistical tests are based on common principles; you do not have to know the names of all statistical tests (there are dozens of them) to comprehend the findings.

▶ *The value of the calculated statistic.* Computers are used to compute a numeric value for the particular statistical test used. The value allows the researchers to draw conclusions about the meaning of the results. The *actual* numeric value of the statistic, however, is not inherently meaningful and need not concern you.

▶ *The significance.* The most important information is whether the results of the statistical tests were significant (not to be confused with important or clinically relevant). If the results were **statistically significant,** it means that, based on the statistical test, the findings are probably reliable and replicable with a new group of people. Research reports also indicate the **level of significance,** which is an index of how probable it is that the findings are reliable. For example, if a report indicates that a finding was significant at the .05 level, this means that only 5 times out of 100 ($5 \div 100 = .05$) would the results be spurious. In other words, 95 times out of 100, similar results would be obtained with other samples from the same population. Readers can therefore have a high degree of confidence—but not total assurance—that the findings are accurate.

Example from the results section of a quantitative study

As shown in Table 4.2, total FIM score was 84.9 . . . on admission, indicating functional dependency, compared with 101.6 . . . on discharge, indicating modified functional independence. A paired *t*-test revealed that mean total FIM scores were significantly higher on discharge [$t(39) = -6.517, p = .0001$] than on admission to the GRU.

In this excerpt, McCloskey indicated that the study participants' average score on the measure of functional ability was significantly better at discharge than on admission. In other words, the average improvement of nearly 17 points on the scale was not likely to

CONSUMER TIP

Be especially alert to the *p* values (probabilities) when reading statistical results. If a *p* value is greater than .05 (e.g., *p* = .08), the results are considered *not* to be statistically significant by conventional standards. Nonsignificant results are sometimes abbreviated NS. Also, be aware that the results are *more* reliable if the *p* value is smaller. For example, there is a higher probability that the results are accurate when *p* = .01 (only 1 in 100 chance of a spurious result) than when *p* = .05 (5 in 100 chances of a spurious result). Researchers sometimes report an exact probability estimate (e.g., *p* = .03), as in the above example, or a probability below conventional thresholds (e.g., *p* < .05—less than 5 in 100). ■

have been a haphazard change, and would be very likely to be replicated with a new sample of elders. In this case, the finding is highly reliable: only one time in 10,000 ($p =$ .0001) would an improvement this great have occurred as a fluke. Note that to comprehend this finding, you do not need to understand what the t statistic is, nor do you need to concern yourself with the actual value of the statistic, -6.517.

In qualitative reports, the researcher often organizes findings according to the major *themes* or categories that were identified in the data. The results section of qualitative reports sometimes has several subsections, with headings corresponding to the themes. Excerpts from the raw data are presented to support and provide a rich description of the thematic analysis. The results section of qualitative reports may also present the researcher's emerging theory about the phenomenon under study, although this may appear in the concluding section of the report.

Example from the results section of a qualitative study

When the daughters began to give care, they had to (re)learn who their mothers had been, who their mother currently was, and how to "be" with the mother and look after her in acceptable ways in private and in public.... The mother–daughter bond grounded the process of learning and relearning. Daughters consistently said things such as "She's still my mom" and "No matter what she does she is still my mom." One daughter said, "It's so hard because she's still my mum, you know, and so maybe that is why ... (drifting). Because she's my mother I can do some stuff easily like let go of, um, arguing with her or something or trying to make her see, see reason where there is none. She's not going to see any reason, you know, like I just have to accept it" (Perry, 2004, p. 59).

In this excerpt, through the use of a direct quote from one study participant, the researcher illustrated the finding that adjusting to the caregiving role was a learning process.

The Discussion

In the discussion section, researchers draw conclusions about the meaning and implications of the findings. This section tries to unravel what the results mean, why things turned out the way they did, and how the results can be used in practice. The discussion in both qualitative and quantitative reports may incorporate the following elements:

▶ *An interpretation of the results.* The interpretation involves the translation of findings into practical, conceptual, or theoretical meaning.
▶ *Implications.* Researchers often offer suggestions for how their findings could be used to improve nursing, and they may also make recommendations on how best to advance knowledge through additional research.
▶ *Study limitations.* The researcher is in the best position possible to discuss study limitations, such as sample deficiencies, design problems, and so forth. Reports that

identify these limitations indicate to readers that the author was aware of these limitations and probably took them into account in interpreting the findings.

Example from a discussion section of a quantitative report

"Improvements were noted in all subscales of the FIM, with some areas demonstrating more improvement than others (self-care, sphincter control, transfers and locomotion). Statistically non-significant improvements were noted in communication; however, participants scored high in this on admission. The inclusion criteria for the study may have also led to this high score in this area, thereby giving little opportunity for improvement." (McCloskey, 2004, p. 191)

As this example illustrates, researchers may speculate in the discussion section about *why* certain findings turned out the way they did.

References

Research journal articles conclude with a list of the books, reports, and journal articles that were referenced in the report. If you are interested in pursuing additional reading on a substantive topic, the reference list of a recent study is an excellent place to begin.

THE STYLE OF RESEARCH JOURNAL ARTICLES

Research reports tell a story. However, the style in which many journal articles are written—especially for quantitative studies—makes it difficult for beginning research consumers to become interested in the story. To unaccustomed audiences, research reports may seem pedantic or bewildering. Four factors contribute to this impression:

▶ *Compactness.* Journal space is limited, so authors compress many ideas and concepts into a short space. Interesting, personalized aspects of the investigation often cannot be reported. And, in qualitative studies, only a handful of supporting quotes can be included.

▶ *Jargon.* The authors of both qualitative and quantitative reports use research terms that are assumed to be part of reader's vocabulary but that may be mystifying.

▶ *Objectivity.* Quantitative researchers often avoid any impression of subjectivity, and so their research stories are told in a way that makes them sound impersonal. For example, most quantitative research reports are written in the passive voice (i.e., personal pronouns are avoided). Use of the passive voice makes a report less lively than use of the active voice, and it tends to give the impression that the researcher did not play an active role in conducting the study. Qualitative reports, by contrast, are more subjective and personal and are written in a more conversational style.

▶ *Statistical information.* In quantitative reports, numbers may intimidate readers who do not have strong mathematic interest or training.

A goal of this textbook is to assist you in understanding the content of research reports and in overcoming anxieties about jargon and statistical information.

READING, SUMMARIZING, AND CRITIQUING RESEARCH REPORTS

Nurses who want to develop an evidence-based practice must be able to read and critically appraise research reports. This section offers some general guidance on reading nursing research reports.

Reading and Summarizing Research Reports

The skills involved in critical appraisal take time to develop. The first step in being able to use research findings in practice is to understand research reports. Your first few attempts to read research reports might be overwhelming, and you may wonder whether being able to understand, let alone appraise, them is a realistic goal. As you progress through this textbook, you will acquire skills to help you evaluate these reports. Some preliminary tips on digesting research reports follow:

▶ Grow accustomed to the style of research reports by reading them frequently, even though you may not yet understand all the technical points. Try to keep the underlying rationale for the style of research reports in mind as you read.

▶ Read from a report that has been photocopied so that you can use a highlighter, write notes in the margins, and so on.

▶ Read journal articles slowly. It may be useful to skim the article first to get the major points and then to read the article more carefully a second time.

▶ On the second or later reading of a journal article, train yourself to become an *active* reader. Reading actively involves constantly monitoring yourself to determine whether you understand what you are reading. If you have comprehension problems, go back and re-read difficult passages or make notes about your confusion so that you can ask someone for clarification. Usually, that "someone" will be your research instructor or a faculty member, but also consider contacting the researchers themselves. The postal and e-mail addresses of the researchers are usually included in the journal article, and researchers are generally more than willing to discuss their research with others.

▶ Keep this textbook with you as a reference while you read articles initially, so that you can look up unfamiliar terms in the glossary or the index.

▶ Try not to get bogged down in (or scared away by) statistical information. Try to grasp the gist of the story without letting symbols and numbers frustrate you.

▶ Until you become accustomed to the style and jargon of research journal articles, you may want to "translate" them mentally or in writing. You can do this by expanding compact paragraphs into looser constructions, by translating jargon into more familiar terms, by recasting sentences into an active voice, and by summarizing findings with words rather than with numbers. As an example, Box 4.2 presents a summary of a fictitious study about the psychological consequences of having an abortion, written

BOX 4.2	Summary of a Fictitious Study for Translation

	The potentially negative sequelae of having an abortion on the psychological adjustment of adolescents have not been adequately studied. The present study sought to determine whether alternative pregnancy resolution decisions have different long-term effects on the psychological functioning of young women.	**Need for the study**
Purpose of the study		
Research design	Three groups of low-income pregnant teenagers attending an inner-city clinic were the <u>subjects</u> in this study: those who delivered and kept the baby; those who delivered and relinquished the baby for adoption; and those who had an abortion. There were 25 subjects in each group. The study <u>instruments</u> included a self-administered <u>questionnaire</u> and a battery of psychological tests measuring depression, anxiety, and psychosomatic symptoms. The instruments were administered upon entry into the study (when the subjects first came to the clinic) and then 1 year after termination of the pregnancy.	**Study population**
Research instruments		**Research sample**
Data analysis procedure	The <u>data</u> were analyzed using <u>analysis of variance (ANOVA)</u>. The ANOVA tests indicated that the three groups did not differ significantly in terms of depression, anxiety, or psychosomatic symptoms at the initial testing. At the <u>posttest</u>, however, the abortion group had significantly higher scores on the depression scale, and these girls were significantly more likely than the two delivery groups to report severe tension headaches. There were no <u>significant</u> differences on any of the <u>dependent variables</u> for the two delivery groups.	**Results**
Implications	The results of this study suggest that young women who elect to have an abortion may experience a number of long-term negative consequences. It would appear that appropriate efforts should be made to follow abortion patients to determine their need for suitable treatment.	**Interpretation**

in the style typically found in research journal articles. Terms that can be looked up in the glossary of this book are underlined, and bolded marginal notes indicate the type of information the author is communicating. Box 4.3 presents a "translation" of this summary, recasting the research information into language that is more digestible.

BOX 4.3   Translated Version of Fictitious Research Study

As researchers, we wondered whether young women who had an abortion had any emotional problems in the long run. It seemed to us that not enough research had been done to know whether any psychological harm resulted from an abortion.

We decided to study this question ourselves by comparing the experiences of three types of teenagers who became pregnant—first, girls who delivered and kept their babies; second, those who delivered the babies but gave them up for adoption; and third, those who elected to have an abortion. All teenagers in our sample were poor, and all were patients at an inner-city clinic. Altogether, we studied 75 girls—25 in each of the three groups. We evaluated the teenagers' emotional states by asking them to fill out a questionnaire and to take several psychological tests. These tests allowed us to assess things such as the girls' degree of depression and anxiety and whether they had any complaints of a psychosomatic nature. We asked them to fill out the forms twice: once when they came into the clinic, and then again a year after the abortion or the delivery.

We learned that the three groups of teenagers looked pretty much alike in terms of their emotional states when they first filled out the forms. But when we compared how the three groups looked a year later, we found that the teenagers who had abortions were more depressed and were more likely to say they had severe tension headaches than teenagers in the other two groups. The teenagers who kept their babies and those who gave their babies up for adoption looked pretty similar 1 year after their babies were born, at least in terms of depression, anxiety, and psychosomatic complaints.

Thus, it seems that we might be right in having some concerns about the emotional effects of having an abortion. Nurses should be aware of these long-term emotional effects, and it even may be advisable to institute some type of follow-up procedure to find out if these young women need additional help.

When you attain a reasonable level of comprehension of a research report, a useful next step is to write a brief (1- to 2-page) synopsis. A synopsis summarizes the study's purpose, research questions, methods, findings, interpretation of the findings, and implications for practice. You do not need to be concerned at this point about critiquing the study's strengths and weaknesses, but rather about succinctly and objectively presenting a summary of what was done and what was learned. By preparing a synopsis, you will become more aware of aspects of the study that you did not understand.

Critiquing Research Reports

A written research **critique** is different from a research summary or synopsis. A research critique is a careful, critical appraisal of a study's strengths and limitations. Critiques usually conclude with the reviewer's summary of the study's merits, recommendations about the value of the evidence, and suggestions for improving the study or the report.

Research critiques of individual studies are prepared for various reasons, and they differ in scope, depending on their purpose. Peer reviewers who are asked to prepare a written critique of a manuscript for a journal editor before acceptance for publication generally critique the following aspects of the study:

▶ *Substantive*—Was the research problem significant to nursing?
▶ *Theoretical*—Were the theoretical underpinnings sound?
▶ *Methodologic*—Were the methods rigorous and appropriate?

▶ *Ethical*—Were the rights of study participants protected?

▶ *Interpretive*—Did the researcher properly interpret data and develop reasonable conclusions?

▶ *Stylistic*—Is the report clearly written, grammatical, and well organized?

In short, peer reviewers provide comprehensive feedback to the researchers and to journal editors about the merit of both the study and the report, and typically offer suggestions for improvements (e.g., for redoing some analyses).

By contrast, critiques designed to guide decisions for evidence-based practice need not be as comprehensive. For example, it is of little significance to practicing nurses that a research report is ungrammatical. A critique on the clinical utility of a study focuses on whether the findings are accurate and clinically meaningful. If the findings cannot be trusted, it makes little sense to incorporate them into practice.

By understanding research methods, you will be in a position to critique the rigor of studies, and this is a primary aim of this book. Most chapters offer guidelines for evaluating various research decisions that will help you to make an overall appraisal of a study. Chapter 17 provides extra guidance on undertaking a critique.

Competent consumers of research must be able to critique not only single, independent studies but also a body of studies on a topic of clinical interest. We describe literature reviews in Chapter 7 and discuss integrative reviews in Chapter 18.

RESEARCH EXAMPLES | **Critical Thinking Activities**

 EXAMPLE 1: Quantitative Research

An abstract for a quantitative nursing study is presented below, followed by some questions to guide critical thinking.

Study
"Insomnia, depression and anxiety disorders and their association with benzodiazepine drug use among the community-dwelling elderly: Implications for mental health nursing" (Voyer, Landreville, Moisan, Tousignant, and Préville, 2005)

Abstract
Benzodiazepine (BZD) drug use among seniors is an important public health issue because the benefit from their use is moderate and of short duration and numerous adverse events have been linked to their use. Furthermore, there is a significant discrepancy between the prevalence of mental health disorders and BZD drug use in the elderly population, which can be attributed to a measurement issue. The goal of this cross-sectional descriptive study was to determine the prevalence of mental health disorders among seniors using BZD and living in the community, basing this information on both a thorough face-to-face interview and a pair of self-reported validated instruments. Among the 216 seniors recruited in our study, nearly 20% were users of BZD, and more than 75% of had been using this drug for more than a year. Thirteen subjects were recognized as depressed according to

Critical Thinking Activities (continued)

a self-report measure, compared with 18 according to the interview. Likewise, 13 seniors were categorized as anxious based on a self-report questionnaire, compared with 39 based on the interview. Among self-reported measures of mental health variables, logistic regression indicated that insomnia increases by 7 the likelihood of using BZD (odds ratio, 7.2) and is the only statistically significant variable associated with BZD consumption. Based on thorough interviews, logistic regression showed that insomnia (odds ratio, 6.9) is still the dominant symptom associated with BZD drugs. In conclusion, our results clearly support the assertion that mental health status is influenced according to how it is measured. Finally, nurses should be aware that not all individuals are capable of expressing their mental health problems using either psychological or emotional terminologies. They may opt for expressing their psychological suffering as a physical symptom such as sleeping problems.

*Critical Thinking Suggestions**
*See the Student Resource CD-ROM for a discussion of these questions.
1. "Translate" the abstract into a summary that is more consumer friendly. (Underline any technical terms and look them up in the glossary.)
2. Also consider the following targeted questions:
   a. What were the independent variables in this study? How were they operationalized?
   b. What was the dependent variable in this study? How was it operationalized?
   c. Was the study experimental or nonexperimental?
   d. Were any of the findings statistically significant?
   e. Would it have been appropriate for the researchers to address the research question using qualitative research methods? Why or why not?
3. If the results of this study are valid and generalizable, what are some of the uses to which the research evidence might be put in clinical practice?

 EXAMPLE 2: Qualitative Research

An abstract for a qualitative nursing study is presented below, followed by some questions to guide critical thinking.

Study
"Prenatal care use among women of low income: A matter of 'taking care of self' " (Sword, 2003)

Abstract
The grounded theory study discussed in this article provides a theoretical explanation of prenatal care use among women of low income. The author recruited 26 women from two communities in Ontario, Canada to participate in an individual or focus group interview and analyzed data using descriptive coding, interpretive coding, and constant comparison. Perceptions of the health care system were identified

(Research Examples continue on page 82)

Critical Thinking Activities (continued)

as important influences on usage behaviour. This broad theme included two sub-themes: (a) program and service attributes, and (b) service provider characteristics. Within each subtheme, both barriers to and facilitative factors for prenatal care became apparent. The author examined relationships among categories to identify a unifying construct. "Taking care of self" emerged as the central phenomenon that explained usage behaviour. Women weigh the pros and cons when deciding whether to access prenatal care, and then take charge, ultimately making a decision in terms of its meaning for self.

Critical Thinking Suggestions

1. "Translate" the abstract into a summary that is more consumer friendly. (Underline any technical terms and look them up in the glossary.)
2. Also consider the following targeted questions:
   a. What was the phenomenon under investigation in this study?
   b. What qualitative research tradition did Sword use in this study? Based on what you've learned thus far about qualitative research traditions, does the selected tradition appear to be appropriate to address the research question?
   c. In this traditional abstract, what main features of the study were summarized?
   d. Would it have been appropriate for the researcher to address the research question using quantitative research methods? Why or why not?
3. If the results of this study are trustworthy, what are some of the uses to which the research evidence might be put in clinical practice?

 EXAMPLE 3: Quantitative Research

Read the abstract for the study by Forchuk and colleagues, "Postoperative Arm Massage," which can be found in Appendix C of this book. "Translate" the abstract into a summary that is more consumer friendly.

 EXAMPLE 4: Qualitative Research

Read the abstract for the study by Milliken and Northcott, "Redefining Parental Identity," which can be found in Appendix D of this book. "Translate" the abstract into a summary that is more consumer friendly.

C H A P T E R   R E V I E W
S u m m a r y   P o i n t s

- The most common types of research reports are theses and dissertations, books, conference presentations (including oral reports and **poster sessions**), and, especially, journal articles.
- Research **journal articles** provide brief descriptions of studies and are designed to communicate the contribution the study has made to knowledge.

▶ Quantitative journal articles (and many qualitative ones) typically follow the **IMRAD format** with the following sections: introduction (explanation of the study problem and its context); method section (the strategies used to address the research problem); results (the actual study **findings**); and discussion (the interpretation of the findings).

▶ Journal articles typically begin with an **abstract** (a brief synopsis of the study) and conclude with references (a list of works cited in the report).

▶ Research reports are often difficult to read because they are dense, concise, and contain a lot of jargon.

▶ Qualitative research reports are written in a more inviting and conversational style than quantitative ones, which are more impersonal and include information on statistical tests.

▶ **Statistical tests** are procedures for testing research hypotheses and evaluating the believability of the findings. Findings that are **statistically significant** are ones that have a high probability (p) of being accurate.

▶ The ultimate goal of this book is to help students to prepare a research **critique**, which is a careful, critical appraisal of the strengths and limitations of a piece of research, often for the purpose of considering the worth of its evidence for nursing practice.

Additional Resources for Review

Chapter 4 of the *Study Guide to Accompany Essentials of Nursing Research*, 6th edition offers various exercises and study suggestions for reinforcing the concepts presented in this chapter. For additional review, see the Student Self-Study Review Questions section of the Student Resource CD-ROM provided with this book.

SUGGESTED READINGS

References for studies cited in the chapter appear at the end of the book.

Methodologic References

Downs, F. S. (1999). How to cozy up to a research report. *Applied Nursing Research, 12,* 215–216.

Sandelowski, M., & Barroso, J. (2002). Finding the findings in qualitative studies. *Journal of Nursing Scholarship, 34,* 213–219.

Tornquist, E. M., Funk, S. G., Champagne, M. T., & Wiese, R. A. (1993). Advice on reading research: Overcoming the barriers. *Applied Nursing Research, 6,* 177–183.

Reviewing the Ethical Aspects of a Nursing Study

On completing this chapter, you will be able to:

▶ Discuss the historical background that led to the creation of various codes of ethics
▶ Understand the potential for ethical dilemmas stemming from conflicts between ethics and requirements for high-quality research evidence
▶ Identify the eight primary ethical principles articulated in the Tri-Council Policy Statement on research ethics and identify procedures for adhering to them
▶ Given sufficient information, evaluate the ethical dimensions of a research report
▶ Define new terms in the chapter

ETHICS AND RESEARCH

Nurses face many ethical issues in their practice. The prolongation of life by artificial means is but one example of situations that have led to discussions about ethics in health care practice. Similarly, the expansion of nursing research has led to ethical concerns about the rights of study participants. Ethics can create particular challenges to nurse researchers because ethical requirements sometimes conflict with the need to produce the highest possible quality evidence for practice. This chapter discusses some of the major ethical principles that should be considered in reviewing studies.

Historical Background

As modern, civilized people, we might like to think that systematic violations of moral principles by researchers occurred centuries ago rather than in recent times, but this is not the case. The Nazi medical experiments of the 1930s and 1940s are the most famous example of recent disregard for ethical conduct. The Nazi program of research involved the use of prisoners of war and racial "enemies" in experiments designed to test the limits of human endurance and human reaction to diseases and untested drugs. The studies were unethical not only because they exposed these people to physical harm and even death but also because the participants could not refuse participation.

There are recent examples from other Western countries. For instance, between 1932 and 1972, a study known as the Tuskegee Syphilis Study, sponsored by the U.S. Public Health Service, investigated the effects of syphilis on 400 men from a poor black community. Medical treatment was deliberately withheld to study the course of the untreated disease. Similarly, Dr. Herbert Green of the National Women's Hospital in Auckland, New Zealand studied women with cervical cancer in the 1980s; patients with carcinoma in situ were not given treatment so that researchers could study the natural progression of the disease. Another well-known case of unethical research involved the injection of live cancer cells into elderly patients at the Jewish Chronic Disease Hospital in Brooklyn in the 1960s without the consent of those patients. There are examples from Canada, too. A world-renowned Canadian psychiatrist attempted to wipe out his patients' memories and insert new thoughts (i.e., to "brain wash" them). Many other examples of studies with ethical transgressions—often less obvious than these examples—have emerged to give ethical concerns the high visibility they have today.

Codes of Ethics

In response to human rights violations, various codes of ethics have been developed. One of the first internationally recognized sets of ethical standards is the **Nuremberg Code,** developed in 1949 after the Nazi atrocities were made public in the Nuremberg trials. Another notable set of international standards is the **Declaration of Helsinki,** which was adopted in 1964 by the World Medical Assembly and most recently revised in 2000. (The ethical principles of the Declaration of Helsinki can be viewed at the World Medical Association website, *http://www.wma.net/e/policy/b3.htm.*)

Most disciplines have established their own **code of ethics.** In Canada, the Canadian Nurses Association (CNA) first published a document entitled *Ethical Guidelines for Nurses in Research Involving Human Participants* in 1983. It was revised in 1994 and again in 2002. The goal of this document is to provide nurses in all areas of professional practice with guidelines relating to research activities. The 2002 guidelines were revised to complement the broader CNA *Code of Ethics for Registered Nurses* (CNA, 2002a). Some nurse ethicists have called for an international code of ethics for nursing research, but nurses in most countries have developed their own professional codes or follow the codes established by their governments. The International Council of Nurses, however, has developed a *Code for Nurses*, which was most recently updated in 2000.

Government Regulations for Protecting Study Participants

Governments throughout the world fund research and establish rules for how such research must be conducted to adhere to ethical principles. Health Canada adopted the *Good Clinical Practice: Consolidated Guidelines* (GCP) in 1997 as the guidelines for certain types of research, namely clinical trial research involving human participants. In addition, Health Canada specified the *Tri-Council Policy Statement: Ethical Conduct for Research Involving Humans* (TCPS) in 1998 as the guidelines to protect human subjects in all types of research (Medical Research Council of Canada, Natural Sciences and Engineering Research Council of Canada, and Social Sciences and Humanities Research Council of Canada, 1998). The TCPS was jointly issued by the Canadian Institute of Health Research (CIHR), the Natural Sciences and Engineering Research Council (NSERC), and the Social Sciences and Humanities Research Council (SSHRC).

The TCPS articulates eight guiding ethical principles on which standards of ethical conduct in research are based. These principles were based on several sources, including past guidelines of the Councils, statements by other Canadian agencies, and input from the international community. An essential component of the GCP and the TCPS is that a research ethics committee, formally known in Canada as a Research Ethics Board (REB), should first review and approve each study that involves human subjects.

CONSUMER TIP

The following websites offer information about various professional codes of ethics and ethical requirements for government-sponsored research:

▶ Canadian policies, from the Tri-Council Policy Statement of the Natural Sciences and Engineering Research Council of Canada (NSERC): *http://www.nserc.ca/programs/ethics*

▶ Canadian Nurses Association: *http://www.cna-nurses.ca/pages/ethics/ethicsframe.htm*

▶ American Nurses Association: *http://www.ana.org/ethics*

▶ Policies from the U.S. National Institutes of Health, Office of Human Subjects Research (OHSR): *http://ohsr.od.nih.gov*

▶ International Council of Nurses: *http://www.icn.ch/icncode.pdf* ■

Ethical Dilemmas in Conducting Research

Research that violates ethical principles is rarely done to be cruel but more typically occurs out of a conviction that knowledge is important and beneficial in the long run. There are situations in which the rights of participants and the demands of the study are put in direct conflict, creating **ethical dilemmas** for researchers. In reading research reports, you need to be aware of such dilemmas. Here are some examples of research questions in which the desire for strong evidence conflicts with ethical considerations:

1. *Research question:* Are nurses equally empathic in their treatment of male and female patients in intensive care units?

   Ethical dilemma: Ethics require that participants be aware of their role in a study. Yet if the researcher informs the nurses in this study that their empathy in treating male and female patients will be scrutinized, will their behaviour be "normal"? If the nurses alter their behaviour because they know research observers are watching, the findings will not be valid.

2. *Research question:* What are the coping mechanisms of parents whose children have a terminal illness?

   Ethical dilemma: To answer this question, the researcher may need to probe into the psychological state of the parents at a vulnerable time in their lives; such probing could be disturbing, yet knowledge of the parents' coping mechanisms might lead to more effective ways of dealing with parents' grief.

3. *Research question:* Does a new medication prolong life in cancer patients?

   Ethical dilemma: The best way to test the effectiveness of an intervention is to administer the intervention to some participants but withhold it from others to see whether differences between the groups emerge. However, if a new drug is untested, the group receiving it may be exposed to potentially hazardous side effects. On the other hand, the group *not* receiving it may be denied a beneficial treatment.

4. *Research question:* What is the process by which adult children adapt to the day-to-day stresses of caring for a parent with Alzheimer's disease?

   Ethical dilemma: In a qualitative study, which would be appropriate for this research question, the researcher sometimes becomes so closely involved with participants that they become willing to share "secrets" or privileged information. Interviews can become confessions—sometimes of unseemly or illegal behaviour. In this example, suppose a woman admitted to abusing her mother physically—how does the researcher respond to that information without undermining a pledge of confidentiality? And, if the researcher reveals the information to appropriate authorities, how can a pledge of confidentiality be given in good faith to other participants?

As these examples suggest, researchers are sometimes in a bind: their goal is to advance knowledge, using the best methods possible, but they must also adhere to the dictates of ethical rules that have been developed to protect participants' rights.

ETHICAL PRINCIPLES FOR PROTECTING STUDY PARTICIPANTS

The ethical framework established by the Tri-Council Policy Statement (1998) is based on a desire to balance the need for research—which is viewed as a fundamental moral commitment to advance human welfare—with the imperative of respecting human dignity. The underlying ethic involves two responsibilities—to establish ethically acceptable research goals and to use suitable means of reaching those goals. The policy statement articulates eight guiding ethical principles: respect for human dignity, respect for free and informed consent, respect for vulnerable persons, respect for privacy and confidentiality, respect of justice and inclusiveness, balancing harms and benefits, minimizing harm, and maximizing benefit. These fundamental principles are briefly described next, followed by a discussion of procedures researchers use to uphold them.

Respect for Human Dignity

A fundamental principle of modern research ethics is respect for human dignity. This principle aspires to protect the interests of study participants, in terms of bodily, psychological, and cultural integrity. The principle of respect for human dignity encompasses the right to self-determination and the right to full disclosure.

Humans are viewed as autonomous agents, capable of controlling their own activities. The principle of **self-determination** means that prospective participants have the right to decide voluntarily whether to participate in a study, without the risk of incurring adverse consequences. It also means that participants have the right to ask questions, to refuse to give information, and to withdraw from the study.

A person's right to self-determination includes freedom from coercion. **Coercion** involves explicit or implicit threats of penalty for failing to participate in a study or excessive rewards for agreeing to participate. The obligation to protect potential participants from coercion requires careful consideration when researchers are in a position of authority or influence over potential participants, as might be the case in a nurse–patient relationship. Coercion can in some cases be subtle. For example, a generous monetary incentive (or **stipend**) offered to encourage the participation of an economically disadvantaged group (e.g., the homeless) might be mildly coercive because such incentives could place undue pressure on prospective participants.

The principle of respect for human dignity also includes people's right to make informed, voluntary decisions about study participation, which requires full disclosure. **Full disclosure** means that the researcher has fully described the nature of the study, the person's right to refuse participation, the researcher's responsibilities, and the likely risks and benefits that would be incurred.

Respect for Free and Informed Consent

The TCPS stipulates that people are generally presumed to have the ability—and the right—to make free and informed decisions. Thus, respect for human dignity implies respect for participants' right to individual consent. **Informed consent** means that participants have adequate information about the research; comprehend the information; and have the power of free choice, that is, to consent voluntarily to participate in the research or to decline participation.

Informed consent is based on the right to self-determination and full disclosure, but in certain circumstances, participants' right to self-determination poses challenges. An important issue concerns some people's inability to make well-informed judgments about the costs and benefits of participation (e.g., children). We discuss the issue of special classes of research participants in the next section.

Adherence to the principle of full disclosure may also be problematic. Full disclosure can sometimes result in two types of biases: (1) biases resulting from inaccurate data and (2) biases stemming from difficulty recruiting a good sample. Suppose we were testing the hypothesis that high school students with a high rate of absenteeism are more likely to be substance abusers than students with good attendance. If we approached potential participants and fully explained the study purpose, some students likely would refuse to participate. Nonparticipation would be selective; in fact, we would expect that those least likely to volunteer would be students who are substance abusers—the group of primary interest. Moreover, by knowing the specific research question, those who do participate might not give candid responses. It might be argued that full disclosure would totally undermine the study.

One technique that researchers sometimes use in such situations is **covert data collection,** or *concealment*—the collection of information without participants' knowledge and thus without their consent. This might happen, for example, if a researcher wanted to observe people's behaviour in a real-world setting and was concerned that doing so openly would change the very behaviour of interest. Researchers might choose to obtain information through concealed methods, such as by observing through a one-way mirror, videotaping participants through hidden equipment, or observing while pretending to be engaged in other activities.

A second, and more controversial, technique is the use of deception. *Deception* can involve either deliberately withholding information about the study or providing participants with false information. For example, we might describe the study of high school students' use of drugs as research on students' health practices, which is a mild form of misinformation.

Deception and concealment are problematic ethically because they interfere with the participants' right to make a truly informed decision about the personal costs and benefits of participation. Some people argue that the use of deception or concealment is never justified. Others, however, believe that if the study involves low risk to participants and if there are anticipated benefits to science and society, deception or concealment may be justified to enhance the validity of the findings.

Another issue relating to full disclosure has emerged recently concerning the collection of data from people over the Internet (e.g., analyzing the content of messages posted to chat rooms, discussion boards, or on listserves). The issue is whether such messages can be used as data without the authors' consent. Some researchers believe that anything posted electronically is in the public domain and therefore can be used without consent for purposes of research. Others, however, feel that the same ethical standards must apply in cyberspace research and that electronic researchers must carefully protect the rights of individuals who are involved in "virtual" communities. Researchers at the University of Toronto have developed useful guidelines for addressing ethical dilemmas arising in research on Internet communities (Flicker, Hans, & Skinner, 2004).

Respect for Vulnerable Persons

Ethical obligations are heightened when the people under study are deemed to be a vulnerable group. **Vulnerable subjects** (a term often used to refer to at-risk study participants) are people with diminished competence or decision-making ability. The TCPS instructs researchers to afford vulnerable groups special protections against exploitation or discrimination.

Groups that are considered to be vulnerable because of diminished competence include children, mentally or emotionally disabled people, and others who are unable to understand information or appreciate the consequences of participation (e.g., comatose patients). The TCPS specifically notes that, in studying such vulnerable groups, researchers must seek to balance two considerations—the vulnerability that arises from their incompetence and the injustice that would arise from excluding them from the study.

Special protections and procedures may also be needed for other groups who do not necessarily lack competence. These include physically disabled people (e.g., the deaf); people who may be at higher-than-average risk of unintended side effects because of their circumstances (e.g., pregnant women); or institutionalized people who may have *diminished autonomy* (e.g., prisoners).

CONSUMER TIP

Some terms introduced in this chapter rarely are used explicitly in research reports. For example, a report almost never calls to the readers' attention that the study participants were *vulnerable subjects.* You need to be sensitive to the special needs of groups that may be unable to act as their own advocates or to assess the costs and benefits of participating in a study.　■

Respect for Privacy and Confidentiality

Researchers demonstrate their respect for human dignity by placing a high value on study participants' privacy. Virtually all research with humans constitutes an intrusion into personal lives, but researchers should ensure that their research is not more intrusive than it needs to be and that participants' privacy is maintained throughout the study. The right to privacy is an internationally recognized ethical principle and has also been enshrined in Canadian law as a constitutional right protected in both federal and provincial statutes.

Participants also have the right to expect that any data they provide will be kept in strictest confidence. The principle of respect for privacy and confidentiality protect access to personal information. When study participants confide personal information to the researchers, or when their behaviour is observed, researchers have an obligation not to share the information with others (even family members or care providers) without the subjects' consent. A promise of **confidentiality** to participants is a pledge that any information they provide will not be publicly reported or made accessible to parties not involved in the research.

Respect for Justice and Inclusiveness

Justice connotes fairness and equality, and so one aspect of the justice principle concerns the equitable distribution of benefits and burdens of research. The selection of study participants should be based on research requirements and not on the vulnerability or compromised position of certain people. Historically, subject selection has been a key ethical concern, with many researchers selecting groups deemed to have lower social standing (e.g., poor people, prisoners, slaves, the mentally retarded) as study participants. The principle of justice imposes particular obligations toward individuals who are unable to protect their own interests (e.g., dying patients) to ensure that they are not exploited for the advancement of knowledge.

Distributive justice also imposes duties to neither neglect nor discriminate against individuals and groups who may benefit from advances in research. During the 1980s and early 1990s, there was growing evidence that women, ethnic or racial minorities, and the elderly were being unfairly excluded from many clinical studies. Section 5 of the TCPS specifically deals with issues of inclusion in research, and section 6 focuses on research involving Aboriginal people. For example, the TCPS stipulates (Article 5.1) that ". . . researchers shall not exclude prospective or actual research subjects on the basis of such attributes as culture, religion, race, mental or physical disability, sexual orientation, ethnicity, sex or age, unless there is a valid reason for doing so" (Medical Research Council of Canada et al., 1998).

The principle of fair treatment covers issues other than subject selection. For example, the right to fair treatment means that researchers must treat people who decline to participate in a study (or who withdraw from the study after agreeing to participate) in a nonprejudicial manner; that they must honour all agreements made with participants (including the payment of any promised stipends); that they demonstrate sensitivity to and respect for the beliefs, habits, and lifestyles of people from different cultures; that they afford participants courteous treatment at all times; and that they avoid situations in which there is a conflict of interest.

Balancing Harms and Benefits

The ethical conduct of research with humans requires a careful analysis of the balance and distribution of harms and benefits of the research. The TCPS indicates that, "Modern research ethics . . . require a favourable harms-benefit balance—that is, that the foreseeable harms should not outweigh anticipated benefits" (Medical Research Council of Canada et al., 1998, p. i.6).

Research is often undertaken under conditions of uncertainty—research involves advancing the frontiers of knowledge, and so it may not be possible to anticipate all possible harms and benefits of participation. This fact imposes special ethical burdens on researchers to undertake studies that address important questions, that use methodologically sound methods, and that are conducted with sensitivity and diligence.

One principle related to a balanced distribution of harms and benefits is that of **beneficence**, which imposes a duty on researchers to maximize net benefits. Human research should be intended to produce benefits for subjects themselves or—a situation that is more common—for other individuals or society as a whole. In most research, the primary benefit concerns the advancement of knowledge, which can be used to promote human health and welfare in the long run.

Another related principle is **nonmaleficence**—researchers' duty to avoid or minimize harm to participants. Participants must not be subjected to unnecessary risks of harm or discomfort, and their participation in a study must be essential to achieving scientifically and societally important aims that could not otherwise be realized. In research with humans, *harm* and *discomfort* can take many forms: they can be physical, emotional, social, or financial. Ethical researchers must use strategies to minimize all types of harms and discomforts, even ones that are temporary.

Clearly, exposing study participants to experiences that result in serious or permanent harm is unacceptable. Ethical researchers must be prepared to terminate their research if they suspect that continuation would result in injury, death, or undue distress to study participants. Although protecting human beings from physical harm may be reasonably straightforward, the psychological consequences of participating in a study are usually subtle and thus require close attention. For example, participants may be asked questions about their personal views, weaknesses, or fears. Such queries might lead people to reveal sensitive personal information. The point is not that researchers should refrain from asking questions but rather that they need to be aware of the nature and scope of the intrusion on people's psyches.

The need for sensitivity may be even greater in qualitative studies, which often involve in-depth exploration into highly personal areas. In-depth probing may expose deep-seated worries and anxieties that study participants had previously repressed. Qualitative researchers, regardless of the underlying research tradition, must thus be especially vigilant in monitoring such problems.

Nonmaleficence also involves ensuring freedom from exploitation. Involvement in a study should not place participants at a disadvantage or expose them to situations for which they have not been prepared. Participants need to be assured that their participation, or information they might provide, will not be used against them. For example, a woman divulging her income should not fear losing public health benefits; a person reporting drug abuse should not fear exposure to criminal authorities.

Study participants enter into a special relationship with researchers, and this relationship should not be exploited. Exploitation might be overt and malicious (e.g., sexual exploitation, use of participants' identification to create a mailing list), but it might also be less flagrant (e.g., getting participants to provide more information in a 1-year follow-up interview, without having warned them of this possibility at the outset). Because nurse researchers may have a nurse–client (in addition to a researcher–participant) relationship, special care may be needed to avoid exploiting that bond. Patients' consent to participate in a study may result from their understanding of the researcher's role as *nurse,* not as *researcher.*

In qualitative research, the risk of exploitation may be especially acute because the psychological distance between investigators and participants typically declines as the study progresses. The emergence of a pseudotherapeutic relationship between researchers and participants is not uncommon, and this imposes additional responsibilities on researchers—and additional risks that exploitation could inadvertently occur. On the other hand, qualitative researchers are typically in a better position than quantitative researchers to do good, rather than just to avoid doing any harm, because of the close relationships they often develop with participants. Beck (2005), for example, documented that participants in one of her studies (the study in Appendix B of this book) expressed a range of benefits they experienced from e-mail exchanges with the researcher during the study.

PROCEDURES FOR PROTECTING STUDY PARTICIPANTS

Now that you are familiar with fundamental ethical principles for conducting research, you need to understand the procedures researchers follow to adhere to them. These procedures should be evaluated in critiquing the ethical aspects of a study.

CONSUMER TIP

When information about ethical considerations is presented in research reports, it almost always appears in the method section, typically in the subsection devoted to data collection procedures but sometimes in a subsection describing the sample. ■

Risk/Benefit Assessments

One of the strategies that researchers use to protect study participants—and that you as a reviewer can use to assess the ethical aspects of a study—is to conduct a **risk/benefit assessment**. Such an assessment is designed to determine whether the benefits of participating in a study are in line with the costs, be they financial, physical, emotional, or social—that is, whether the *risk/benefit* ratio is acceptable. Box 5.1 summarizes major costs and benefits of research participation.

CONSUMER TIP

In your evaluation of the risk/benefit ratio of a study, you might consider whether you yourself would have felt comfortable being a study participant. ■

BOX 5.1   Potential Benefits and Risks of Research to Participants

Major Potential Benefits to Participants

▶ Access to an intervention that might otherwise be unavailable to them
▶ Comfort in being able to discuss their situation or problem with a friendly, objective person
▶ Increased knowledge about themselves or their conditions, either through opportunity for introspection and self-reflection or through direct interaction with researchers
▶ Escape from a normal routine, excitement of being part of a study
▶ Satisfaction that information they provide may help others with similar problems or conditions
▶ Direct monetary or material gain through stipends or other incentives

Major Potential Risks to Participants

▶ Physical harm, including unanticipated side effects
▶ Physical discomfort, fatigue, or boredom
▶ Psychological or emotional distress resulting from self-disclosure, introspection, fear of the unknown, discomfort with strangers, fear of eventual repercussions, anger or embarrassment at the type of questions being asked
▶ Social risks, such as the risk of stigma, adverse effects on personal relationships, loss of status
▶ Loss of privacy
▶ Loss of time
▶ Monetary costs (e.g., for transportation, child care, time lost from work)

The risk/benefit ratio should also be considered in terms of whether the risks to research participants are commensurate with the benefit to society and to nursing. The degree of risk to be taken by participants should never exceed the potential humanitarian benefits of the knowledge to be gained. Thus, an important question in assessing the overall risk/benefit ratio is whether the study focuses on a significant topic that has the potential to improve patient care.

All research involves some risks, but in many cases, the risk is minimal. **Minimal risk** is defined as risks anticipated to be no greater than those ordinarily encountered in daily life or during routine tests or procedures. When the risks are not minimal, researchers must proceed with caution, taking every step possible to reduce risks and maximize benefits.

Example of risk/benefit assessment

Hentz (2002) studied the phenomenon of *body memory* following the loss of a loved one. Here is how she described risks and benefits: "One of the benefits for the participants was the ability to share experiences with someone interested and concerned. The other benefit was in knowing that the participants' stories may help others facing similar experiences. The actual interview often evoked strong emotions; however, many of the participants commented that they felt better having told their stories. Having their stories heard and acknowledged was experienced by participants as therapeutic." (p. 165)

Informed Consent

A particularly important procedure for safeguarding human subjects and protecting their right to self-determination involves obtaining evidence of their informed consent. Researchers usually document the informed consent process by having participants sign a **consent form,** an example of which is shown in Figure 5.1. This form includes information about the study purpose, specific expectations regarding participation (e.g., how much time will be involved), the voluntary nature of participation, and potential costs and benefits.

Researchers rarely obtain written informed consent when the primary means of data collection is through self-administered questionnaires. Researchers generally assume **implied consent** (i.e., that the return of the completed questionnaire reflects respondents' voluntary consent to participate). This assumption, however, is not always warranted (e.g., if patients feel that their treatment might be affected by failure to cooperate).

In some qualitative studies, especially those requiring repeated contact with participants, it is difficult to obtain a meaningful informed consent at the outset. Qualitative researchers do not always know in advance how the study will evolve. Because the research design emerges during data collection and analysis, researchers may not know the exact nature of the data to be collected, what the risks and benefits will be, nor how much of a time commitment will be required. Thus, in a qualitative study, consent may be viewed as an ongoing, transactional process, referred to as **process consent**. In process consent, researchers continuously renegotiate the consent,

I, _____ agree to take part in a nursing study about the use of research findings in postoperative pain management. I understand that participation in the study may involve one or two interviews with a researcher, which will be tape recorded, and that the recording will be typed into a written record. I will be answering questions about:

▶ My experiences with and beliefs about pain management
▶ My experiences using research evidence
▶ Factors that I believe make it easier or more difficult to use current research or to follow current pain management practices
▶ factors that I think influence pain management practices in a unit and a hospital

I may also be completing short questions and scales (e.g., answering questions using ratings of 1 to 5 or more) about research use and factors thought to influence it. Alternatively I may only be completing scales and questionnaires.

I have been told that the interviews will take about 30 to 60 minutes and occur at a convenient time and place in my off-duty hours or with the unit manager's agreement during work hours.

I have been told that I may refuse to answer questions, stop the interview at any time, or withdraw from the study. I do not have to answer any questions or discuss any subject in the interview if I do not want to. My name will not appear on the questionnaires, and my specific answers will remain confidential. I will not be identified in any report or presentation that may arise from the study. Taking part in this study or dropping out will not affect my employment.

While I may not benefit directly from the study, the information gained may assist nurses with both research use and pain management for postoperative patients.

I have been told that the data (typed records of interviews, taped interviews, observations, results or questionnaires) will be preserved using record management standards that protect the privacy of the participants in the project and that guard against the disclosure of individual information. It has also been explained to me that the data may be used for other research studies in the future. If this is done, proper ethical review will be obtained to ensure that the same practices of confidentiality are observed as within this study.

The above research procedures have been explained to me. Any questions have been answered to my satisfaction. I have been given a copy of this form to keep.

_____   _____   _____
(Signature of Participant)   (Date)   (Printed Name)

_____   _____   _____
(Signature of Witness)   (Date)   (Printed Name)

If you have any questions about this study please contact:

Dr. Carole Estabrooks (Principal Investigator) or   **Telephone:** (780) 555-1234
Dr. Profetto-McGrath (Research Associate)   **Telephone:** (780) 555-4321

FIGURE 5.1 Sample consent form.

allowing participants to play a collaborative role in the decision-making process regarding their ongoing participation.

Example of informed consent in a quantitative study

Davison, Goldenberg, Gleave, and Degner (2003) studied the effect of providing individualized information to men and their partners to facilitate treatment decision making relating to prostate cancer. The first researcher (Davison) provided an explanation of the study purpose and obtained written informed consent from each participant who had made an appointment at the Prostate Centre to obtain information.

Example of process consent

Wuest, Ford-Gilboe, Merritt-Gray, & Berman (2003) studied the health promotion processes of single-parent families after leaving abusive partners/fathers. Tape-recorded interviews were conducted with 36 mothers in a location of their choice; each woman gave informed consent before participation. As data analysis proceeded, the researchers conducted second interviews with each family. On repeat interviews, consent was reconfirmed.

Confidentiality Procedures

Participants' right to privacy is protected either through anonymity or through other confidentiality procedures. **Anonymity** occurs when even the researcher cannot link a participant with his or her data. For example, if a researcher distributed questionnaires to a group of nursing home residents and asked that they be returned without any identifying information, the responses would be anonymous. As another example, if a researcher reviewed hospital records from which all identifying information (e.g., name, address, and so forth) had been expunged, anonymity would again protect people's right to privacy.

Example of anonymity

DuMont and Parnis (2003) studied nurses' opinions and practices related to the collection of forensic evidence in the context of sexual assault cases. An anonymous questionnaire was distributed to all nurses working in sexual assault care centres in Ontario. The cover letter explicitly described procedures designed to ensure anonymity.

In situations in which anonymity is impossible, researchers implement other confidentiality procedures. These include securing individual confidentiality assurances from everyone involved in collecting or analyzing research data; maintaining identifying information in locked files to which few people have access; substituting **identification (ID) numbers** for participants' names on study records and computer files to prevent any accidental *breach of confidentiality*; and reporting only aggregate data for groups of participants or taking steps to disguise a person's identity in a research report.

Extra precautions are often needed to safeguard participants' privacy in qualitative studies. Anonymity is rarely possible in qualitative research because researchers usually meet with participants personally. Moreover, because of the in-depth nature of many qualitative studies, there may be a greater invasion of privacy than is true in quantitative research. Researchers who spend time in participants' homes may, for example, have difficulty segregating the public behaviours participants are willing to share from the private behaviours that unfold unwittingly during data collection. A final issue is adequately disguising participants in research reports to avoid a breach of confidentiality. Because the number of respondents is small and because rich descriptive information is presented in research reports, qualitative researchers need to take extra precautions to safeguard participants' identity. This may mean more than simply using a fictitious name—it may also mean withholding information about the characteristics of the informant, such as age and occupation.

Example of confidentiality procedures in a qualitative study

Spiers (2002) described interpersonal contexts in which care was negotiated between home care nurses and their patients. Her qualitative study was based on an analysis of 31 videotaped home visits. The video portion of the tapes was not altered, in as much as the researcher wanted to analyze facial expressions. However, any audio containing names or other identifying information was removed in dubbed tapes. Pseudonyms were used in the transcripts.

CONSUMER TIP

As a means of enhancing both personal and institutional privacy, research reports frequently avoid giving explicit information about the locale of the study. For example, the report might state that data were collected in a 200-bed, private, for-profit nursing home, without mentioning its name or location. ■

Debriefings and Referrals

Researchers can often show their respect for study participants—and proactively minimize emotional risks—by carefully attending to the nature of the interactions they have with them. For example, researchers should always be gracious and polite, should phrase questions tactfully, and should be sensitive to cultural and linguistic diversity.

There are also more formal strategies that researchers can use to communicate their respect and concern for participants' well-being. For example, it is sometimes advisable to offer **debriefing** sessions after data collection is completed to permit participants to ask questions or air complaints. Debriefing is especially important when the data collection has been stressful or when ethical guidelines had to be "bent" (e.g., if any deception was used in explaining the study). Researchers can also demonstrate their interest in participants by offering to share findings with them once the data have been analyzed (e.g., by mailing them a summary or advising them of an appropriate website). Finally, in some situations, researchers may need to assist study participants by making referrals to appropriate health, social, or psychological services.

Example of referrals

Neufeld and Harrison (2003) studied appraisals of support among women caring for a family member with dementia. The research involved a series of interviews over an 18-month period with the women caregivers. Referrals to mental health or other support services were available to study participants who expressed a need.

Treatment of Vulnerable Groups

Adherence to ethical standards is often straightforward. The rights of special vulnerable groups, however, often need to be protected through additional procedures and heightened sensitivity. You should pay particular attention to the ethical dimensions of a study when people who are vulnerable are involved. Some safeguards that can be used with vulnerable groups include the following:

▶ *Children.* Legally and ethically, children do not have the competence to give their informed consent; therefore, the informed consent of children's parents or legal guardians should be obtained. However, it is advisable—especially if the child is at least 7 years old—to obtain the child's assent as well. **Assent** refers to the child's affirmative agreement to participate. If the child is mature enough to understand the basic information in an informed consent form (e.g., a 13-year-old), researchers should obtain written consent from the child as well, as evidence of respect for the child's right to self-determination.

▶ *Mentally or emotionally disabled people.* People whose disability makes it impossible for them to make an informed decision about participation (e.g., people affected by cognitive impairment or mental illness) also cannot provide informed consent. In such cases, researchers obtain written consent from the person's legal guardian, but informed consent from prospective participants should be sought as a supplement to consent from guardians whenever possible.

▶ *Physically disabled people.* For certain physical disabilities, special procedures for obtaining consent may be required. For example, with deaf people, the entire consent process may need to be in writing. For people who cannot read or write or who have a physical impairment preventing them from writing, alternative procedures for documenting informed consent (e.g., videotaping the consent proceedings) can be used.

▶ *Terminally ill people.* Terminally ill people who participate in a study can seldom expect to benefit personally from the research, and thus the risk/benefit ratio needs to be carefully evaluated. Researchers must also take steps to ensure that if terminally ill people participate in the study, their health care and comfort are not compromised.

▶ *Institutionalized people.* Nurses often conduct studies with hospitalized or institutionalized people, who may feel pressured into participating or may believe that their treatment would be jeopardized by failure to cooperate. Prison inmates, who have lost their autonomy in many spheres of activity, may similarly feel constrained in their ability to give free consent. Researchers studying institutionalized groups need to place special emphasis on the voluntary nature of participation.

▶ *Pregnant and breastfeeding women.* The TCPS notes that when researchers are contemplating research with pregnant women, they must take into consideration the benefits and harms not only for the pregnant woman but also for her embryo or foetus, and similar concerns arise in connection with breastfeeding mothers and their infants. Special care should be taken in research with pregnant women or new mothers, who might be at heightened physical and psychological risk.

Example of research with a vulnerable group

Rennick, Morin, Kim, Johnston, Dougherty, and Platt (2004) conducted a study design to identify children at high risk for psychological problems following hospitalization in a paediatric intensive care unit. Children were categorized as being at high or low risk for developing persistent psychological sequelae based on illness severity and number of invasive procedures to which they were exposed. All parents provided written consent for their children to participate, and all children gave written or verbal assent.

Research Ethics Boards and External Reviews

It is sometimes hard for researchers to be objective in assessing risks and benefits or in developing procedures to protect human rights. Researchers' commitment to a topic area or their desire to conduct a rigorous study may cloud their judgment. Because of this possibility, the ethical dimension of a study is usually subjected to external review.

Canada, like most other Western countries, has developed a model of ethics review for research using human subjects. The model involves the review of proposed research plans, using the ethical guidelines outlined in the TCPS, by independent **Research Ethics Boards (REBs)** before the study gets underway. REBs are established in the institutions where research is conducted, such as in hospitals and universities. The REBs are mandated to reject, propose modifications to, or terminate any research conducted within the institution or by members affiliated with it, if ethical transgressions are noted. The guidelines in the TCPS are considered a *minimum* standard for the ethical conduct of research. Each REB must consist of at least five members, and at least one person must be unaffiliated with the institution where the REB is housed.

Example of REB approval

Watt-Watson, Chung, Chan, and McGillion (2004) studied pain management, levels of pain, and other pain-related outcomes in patients at four points in time after discharge following ambulatory same-day surgery. The researchers obtained approval for their study by the University Research Services offices (University of Toronto) and the Research Ethics Board of the hospital involved.

Not all studies are reviewed by REBs or other formal committees. Nevertheless, researchers have a responsibility to ensure that their research plans are ethically acceptable, and it is a good practice for researchers to solicit external advice even when they are not required to do so.

CONSUMER TIP

Research reports may use alternate terms such as ethical review by *human subjects committees* or *Institutional Review Boards (IRB)*. ■

OTHER ETHICAL ISSUES

When critiquing the ethical dimensions of a study, a prime consideration is the researchers' treatment of human study participants. Two other ethical issues also deserve mention: the treatment of animals in research and research misconduct.

Ethical Issues in Using Animals in Research

A small but growing number of nurse researchers use animals rather than human beings as their subjects, typically focusing on biophysiologic phenomena. Despite some opposition to such research by animal rights activists, researchers in health fields likely will continue to use animals to explore basic physiologic mechanisms and to test experimental interventions that could pose risks (as well as offer benefits) to humans.

Ethical considerations are clearly different for animals and humans (e.g., the concept of *informed consent* is not relevant for animals). In Canada, researchers who use animals in their studies must adhere to the policies and guidelines of the Canadian Council on Animal Care (CCAC). The CCAC guidelines, articulated in the two-volume *Guide to the Care and Use of Experimental Animals* (*http://www.ccac.ca*), establish principles for the proper care and treatment of animals used in biomedical and behavioural research. These principles cover such issues as the transport of animals, alternatives to using animals, pain and distress in animal subjects, researcher qualifications, the use of appropriate anaesthesia, and euthanizing animals under certain conditions during or after the study.

Holtzclaw and Hanneman (2002), in discussing the use of animals in nursing research, noted several important considerations. First, there must be a compelling reason to use an animal model—not simply convenience or novelty. Second, the study procedures should be humane, well planned, and well funded. They noted that animal studies require serious ethical and scientific consideration to justify their use.

Explicit instances of animal cruelty in health care research are rare but have been reported. For example, during the 1980s, a physiologist at the University of Western Ontario was accused of cruelty in a study in which a baboon was kept for several months in a restraining chair. The study was supported by the Canadian Medical Research Council.

Example of animal research

Bartfay and Bartfay (2002) conducted a study to explore the link between iron overload and heart failure using a murine model. Twenty mice were housed in cages (5 per cage) in a temperature- and humidity-controlled room with 12-hour light–dark cycles and given access to food and water. Half the mice were assigned to an iron-overload condition, and the other half received a placebo. The researchers specifically noted that the study had institutional approval and that it conformed to the standards for animal treatment issued by the CCAC and by the Province of Ontario.

Research Misconduct

Millions of movie-goers watched breathlessly as Dr. Richard Kimble (Harrison Ford) exposed the fraudulent scheme of a medical researcher in the film *The Fugitive*. This film reminds us that ethics in research involves not only the protection of the rights of human and animal subjects but also protection of the public trust.

The issue of **research misconduct** (or *scientific misconduct*) has received increasing attention in recent years as incidents of researcher fraud and misrepresentation have come to light. In Canada, the three major federal funding sources (CIHR, NSERC, and SSHRC) have issued a TCPS on integrity in research and scholarship, updated in April 2003. The Councils hold researchers accountable for adhering to five principles, which cover issues such as conflicts of interest, proper acknowledgment of scholarly contributions, and obtaining permissions for use of information (*http://www.sshrc.ca/web/apply/policies/integrity_e.asp*). The policy statement articulates three fundamental aspects of research integrity: (1) *truthfulness* in describing the manner is which data are collected, analyzed, and reported;

(2) *scrupulousness* in crediting sources of original research concepts and information; and (3) *probity* in the use of research funds.

Definitions of research misconduct, including that offered by the TCPS, usually include transgressions such as fabrication, falsification, and plagiarism. *Fabrication* involves making up study results and reporting them. *Falsification* involves manipulating research materials, equipment, or processes; it also involves changing or omitting data, or distorting results such that the research is not accurately represented in research reports. *Plagiarism* involves the appropriation of someone's ideas or results without giving due credit. In addition to these three main forms, research misconduct covers many other issues, such as improprieties of authorship, poor data management, conflicts of interest, inappropriate financial arrangements, failure to comply with governmental regulations, and unauthorized use of confidential information. The TCPS notes that misconduct does *not* include honest error or honest differences in interpretations or judgments of data.

Example of research misconduct

In the 1990s, public trust in medical research was eroded by the revelation that data obtained for the National Surgical Adjuvant Breast and Bowel Project from participants enrolled at Saint-Luc Hospital in Montreal were falsified (see Weijer, Shapiro, Fuks, Glass, & Skrutkowska, 1995).

In reading research reports, you are not likely to be able to detect research misconduct. Awareness of this issue is, however, critical to being an astute consumer of research.

CRITIQUING THE ETHICS OF RESEARCH STUDIES

Guidelines for critiquing the ethical aspects of a study are presented in Box 5.2. A person serving on an REB or similar committee should be provided with sufficient information to answer all these questions. Research reports, however, do not always include detailed information about ethical procedures because of space constraints in journals. Thus, it may not always be possible to critique researchers' adherence to ethical guidelines. Nevertheless, we offer a few suggestions for considering the ethical aspects of a study.

Many research reports do acknowledge that the study procedures were reviewed by an REB or a human subjects committee of the institution with which the researchers are affiliated. When a research report specifically mentions a formal external review, it is generally safe to assume that a panel of concerned people thoroughly reviewed the ethical issues raised by the study.

BOX 5.2   Questions for Critiquing the Ethical Aspects of a Study

1. Was the study approved and monitored by a Research Ethics Board or other similar ethics review committees?
2. Were study participants subjected to any physical harm, discomfort, or psychological distress? Did the researchers take appropriate steps to remove or prevent harm?
3. Did the benefits to participants outweigh any potential risks or actual discomfort they experienced? Did the benefits to society outweigh the costs to participants?
4. Was any type of coercion or undue influence used to recruit participants? Did they have the right to refuse to participate or to withdraw without penalty?
5. Were participants deceived in any way? Were they fully aware of participating in a study, and did they understand the purpose and nature of the research?
6. Were appropriate informed consent procedures used with all participants? If not, were there valid and justifiable reasons?
7. Were adequate steps taken to safeguard the privacy of participants? How were the data kept anonymous or confidential?
8. Were vulnerable groups involved in the research? If yes, were special precautions instituted because of their vulnerable status?
9. Were groups omitted from the inquiry without a justifiable rationale (e.g., women, minorities)?

You can also come to some conclusions based on a description of the study methods. There may be sufficient information to judge, for example, whether study participants were subjected to physical or psychological harm or discomfort. Reports do not always specifically state whether informed consent was secured, but you should be alert to situations in which the data might have been gathered without explicit consent (e.g., if data were gathered unobtrusively).

In thinking about the ethical aspects of a study, you should also consider who the study participants were. For example, if the study involved vulnerable groups, there should be more information about protective procedures. You might also need to attend to who the study participants were *not*. For example, there has been considerable concern about the omission of certain groups (e.g., minorities) from clinical research.

It is often especially difficult to determine whether the participants' privacy was safeguarded unless the researcher specifically mentions pledges of confidentiality or anonymity. A situation requiring special scrutiny arises when data are collected from two people simultaneously (e.g., a husband and wife who are jointly interviewed) or when interviews in participants' homes occur with other family members present.

CONSUMER TIP

Consumers, like researchers, face the issue of ethical dilemmas. As a reviewer assessing the quality of research evidence for nursing practice, you must be critical of methodologic weaknesses—yet some weaknesses may reflect the researcher's need to conduct research ethically. ■

RESEARCH EXAMPLES   Critical Thinking Activities

 EXAMPLE 1: Quantitative Research

Aspects of a quantitative nursing study, featuring key terms and ethical concepts discussed in this chapter, are presented below, followed by some questions to guide critical thinking.

Study
"Prevalence and correlates of *Chlamydia* infection in Canadian street youth" (Shields, Wong, Mann, Jolly, Haase, Mahaffey, Moses, Morin, Patrick, Predy, Rossi, & Sutherland, 2004)

Study Purpose
The purpose of the study was to document the prevalence of *Chlamydia* species infection among Canadian street youth and to identify background factors associated with increased risk of infection.

Research Method
Nurses who had experience working with street youth recruited a total of 1355 youth aged 15 to 24 years in seven large urban centers throughout Canada. Information about their sexual activity and lifestyles was collected through nurse-administered questionnaires. Participants also provided a urine sample to test for *Chlamydia trachomatis*.

Ethics-Related Procedures
Recruitment of participants occurred through drop-in centers, which provided an environment suitable for confidential discussions. Youth who were intoxicated (on drugs or alcohol) were excluded from the study. Informed consent was obtained from each youth before participation in the study. The youth were advised that they could withdraw from the study at any point and that, if they chose to do so, their questionnaire would be destroyed. Questionnaires were assigned an identification number—names were never attached to them. Test results for the urine sample were linked to the questionnaires by this ID number. Youth were strongly encouraged to return to the drop-in center to learn their test results, and those who tested positive were given a dose of azithromycin. A food voucher was offered to each youth as an incentive to participate in the study. The study design, procedures, and questionnaire were approved by local universities or hospital REBs in each city where the study took place.

Key Findings
▶ The prevalence rate of *Chlamydia* species infection was 8.6%, a high prevalence rate compared with the general population of youth. Higher prevalence rates were found in females (10.9%) than in males (7.3%).
▶ Among females, factors associated with higher risk of infection included being Aboriginal and having been in foster care.

Critical Thinking Activities (continued)

*Critical Thinking Suggestions**

*See the Student Resource CD-ROM for a discussion of these questions.

1. Answer questions 1 through 8 from Box 5.2 regarding this study.

2. Also consider the following targeted questions, which may assist you in further assessing the ethical aspects of the study:

    a. Could the data in this study have been collected anonymously? Why do you think anonymity was not used?

    b. Parental consent was apparently not obtained in this study—should it have been?

    c. Comment on the appropriateness of the recruitment incentive.

    d. If you had a young cousin or other relative who was living on the streets, how would you feel about his or her participating in the study?

3. If the results of this study are valid and reliable, what are some of the uses to which the findings might be put in clinical practice?

 EXAMPLE 2: Qualitative Research

Aspects of a qualitative nursing study, featuring key terms and ethical concepts discussed in this chapter, are presented below, followed by some questions to guide critical thinking.

Study

"'Like, what am I supposed to do?': Adolescent girls' health concerns in their dating relationships" (Banister, Jakubec, & Stein, 2003)

Study Purpose

The study explored the health-related concerns of girls aged 15 and 16 years in their dating relationships.

Research Methods

Study participants were recruited at five sites (four schools—including a First Nations school—and a youth clinic) that were known to have large numbers of at-risk adolescents (e.g., at-risk for unplanned pregnancy, school drop-out). A total of 40 girls, aged 15 and 16 years, were interviewed in a group format, with five groups of 8 girls. Four group interviews, lasting about 90 minutes each, were conducted with each group. Group sessions were audiotaped and transcribed, and researchers also took observational notes during these sessions. The group interviews addressed such issues as sexuality, drug and alcohol use, and violence and physical abuse.

Ethics-Related Procedures

Banister and her colleagues obtained written informed consent from each participant before data collection. The researchers informed each girl that her participation was voluntary and that she could withdraw from the study at any time. The

(Research Examples continue on page 106)

Critical Thinking Activities (continued)

researchers also alerted participants to the limits of confidentiality within a group setting. To reduce the risk of breach of confidentiality, each group was encouraged to create its own "code of conduct," which served to illustrate the importance of respecting the principles of confidentiality within the group. The REB at the researchers' university reviewed and approved the study. In addition, the youth clinic, school district, and the Chief of the band associated with the First Nations school also reviewed the study and consented to its being conducted in their communities.

Key Findings
▶ Participants indicated that, to avoid behaviours risky to their health, they had to negotiate power relationships with partners and peers.
▶ The girls' desire for a dating partner often outweighed their desire to avoid health threats such as substance abuse and violence.

Critical Thinking Suggestions
1. Answer questions 1 through 8 from Box 5.2 regarding this study.
2. Also consider the following targeted questions, which may assist you in further assessing the ethical aspects of the study:
   a. What ethical dilemma might the researchers face if participants told them of instances of physical abuse?
   b. Could the data in this study have been collected anonymously? Why do you think anonymity was not used?
   c. If you had an adolescent cousin or other relative, how would you feel about her participating in the study?
3. If the results of this study are trustworthy, what are some of the uses to which the findings might be put in clinical practice?

 EXAMPLE 3: Quantitative Research

1. Read the method section from the study by Feeley and colleagues ("Mother–VLBW Infant Interaction") in Appendix A of this book and then answer the relevant questions in Box 5.2.
2. Also consider the following targeted questions, which may further sharpen your critical thinking skills and assist you in assessing ethical aspects of the study:
   a. Did this report provide detailed information about the researchers' efforts to protect participants' rights? Was any information missing? If so, was the absence of this information critical in your ability to draw conclusions about the ethical aspects of this study?
   b. Where was information about ethical issues located in this report?
   c. If you had a woman friend or family member with a VLBW infant, how would you feel about her participating in the study?

Critical Thinking Activities (continued)

 EXAMPLE 4: Qualitative Research

1. Read the method section from Beck's study ("Birth Trauma") in Appendix B of this book and then answer the relevant questions in Box 5.2.

2. Also consider the following targeted questions, which may further sharpen your critical thinking skills and assist you in assessing ethical aspects of the study:

    a. Where was information about the ethical aspects of this study located in the report?

    b. What additional information regarding the ethical aspects of the study could Beck have included in this article?

    c. If you had a woman friend or family member who had experienced birth trauma, how would you feel about her participating in the study?

CHAPTER REVIEW
Summary Points

▶ Because research has not always been conducted ethically, and because of the **ethical dilemmas** researchers often face in designing studies that are both ethical and methodologically rigorous, **codes of ethics** have been developed to guide researchers.

▶ In Canada, the Tri-Council Policy Statement on ethical conduct for research with humans set forth eight key ethical principles: respect for human dignity, respect for free and informed consent, respect for vulnerable persons, respect for privacy and confidentiality, respect of justice and inclusiveness, balancing harms and benefits, minimizing harm, and maximizing benefit.

▶ *Respect for human dignity* includes the participants' right to **self-determination**, which means participants have the freedom to control their own actions, including the right to refuse to participate in the study or to answer certain questions.

▶ **Informed consent** is intended to provide prospective participants with information needed to make a reasoned and voluntary decision about participation in a study.

▶ **Full disclosure** means researchers have fully described the study, including risks and benefits, to prospective participants. When full disclosure poses the risk of biased results, researchers sometimes use **covert data collection** or *concealment* (the collection of data without the participants' knowledge or consent) or *deception* (withholding information from participants or providing false information).

▶ **Vulnerable subjects** require additional protection as participants. They may be vulnerable because they are not able to make a truly informed decision about study participation (e.g., children); because of diminished autonomy (e.g., prisoners); or because their circumstances heighten the risk of physical or psychological harm (e.g., pregnant women).

▶ The principle of *justice* includes the right to fair and equitable treatment and to an inclusionary approach to recruitment of participants.

▶ **Beneficence** involves the performance of some good, and the protection of participants from harm and exploitation (**nonmaleficence).**

❱ Various procedures have been developed to safeguard study participants' rights, including the performance of a risk/benefit assessment, the implementation of informed consent procedures, and efforts to safeguard participants' confidentiality.

❱ In a **risk/benefit assessment**, the individual benefits of participation in a study (and societal benefits of the research) are weighed against the costs to individuals.

❱ Informed consent normally involves the signing of a **consent form** to document voluntary and informed participation. In qualitative studies, consent may need to be continually renegotiated with participants as the study evolves, through **process consent** procedures.

❱ Privacy can be maintained through **anonymity** (wherein not even researchers know the participants' identity) or through formal **confidentiality** procedures that safeguard the information participants provide.

❱ Researchers sometimes offer **debriefing** sessions after data collection to provide participants with more information or an opportunity to air complaints.

❱ External review of the ethical aspects of a study by a **Research Ethics Board (REB)** or other human subjects committee is highly desirable and may be required by either the agency funding the research or the organization from which participants are recruited.

❱ Ethical conduct in research involves not only protection of the rights of human and animal subjects but also efforts to maintain high standards of integrity and avoid such forms of **research misconduct** as plagiarism, fabrication of results, or falsification of data.

Additional Resources for Review

Chapter 5 of the *Study Guide to Accompany Essentials of Nursing Research,* 6th edition offers various exercises and study suggestions for reinforcing the concepts presented in this chapter. For additional review, see the Student Self-Study Review Questions section of the Student Resource CD-ROM provided with this book.

SUGGESTED READINGS

References for studies cited in the chapter appear at the end of the book.

References on Research Ethics

Canadian Nurses Association. (2002a). *Code of ethics for registered nurses.* Ottawa, ON: Author.

Canadian Nurses Association. (2002b). *Ethical guidelines for nurses in research involving human subjects.* Ottawa, ON: Author.

Flicker, S., Haans, D., & Skinner, H. (2004). Ethical dilemmas in research on Internet communities. *Qualitative Health Research, 14,* 124–134.

Holtzclaw, B. J., & Hanneman, S. K. (2002). Use of nonhuman biobehavioral models in critical care nursing research. *Critical Care Nursing Quarterly, 24,* 30–40.

Medical Research Council of Canada, Natural Sciences and Engineering Research Council of Canada, and Social Sciences and Humanities Research Council of Canada. (1998, with 2000, 2002 updates). *Tri-council policy statement: Ethical conduct for research involving humans.* Ottawa, ON: Minister of Supply and Services.

Silva, M. C. (1995). *Ethical guidelines in the conduct, dissemination, and implementation of nursing research.* Washington, DC: American Nurses Association.

Weijer, C., Shapiro, S., Fuks, A., Glass, K. C., & Skrutkowska, M. (1995). Monitoring clinical research: An obligation unfulfilled. *Canadian Medical Association Journal, 152,* 1973–1980.

Preliminary Steps in the Research Process

Scrutinizing Research Problems, Research Questions, and Hypotheses

STUDENT OBJECTIVES

On completing this chapter, you will be able to:

▶ Describe the process of developing and refining a research problem
▶ Distinguish statements of purpose and research questions for quantitative and qualitative studies
▶ Describe the function and characteristics of research hypotheses and distinguish different types of hypotheses
▶ Critique statements of purpose, research questions, and hypotheses in research reports with respect to their placement, clarity, wording, and significance
▶ Define new terms in the chapter

RESEARCH PROBLEMS AND RESEARCH QUESTIONS

A study begins as a problem that a researcher would like to solve or as a question that he or she would like to answer. This chapter discusses the formulation and evaluation of research problems, research questions, and hypotheses. We begin by clarifying some related terms.

Basic Terms Relating to Research Problems

At the most general level, researchers select a *topic* or a phenomenon on which to focus. Patient compliance, coping with disability, and pain management are examples of research topics. Within these broad topic areas are many potential research problems. In this section, we illustrate various terms as we define them using the topic *side effects in patients undergoing chemotherapy.*

A **research problem** is a perplexing or troubling condition. Both qualitative and quantitative researchers identify a research problem within a broad topic area of interest. The purpose of disciplined research is to "solve" the problem—or to contribute to its solution—by accumulating relevant information. A **problem statement** articulates the problem to be addressed. Table 6.1 presents a problem statement related to the topic of side effects in chemotherapy patients.

TABLE 6.1	Example of Terms Relating to Research Problems
TERM	**EXAMPLE**
Topic/focus	Side effects of chemotherapy
Research problem	Nausea and vomiting are common side effects among patients on chemotherapy, and interventions to date have been only moderately successful in reducing these effects. New interventions that can reduce or prevent these side effects need to be identified.
Statement of purpose	The purpose of the study is to test an intervention to reduce chemotherapy-induced side effects—specifically, to compare the effectiveness of patient-controlled and nurse-administered antiemetic therapy for controlling nausea and vomiting in patients on chemotherapy.
Research question	What is the relative effectiveness of patient-controlled antiemetic therapy versus nurse-controlled antiemetic therapy with regard to (a) medication consumption and (b) control of nausea and vomiting in patients on chemotherapy?
Hypotheses	(1) Participants receiving antiemetic therapy by a patient-controlled pump report less nausea than participants receiving the therapy by nurse administration; (2) participants receiving antiemetic therapy by a patient-controlled pump vomit less than participants receiving the therapy by nurse administration; (3) participants receiving antiemetic therapy by a patient-controlled pump consume less medication than participants receiving the therapy by nurse administration.
Aims/objectives	This study has as its aim the following objectives: (1) to develop and implement two alternative procedures for administering antiemetic therapy for patients receiving moderate emetogenic chemotherapy (patient controlled versus nurse controlled); (2) to test three hypotheses concerning the relative effectiveness of the alternative procedures on medication consumption and control of side effects; and (3) to use the findings to develop recommendations for possible changes to therapeutic procedures.

Research questions are the specific queries researchers want to answer in addressing a research problem. Research questions guide the types of data to be collected in the study. Researchers who make specific predictions regarding the answers to research questions pose **hypotheses** that are tested empirically. Examples of both research questions and hypotheses are presented in Table 6.1.

In a research report, you might also encounter other related terms. For example, many reports include a **statement of purpose** (or purpose statement), which is the researcher's summary of the overall goal. A researcher might also identify several specific *research aims* or *objectives*—the specific accomplishments the researcher hopes to achieve by conducting the study. The objectives include obtaining answers to research questions but may also encompass some broader aims (e.g., developing recommendations for changes to nursing practice based on the study results), as illustrated in Table 6.1.

Research Problems and Paradigms

Some research problems are better suited for studies using qualitative versus quantitative methods. Quantitative studies usually involve concepts that are well developed, about which there is an existing body of literature, and for which reliable methods of measurement have been developed. For example, a quantitative study might be undertaken to determine whether postpartum depression is higher among women who return to work 6 months after delivery than among those who stay home with their babies. There are relatively accurate measures of postpartum depression that would yield quantitative information about the level of depression in a sample of employed and nonemployed postpartum women.

Qualitative studies are often undertaken because some aspect of a phenomenon is poorly understood, and the researcher wants to develop a rich, comprehensive, and context-bound understanding of it. In the example of postpartum depression, qualitative methods would not be well suited to comparing levels of depression among two groups of women, but they would be ideal for exploring, for example, the *meaning* of postpartum depression among new mothers. In evaluating a research report, an important consideration is whether the research problem fits the chosen paradigm and its associated methods.

Sources of Research Problems

Where do ideas for research problems come from? At a basic level, research topics originate with researchers' interests. Because research is a time-consuming enterprise, curiosity about and interest in a topic are essential to the success of the project.

Research reports rarely indicate the source of a researcher's inspiration for a study, but a variety of sources can fuel a researcher's curiosity, including the following:

- ▶ *Clinical experience.* The nurse's everyday experience is a rich source of ideas for research topics. Problems that need immediate solution have high potential for clinical significance.
- ▶ *Nursing literature.* Ideas for studies often come from reading the nursing literature. Research reports may suggest problem areas indirectly by stimulating the reader's imagination and directly by explicitly stating what additional research is needed.

▶ *Social issues.* Topics are sometimes suggested by global social or political issues of relevance to the health care community. For example, the feminist movement has raised questions about such topics as gender equity and domestic violence.

▶ *Theories.* Theories from nursing and other related disciplines are another source of research problems. Researchers ask, If this theory is correct, what would I predict about people's behaviours, states, or feelings? The predictions can then be tested through research.

▶ *Ideas from external sources.* External sources and direct suggestions can sometimes provide the impetus for a research idea. For example, ideas for studies may emerge from reviewing a funding agency's research priorities or from brainstorming with other nurses.

It should be noted that researchers who have developed a program of research on a topic area may get inspiration for "next steps" from their own findings, or from a discussion of those findings with others.

Example of a problem source for a qualitative study

Beck (one of this book's authors) has developed a strong research program on postpartum depression. In 2001, Beck was invited to deliver the keynote address at an international conference in New Zealand. She was asked to speak about perinatal anxiety disorders and, in preparing for her talk, came across some articles on posttraumatic stress disorder (PTSD) after childbirth. In her keynote address, in which she described the continuum of perinatal anxiety disorders, Beck briefly touched on PTSD due to birth trauma. At the same conference, a woman named Sue Watson did a presentation on PTSD after childbirth. She was the chairperson of Trauma and Birth Stress (TABS), a charitable trust in New Zealand dedicated to supporting women who have experienced birth trauma and the resulting PTSD. Watson had herself suffered from PTSD following the birth of her first baby. Her powerful presentation alerted Beck to the devastating effects that birth trauma can have on mothers. Beck then approached Watson to discuss the possibility of conducting a phenomenological study on birth trauma and PTSD with some of the mothers who belonged to TABS. Watson was immediately supportive and helped to recruit mothers into Beck's study. Beck's report on this study is reprinted in Appendix B.

Development and Refinement of Research Problems

The development of a research problem is a creative process. Researchers often begin with interests in a broad topic area, and then develop the topic into a more specific researchable problem. For example, suppose a nurse working on a medical unit begins to wonder why some patients complain about having to wait for pain medication when certain nurses are assigned to them. The general topic is discrepancy in patient complaints about pain medications administered by different nurses. The nurse might ask, What accounts for this discrepancy? This broad question may lead to other questions, such as, How do the two groups of nurses differ? or What characteristics do the complaining patients share? At this point, the nurse may observe that the cultural or ethnic background of the patients and nurses could be a relevant factor. This may direct the nurse to a review of the literature for studies concerning ethnic groups and their relationship to nursing behaviours, or it may provoke a discussion of these observations with peers. These efforts may result in several research questions, such as the following:

▶ What is the essence of patient complaints among patients of different ethnic backgrounds?

▶ How are complaints by patients of different ethnic backgrounds expressed by patients and perceived by nurses?

▶ Is the ethnic background of nurses related to the frequency with which they dispense pain medication?

▶ Is the ethnic background of patients related to the frequency and intensity of their complaints of having to wait for pain medication?

▶ Does the number of patient complaints increase when the patients are of dissimilar ethnic backgrounds as opposed to when they are of the same ethnic background as the nurse?

▶ Do nurses' dispensing behaviours change as a function of the similarity between their own ethnic background and that of patients?

These questions stem from the same general problem, yet each would be studied differently; for example, some suggest a qualitative approach, and others suggest a quantitative one. A quantitative researcher might become curious about nurses' dispensing behaviours, based on some evidence in the literature regarding ethnic differences. Both ethnicity and nurses' dispensing behaviours are variables that can be reliably measured. A qualitative researcher who noticed differences in patient complaints would likely be more interested in understanding the *essence* of the complaints, the patients' *experience* of frustration, the *process* by which the problem was resolved, or the full *nature* of the nurse–patient interactions regarding the dispensing of medications. These are aspects of the research problem that would be difficult to measure quantitatively. Researchers choose a problem to study based on several factors, including its inherent interest to them and its fit with a paradigm of preference.

COMMUNICATING THE RESEARCH PROBLEM, PURPOSE, AND QUESTIONS

Researchers communicate their objectives in various ways in research reports. This section discusses the wording and placement of problem statements, statements of purpose, and research questions; the following major section discusses hypotheses.

Problem Statements

A problem statement is an expression of a dilemma or disturbing situation that needs investigation. A problem statement identifies the nature of the problem that is being addressed in the study and, typically, its context and significance. Generally, the problem statement should be broad enough to include central concerns but narrow enough in scope to serve as a guide to study design.

Example of a problem statement from a quantitative study

"One of the major issues facing gerontological nursing practice today is how to best care for the growing population of seniors increasingly obtaining non-acute care in acute care settings. Many jurisdictions, particularly those with a shortage of nursing home beds, have large populations of seniors virtually living in their hospitals yet very little study has been undertaken of the way in which these patients are managed...In Canada, in 1998, while 12.3% of the population was over 65 years, they accounted for 47% of healthcare spending. The proportion of elderly people...will increase to 23.5% over the next 20 years...thus increasing the strain on a healthcare sector already suffering cutbacks in hospitals and acute-care beds....The strain on acute care resources is exacerbated by the inappropriateness of utilizing acute care beds for non-acute patients and the delayed discharge of elderly" (Ostry, Tomlin, Cvitkovich, Ratner, Park, Tate, & Yassi, 2004, pp. 143–144).

In this example, the general topic is care for the elderly, but the investigators narrowed the scope of their inquiry to studying elders' use of acute care hospital resources. This problem statement asserted the nature of the problem (costly and inappropriate use of acute care resources for elders) and its significance (growing numbers of elderly people in Canada). It also provided a justification for conducting a new study: little research has been conducted into how these patients are managed.

The problem statement for a qualitative study similarly expresses the nature of the problem, its context, and its significance.

Example of a problem statement from a qualitative study

"Canada is a multicultural society. The 2001 census indicated about 327,550 Filipino Canadians live in Canada, of which 14,170 reside in the western city where this study was conducted....Filipino Canadians are employed in this city's hospitals, but most nursing care is provided by non-Filipino nurses. Information to enable nurses to give culturally safe nursing care is lacking" (Pasco, Morse, & Olson, 2004, p. 239).

As in the previous example, the researchers articulated the nature of the problem and a justification for conducting a new study. Qualitative studies that are embedded in a particular research tradition generally incorporate terms and concepts in their problem statements that foreshadow their tradition of inquiry. For example, the problem statement in a grounded theory study might refer to the need to develop deeper understandings of social processes. A problem statement for a phenomenological study might note the need to know more about people's experiences or the meanings they attribute to those experiences. And an ethnographer might indicate the desire to describe how cultural forces affect people's behaviour.

HOW-TO-TELL TIP

How can you tell a problem statement? Problem statements appear in the introduction to a research report—indeed, the first sentence of a research report is often the starting point of a problem statement. However, problem statements are often interwoven with a review of the literature, which provides context by documenting knowledge gaps. Problem statements are rarely explicitly labelled as such and must therefore be ferreted out. ■

Statements of Purpose

Many researchers first articulate their goals as a broad statement of purpose, worded declaratively. The purpose statement captures, in a sentence or two, the essence of the study and establishes the general direction of the inquiry. The word *purpose* or *goal* usually appears in a purpose statement (e.g., "The purpose of this study was . . ." or "The goal of this study was . . ."), but sometimes the word *intent, aim,* or *objective* is used instead.

In a quantitative study, a well-worded statement of purpose identifies the key study variables and their possible interrelationships as well as the population of interest.

Example of a statement of purpose from a quantitative study

The purpose of this study was to determine whether sending an information pamphlet to patients 2 weeks before a positron emission tomography (PET) test significantly reduces patient anxiety about the test (Westerman, Aubrey, Gauthier, Aung, Beanlands, Ruddy, Davies, De Kemp, & Woodend, 2004).

This statement identifies the population of interest (patients scheduled for a PET test), the independent variable (receipt of an information pamphlet), and the dependent variable (patient anxiety).

In qualitative studies, the statement of purpose indicates the nature of the inquiry, the key phenomenon under investigation, and the group or community under study.

Example of a statement of purpose from a qualitative study

The purpose of this study was to explore the hope-fostering strategies of elderly patients with advanced cancer receiving palliative home care (Duggleby & Wright, 2004).

This statement indicates that the phenomenon of interest is hope-fostering strategies and that the group under study is elderly cancer patients receiving palliative home care.

Researchers typically use verbs in their statements of purpose that suggest how they sought to solve the problem, or what the state of knowledge on the topic is. A study whose purpose is to *explore* or *describe* a phenomenon is likely to focus on a little-researched topic, often involving a qualitative approach. A statement of purpose for a qualitative study may also imply a flexible design through the use of verbs such as *understand* or *discover.* Creswell (1998) notes that qualitative researchers often "encode" the tradition of inquiry not only through their choice of verbs but also through the use of certain terms or "buzz words" associated with those traditions, as follows:

▶ *Grounded theory:* Processes; social structures; social interactions
▶ *Phenomenological studies:* Experience; lived experience; meaning; essence
▶ *Ethnographic studies:* Culture; roles; myths; cultural behaviour

Quantitative researchers also suggest the nature of the inquiry through their selection of verbs. A purpose statement indicating that the purpose is to *test* the effectiveness of an intervention or to *compare* two alternative nursing strategies suggests a study with a more established knowledge base, using a design with tight controls. Note that researchers' choice of verbs in a statement of purpose should connote a certain degree of objectivity. A statement of purpose indicating that the intent of the study was to *prove, demonstrate,* or *show* something suggests a bias.

Research Questions

Research questions are, in some cases, direct rewordings of statements of purpose, phrased interrogatively rather than declaratively. The research questions for the examples cited in the previous section might be as follows:

▶ Does sending an information pamphlet to patients 2 weeks before a positron emission tomography (PET) test reduce patient anxiety?
▶ What are the hope-fostering strategies of elderly patients with advanced cancer receiving palliative home care?

Questions that are simple and direct invite an answer and help to focus attention on the kinds of data needed to provide that answer. Some research reports thus omit a statement of purpose and state only the research question. Other researchers use a set of research questions to clarify or amplify the purpose statement.

In a quantitative study, research questions identify the key variables (most often, the independent and dependent variables), the relationships among them, and the population under study.

Example of a research question from a quantitative study

Does nurses' level of education (diploma/baccalaureate versus master's/doctoral) affect their perceptions of their collaboration with other health professionals (Miller, 2004)?

In this example, the independent variable is the nurses' highest level of education; the dependent variable is the nurses' perceptions of their interprofessional collaboration.

Researchers in the various qualitative traditions differ in the types of questions they believe to be important. Grounded theory researchers are likely to ask *process* questions, phenomenologists tend to ask *meaning* questions, and ethnographers generally ask *descriptive* questions about cultures. The terms associated with the various traditions, discussed earlier in connection with purpose statements, may also be incorporated into the research questions.

Example of a research question from a phenomenological study

What is the experience of patients with a severe and persistent psychiatric disorder when placed in seclusion in a psychiatric unit of a hospital (Holmes, Kennedy, & Perron, 2004)?

Not all qualitative studies are rooted in specific research traditions, however. Many researchers use naturalistic methods to describe or explore phenomena without focusing on cultures, meaning, or social processes.

Example of a research question from a descriptive qualitative study

How do bereaving family caregivers of patients who have had advanced cancer perceive the effects of home-based caregiving on their bereavement (Koop & Strang, 2003)?

In qualitative studies, research questions sometimes evolve over the course of the study. Researchers begin with a *focus* that defines the general boundaries of the inquiry, but the boundaries are not cast in stone—they "can be altered and, in the typical naturalistic inquiry, will be" (Lincoln & Guba, 1985, p. 228). Naturalists thus begin with a research question in mind but are sufficiently flexible that the question can be modified as new information makes it relevant to do so.

CONSUMER TIP

Researchers most often state their purpose or research questions at the end of the introduction or immediately after the review of the literature. Sometimes, a separate section of a research report—typically located just before the method section—is devoted to stating the research problem formally and might be labelled "Purpose," "Statement of Purpose," "Research Questions," or, in quantitative studies, "Hypotheses." ▪

RESEARCH HYPOTHESES IN QUANTITATIVE RESEARCH

In quantitative studies, researchers may present a statement of purpose and then one or more hypotheses. A hypothesis is a tentative prediction about the relationship between two or more variables in the population under study. In a qualitative study, the researcher does not begin with a hypothesis, in part because there is generally too little known about the topic to justify a hypothesis and in part because qualitative researchers want their inquiry to be guided by participants' viewpoints rather than by their own *a priori* hunches (although findings from qualitative studies may *lead to* the formulation of hypotheses). Thus, our discussion here focuses on hypotheses in quantitative research.

Function of Hypotheses in Quantitative Research

A hypothesis translates a research question into a statement of expected outcomes. For instance, the research question might ask, Does therapeutic touch affect patients' muscle tension levels? The researcher might hypothesize as follows: The muscle tension levels of patients treated with therapeutic touch is lower than the muscle tension levels of patients treated with physical touch.

Hypotheses sometimes emerge from a theory. Scientists reason from theories to hypotheses and test those hypotheses in the real world. The validity of a theory is never examined directly, but it can be evaluated through hypothesis testing. For example, the theory of reinforcement maintains that behaviour that is positively reinforced (rewarded) tends to be learned (repeated). The theory is too abstract to test, but hypotheses based on the theory can be tested. For instance, the following hypotheses are deduced from reinforcement theory

▶ Elderly patients who are praised (reinforced) for self-feeding require less assistance in feeding than patients who are not praised.
▶ Paediatric patients who are given a reward (e.g., permission to watch television) when they cooperate during nursing procedures are more compliant during those procedures than nonrewarded peers.

Both of these propositions can be tested in the real world. The theory gains support if the hypotheses are confirmed.

Even in the absence of a theory, hypotheses can offer direction and suggest explanations. For example, suppose we hypothesized that widowers experience more psychological distress in the 6 months after the death of their spouse than widows. This prediction could be based on theory (e.g., role expectation theory), earlier studies, or personal observations.

The development of predictions in and of itself forces researchers to think logically, to exercise critical judgment, and to tie together earlier findings.

Now let us suppose the above hypothesis is not confirmed by the evidence collected; that is, we find that men and women experience comparable levels of emotional distress in the 6 months after their spouses' death.

The failure of data to support a prediction forces investigators to analyze theory or previous research critically, to review limitations of the study's method carefully, and to explore alternative explanations for the findings.

The use of hypotheses in quantitative studies tends to induce critical thinking and, hence, to facilitate interpretation of the data.

To further illustrate the utility of hypotheses, suppose the researcher conducted the study guided only by the research question, Is there a relationship between a person's gender and the degree of distress experienced after losing a spouse? Investigators without a hypothesis are, apparently, prepared to accept any results. The problem is that it is almost always possible to explain something superficially after the fact, no matter what the findings are. Hypotheses guard against superficiality and minimize the possibility that spurious results will be misconstrued.

CONSUMER TIP

Some quantitative research reports explicitly state the hypotheses that guided the study, but most do not. The absence of a hypothesis sometimes is appropriate, but it often is an indication that researchers have failed to consider critically the implications of theory or existing knowledge or have failed to disclose the hunches that may have influenced their methodologic decisions. ■

Characteristics of Testable Hypotheses

Testable research hypotheses state the expected relationship between the independent variable (the presumed cause or antecedent) and the dependent variable (the presumed effect) within a population.

Example of a research hypothesis

Among women who have had a breast cancer diagnosis, those who initially used an avoidance coping strategy have poorer psychological adjustment 3 years later than women low on avoidance (Hack & Degner, 2004).

In this example, the independent variable is the persons' coping strategy (low versus high on avoidance), and the dependent variable is long-term psychological adjustment. The hypothesis predicts that these two variables are related within the population of women with a breast cancer diagnosis—poorer adjustment is expected among those with higher avoidance.

Unfortunately, researchers sometimes state hypotheses that fail to make a relational statement, and such hypotheses are not testable. Consider, for example, the following prediction: "Pregnant women who receive prenatal instruction by a nurse regarding post-partum experiences are not likely to experience postpartum depression." This statement expresses no anticipated relationship; in fact, there is only one variable (postpartum depression), and a relationship by definition requires at least two variables.

When a hypothesis does not state an anticipated relationship, it cannot be tested. In our example, how would we know if the hypothesis was supported—what absolute standard could be used to decide whether to accept or reject the hypothesis? To illustrate more concretely, suppose we asked a group of mothers who received prenatal instruction the following question 2 months after delivery: Overall, how depressed have you been since you gave birth? Would you say (1) extremely depressed, (2) moderately depressed, (3) somewhat depressed, or (4) not at all depressed?

Based on responses to this question, how could we compare the actual outcome with the predicted outcome? Would *all* the women in the sample have to say they were "not at all depressed"? Would the prediction be supported if 51% of the women said they were "not at all depressed" *or* "somewhat depressed"? There is no adequate way of testing the accuracy of the prediction.

A test is simple, however, if we modify the prediction to the following: Pregnant women who receive prenatal instruction are less likely to experience postpartum depression than pregnant women with no prenatal instruction. Here, the dependent variable is the women's depression and the independent variable is their receipt or nonreceipt of prenatal instruction. The relational aspect of the prediction is embodied in the phrase *less ... than*. If a hypothesis lacks a phrase such as *more than, less than, greater than, different from, related to, associated with*, or something similar, it is not amenable to testing in a quantitative study. To test this revised hypothesis, we could ask two groups of women with different prenatal instruction experiences to respond to the question on depression and then compare the groups' responses. The absolute degree of depression of either group would not be at issue.

Hypotheses should be based on justifiable rationales. The most defensible hypotheses follow from previous research findings or are deduced from a theory. When a relatively new area is being investigated, researchers may have to turn to logical reasoning or personal experience to justify predictions.

 CONSUMER TIP

Hypotheses are typically fairly easy to identify because researchers make statements such as, "The study tested the hypothesis that..." or, "It was predicted that...". ■

Wording Hypotheses

A hypothesis can predict the relationship between a single independent variable and a single dependent variable (a *simple hypothesis*), or it can predict a relationship between two or more independent variables or two or more dependent variables (a *complex hypothesis*). In the following examples, independent variables are indicated as IVs and dependent variables are identified as DVs:

Example of a simple hypothesis

Greater critical thinking ability (IV) is associated with more liberal attitudes toward women's roles in society (DV) (Loo & Thorpe, 2005).

Example of a complex hypothesis

Intermediate care facilities that have low staffing levels and less supportive work environments (IVs) have higher rates of staff injuries (DV) than facilities with better staffing levels and work environments (Yassi, Cohen, Cvitkovich, Park, Ratner, Ostry, Village, & Polla, 2004).

Hypotheses can be stated in various ways as long as the researcher specifies or implies the relationship that will be tested. Here is an example about the effect of postpartum exercise:

1. Low levels of exercise are associated with greater weight retention than high levels of exercise.
2. There is a relationship between level of exercise and weight retention.
3. The greater the level of exercise, the lower the weight retention.
4. Women with different levels of exercise differ with regard to weight retention.
5. Weight retention decreases as the woman's level of exercise increases.
6. Women who exercise have lower weight retention than women who do not.

Other variations are also possible. The important point to remember is that the hypothesis specifies the independent variable (here, level of exercise postpartum), the dependent variable (weight retention), and the anticipated relationship between them.

Hypotheses usually should be worded in the present tense. Researchers make a prediction about a relationship in the population—not just about a relationship that will be revealed in a particular sample of study participants.

Hypotheses can be either directional or nondirectional. A **directional hypothesis** is one that specifies not only the existence but also the expected direction of the relationship between variables. In the six versions of the hypothesis above, versions 1, 3, 5, and 6 are directional because there is an explicit prediction that women who do not exercise postpartum are at greater risk of weight retention than women who do. A **nondirectional hypothesis,** by contrast, does not stipulate the direction of the relationship, as illustrated in versions 2 and 4. These hypotheses predict that a woman's level of exercise and weight retention are related, but they do not stipulate whether the researcher thinks that exercise is related to more weight retention, or less.

Hypotheses based on theory are usually directional because theories provide a rationale for expecting variables to relate in certain ways. Existing studies also offer a basis for specifying directional hypotheses. When there is no theory or related research, when findings from prior studies are contradictory, or when researchers' own experience leads to ambivalent expectations, nondirectional hypotheses may be appropriate. Some people argue, in fact, that nondirectional hypotheses are preferable because they connote impartiality. Directional hypotheses, it is said, imply that researchers are intellectually committed to certain outcomes, and such commitment might lead to bias. This argument fails to recognize that researchers typically *do* have hunches about the outcomes, whether they state those expectations explicitly or not. We prefer directional hypotheses—when there is a reasonable basis for them—because they clarify the study's framework and demonstrate that researchers have thought critically about the phenomena under study.

Another distinction is the difference between research and null hypotheses. **Research hypotheses** (also referred to as *substantive hypotheses*) are statements of actual expected relationships between variables. All hypotheses presented thus far are research hypotheses that indicate researchers' true expectations.

For statistical analyses, the logic of statistical inference requires that hypotheses be expressed as though no relationship were expected. **Null hypotheses** (or *statistical hypotheses*) state that there is no relationship between the independent variables and dependent variables. The null form of the hypothesis used in our preceding example would be: Mothers' exercise levels postpartum are unrelated to their weight retention. A null hypothesis might be compared to the assumption of innocence of an accused criminal in the Canadian justice system; the variables are assumed to be "innocent" of any relationship until they can be shown to be "guilty" through statistical procedures. The null hypothesis is the formal statement of this presumed innocence.

Research reports typically present research rather than null hypotheses. When statistical tests are performed, the underlying null hypotheses are assumed without being stated. If the researcher's actual research hypothesis is that no relationship among variables exists, the hypothesis cannot be adequately tested using traditional statistical procedures. This issue is explained in Chapter 15.

CONSUMER TIP

When researchers use statistical tests (and this is almost always the case in quantitative studies), it means that there were underlying hypotheses—*whether the researchers explicitly stated them or not*—because statistical tests are designed to test hypotheses.   ■

Hypothesis Testing and Proof

Hypotheses are never *proved* (or *disproved*) through hypothesis testing; rather, they are *accepted* or *rejected*. Findings are always tentative. Certainly, if the same results are replicated in numerous studies, greater confidence can be placed in the conclusions. Hypotheses come to be increasingly supported with mounting evidence.

Let us look more closely at why this is so. Suppose we hypothesized that height and weight are related—which, indeed, they are in a general population. We predict that, on average, tall people weigh more than short people. We would then obtain height and weight measurements from a sample and analyze the data. Now suppose we happened by chance to choose a sample that consisted of short, fat people, and tall, thin people. Our results might indicate that there was no significant relationship between a person's height and weight. Would we then be justified in stating that this study *proved* or *demonstrated* that height and weight are unrelated?

As another example, suppose we hypothesized that tall people are better nurses than short people. This hypothesis is used here only to illustrate a point because, in reality, we would expect no relationship between height and a nurse's job performance. Now suppose that, by chance again, we draw a sample of nurses in which tall nurses received better job evaluations than short ones. Can we conclude definitively that height is related to nursing performance? These two examples demonstrate the difficulty of using observations from a sample to generalize to the population from which a sample has been drawn. Other problems, such as the accuracy of the measures, prohibit researchers from concluding with finality that hypotheses are proved.

CRITIQUING RESEARCH PROBLEMS, RESEARCH QUESTIONS, AND HYPOTHESES

In critiquing research reports, you will need to evaluate whether researchers have adequately communicated their research problem. The researchers' description of the problem, statement of purpose, research questions, and hypotheses set the stage for the description of what was done and what was learned. Ideally, you should not have to dig too deeply to decipher the research problem or to discover the questions.

Critiquing the Substance of a Research Problem

A critique of the research problem involves multiple dimensions. Substantively, you need to consider whether the problem has significance for nursing. The following issues are relevant in considering the significance of a study problem:

1. *Implications for nursing practice.* A primary consideration in evaluating the significance of a research problem is whether it has the potential to produce evidence for improving nursing practice: Are there practical applications that might stem from research on the problem? Will more knowledge about the problem improve nursing practice? Will the findings challenge (or lend support to) assumptions about nursing? If the answer to such questions is no, the significance of the problem is bound to be low.
2. *Extension of knowledge base.* Studies that build in a meaningful way on the existing knowledge base are well poised to make contributions to evidence-based nursing practice. Researchers who develop a systematic *program of research*, building on their own earlier findings, are especially likely to make significant contributions. For example, Beck's series of studies relating to postpartum depression (e.g., Beck, 1993, 1996,

2001; Beck & Gable, 2002, 2003) have influenced women's health care worldwide. As another example, Sloan and an interdisciplinary team of colleagues (Sloan, Scott-Findlay, Nemecek, Blood, Trylinski, Whittaker, El Sayed, Clinch, & Khoo, 2004) have developed a line of research that focuses on the interactions of patients with cancer and the health care system.

3. *Promotion of theory development.* Studies that test or develop a theory often have a better chance of contributing to knowledge than studies that do not have a conceptual context. For example, Marilyn Ford-Gilboe and colleagues have undertaken numerous studies to develop, refine, and test the Developmental Model of Health and Nursing, which we will describe in Chapter 8 (e.g., Black & Ford-Gilboe, 2004; Bluvol & Ford-Gilboe, 2004; Fulford & Ford-Gilboe, 2004; Monteith & Ford-Gilboe, 2002; Sgarbossa & Ford-Gilboe, 2004).

4. *Correspondence to research priorities.* Research priorities have been established by research scholars, agencies that fund nursing research (such as the Canadian Institutes of Health Research), and professional nursing organizations. Research problems stemming from such priorities have a high likelihood of yielding important new evidence for nurses because they reflect expert opinion about areas of needed research. As an example, Loiselle, Semenic, and Côté (2005) conducted a systematic research dissemination project based on findings relating to breastfeeding information and support offered by hospitals and community health centers in the Montreal region (Loiselle, Semenic, Côté, Lapointe, & Gendron, 2001). This project corresponds to a research and public health priority identified by the Ministry of Health and Social Services and the Conseil Québecois de la Recherche Sociale (CQRS).

When critiquing a study, you need to consider whether the research problem was meaningfully based on prior research, has a relationship to a theoretical context, addresses a current research priority, and, most importantly, can contribute useful evidence for nursing practice.

Critiquing Other Aspects of Research Problems

Another dimension in critiquing the research problem concerns methodologic issues—in particular, whether the research problem is compatible with the chosen research paradigm and its associated methods. You should also evaluate whether the statement of purpose or research questions have been properly worded and lend themselves to empirical inquiry.

In a quantitative study, if the research report does not contain explicit hypotheses, you need to consider whether their absence is justified. If there are hypotheses, you should evaluate whether the hypotheses are logically connected to the research problem and whether they are consistent with available knowledge or relevant theory. The wording of the hypothesis should also be assessed. The hypothesis is a valid guidepost to scientific inquiry only if it is testable. To be testable, the hypothesis must contain a prediction about the relationship between two or more measurable variables.

Specific guidelines for critiquing research problems, research questions, and hypotheses are presented in Box 6.1.

BOX 6.1 Guidelines for Critiquing Research Problems, Research Questions, and Hypotheses

1. What is the research problem? Is it easy to locate and clearly stated?
2. Does the problem have significance for nursing? How might the research contribute to nursing practice, administration, education, or policy?
3. Is there a good fit between the research problem and the paradigm within which the research was conducted? Is there a good fit with the qualitative research tradition?
4. Does the report formally present a statement of purpose, research question, and/or hypotheses? Is this information communicated clearly and concisely, and is it placed in a logical and useful location?
5. Are purpose statements or questions worded appropriately? (For example, are key concepts/variables identified and the population of interest specified? Are verbs used appropriately to suggest the nature of the inquiry and/or the research tradition?)
6. If there are no formal hypotheses, is their absence justified? Are statistical tests used in analyzing the data despite the absence of stated hypotheses?
7. Do hypotheses (if any) flow from a theory or previous research? Is there a justifiable basis for the predictions?
8. Are hypotheses (if any) properly worded—do they state a predicted relationship between two or more variables? Are they directional or nondirectional, and is there a rationale for how they were stated? Are they presented as research or as null hypotheses?

RESEARCH EXAMPLES   Critical Thinking Activities

 EXAMPLE 1: Quantitative Research

Aspects of a quantitative nursing study, featuring terms and concepts discussed in this chapter, are presented below, followed by some questions to guide critical thinking.

Study
"Children at risk of injury" (Bruce, Lake, Eden, & Denney, 2004)

Research Problem
"In Canada, almost 10 children out of 100,000 died annually between 1991 and 1995 as a result of injury (intentional and unintentional), claiming the lives of 2,665 children for that time period (UNICEF, 2001). Although much attention and research have emerged about the preventable nature of childhood injuries, unintentional injury remains the leading cause of mortality and morbidity in children. In addition to the demand on health care resources, childhood injuries have far-reaching consequences for both the child and the family. Researchers have explored several individual children and parent factors; however, results have failed to demonstrate any significant findings that could explain childhood injuries." (p. 121)

(Research Examples continue on page 128)

Critical Thinking Activities (continued)

Statement of Purpose

The aim of the study was to examine factors that influence parents' injury prevention activities. More specifically, the purpose was to determine whether there was a relationship between parents' risk perceptions, their preventative actions, children's injury behaviour, and the prevalence of childhood injury.

Hypotheses

The researchers posed several specific hypotheses, including the following:

▶ The prevalence of childhood injuries is higher among families in which parents have low perceptions of risk of injury and hazard than among parents with higher perceptions.

▶ Parenting stress is higher among parents with injured than noninjured children.

▶ Prevalence of childhood injuries is higher among children with risky behaviours.

Method

Data for the study were collected from 228 families of children aged 2 to 5 years who were seeking treatment in the emergency department of a paediatric tertiary care center. Families were categorized as having injured or uninjured children. Questionnaire packets were completed by parents while they were in the waiting area.

Key Findings

▶ Parental risk perception was not related to whether the child was injured or uninjured; thus, the first hypothesis was not confirmed.

▶ Parenting stress was higher among parents of noninjured children, contrary to the second hypothesis.

▶ Children who were reported by their parents to engage in risk behaviours were more likely to be in the injured group, consistent with the third hypothesis.

Critical Thinking Suggestions*

*See the Student Resource CD-ROM for a discussion of these questions.

1. Answer questions 2 to 5 and 8 from Box 6.1 regarding this study.

2. Also consider the following targeted questions, which may assist you in further assessing aspects of the study:

    a. Where in the research report do you think the researchers would have presented the hypotheses? Where in the research report would the outcomes of the hypothesis tests be placed?

    b. What clues does the summary give you that this study is quantitative?

    c. Would it have been possible to state the three hypotheses as a single hypothesis? If yes, state what it would be.

    d. Develop a research question for a phenomenological or grounded theory study (or both) relating to the same general topic area as this study.

3. If the results of this study are valid and reliable, what are some of the uses to which the findings might be put in clinical practice?

EXAMPLE 2: Qualitative Research

Aspects of a qualitative nursing study, featuring terms and concepts discussed in this chapter, are presented below, followed by some questions to guide critical thinking.

Study
"Relationships between families and registered nurses in long-term-care facilities: A critical analysis" (Ward-Griffin, Bol, Hay, and Dashnay, 2003)

Research Problem
"Over the past decade the citizens of the province of Ontario have experienced an upheaval in health care. Years of restructuring and underfunding have created gaps in health care that have led to increased reliance on family members to provide care to elderly persons. There has been a significant movement towards the sharing of care between unpaid caregivers and paid health-care professionals in hospitals nursing homes, and the community.... Although much has been written about the relationships between these two groups of caregivers and about the benefits, to both family and staff, of "sharing the caring",... this dyadic relationship has undergone little empirical analysis." (p. 151)

Statement of Purpose
The purpose of the study was to critically examine relationships between families and registered nurses caring for residents of a long-term care facility.

Research Questions
The researchers identified four specific research questions: (1) How do families and nurses describe their relationship? (2) What strategies do families and nurses use to negotiate their caregiving work? (3) What are the consequences of the negotiation process? and (4) What factors influence the negotiation process?

Method
An ethnographic method was used to study 17 family-nurse dyads in a long-term care facility for war veterans in the province of Ontario. Data were collected primarily through in-depth interviews with 34 family members and nurses.

Key Findings
The analysis revealed four types of family-nurse relationships—conventional, competitive, collaborative, and "carative"—each reflecting distinct roles of nurse and family, negotiating strategies, and consequences. Both intrinsic and extrinsic factors were found to influence the development of certain types of relationships.

Critical Thinking Suggestions
1. Answer questions 2 to 6 from Box 6.1 regarding this study.
2. Also consider the following targeted questions, which may assist you in further assessing aspects of the study:

(Research Examples continue on page 130)

Critical Thinking Suggestions (continued)

    a. Where in the research report do you think the researchers placed the statement of purpose and research questions?

    b. What clues does the summary give you that this study is qualitative?

    c. Could the findings from this study be used to generate hypotheses?

3. If the results of this study are trustworthy, what are some of the uses to which the findings might be put in clinical practice?

 EXAMPLE 3: Quantitative Research

1. Read the abstract and the introduction from the study by Feeley and colleagues ("Mother–VLBW Infant Interaction") in Appendix A of this book and then answer the relevant questions in Box 6.1.

2. Also consider the following targeted questions, which may further sharpen your critical thinking skills and assist you in assessing aspects of the study:

    a. Would you describe the hypotheses in this study as simple or complex?

    b. State the researchers' research hypotheses as null hypotheses.

 EXAMPLE 4: Qualitative Research

1. Read the abstract and the introduction from Beck's study ("Birth Trauma") in Appendix B of this book, and then answer the relevant questions in Box 6.1.

2. Also consider the following targeted questions, which may further sharpen your critical thinking skills and assist you in assessing aspects of the study:

    a. Do you think that Beck provided sufficient rationale for the significance of her research problem?

    b. Do you think that Beck needed to include research questions in her report, or was the purpose statement clear enough to stand alone?

CHAPTER REVIEW
Summary Points

▶ **A research problem** is a perplexing or enigmatic situation that a researcher wants to address through disciplined inquiry. Sources of ideas for nursing research problems include clinical experience, relevant literature, social issues, and theory.

▶ Researchers usually identify a broad topic or focus, then narrow the scope of the problem and identify questions consistent with a paradigm of choice.

▶ A **statement of purpose** summarizes the overall goal of the study; in both qualitative and quantitative studies, the purpose statement identifies the key concepts (variables) and the study group or population.

▶ A **research question** states the specific query the researcher wants to answer to address the research problem.

▶ A **hypothesis** is a statement of a predicted relationship between two or more variables. A testable hypothesis states the anticipated association between one or more independent and one or more dependent variables.

▶ A **directional hypothesis** specifies the expected direction or nature of a hypothesized relationship; **nondirectional hypotheses** predict a relationship but do not stipulate the form that the relationship will take.

▶ **Research hypotheses** predict the existence of relationships; **null hypotheses** express the absence of any relationship.

▶ Hypotheses are never proved or disproved in an ultimate sense—they are accepted or rejected, supported or not supported by the data.

Additional Resources for Review

Chapter 6 of the *Study Guide to Accompany Essentials of Nursing Research,* 6th edition offers various exercises and study suggestions for reinforcing the concepts presented in this chapter. For additional review, see the Student Self-Study Review Questions section of the Student Resource CD-ROM provided with this book.

SUGGESTED READINGS

References for studies cited in the chapter appear at the end of the book.

Methodologic References

Creswell, J. W. (1998). *Qualitative inquiry and research design: Choosing among five traditions.* Thousand Oaks, CA: Sage Publications.

Kerlinger, F. N., & Lee, H. B. (2000). *Foundations of behavioral research* (4th ed.). Orlando, FL: Harcourt College.

Lincoln, Y. S., & Guba, E. G. (1985). *Naturalistic inquiry.* Newbury Park, CA: Sage Publications.

Polit, D. F., & Hungler, B. P. (2004). *Nursing research: Principles and methods* (7th ed.). Philadelphia: Lippincott Williams & Wilkins.

Finding and Reviewing Studies in the Literature

STUDENT OBJECTIVES

On completing this chapter, you will be able to:

▌ Describe several purposes of a research literature review
▌ Identify bibliographic aids for retrieving nursing research reports, and locate references for a research topic
▌ Identify appropriate information to include in a research literature review
▌ Understand the steps involved in writing a literature review
▌ Evaluate the style, content, and organization of a traditional literature review
▌ Define new terms in the chapter

PURPOSES AND USES OF LITERATURE REVIEWS

Literature reviews serve a number of important functions in the research process—and they also play a critical role for nurses seeking to develop an evidence-based practice. This chapter presents information on locating research reports, organizing and preparing a written review, and critiquing reviews prepared by others.

Researchers and Literature Reviews

For researchers, familiarity with relevant research literature can help in various ways, such as with the following:

▶ Identifying a research problem and refining research questions or hypotheses
▶ Getting oriented to what is known and not known about a topic, to learn what research can best make a contribution
▶ Determining gaps or inconsistencies in a body of research
▶ Identifying relevant theoretical or conceptual frameworks (or suitable research methods) for a research problem
▶ Gaining insights for interpreting study findings and developing implications

Literature reviews can inspire new research ideas and help to lay the foundation for studies. A literature review is a crucial early task for most quantitative researchers. As previously noted, however, qualitative researchers have varying opinions about literature reviews, with some deliberately avoiding a literature search before entering the field. Some viewpoints are associated with qualitative research traditions. In grounded theory studies, researchers typically begin to collect data before examining the literature. As the data are analyzed and the grounded theory takes shape, researchers then turn to the literature, seeking to relate prior findings to the theory. Phenomenologists, by contrast, often undertake a search for relevant materials at the outset of a study. Ethnographers, although they often do not perform a thorough up-front literature review, often review the literature to help shape their choice of a cultural problem before going into the field.

Researchers usually summarize relevant literature in the introduction to research reports, regardless of when they perform the literature search. The literature review provides readers with a background for understanding current knowledge on a topic and illuminates the significance of the new study. Written reviews thus serve an integrative function and facilitate the accumulation of evidence on a problem.

Nonresearchers and Literature Reviews

Research reviews are not prepared solely in the context of doing a study. Nursing students and nurses in a variety of roles also review and synthesize evidence on a topic. The specific purpose of the review varies depending on the reviewer's role. Here are a few examples:

▶ Acquiring knowledge on a topic
▶ Evaluating current practices, and making recommendations for change
▶ Developing evidence-based clinical protocols and interventions to improve clinical practice
▶ Developing or revising nursing curricula
▶ Developing policy statements and practice guidelines

Thus, both consumers and producers of nursing research need to acquire skills for preparing and critiquing written summaries of knowledge on a problem.

LOCATING RELEVANT LITERATURE FOR A RESEARCH REVIEW

The ability to identify and locate documents on a research topic is an important skill. It is also a skill that requires adaptability—rapid technologic changes, such as the expanding use of the Internet, are making manual methods of finding information from print resources obsolete, and more sophisticated methods of searching the literature are being introduced continuously. We urge you to consult with librarians at your institution for updated guidance.

CONSUMER TIP

Locating all relevant information on a research question is a bit like being a detective. The various electronic and print literature retrieval tools are a tremendous aid, but there inevitably needs to be some digging for, and a lot of sifting and sorting of, the clues to knowledge on a topic. Be prepared for sleuthing! ■

One caveat should be mentioned. You may be tempted to do a literature search through an Internet search engine, such as Yahoo or Google. Such a search might yield a lot of information, such as summaries for lay persons, press releases, connections to advocacy groups, and so on. Such Internet searches, however, are unlikely to give you comprehensive bibliographic information on the *research* literature on your topic—and you might become frustrated with searching through the vast number of websites now available.

Electronic Literature Searches

Almost all college and university libraries offer students the capability of performing their own searches of **electronic databases**—huge bibliographic files that can be accessed by computer. Most of the electronic databases of interest to nurses can be accessed either through an **online search** (i.e., by directly communicating with a host computer over the Internet) or by CD-ROM (compact disks that store the bibliographic information). Several competing commercial vendors (e.g., Aries Knowledge Finder, Ovid, SilverPlatter) offer information retrieval services for bibliographic databases. Their programs are user-friendly—they are menu driven with on-screen support, and retrieval usually can proceed with minimal instruction. Some of these service providers offer free trial services that allow you to test an online service before subscribing, and some offer discount rates for students.

Major electronic databases that contain references on nursing studies include the following:

▶ CINAHL (Cumulative Index to Nursing and Allied Health Literature)
▶ MEDLINE (Medical Literature On-Line)
▶ Cochrane Database
▶ EMBASE (the Excerpta Medica database)
▶ PsycINFO (Psychology Information)

Most nursing school libraries subscribe to CINAHL, one of the most useful databases for nurses. The CINAHL database (*http://www.cinahl.com*) is described more fully in the next section. The MEDLINE database, perhaps the second most important database for nurse researchers, can be accessed free of charge through PubMed (*http://www. ncbi.nlm.nih.gov/PubMed*).

Several other types of electronic resources should be mentioned. First, books and other holdings of libraries can almost always be scanned electronically using *online catalogue systems*, and the catalogue holdings of libraries across the country can be reviewed over the Internet. Finally, it may be useful to search through Sigma Theta Tau International's Registry of Nursing Research on the Internet at *http://www.stti.iupui.edu/VirginiaHendersonLibrary/*. This registry is an electronic research database with more than 12,000 studies that can be searched by **key words**, variables, and researchers' names. The registry provides access to studies that have not yet been published, which cuts down on the publication lag time; however, caution is needed because these studies have not been critiqued by external reviewers. Electronic publishing in general is expanding at a rapid pace; librarians and faculty should be consulted for useful websites.

CONSUMER TIP

It is rarely possible to identify all relevant studies exclusively through literature retrieval mechanisms. An excellent method of identifying additional references is to find recently published studies and examine their references. Researchers usually know about other relevant studies and cite them to provide context for their own work. ▬

The CINAHL Database

This section illustrates some of the features of an electronic search, through the use of the CINAHL database. Our illustrated example relied on the online Ovid Search, but similar features are available through other software programs.

The CINAHL database covers references to more than 1200 English- and foreign-language nursing journals, as well as to books, dissertations, and selected conference proceedings in nursing and allied health fields. The database covers materials dating from 1982 to the present and has about 1 million records. In addition to providing bibliographic information (i.e., the author, title, journal, year of publication, volume, and page numbers of a reference), abstracts are available for almost 1000 journals.

Most searches are likely to begin with a **subject search**—a search for references relating to a specific topic. For this type of search, you would type in a word or phrase that captures the essence of the topic, and the computer would then proceed with the search. Fortunately, through *mapping* capabilities, most retrieval software translates

CONSUMER TIP

If you want to identify all major research reports on a topic, you need to be flexible and to think broadly about the key words and subject headings that could be related to your topic. For example, if you are interested in anorexia nervosa, you should search for anorexia, eating disorders, and weight loss, and perhaps appetite, eating behaviour, nutrition, bulimia, body weight changes, and body image. ▬

(maps) the topic you type into the most plausible CINAHL subject heading. An important alternative to a subject search is a **textword search** that looks for your specific words in text fields of each record, including the title and the abstract. (If you know the name of a researcher who has worked on a specific research topic, an **author search** might be productive.)

After you have typed in your topic, the computer will tell you how many "hits" there are in the database (i.e., matches against your topic). In most cases, the number of hits initially will be large, and you will want to constrain the search to ensure that you retrieve only the most relevant references. You can limit your search in a number of ways. For example, you might want only references published in nursing journals; only those that are for studies; only those published in certain years (e.g., 2000 or later); or only those with participants in certain age groups (e.g., infants).

To illustrate with a concrete example, suppose we were interested in recent research on postoperative pain, which is the term we enter in a subject search. Here is an example of how many hits there were on successive restrictions to the search for studies on therapies for postoperative pain, using the CINAHL database current to November 28, 2004:

Search Topic/Restriction	*Hits*
Postoperative pain	2164
Restrict to therapy subheadings	1249
Limit to research reports with abstracts in English-language journals	391
Limit to core nursing journals	107
Limit to 2000 to 2004 publications	43

This narrowing of the search—from 2164 initial references on postoperative pain to 43 references for recent nursing research reports on postoperative pain therapies—took less than a minute to perform. Next, we would display the 43 references on the monitor, and we could then print full bibliographic information for the ones that appeared especially promising. An example of an abridged CINAHL record entry for a study identified through this search on postoperative pain is presented in Figure 7.1, a study by Forchuk and colleagues. The entry shows an accession number—the unique identifier for each record in the database—that can be used to order the full text of the report. Then the authors, their contact information, and the title of the study are displayed, followed by source information. The source indicates the following:

Name of the journal (*Cancer Nursing*)
Volume (27)
Issue (1)
Page numbers (25–33)
Year and month of publication (2004, Jan–Feb)
Number of cited references (34 ref.)

The printout shows all the CINAHL subject headings for this entry, any one of which could have been used to retrieve this reference through a subject search. Note that the subject headings include substantive topics (e.g., breast neoplasms, postoperative pain), methodologic topics (e.g., descriptive statistics, interviews), and headings relating to the group under study (e.g., female). Next, any formal instruments used in the study are noted

Accession Number
2004052949

Authors
Forchuk C, Baruth P, Prendergast M, Holliday R, Bareham R, Brimner S, Schulz V, Chan YCI, Yammine N.

Institution
University of Western Ontario; *cforchuk@uwo.ca*

Title
Postoperative arm massage: A support for women with lymph node dissection

Source
Cancer Nursing, *27*(1):25–33, 2004 Jan-Feb, (34 ref)

CINAHL Subject Headings

Adult
Aged
Arm Circumference / ev [Evaluation]
*Breast Neoplasms / su [Surgery]
Cancer Patients
Checklists
Clinical Assessment Tools
Clinical Trials
Coefficient Alpha
Convenience Sample
Descriptive Statistics
Family Relations
Female
Functional Assessment

Health Care Costs / ev [Evaluation]
Health Services / ut [Utilization]
Interrater Reliability
Interviews
*Lymph Node Excision
Lymphedema
*Massage
Middle Age
Pain Measurement
*Postoperative Care
*Postoperative Pain / th [Therapy]
Purposive Sample
Range of Motion / ev [Evaluation]
Significant Other
Stress Psychological / ev [Evaluation]
T-Tests

Instrumentation
Shoulder Pain and Disability Index (SPADI)

Abstract
Purpose/objective: To evaluate the usefulness of arm massage from a significant other following lymph node dissection surgery. **Design:** Randomized clinical trial with a pretest-posttest design. Data were collected before surgery, within 24 hours after surgery, within 10 to 14 days post surgery, and 4 months after surgery. **Sample:** 59 women aged 21 to 78 years undergoing lymph node dissection surgery who had a significant other with them during the postoperative period. **Methods:** Subjects were randomly assigned to intervention and control groups. Subjects' significant others in the intervention group were first taught, then performed arm massage as a postoperative support measure. **Research main variables:** Variables included postoperative pain, family strengths and stressors, range of motion, and healthrelated costs. **Findings:** Participants reported a reduction in pain in the immediate postoperative period and better shoulder function. **Conclusion:** Arm massage decreased pain and discomfort related to surgery, and promoted a sense of closeness and support amongst subjects and their significant other. **Implication for nursing practice:** Postoperative message therapy for women with lymph node dissection provided therapeutic benefits for patients and their significant other. Nurses can offer effective alternative interventions along with standard procedures in promoting optimal health.

ISSN
0162-220X

Language
English

FIGURE 7.1 Example of a printout from a CINAHL search.

under Instrumentation; in this case, the Shoulder Pain and Disability Index, or SPADI, is cited. Then the study abstract is presented. Based on the abstract, you would decide whether this study was pertinent to your literature review; if so, the full research report could be obtained. Reports in the CINAHL database can be ordered by mail or fax; therefore, it is not necessary for your library to subscribe to the referenced journal. Moreover, many of the retrieval service providers, such as Ovid, offer *full-text* online services, which would enable you to download documents from certain journals. (Note that this study by Forchuk and colleagues appears in its entirety in Appendix C of this book.)

CONSUMER TIP

If your topic includes independent and dependent variables, you may need to do searches for each. For example, if you were interested in learning about the effect of stress on the health beliefs of acquired immunodeficiency syndrome (AIDS) patients, you might want to read about the effects of stress (in general) and about people's health beliefs (in general). Moreover, you might also want to learn something about patients with AIDS and their problems. If you are searching for references electronically, you can combine searches, so that the references for two independent searches can be linked (e.g., the computer can identify those references that have both stress and health beliefs as subject headings or textwords). ■

Example of a literature search

Fortin, Lapointe, Hudon, Vanasse, Ntetu, and Maltais (2004) published a literature review on the relationship between multimorbidity and quality of life of patients in primary care settings. They conducted computerized searches of the MEDLINE and EMBASE databases, using the following key words: multimorbidity, comorbidity, chronic disease, quality of life, and health-related quality of life.

PREPARING WRITTEN REVIEWS OF RESEARCH EVIDENCE

Identifying references, using the guidelines and tools described in the previous section, is an early step in preparing a written review of research literature. Subsequent steps are summarized in Figure 7.2.

Retrieving and Screening References

As Figure 7.2 shows, after identifying promising references, you need to retrieve the full reports. In addition to obtaining reports through your library or through CINAHL or other electronic databases, many nursing journals (e.g., *CJNR*) are now available online.

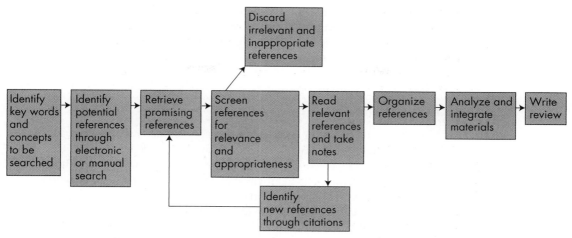

FIGURE 7.2 Flow of tasks in a literature review.

The next step is to screen reports for relevance and appropriateness. The report's *relevance*, which concerns whether it really focuses on the topic of interest, usually can be judged quickly by reading the introduction. *Appropriateness* concerns the nature of the information in the report. The most important information for a research review comes from reports that describe study findings. You should rely primarily on **primary source** research reports, which are descriptions of studies written by the researchers who conducted them. **Secondary source** research articles are descriptions of studies prepared by someone other than the original researcher. Literature review articles are secondary sources. Recent review articles are a good place to begin a literature search because they summarize current knowledge, and the reference lists are helpful. However, secondary descriptions of studies should not be considered substitutes for primary sources.

Examples of primary and secondary sources on breast cancer

Primary source—an original study based on data from 76 women during adjuvant breast cancer chemotherapy that examined weight and body composition changes over the course of the women's treatment (Ingram & Brown, 2004).
    Secondary source—a review article on research relating to prophylactic bilateral mastectomy for breast cancer prevention (Metcalfe, 2004).

For some literature reviews, it may be important to find references from the conceptual literature (i.e., references on a theory or conceptual model). In the conceptual literature, a primary source is a description of a theory written by the theory's developer, and a secondary source is a discussion or critique of the theory.

In addition to empirical and conceptual references, you may find in your search various nonresearch references, including opinion articles, case reports, anecdotes, and clinical descriptions. Such materials may serve to broaden understanding of a research problem, demonstrate a need for research, or describe aspects of clinical practice. They may thus play important roles in formulating research ideas, but they have limited utility in written research reviews because they do not address the central question: What is the current state of *knowledge* on this problem?

Abstracting and Recording Notes

Once you judge a reference to be relevant and appropriate, you should read the entire report carefully and critically, using guidelines that are provided throughout this book.
It is useful to work with photocopied articles, so that you can highlight or underline critical information. Even with a copied article, we recommend taking notes or writing a summary of the study's strengths and limitations. A formal protocol, such as the one presented in Figure 7.3, is sometimes helpful for recording information in a systematic fashion. Although many of the terms on this protocol are probably not familiar to you at this point, you will learn their meaning as you progress through this book.

Organizing the Evidence

Organization is crucial in preparing a written review. When literature on a topic is extensive, it is useful to summarize information in a table. The table could include columns with headings such as Author, Sample, Design, Data Collection Approach, and Key Findings. Such a table provides a quick overview that allows you to make sense of a mass of information.

Example of tabular organization

Dennis and Stewart (2004) reviewed the literature relating to biologic interventions to treat postpartum depression. Their review included several tables that summarized research relating to this topic. For example, their first table summarized nine studies, and the column headings were: Study, Design, Participants, and Intervention.

Most writers find it helpful to work from an outline—a written one if the review is lengthy and complex, a mental one for short reviews. The important point is to work out a structure before starting to write so that the review has a meaningful flow. Although the specifics of the organization differ from topic to topic, the overall goal is to structure the review in such a way that the presentation is logical, demonstrates meaningful integration, and leads to a conclusion of what is known and not known about the topic.

After the organization of topics has been determined, you should review your notes or protocols. This not only helps refresh your memory about material read earlier but also lays the groundwork for decisions about where a particular reference fits in the outline. If certain references do not seem to fit anywhere, they may need to be put aside; remember that the number of references is less important than their relevance and the overall organization of the review.

Citation: Authors: _____
Title: _____
Journal: _____
Year: _____ Volume: _____ Issue: _____ Pages: _____

Type of Study: ☐ Quantitative ☐ Qualitative ☐ Both

Location/setting: _____

Key Concepts/ Concepts: _____
Variables: Intervention/Independent Variable: _____
Dependent Variable: _____
Controlled Variables: _____

Design Type: ☐ Experimental ☐ Quasi-experimental ☐ Preexperimental ☐ Nonexperimental
Specific Design: _____
Descrip. of Intervention: _____

☐ Longitudinal/prospective ☐ Cross-sectional   No. of data collection points: _____
Comparison group(s): _____

Qual. Tradition: ☐ Grounded theory ☐ Phenomenology ☐ Ethnography ☐ Other: _____

Sample: Size: _____ Sampling method: _____
Sample characteristics: _____

Data Sources: Type: ☐ Self-report ☐ Observational ☐ Biophysiologic ☐ Other: _____
Description of measures: _____

Data Quality: _____

Statistical Tests: Bivariate: ☐ t test ☐ ANOVA ☐ Chi-square ☐ Pearson's r ☐ Other: _____
Multivariate: ☐ Multiple regression ☐ MANOVA ☐ ANCOVA ☐ Other: _____

Findings: _____
_____
_____

Recommendations: _____
_____

Strengths: _____
_____

Weaknesses: _____
_____

FIGURE 7.3 Example of a literature review protocol.

CONSUMER TIP

An important principle in organizing a review is to figure out a way to cluster and compare studies. For example, you could contrast studies that have similar findings with studies that have conflicting or inconclusive findings, making sure to analyze why discrepancies may have occurred. Other reviews might have sample characteristics as an organizing scheme if findings vary according to such characteristics (e.g., if results differ for male and female participants). Doing a research review is a bit like doing a qualitative study—you must search for important *themes* in the findings. ■

Writing a Literature Review

Research reviews tend to be written in a particular style and typically include specific types of information.

CONTENT OF A RESEARCH REVIEW

A written research review should provide a thorough, objective summary of the current state of evidence on a topic. A literature review should be neither a series of quotes nor a series of abstracts. The key tasks are to summarize and evaluate the evidence so as to reveal the state-of-the-art of knowledge of a topic—not simply to describe what researchers have done. The review should point out both consistencies and contradictions in the literature and offer possible explanations for inconsistencies (e.g., different conceptualizations or data collection methods).

Although important studies should be described in some detail, it is not necessary to provide extensive coverage for every reference. Reports with similar findings sometimes can be summarized together.

Example of grouped studies

In their literature review for a study focusing on the stress experienced by nurses in their work environments following health care reform in the 1990s, Peter, Macfarlane, and O'Brien-Pallas (2004, p. 357) summarized several studies that examined health care restructuring as follows: "Higher stress, emotional exhaustion, and the lowered morale and satisfaction of nurses were found in several studies (Shamian & Lightstone 1997, Corey-Lisle et al. 1999, Burke & Greenglass 2000, . . . Denton et al. 2002)."

The literature should be summarized in your own words. The review should demonstrate that consideration has been given to the cumulative significance of the body of research. Stringing together quotes from various documents fails to show that previous research on the topic has been assimilated and understood.

Reviews should be as objective as possible. Studies that conflict with personal values or hunches should not be omitted. Also, the review should not deliberately ignore a study because its findings contradict other studies. Inconsistent results should be analyzed and the supporting evidence evaluated objectively.

The literature review should conclude with a critical summary that recaps key study findings and indicates how credible they are; it should also make note of gaps in the research. The summary thus requires critical judgment about the extensiveness and dependability of evidence on a topic.

As you progress through this book, you will become increasingly proficient in critically evaluating research reports. We hope you will understand the mechanics of writing a research review when you have completed this chapter, but we do not expect that you will be in a position to write a state-of-the-art review until you have acquired more skills in research methods.

STYLE OF A RESEARCH REVIEW

Students preparing their first written research review often have trouble adjusting to the standard style of research reviews. One issue is that students sometimes accept research results without criticism or reservation, reflecting a common misunderstanding about the conclusiveness of research. You should keep in mind that no hypothesis or theory can be proved or disproved by empirical testing, and no research question can be definitely answered in a single study. The problem is partly a semantic one: hypotheses are not proved, they are supported by research findings; theories are not verified, but they may be tentatively accepted if a substantial body of evidence demonstrates their legitimacy. When describing study findings, you should generally use phrases indicating tentativeness of the results, such as the following:

▶ Several studies have *found* . . .
▶ Findings thus far *suggest* . . .
▶ Results from a landmark study *indicated* . . .
▶ The data *supported* the hypothesis . . .
▶ There *appears* to be strong evidence that . . .

A related stylistic problem among novice reviewers is an inclination to intersperse opinions (their own or someone else's) into the review. The review should include opinions sparingly and should be explicit about their source. Your own opinions do not belong in a review, except for assessments of study quality.

The left-hand column of Table 7.1 presents examples of stylistic flaws. The right-hand column offers recommendations for rewording the sentences to conform to a more acceptable form for a research literature review. Many alternative wordings are possible.

LENGTH OF A RESEARCH REVIEW

There are no formulas for how long a review should be. The length depends on several factors, including the complexity of the research question, the extent of prior research, and the purpose for which the review is being prepared. Literature reviews prepared for proposals (e.g., proposals to undertake a study or to test a clinical innovation) tend to be fairly comprehensive. Reviews in theses and dissertations are also lengthy. In these cases, the literature review serves both to summarize knowledge and to document the reviewer's capability.

Because of space limitations in journal articles, literature reviews that appear within research reports are concise. Literature reviews in the introduction to research reports

TABLE 7.1 Examples of Stylistic Difficulties for Research Reviews

INAPPROPRIATE STYLE OR WORDING	RECOMMENDED CHANGE
1. It is known that unmet expectations engender stress.	Dr. A. Cassard, an expert on stress and anxiety, has found that unmet expectations engender stress (Cassard, 2005).
2. Women who do not participate in childbirth preparation classes tend to manifest a high degree of stress during labor.	Studies have found that women who participate in preparation for childbirth classes manifest less stress during labor than those who do not (Klotz, 2003; Weller, 2004; McTygue, 2005).
3. Studies have proved that doctors and nurses do not fully understand the psychobiologic dynamics of recovery from a myocardial infarction.	Studies by Lowe (2004) and Martin (2003) suggest that doctors and nurses do not fully understand the psychobiologic dynamics of recovery from a myocardial infarction.
4. Attitudes cannot be changed quickly.	Attitudes have been found to be relatively enduring attributes that cannot be changed quickly (Geair, 2003; Casey, 2004).

NOTE: All references are fictitious.

demonstrate the need for the new study and provide a context for the research questions. The literature review sections of qualitative reports tend to be especially brief. However, there are stand-alone research reviews in nursing journals that are more extensive than those appearing in the introductions of research reports. We discuss such reviews next.

READING AND USING EXISTING RESEARCH REVIEWS

Most of this chapter provides guidance on how to conduct a literature review—how to locate and screen references, what type of information to seek, and how to organize and write a review. However, practicing nurses may not need to perform a full-fledged review if a comprehensive and recent literature review on the topic of interest has been published. Several different types of *integrative reviews* that can be used to support evidence-based nursing practice are briefly described in this section. Further information about conducting and critiquing integrative reviews is provided in Chapter 18.

Traditional Narrative Reviews

A traditional narrative literature review synthesizes and summarizes, in a narrative fashion, a body of research literature. The information offered in this chapter has been designed to help you prepare such a review.

Narrative integrative reviews are frequently published in nursing journals, especially in nursing specialty journals. These reviews may have a number of different purposes, including providing practitioners with state-of-the-art research-based information; providing a foundation for the development of innovations for clinical practice; and developing an agenda for further research.

Example of a narrative research review

Epstein, Stinson, & Stevens (2005) conducted a critical review of studies that examined the effect of camp on the health-related quality of life in children with chronic illnesses. Using CINAHL, MEDLINE, and PsycINFO databases, they identified 18 studies that met specified criteria. The studies in the review involved a total of 1270 children aged 6 to 25 years.

Meta-analysis

Meta-analysis is a technique for integrating quantitative research findings statistically. Meta-analysis treats the findings from a study as one piece of datum. The findings from multiple studies on the same topic are then combined to create a data set that can be analyzed in a manner similar to that obtained from individuals. Thus, instead of study participants being the **unit of analysis** (the most basic entity on which the analysis focuses), individual studies are the unit of analysis in a meta-analysis. Typically, the meta-analyst takes information about the strength of the relationship between the independent and dependent variables from each study, quantifies that information, and then essentially takes an average across all studies.

Traditional narrative research reviews have some shortcomings that make meta-analyses appealing. For example, if there are many studies and results are inconsistent, it may be difficult to draw conclusions in a narrative review. Furthermore, integration in narrative reviews can be subject to reviewer biases. Another advantage of meta-analysis is that it can take into account the quality of the studies being combined. Meta-analysis provides a convenient and objective method of integrating a large body of findings and of observing patterns and relationships that might otherwise have gone undetected. Meta-analysis can thus serve as an important tool in evidence-based practice. Because of this fact, we discuss meta-analyses at greater length in the final chapter.

Example of a meta-analysis

Taylor-Piliae and Froelicher (2004) conducted a meta-analysis to integrate findings on the effectiveness of Tai Chi exercise in improving aerobic capacity. They integrated results from seven studies. The aggregated evidence suggested that Tai Chi may be effective, especially when the classical Yang style of Tai Chi is performed for 1 year by sedentary adults. (This study appears in its entirety in Appendix F of the *Study Guide to Accompany Essentials of Nursing Research*, 6th edition.)

Qualitative Metasynthesis

A qualitative **metasynthesis** involves integrating qualitative research findings on a specific topic that are themselves interpretive syntheses of data (Sandelowski & Barroso, 2003). A metasynthesis is more than just a summary of findings—it involves interpretation of those findings, and this is where a metasynthesis differs from a meta-analysis. A metasynthesis is less about reducing data and more about amplifying and interpreting data. Sandelowski, Docherty, and Emden (1997) warn researchers that qualitative metasynthesis is a complex process that involves "carefully peeling away the surface layers of studies to find their hearts and souls in a way that does the least damage to them" (p. 370). Various methods have been used to synthesize qualitative findings, but to date, no firm guidelines exist.

Example of a qualitative metasynthesis

Paterson, Canam, Joachim, and Thorne (2003) conducted a metasynthesis of studies of the experience of fatigue in chronic illness. Their metasynthesis used findings from 35 published and unpublished studies from the nursing, allied health, and social science literature from 1980 to 2001. They focused their inquiry on the embedded assumptions that have influenced the way researchers have made sense of their findings about fatigue in chronic illness. The four key assumptions they found are (a) fatigue as exclusively attributed to disease; (b) fatigue as a unitary phenomenon; (c) fatigue as inherently problematic; and (d) fatigue in isolation from the context in which it occurred.

Critiquing Research Reviews

Some nurses never prepare a written research review, and perhaps you will never be required to do one. Most nurses, however, do *read* research reviews (including the literature review sections of research reports), and they should be prepared to evaluate such reviews critically. You may find it difficult to critique a research review because you are probably a lot less familiar with the topic than the writer. You may thus not be able to judge whether the author has included all relevant literature and has adequately summarized knowledge on that topic. Many aspects of a research review, however, are amenable to evaluation by readers who are not experts on the topic. Some suggestions for critiquing written research reviews are presented in Box 7.1. Additionally, when a literature review—whether it be a traditional review, a meta-analysis, or a metasynthesis—is published as a stand-alone article, it should include information that will help you understand its scope and evaluate its thoroughness. This is discussed in more detail in Chapter 18.

In assessing a written literature review, the overarching question is whether the review adequately summarizes the current state of research evidence. If the review is written as part of an original research report, an equally important question is whether the review lays a solid foundation for the new study.

BOX 7.1   Guidelines for Critiquing Literature Reviews

1. Does the review seem thorough—does it include all or most of the major studies on the topic? Does it include recent research? Are studies from other related disciplines included, if appropriate?
2. Does the review rely on appropriate materials (e.g., mainly on research reports, using primary sources)?
3. Is the review merely a summary of existing work, or does it critically appraise and compare key studies? Does the review identify important gaps in the literature?
4. Is the review well organized? Is the development of ideas clear?
5. Does the review use appropriate language, suggesting the tentativeness of prior findings? Is the review objective? Does the author paraphrase, or is there an overreliance on quotes from original sources?
6. If the review is part of a research report for a new study, does the review support the need for the study? If it is a critical integrative review designed to summarize evidence for clinical practice, does the review draw appropriate conclusions about practice implications?

RESEARCH EXAMPLES   **Critical Thinking Activities**

 EXAMPLE 1: Quantitative Research

Aspects of a quantitative nursing study, featuring terms and concepts discussed in this chapter, are presented below, followed by some questions to guide critical thinking.

Study
"Efficacy of therapeutic touch in treating pregnant inpatients who have a chemical dependency" (Larden, Palmer, & Janssen, 2004)

Statement of Purpose
The purpose of the study was to determine whether, among pregnant women hospitalized for treatment of their chemical dependency, those given daily therapeutic touch (TT) would experience lower anxiety and lower levels of withdrawal symptoms than those who received either standard care or daily companionship by nurses.

Method
Fifty-four pregnant women admitted to a chemical dependency treatment ward in Vancouver were put into one of three groups, at random: a TT group, a daily companionship group, and a standard care group. Anxiety and withdrawal symptoms were measured daily over a 7-day period.

Literature Review From the Report (Excerpt)
"Empirical research has demonstrated that TT has significantly reduced anxiety in cardiovascular patients (Heidt, 1981; Quinn, 1984), the elderly (Lin & Taylor,

(Research Examples continue on page 148)

Critical Thinking Activities (continued)

1998, Simington & Laing, 1993), middle-aged psychiatric patients (Gagne & Toyne, 1994), burn patients (Turner, Clark, Gauthier, & Williams, 1998), people with terminal cancer (Giasson & Bouchard, 1998), and female volunteers (LaFreniere et al., 1999). TT has not been found to significantly lower anxiety scores in two studies in which only healthy participants were recruited (Engle & Graney, 2000; Olson & Sneed, 1995).

TT has also been found to significantly lessen a variety of types of pain, such as tension headaches (Keller & Bzdek, 1986) and musculoskeletal pain in the elderly. Two meta-analyses of TT (Peters, 1999; Winstead-Fry & Kijek, 1999) concluded that TT could produce a moderate effect on physiological and psychological outcomes. Heterogeneity of study methods, underreporting of data, and inadequate description of study samples and the TT intervention limited the validity of the conclusions from these studies. . . .

One small pilot study examining the efficacy of TT as a complementary therapy in prolonged periods of abstinence in people who abuse alcohol and other drugs (Hagemaster, 2000) reported a trend . . . toward decreased depression among participants treated with TT. There is no published research investigating the effect of TT on pregnant women with chemical dependency" (p. 322).

Key Findings
▶ Anxiety scores were significantly lower among the women in the TT group on days 1, 2, and 3 of treatment.
▶ There were no statistically significant group differences with respect to withdrawal symptoms.

Critical Thinking Suggestions*
*See the Student Resource CD-ROM for a discussion of these questions.
1. Answer the questions from Box 7.1 regarding this study.
2. Also consider the following targeted questions, which may assist you in further assessing aspects of the study:
   a. What was the independent variable in this study? Did the literature review cover findings from prior studies about this variable?
   b. What were the dependent variables in this study? Did the literature review cover findings from prior studies about these variables and its relationship with the independent variable?
   c. In performing the literature review, what key words might Larden and colleagues have used to search for prior studies?
   d. Using the key words, perform a computerized search to see if you can find a recent relevant study to augment the review.
3. If the results of this study are valid and reliable, what are some of the uses to which the findings might be put in clinical practice?

Critical Thinking Activities (continued)

 EXAMPLE 2: Qualitative Research

Aspects of a qualitative nursing study, featuring terms and concepts discussed in this chapter, are presented below, followed by some questions to guide critical thinking.

Study
"A different way of being: Adolescents' experiences with cancer" (Woodgate, 2005)

Statement of Purpose
The purpose of the study was to understand the impact that cancer and its symptoms have on adolescents' sense of self.

Method
This qualitative study involved in-depth interviews with 15 male and female adolescents between 12 and 18 years of age who were in treatment for cancer in a western Canadian city. Researchers also observed the adolescents in the inpatient and outpatient units during various periods.

Literature Review From the Report (Excerpt)
"Childhood cancer can best be described as a powerful life event that causes children and families to face many challenges including uncertainty, changes and restrictions in the daily routine, increased psychological and physical work, lengthy and intense treatment regimens, and multiple losses.[1–3] One of the more stressful challenges for children and families is unmanageable symptoms.[4–9] In addition to these challenges, the adolescent children with cancer are confronted with their own unique challenges. They must deal with not only events specific to the diagnosis and adverse treatment effects of a life-threatening illness but also complex developmental challenges and demands.[10–13] (. . .)

The many challenges and stressors faced by adolescents with cancer have led to a concern for their psychosocial well-being. Accordingly, researchers within the last 2 decades have studied their psychosocial functioning with attention to evaluating selective psychosocial dimensions including emotional adjustment, coping methods or styles, and sociobehavioral support and adjustment.[14–17] To date, findings have been conflicting. At best one can conclude from this body of work that although having cancer does not always lead to adjustment difficulties in adolescents, it nonetheless puts them at greater risk for psychosocial difficulties.[18]

Researchers have also increasingly focused on examining the impact of cancer stressors on the sense of self in adolescents. . . . Research directed at the study of a sense of self in adolescents with cancer has mainly involved adolescents completing standardized questionnaires that assess both global or general self esteem and also perceived competence in a specific area such as intellectual and school status.[20, 24–27] Much of this research is based on the premise that adolescents with a history of cancer are at greater risk for lower self-esteem levels than are healthy

(Research Examples continue on page 150)

Critical Thinking Activities (continued)

peers because of the effects of cancer on the developing self. Although differences have been reported in the self-esteem ratings between adolescents with cancer and healthy adolescents,[25] the majority of findings have shown that self-esteem ratings of adolescents with cancer are for the most part within normal range.

Although the potential for increased emotional distress and psychosocial difficulties in adolescents with cancer has been documented, there is still much to learn. Especially needed is an understanding of how adolescents with cancer view themselves as they progress through the cancer trajectory" (p. 9).

Key Findings
Adolescents experienced changes in their lived bodies because of their cancer symptoms, and this, in turn, impacted their sense of self and way of being in the world. Although they spoke of the significance that cancer had on their lives, they described themselves as "still being pretty much the same person."

Critical Thinking Suggestions
1. Answer the questions from Box 7.1 regarding this study.
2. Also consider the following targeted questions, which may assist you in further assessing aspects of the study:
   a. What was the central phenomenon that the researchers focused on in this study? Was that phenomenon adequately covered in the literature review?
   b. In performing the literature review, what key words might the researchers have used to search for prior studies?
   c. Using the key words, perform a computerized search to see if you can find a recent relevant study to augment the review.
3. If the results of this study are trustworthy, what are some of the uses to which the findings might be put in clinical practice?

 EXAMPLE 3: Quantitative Research

1. Read the introduction from the study by Feeley and colleagues ("Mother–VLBW Infant Interaction") in Appendix A of this book and then answer the questions in Box 7.1.
2. Also consider the following targeted questions, which may further sharpen your critical thinking skills and assist you in assessing aspects of the study:
   a. What were the independent variables and the dependent variables in this study? Did the literature review cover findings from prior studies about these variables and their interrelationships?
   b. In performing the literature review, what key words might have been used to search for prior studies?
   c. Using the key words, perform a computerized search to see if you can find a recent relevant study to augment the review.

Critical Thinking Activities (continued)

 EXAMPLE 4: Qualitative Research

1. Read the abstract and the introduction to Beck's study ("Birth Trauma") in Appendix B of this book and then answer the relevant questions in Box 7.1.

2. Also consider the following targeted questions, which may further sharpen your critical thinking skills and assist you in assessing aspects of the study:

   a. What was the central phenomenon that Beck focused on in this study? Was that phenomenon adequately covered in the literature review?

   b. In what sections of the report did Beck discuss prior research?

   c. In performing her literature review, what key words might Beck have used to search for prior studies?

   d. Using the key words, perform a computerized search to see if you can find a recent relevant study to augment the review.

CHAPTER REVIEW

Summary Points

▶ A research **literature review** is a written summary of the state of knowledge on a research problem.

▶ Researchers undertake literature reviews to determine knowledge on a topic of interest, to provide a context for a study, and to justify the need for a study; consumers review and synthesize evidence-based information to gain knowledge and improve nursing practice.

▶ **Electronic databases,** which are important tools for locating references, usually can be accessed through an **online search** or by way of CD-ROM. For nurses, the **CINAHL database** is especially useful.

▶ Most database searches begin with a **subject search**, but a **textword search** and an **author search** are other possibilities.

▶ In writing a research review, reviewers should carefully organize the relevant materials, which should consist primarily of **primary source** research reports.

▶ The role of reviewers is to point out what has been studied to date, how adequate and dependable those studies are, and what gaps exist in the body of research.

▶ Nurses need to have skills in using and critiquing research reviews prepared by others, including traditional narrative reviews, **meta-analyses** (the integration of study findings using statistical procedures), and qualitative **metasyntheses** (integrations of qualitative research findings that produce new interpretations.)

Additional Resources for Review

Chapter 7 of the *Study Guide to Accompany Essentials of Nursing Research,* 6th edition offers various exercises and study suggestions for reinforcing the concepts presented in this chapter. For additional review, see the Student Self-Study Review Questions section of the Student Resource CD-ROM provided with this book.

SUGGESTED READINGS

* References for studies cited in the chapter appear at the end of the book.

Methodologic References

Fink, A. (1998). *Conducting research literature reviews: From paper to the Internet.* Thousand Oaks, CA: Sage Publications.

Martin, P. S. (1997). Writing a useful literature review for a quantitative research project. *Applied Nursing Research, 10,* 159–162.

Sandelowski, M., & Barroso, J. (2003). Creating metasummaries of qualitative findings, *Nursing Research, 52,* 226–233.

Sandelowski, M., Docherty, S., & Emden, C. (1997). Qualitative metasynthesis: Issues and techniques. *Research in Nursing & Health, 20,* 365–371.

8

Examining the Conceptual/Theoretical Basis of a Study

STUDENT OBJECTIVES

On completing this chapter, you will be able to:

▶ Identify the major characteristics of theories, conceptual models, and frameworks

▶ Identify several conceptual models of nursing and other models used by nurse researchers

▶ Describe how theory and research are linked in quantitative and qualitative studies

▶ Critique the appropriateness of a theoretical framework—or its absence—in a study

▶ Define new terms in the chapter

THEORIES, MODELS, AND FRAMEWORKS

Theories and conceptual models are the primary mechanisms by which researchers organize findings into a broader conceptual context. Different terms are associated with conceptual contexts for research, including *theories, models, frameworks, schemes,* and *maps.* There is overlap in how these terms are used, partly because they are used differently by different writers. We provide guidance in distinguishing them but note that our definitions are not universal.

Theories

Classically, **theory** is defined as an abstract generalization that offers a systematic explanation about how phenomena are interrelated. Traditionally, a theory embodies at least two concepts that are related in a manner that the theory purports to explain. As classically defined, theories consist of concepts and a set of propositions that form a logically interrelated system, providing a mechanism for deducing new statements from original propositions. To illustrate, consider the theory of reinforcement, which posits that behaviour that is reinforced (i.e., rewarded) tends to be repeated and learned. This theory consists of concepts (reinforcement and learning) and a proposition stating the relationship between them. The proposition lends itself to hypothesis generation—for example, we could deduce that hyperactive children who are praised when they are engaged in quiet play exhibit less acting-out behaviours than similar children who are not praised. This prediction, as well as many others based on the theory of reinforcement, could then be tested in a study.

Others use the term *theory* less restrictively to refer to a broad characterization of a phenomenon. Some authors specifically refer to this type of theory as **descriptive theory**—a theory that accounts for (i.e., thoroughly describes) a single phenomenon. Descriptive theories are inductive, empirically driven abstractions that "describe or classify specific dimensions or characteristics of individuals, groups, situations, or events by summarizing commonalities found in discrete observations" (Fawcett, 1999, p. 15). Such theories play an especially important role in qualitative studies.

Both classical and descriptive theories serve to make research findings meaningful and interpretable. Theories allow researchers to knit together observations into an orderly system. Theories also serve to explain research findings: theory may guide researchers' understanding not only of the "what" of natural phenomena but also of the "why" of their occurrence. Finally, theories help to stimulate research and the extension of knowledge by providing both direction and impetus.

Theories are abstractions that are created and invented by humans—they are not just "out there" waiting to be discovered. Theory development depends not only on observable facts but also on the theorist's ingenuity in pulling those facts together and making sense of them. Because theories are created, it follows that they are tentative. A theory can never be proved—a theory simply represents a theorist's best efforts to describe and explain phenomena. Through research, theories evolve and are sometimes discarded.

Theories are sometimes classified by their level of generality. **Grand theories** (or **macro-theories**) purport to explain large segments of the human experience. Some sociologists, such as Talcott Parsons, developed general theoretical systems to account for broad classes of social functioning. Within nursing, theories are more restricted in scope, focusing on a narrow range of phenomena. Theories that explain a portion of the human experience are sometimes referred to as **middle-range theories**. For example, there are middle-range theories to explain such phenomena as stress and infant attachment.

Models

A **conceptual model** deals with abstractions (concepts) that are assembled because of their relevance to a common theme. Conceptual models provide a perspective about interrelated phenomena, but they are more loosely structured than theories and do not link concepts in a logically derived deductive system. A conceptual model broadly presents an understanding of a phenomenon and reflects the philosophical views of the model's designer. There are many conceptual models of nursing that offer broad explanations of the nursing process. Conceptual models are not directly testable by researchers in the same way that theories are, but like theories, conceptual models can serve as springboards for generating hypotheses.

Some writers use the term **model** for mechanisms representing phenomena with a minimal use of words. Words that define a concept can convey different meanings to different people; thus, a visual or symbolic representation of a phenomenon can sometimes express abstract ideas in a more understandable form. Two types of models that are used in research contexts are schematic models and statistical models.

Statistical models, not elaborated on here, are mathematic equations that express the nature and magnitude of relationships among a set of variables. These models are tested using sophisticated statistical methods. A **schematic model** (or **conceptual map**) represents a phenomenon of interest in a diagram. Concepts and the linkages between them are represented through boxes, arrows, or other symbols, as in Figure 8.1. This model is the Developmental Model of Health and Nursing, or DMHN (Ford-Gilboe, 2002). The DMHN is a strengths-oriented model that focuses on how families and their members develop strategies needed to support a healthy lifestyle, with an emphasis on the family's role in shaping patterns of response to health situations. According to the model, a person's health status (and quality of life) is affected by a multiplicity of factors, including contextual factors, nursing actions, and individual and family behaviours. The central concept in

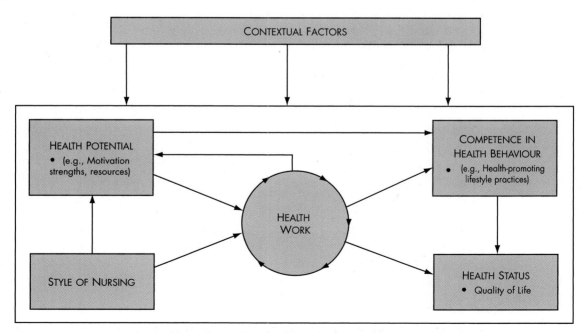

FIGURE 8.1 Schematic model: The Developmental Model of Health and Nursing. (Adapted from Fulford & Ford-Gilboe, 2004; Landenbach & Ford-Gilboe, 2004; Sgarbossa & Ford-Gilboe, 2004.)

the DMHN is *health work*, which is a process through which families learn to manage health situations, problem-solve, and develop growth-seeking behaviours.

Frameworks

A **framework** is the conceptual underpinnings of a study. Not every study is based on a theory or model, but every study has a framework. In a study based on a theory, the framework is the **theoretical framework**; in a study rooted in a specified conceptual model, the framework is often called the **conceptual framework**. (However, the terms *conceptual framework, conceptual model,* and *theoretical framework* are often used interchangeably.)

The framework for a study is often implicit (i.e., not formally acknowledged or described). World views and views on nursing shape how concepts are defined and operationalized. As noted in Chapter 2, researchers undertaking a study should make clear the conceptual definition of their key variables, thereby providing information about the study's framework.

Example of conceptual and operational definitions

As previously noted, the central concept in the Developmental Model of Health and Nursing, is *health work*. Ford-Gilboe and her colleagues have developed both conceptual and operational definitions of this construct:

Conceptual definition: Health work is a universal process whereby families develop or learn ways of coping with health situations and using strengths and resources to achieve goals for healthy individual and family development (Ford-Gilboe, 2002).

Operational definition: Health work is observed in the problem-solving (coping) and goal attainment activities of the family. The construct is measured using a 21-question rating scale that was developed to measure the degree to which families engage in health work, the Health Options Scale, or HOS (Ford-Gilboe, 2002; Laudenbach & Ford-Gilboe, 2004).

In most qualitative studies, the frameworks are part of the research tradition within which the study is embedded. For example, ethnographers generally begin their work within a theory of culture. *Grounded theory* researchers incorporate sociologic principles into their framework and their approach to looking at phenomena. The questions that most qualitative researchers ask and the methods they use to address those questions inherently reflect certain theoretical formulations.

CONCEPTUAL MODELS AND THEORIES USED BY NURSE RESEARCHERS

Nurse researchers have used both nursing and nonnursing frameworks to provide conceptual contexts for their studies. This section briefly discusses some of the more prominent frameworks that have appeared in nursing research studies.

Conceptual Models of Nursing

Nurse theorists have developed a number of conceptual models of nursing that constitute formal explanations of what nursing is. Four concepts are central to models of nursing: person, environment, health, and nursing (Fawcett, 1995). The various nursing models define these concepts differently and link them in diverse ways. Moreover, the various models emphasize different processes as being central to nursing. For example, Sister Callista Roy's Adaptation Model identifies adaptation of patients as a critical phenomenon (Roy & Andrews, 1999). Martha Rogers (1986), by contrast, emphasizes the centrality of the individual as a unified whole, and her model views nursing as a process in which individuals are aided in achieving maximum well-being within their potential. The conceptual models were not developed primarily as a base for nursing research. Nevertheless, nurse researchers have turned to these conceptual frameworks for inspiration in formulating research questions and hypotheses.

In Canada, nursing education, practice, and research have been especially influenced by Moyra Allen's model of nursing, which has come to be known as the **McGill Model of Nursing** (Allen & Warner, 2002). This model focuses on the health-promoting interactions of nurses with individuals and families. The goal of nursing is to work with and actively promote patient and family strengths toward achievement of life goals. Health promotion is viewed as a collaborative process in which nurses help families explore health issues and develop healthy lives. In the McGill Model, the goal of nursing is to acknowledge the capabilities and strengths that clients and their families possess and to actively work with them to maintain, strengthen, and develop their health potential.

The previously discussed Developmental Model of Health and Nursing (Figure 8.1) represents a theoretical extension and refinement of the McGill Model of Nursing. In the model, family health work is supported by the family's health potential—the strengths, motivation, and resources of the family unit and its members. Health potential can, in turn, be affected by nursing actions. Although little research has been conducted to explore the relationship between nursing care and family health work, other aspects of the model have been subjected to formal testing, and results are promising.

Example of a study using the DMHN

Monteith and Ford-Gilboe (2002) used the DMHN as the framework for a study of health promotion in families with preschool children. They tested the relationships among the mothers' resilience, family health work, and the mothers' health-promoting lifestyle practices. Mothers' *resilience*—the capacity to adapt, change and grow despite ongoing stress—was viewed as an aspect of health potential (the upper left-hand box in the model). One of their specific hypotheses based on the model was: There is a positive relationship between mother's resilience and family health work. The data supported this hypothesis, as well as other hypotheses predicted by the model.

Table 8.1 lists several other conceptual models of nursing, together with a study for each that claimed the model as its framework.

TABLE 8.1 Selected Conceptual Models of Nursing Used by Nurse Researchers

THEORIST	NAME OF MODEL/THEORY	KEY THESIS OF MODEL	RESEARCH EXAMPLE
F. Moyra Allen, 2002	McGill Model of Nursing	Nursing is the science of health-promoting interactions. Health promotion is a process of helping people cope and develop; the goal of nursing is to actively promote patient and family strengths and the achievement of life goals.	Cossette, Frasure-Smith, and Lespérance (2002) included elements of the McGill Model in their study to document the types of nursing approaches that were associated with reductions in psychological distress among patients after myocardial infarction.
Madeline Leininger, 1991	Theory of Culture Care Diversity	Caring is a universal phenomenon but varies transculturally.	Van den Brink (2003) incorporated Leininger's theory into a study of diversity and universality of care values relevant to the care of elderly Turkish patients in the Netherlands.
Betty Neuman, 2001	Health Care Systems Model	Each person is a complete system; the goal of nursing is to assist in maintaining client system stability.	Skillen, Anderson, and Knight (2001) conducted a study of nurse case managers' reported use of assessment skills using concepts from Neuman as an organizing framework.
Dorothea Orem, 2003	Self-Care Model	Self-care activities are what people do on their own behalf to maintain health and well-being; the goal of nursing is to help people meet their own therapeutic self-care demands.	Kreulen and Braden (2004) developed a model of relationships between self-help–promoting nursing interventions and health status outcomes, using concepts from Orem's model.
Rosemary Rizzo Parse, 1999	Theory of Human Becoming	Health and meaning are co-created by indivisible humans and their environment; nursing involves having clients share views about meanings.	Jonas-Simpson (2003) studied older women's experience of *being listened to* within the context of Parse's theory.
Martha Rogers, 1986	Science of Unitary Human Beings	The individual is a unified whole in constant interaction with the environment; nursing helps individuals achieve maximum well-being within their potential.	Wright (2004) studied the relationship between trust and power in adults (as a way of illuminating nurse–client relationships), using Rogers' theory.
Sr. Callista Roy	Adaptation Model	Humans are adaptive systems that cope with change through adaptation; nursing helps to promote client adaptation during health and illness.	Shyu, Liang, Lu, and Wu (2004) tested Roy's model in their study of environmental barriers and mobility among elders in Taiwan.

Other Models Developed by Nurses

In addition to conceptual models that describe and characterize the nursing process, nurses have developed other models and theories that focus on specific phenomena of interest to nurses. One example is Nola Pender's Health Promotion Model (2001), which is designed to explain participation in health-promoting behaviours. According to this model, a person's decision to engage in health-promoting behaviours is affected by a number of cognitive/perceptual factors (e.g., the person's beliefs about the importance of health) and is modified indirectly by other factors (e.g., gender).

Another example is Mishel's Uncertainty in Illness Theory (1988), which focuses on the concept of uncertainty—the inability of a person to determine the meaning of illness-related events. According to this theory, a situation appraised as uncertain will mobilize individuals to use their resources to adapt to the situation. Mishel's conceptualization of uncertainty has been used as a framework for both qualitative and quantitative studies.

Example of a study based on uncertainty theory

Guided by Mishel's Uncertainty in Illness Theory, Bérubé and Loiselle (2003) studied relationships among uncertainty, hope, and coping in people with a spinal cord injury.

Other Models Used by Nurse Researchers

Many concepts of interest to nurse researchers are not unique to nurses, and therefore nursing studies are sometimes linked to frameworks outside the nursing profession. Four conceptual models that have been used frequently in nursing studies are as follows:

▶ *Lazarus and Folkman's Theory of Stress and Coping.* This theory, which explains methods of dealing with stress, posits that coping strategies are learned, deliberate responses to stressors and are used to adapt to or change the stressors. According to this theory, people's perception of mental and physical health is related to the ways they evaluate and cope with life stress (Lazarus & Folkman, 1984). An example of a Canadian nursing study that used this theory as its framework is Low and Gutman's (2003) study of discrepancies between the perceptions of patients with chronic obstructive pulmonary disease and their spouses regarding the patients' health-related quality of life.

▶ *Azjen's Theory of Planned Behavior* (TPB). The TPB, an extension of a theory called the Theory of Reasoned Action (TRA) (Azjen & Fishbein, 1980), provides a framework for understanding the relationships among a person's attitudes, intentions, and behaviours. According to the TPB, behavioural intentions are the best predictor of a person's actual behaviour, and behavioural intentions are a function of attitude toward performing the behaviour, perceived control over the behaviour, and subjective norms—the person's belief in whether others think the behaviour should be performed (Azjen, 1988). The TPB and TRA have been used in many Canadian nursing studies, including a study of neonatal nurses' behaviours preventing overstimulation in preterm infants (Aïta & Goulet, 2003) and a study of adolescents' attitudes toward breastfeeding (Goulet, Lampron, Marcil, & Ross, 2004). A research example using the TPB is described in greater detail at the end of this chapter.

▶ *Bandura's Social Cognitive Theory.* Social Cognitive Theory (Bandura, 1997) offers an explanation of human behaviour using the concepts of self-efficacy, outcome expectations, and incentives. Self-efficacy expectations involve people's belief in their own capacity to carry out particular behaviours (e.g., smoking cessation). Self-efficacy expectations determine the behaviours a person chooses to perform, their degree of perseverance, and the quality of the performance. Many nurses have applied this theory to their research, including Babenko-Mould, Andrusyszen, and Goldenberg (2004), who studied the effects of computer-based clinical conferencing on nursing students' self-efficacy, and Hamilton and Haennel (2004), who studied the self-efficacy of patients in cardiac rehabilitation in relation to their functional ability and health-related quality of life.

▶ *Becker's Health Belief Model* (HBM). The HBM is a framework for explaining health-related behaviour, such as health care use and compliance with a medical regimen. According to the model, health-related behaviour is influenced by a person's perception of a threat posed by a health problem as well as by the value associated with actions aimed at reducing the threat (Becker, 1976). Nurse researchers have used the HBM extensively—for example, Wyatt and Ratner (2004) used the HBM as the framework of their study of women's information needs and knowledge deficits regarding acute myocardial infarction.

The use of theories and conceptual models from other disciplines such as psychology (**borrowed theories**) has not been without controversy; some commentators advocate the development of unique nursing theories. However, nursing research is likely to continue on its current path of conducting studies within a multidisciplinary and multitheoretical perspective. Moreover, when a borrowed theory is tested and found to be empirically adequate in health-relevant situations of interest to nurses, it becomes **shared theory**.

 CONSUMER TIP

Among nursing studies that are linked to a conceptual model or theory, about half are based on borrowed or shared theories. Among the models of nursing, those of Allen, Roy, Orem, and Rogers are especially likely to be used as the basis for research. ■

TESTING, USING, AND DEVELOPING THEORY THROUGH RESEARCH

The relationship between theory and research is a reciprocal one. Theories and models are built inductively from observations, and research findings provide an important source of observations. Concepts and relations that are validated in studies can be the foundation for theory development. The theory, in turn, must be tested by subjecting deductions from it (hypotheses) to further empirical inquiry. Thus, research plays a dual and continuing role in theory building and testing. Theory can guide and generate ideas for research; research can assess the worth of the theory and provide a foundation for new ones.

Theories and Qualitative Research

Qualitative research traditions provide researchers with an overarching framework and theoretical grounding, although different traditions involve theory in different ways. Morse (2004) has developed a useful paper that discusses the derivation and kinds of concepts that qualitative inquiry generates.

Sandelowski (1993) makes a distinction between **substantive theory** (inductively derived conceptualizations of the target phenomena under study) and theory that reflects a conceptualization of human inquiry. Some qualitative researchers insist on an atheoretical stance regarding the phenomenon of interest, with the goal of suspending *a priori* conceptualizations (substantive theories) that might bias their collection and analysis of data. For example, phenomenologists are generally committed to theoretical naïveté, and explicitly try to hold preconceived views of the phenomenon in check. Nevertheless, phenomenologists are guided in their inquiries by a framework or philosophy that focuses their analysis on certain aspects of a person's lifeworld. That framework is based on the premise that human experience is an inherent property of the experience itself, not constructed by an outside observer.

Ethnographers bring a strong cultural perspective to their studies, and this perspective shapes their initial fieldwork. Fetterman (1998) has observed that most ethnographers adopt one of two cultural theories: *ideational theories*, which suggest that cultural conditions and adaptation stem from mental activity and ideas, or *materialistic theories*, which view material conditions (e.g., resources, money, production) as the source of cultural developments.

The theoretical underpinning of grounded theory studies is *symbolic interactionism*, which stresses that behaviour is developed through ongoing processes of negotiation within human interactions. Similar to phenomenologists, however, grounded theory researchers attempt to hold prior substantive theory (existing conceptualizations about the

Example of theory in a grounded theory study

Fergus, Gray, Fitch, Labrecque, and Phillips (2002) examined the understudied topic of patient-provided support for spouse caregivers in the context of prostate cancer. Based on three rounds of interviews with 34 men with prostate cancer and their caregiving wives, the researchers identified *active consideration* as a central process. Active consideration encompassed four dimensions: easing spousal burden, keeping us up, maintaining connection, and considering spouse. The researchers used their findings as the basis for developing a theory expounding on the double bind of being both a patient and an agent.

phenomenon) in abeyance until their own substantive theory emerges. Once the theory takes shape, grounded theorists use previous literature for comparison with the emerging categories of the theory. The goal of grounded theory is to use the data, grounded in reality, to provide an explanation of events as they occur in reality—not as they have been conceptualized in preexisting theories. Grounded theory methods are designed to facilitate the generation of theory that is *conceptually dense*, that is, has many conceptual patterns and relationships.

In grounded theory studies, substantive theory is produced "from the inside," but theory can also enter a qualitative study "from the outside." Some qualitative researchers use existing theory or models as an interpretive framework. For example, a number of qualitative nurse researchers acknowledge that the philosophical roots of their studies lie in conceptual models of nursing such as those developed by Neuman, Parse, and Rogers.

Example of existing theory as an interpretive framework in a qualitative study

Bournes (2002) studied the structure of the experience of *having courage* as an aspect of human becoming (Parse's theory) among people with spinal cord injuries.

Another strategy that can lead to theory development involves an integrative review of qualitative studies on a specific topic, that is, a metasynthesis. In such integrative reviews, qualitative studies are combined to identify their essential elements. Findings from different sources are then used for theory building. Paterson (2001, 2003), for example, used the results of 292 qualitative studies that described the experiences of adults with chronic illness to develop the Shifting Perspectives Model of Chronic Illness. This model depicts living with chronic illness as an ongoing, constantly shifting process in which individuals' perspectives change in the degree to which illness is in the foreground or background in their lives.

Theories and Quantitative Research

Quantitative researchers, like qualitative researchers, link research to theory or models in several ways. The classic approach is to test hypotheses deduced from an existing theory. The process of theory testing begins when a researcher extrapolates the implications of the theory or conceptual model for a problem of interest. The researcher asks: If this theory or model is correct, what kinds of behaviour or outcomes would I expect to find in specified situations? Through such questioning, the researcher deduces implications of the theory in the form of research hypotheses, that is, predictions about how variables would be related if the theory were correct. For example, a researcher might conjecture that, if Orem's Self-Care Model is valid, nursing effectiveness could be enhanced in environments more conducive to self-care (e.g., a birthing room versus a delivery room). Comparisons between the observed outcomes of research and the relationship predicted by the hypotheses are the focus of the testing process. Studies that have tested the DMNH provide examples of this type of theory—research link. These studies involved the development of specific hypotheses derived from the model, the collection of data using measures that operationalized the key constructs of the model, and formal testing of the hypotheses using statistical procedures (e.g., Black & Ford-Gilboe, 2004; Bluvol & Ford-Gilboe, 2004; Sgarbossa & Ford-Gilboe, 2004).

Researchers sometimes base a new study on a theory or model in an effort to explain findings from previous research. For example, suppose that several researchers discovered that nursing home patients demonstrate greater levels of depression and noncompliance with nursing staff around bedtime than at other times. These descriptive findings are provocative, but they shed no light on the cause of the problem and consequently suggest no way to improve it. Several explanations, rooted in models such as Lazarus and Folkman's model or one of the models of nursing, may be relevant in explaining the behaviour and moods of the nursing home patients. By directly testing the theory in a new study (i.e., deducing hypotheses derived from the theory), a researcher could gain some understanding of why bedtime is a vulnerable period for the elderly in nursing homes.

CONSUMER TIP

When a quantitative study is based on a theory or conceptual model, the research report usually states this fact fairly early—often in the first paragraph, or even in the title. Many studies also have a subsection of the introduction called "Conceptual Framework" or "Theoretical Framework." The report usually includes a brief overview of the theory so that even readers with no background in the theory can understand, in a general way, the conceptual context of the study.   ▄

Tests of a theory sometimes take the form of testing a theory-based intervention. If a theory is correct, it has implications for strategies to influence people's attitudes or behaviours, including health-related ones. The impetus for an intervention may be a theory developed in a qualitative study. The actual tests of the effectiveness of the intervention—which are also indirect tests of the theory—are done in structured quantitative research.

Example of using theory in an intervention study

Côté and Pepler (2002, 2005) developed an intervention designed to enhance the coping skills of acutely ill HIV-positive men, as described in Chapter 1. The cognitive coping skills intervention was based on concepts from the McGill Model of Nursing and from Lazarus and Folkman's theory of stress. The researchers noted that the McGill Model of Nursing "includes the objectives to engage the individual in a learning process to acquire coping strategies and improve quality of life" (2002, p. 238).

A few nurse researchers have begun to adopt a useful strategy for furthering knowledge through the direct testing of two competing theories in a single study. Almost all phenomena can be explained in alternative ways. Researchers who directly test alternative explanations, using a single sample of participants, are in a position to make powerful comparisons about the utility of the competing theories.

It should also be noted that many researchers who cite a theory or model as their framework are not directly *testing* the theory. Silva (1986), in her analysis of 62 studies that used 5 nursing models, found that only 9 were direct and explicit tests of the models cited by the researchers. She found that the most common use of nursing models in empirical studies was to provide an organizing structure. In such an approach, researchers begin with a broad conceptualization of nursing (or stress, uncertainty, and so on) that is consistent with that of the model. The researchers *assume* that the models they espouse are valid, and then use the model's constructs to provide a broad organizational or interpretive context. Using models in this fashion can serve a valuable organizing purpose, but such studies offer little evidence about the validity of the theory itself. To our knowledge, Silva's study has not been replicated with a more recent sample of studies. However, our sense is that, even today, many quantitative studies that cite models and theories are using them primarily as organizational or interpretive tools.

Example of using a model as an organizing structure

Gagnon and Grenier (2004) undertook a study designed to identify, validate, and rank indicators of quality of care related to the empowerment of patients with a chronic complex illness. Their study was theoretically grounded in (but did not test) the empowerment theory of Zimmerman.

CRITIQUING CONCEPTUAL AND THEORETICAL FRAMEWORKS

You will find references to theories and conceptual frameworks in some of the studies you read. It is often challenging to critique the theoretical context of a published research report (or the absence of one), but we offer a few suggestions.

In a qualitative study in which a grounded theory is presented, you will not be given enough information to refute the proposed descriptive theory; only evidence supporting the theory is presented. However, you can determine whether the theory seems logical, whether the conceptualization is insightful, and whether the evidence is solid and convincing. In a phenomenological study, you should look to see whether the researcher addresses the philosophical underpinnings of the study. The researcher should briefly discuss the philosophy of phenomenology on which the study was based.

Critiquing a theoretical framework in a quantitative report is also difficult because most of you are not likely to be familiar with the cited models. Some suggestions for evaluating the conceptual basis of a quantitative study are offered in the following discussion and in Box 8.1.

The first task is to determine whether the study does, in fact, have a theoretical or conceptual framework. If there is no mention of a theory or conceptual model, you should

BOX 8.1   Guidelines for Critiquing Theoretical and Conceptual Frameworks

1. Does the report describe an explicit theoretical or conceptual framework for the study? If not, does the absence of a framework detract from the usefulness or significance of the research?
2. Does the report adequately describe the major features of the theory or model so that readers can understand the conceptual basis of the study?
3. Is the theory or model appropriate for the research problem? Would a different framework have been more fitting?
4. Is the theory or model used as the basis for generating hypotheses that were tested, or is it used as an organizational or interpretive framework? Was this appropriate?
5. Do the research problem and hypotheses (if any) naturally flow from the framework, or does the purported link between the problem and the framework seem contrived? Are deductions from the theory logical?
6. Are the concepts adequately defined in a way that is consistent with the theory?
7. Is the framework based on a conceptual model of nursing or on a model developed by nurses? If it is borrowed from another discipline, is there adequate justification for its use?
8. Did the framework guide the study methods? For example, was the appropriate research tradition used if the study was qualitative? If quantitative, do the operational definitions correspond to the conceptual definitions? Were hypotheses tested statistically?
9. Does the researcher tie the findings of the study back to the framework at the end of the report? How do the findings support or undermine the framework? Are the findings interpreted within the context of the framework?

consider whether the study's contribution to knowledge is diminished by the absence of such a framework. Nursing has been criticized for producing many pieces of isolated research that are difficult to integrate because of the absence of a theoretical foundation, but sometimes the research is so pragmatic that it does not need a theory to enhance its utility. For example, research designed to determine the optimal frequency of turning patients has a utilitarian goal; it is difficult to see how a theory would enhance the value of the findings.

CONSUMER TIP

In most quantitative nursing studies, the research problem is *not* linked to a specific theory or conceptual model. Thus, students may read many studies before finding a study with an explicit theoretical underpinning. ■

If the study does involve an explicit framework, you would then ask whether the particular framework is appropriate. You may not be able to challenge the researcher's use of a specific theory or to recommend an alternative because that would require theoretical grounding. However, you can evaluate the logic of using a particular theory and assess whether the link between the problem and the theory is genuine. Does the researcher present a convincing rationale for the framework used? Do the hypotheses flow from the theory? Will the findings contribute to the validation of the theory? Does the researcher interpret the findings within the context of the framework? If the answer to such questions is no, you may have grounds for criticizing the study's framework, even though you may not be in a position to articulate how the conceptual basis of the study could be improved.

CONSUMER TIP

Some studies (in nursing as in any other discipline) claim theoretical linkages that are not justified. This is most likely to occur when researchers first formulate the research problem and then find a theoretical context to fit it. An after-the-fact linkage of theory to a research question *may* prove useful, but it is usually problematic because the researcher will not have taken the nuances of the theory into consideration in designing the study. If a research problem is truly linked to a conceptual framework, then the design of the study, the measurement of key constructs, and the analysis and interpretation of data will flow from that conceptualization. ■

RESEARCH EXAMPLES · Critical Thinking Activities

EXAMPLE 1: Quantitative Research

Aspects of a quantitative nursing study, featuring key terms and concepts discussed in this chapter, are presented below, followed by some questions to guide critical thinking.

Study
"Factors influencing the breastfeeding decisions of long-term breastfeeders" (Rempel, 2004)

Statement of Purpose
The purpose of the study was to understand mothers' decisions regarding long-term breastfeeding, using the Theory of Planned Behavior (TPB) to explain intended and actual breastfeeding duration.

Method
A sample of 317 primigravidas from Ontario participated in the study and provided data through self-administered questionnaires or interviews prenatally and then at 1, 2, 4, 6, 9, and 12 months postpartum. This research focused primarily on a group of 80 women who were still engaged in any amount of breastfeeding at 9 months postpartum, with the focus on understanding factors that predicted continued breastfeeding 3 months later.

Theoretical Framework
The TPB posits that breastfeeding duration can be predicted primarily by breastfeeding intentions. These, in turn, are a function of three main factors: (1) the mothers' attitudes toward breastfeeding; (2) subjective norms—the degree to which mothers believe that significant others approve of them breastfeeding; and (3) perceived control—the degree of control mothers feel they have over continuing to breastfeed. Rempel tested the hypothesis that these three TPB factors would explain the prenatal breastfeeding intentions of the full sample of 317 women. She

Critical Thinking Activities (continued)

also predicted that the explanatory power of subjective norms would become increasingly important in predicting long-term duration among the 80 women who were still breastfeeding at 9 months postpartum.

Key Findings
▶ Although breastfeeding attitudes did predict breastfeeding intentions for the entire sample of women, consistent with the TPB, attitudes did not explain decisions to continue breastfeeding beyond 9 months postpartum.
▶ Perceived control over breastfeeding helped to explain long-term breastfeeding.
▶ Subjective norms significantly affected breastfeeding decisions of long-term breastfeeders. The longer mothers continued to breastfeed, the less support they perceived from others for breastfeeding.

Critical Thinking Suggestions*
*See the Student Resource CD-ROM for a discussion of these questions.
1. Answer questions 1 and 3 through 8 from Box 8.1 regarding this study.
2. Also consider the following targeted questions, which may assist you in further assessing aspects of the study:
   a. Is there another model or theory that was described in this chapter that could have been used to study breastfeeding duration? If yes, would this model have been a better choice for a framework than the TPB?
   b. Nurse researchers in several countries, including the United States and China, have tested the TPB for explaining breastfeeding duration and have found support for the theory. What does this suggest about the cross-cultural utility of the TPB?
   c. Were Rempel's findings consistent with the Theory of Planned Behavior?
3. If the results of this study are valid and reliable, what are some of the uses to which the findings might be put in clinical practice?

 EXAMPLE 2: Qualitative Research

Aspects of a qualitative nursing study, featuring terms and concepts discussed in this chapter, are presented below, followed by some questions to guide critical thinking.

Study
"Quality of life for women living with a gynecologic cancer" (Pilkington & Mitchell, 2004)

Statement of Purpose
The purpose of the study was to enhance understanding about quality of life from the perspective of women living with a gynecologic cancer.

Method
The study participants were 14 Canadian women diagnosed with a gynecologic cancer. The in-depth interviews (lasting from 20 minutes to more than 2 hours)

(Research Examples continue on page 168)

Critical Thinking Activities (continued)

were audiotaped and transcribed for analysis. Among the questions asked were the following: What enhances or diminishes your quality of life? and What does quality of life mean to you?

Theoretical Framework

Parse's Human Becoming Theory provided the theoretical perspective for the study and guided the descriptive exploratory methods used. The researchers noted that Parse's theory views humans as unitary beings who participate with others and the universe in shaping their unique lives. The Human Becoming Theory has three principles that center on the themes of meaning, rhythmicity, and transcendence. The *meaning* principle posits that humans co-create personal reality in the process of choosing and living value priorities. The *rhythmicity* principle concerns the paradoxical patterns of relating that humans co-create with the universe. The *transcendence* principle specifies how humans always move with possibilities in a continuous process of becoming—a process of lived health and quality of life. In this view, quality of life signifies *what life is like* from the perspective of the person who is living the life. These concepts were the underpinning of the researchers' exploratory interviews. For example, one of their objectives was to describe the hopes, dreams, plans, and concerns of the women related to quality of life (transcendence), and another was to describe patterns of relating linked with quality of life (rhythmicity).

Key Findings

The findings consisted of four broad themes that describe quality of life from the participants' perspectives. The four themes were synthesized into the following description: "Quality of life is treasuring loving expressions while affirming personal worth, as consoling immersions amid torment emerge with expanding fortitude for enduring" (p. 149).

Critical Thinking Suggestions

1. Answer questions 1 and 3 through 9 from Box 8.1 regarding this study.
2. Also consider the following targeted questions, which may assist you in further assessing aspects of the study:
    a. Was this study a test of Parse's theory?
    b. Did Pilkington and Mitchell operationalize Parse's concepts in this study?
    c. In what way was the use of theory different in this study than in the previous study by Rempel?
3. If the results of this study are trustworthy, what are some of the uses to which the findings might be put in clinical practice?

 EXAMPLE 3: Quantitative Research

1. Read the Introduction and Results section from the study by Feeley and colleagues ("Mother—VLBW Infant Interactions") in Appendix A of this book, and then answer the questions in Box 8.1.
2. Also consider the following targeted questions, which may further sharpen your critical thinking skills and assist you in assessing aspects of the study's merit:

Critical Thinking Activities (continued)

a. The report refers to "a model that included six infant, mother, and contextual factors." To what type of model are the researchers referring?

b. Would a schematic model have helped readers to better understand the framework? Attempt to draw one that captures major variables in this study.

 EXAMPLE 4: Qualitative Research

1. Read the introduction and results section of Beck's study ("Birth Trauma") in Appendix B of this book and then answer the relevant questions in Box 8.1.

2. Also consider the following targeted questions, which may further sharpen your critical thinking skills and assist you in assessing aspects of the study:

a. Do you think that a schematic model would have helped to present the findings in this report?

b. Does Beck present convincing evidence to support her use of the philosophy of phenomenology?

CHAPTER REVIEW
Summary Points

▶ A **theory** is a broad characterization of phenomena. As classically defined, a theory is an abstract generalization that systematically explains the relationships among phenomena. **Descriptive theory** thoroughly describes a phenomenon.

▶ The overall objective of theory is to make research findings meaningful, summarize existing knowledge into coherent systems, stimulate and provide direction to new research, and explain the nature of relationships among variables.

▶ The basic components of a theory are concepts; classically defined theories consist of a set of propositions about interrelationships among concepts, arranged in a logical system that permits new statements to be derived from them.

▶ Concepts are also the basic elements of **conceptual models**, but the concepts are not linked to one another in a logically ordered, deductive system.

▶ **Schematic models** (or **conceptual maps**) are symbolic representations of phenomena that depict a conceptual model through the use of symbols or diagrams.

▶ **A framework** is the conceptual underpinnings of a study. In many studies, the framework is implicit and not fully explicated.

▶ Several conceptual models of nursing have been developed and have been used in nursing research (e.g., Moyra Allen's McGill Model of Nursing). The concepts that are central to models of nursing are person, environment, health, and nursing.

▶ Nonnursing models used by nurse researchers (e.g., Lazarus and Folkman's Theory of Stress and Coping) are referred to as **borrowed theories**; when the appropriateness of borrowed theories for nursing inquiry is confirmed, the theories become **shared theories**.

▶ In some qualitative research traditions (e.g., phenomenology), the researcher strives to suspend previously held substantive conceptualizations of the phenomena under study, but nevertheless there is a rich theoretical underpinning associated with the tradition itself.

❱ Some qualitative researchers specifically seek to develop *grounded theories*, data-driven explanations to account for phenomena under study (**substantive theories**) through inductive processes.

❱ In classical applications of theory, quantitative researchers test hypotheses deduced from a theory. A particularly fruitful approach involves testing two competing theories in one study.

❱ In both qualitative and quantitative studies, researchers sometimes use a theory or model as an organizing framework or as an interpretive tool.

❱ Researchers sometimes develop a problem, design a study, and *then* look for a conceptual framework; such an after-the-fact selection of a framework is less compelling than the systematic testing of a particular theory.

Additional Resources for Review

Chapter 8 of the *Study Guide to Accompany Essentials of Nursing Research,* 6th edition offers various exercises and study suggestions for reinforcing the concepts presented in this chapter. For additional review, see the Student Self-Study Review Questions section of the Student Resource CD-ROM provided with this book.

SUGGESTED READINGS

References for studies cited in the chapter appear at the end of the book.

Theoretical References

Allen, F. M., & Warner, M. (2002). A developmental model of health and nursing. *Journal of Family Issues, 8,* 96–135.

Azjen, I. (1988). *Attitudes, personality, and behavior.* Chicago, IL: Dorsey Press.

Azjen, I., & Fishbein, M. (1980). *Understanding attitudes and predicting social behavior.* Englewood Cliffs, NJ: Prentice Hall.

Bandura, A. (1997). *Self-efficacy: The exercise of control.* New York: W. H. Freeman.

Becker, M. (1976). *Health belief model and personal health behavior.* Thorofare, NJ: Slack.

Fawcett, J. (1995). *Analysis and evaluation of conceptual models of nursing* (3rd ed.). Philadelphia: F. A. Davis.

Fawcett, J. (1999). *The relationship between theory and research* (3rd ed.). Philadelphia: F. A. Davis.

Fetterman, D. M. (1998). *Ethnography: Step by step* (2nd ed.). Newbury Park, CA: Sage Publications.

Ford-Gilboe, M. (2002). Developing knowledge about family health promotion by testing the Developmental Health Model. *Journal of Family Nursing, 8,* 140–156.

Lazarus, R. S., & Folkman, S. (1984). *Stress, appraisal, and coping.* New York: Springer.

Leininger, M. (1991). *Culture care diversity and universality: A theory of nursing.* New York: National League for Nursing.

Mishel, M. H. (1988). Uncertainty in illness. *Image—The Journal of Nursing Scholarship, 20,* 225–232.

Morse, J. M. (2004). Constructing qualitative derived theory: Concept construction and concept typologies. *Qualitative Health Research, 14,* 1387–1395.

Neuman, B., & Fawcett, J. (2001). *The Neuman systems model* (4th ed.). Englewood, NJ: Prentice Hall.

Orem, D. E., Taylor, S. G., Renpenning, K. M., & Eisenhandler, S. A. (2003). *Self-care theory in nursing: Selected papers of Dorothea Orem.* New York: Springer.

Parse, R. R. (1999). *Illuminations: The human becoming theory in practice and research.* Sudbury, MA: Jones & Bartlett.

Reed, P. G., Shearer, N., & Nicoll, L. H. (2003). *Perspectives on nursing theory* (4th ed.). Philadelphia: Lippincott Williams & Wilkins.

Rogers, M. E. (1986). Science of unitary human beings. In V. Malinski (Ed.), *Explorations on Martha Rogers' science of unitary human beings.* Norwalk, CT: Appleton-Century-Crofts.

Roy, C. Sr., & Andrews, H. A. (1999). *The Roy Adaptation Model* (2nd ed.). Englewood, NJ: Prentice Hall.

Sandelowski, M. (1993). Theory unmasked: The uses and guises of theory in qualitative research. *Research in Nursing & Health, 16,* 213–218.

Silva, M. C. (1986). Research testing nursing theory: State of the art. *Advances in Nursing Science, 9,* 1–11.

Designs for Nursing Research

Scrutinizing Quantitative Research Design

STUDENT OBJECTIVES

On completing this chapter, you will be able to:

▶ Discuss decisions that are embodied in a research design for a quantitative study
▶ Describe and evaluate experimental, quasi-experimental, preexperimental, and nonexperimental designs
▶ Distinguish between and evaluate cross-sectional and longitudinal designs
▶ Identify and evaluate alternative methods of controlling extraneous variables
▶ Understand various threats to the validity of quantitative studies
▶ Evaluate a quantitative study in terms of its overall research design and methods of controlling extraneous variables
▶ Define new terms in the chapter

DIMENSIONS OF RESEARCH DESIGN IN QUANTITATIVE STUDIES

The research design of a quantitative study incorporates key methodologic decisions about the fundamental form of a study and spells out the researcher's strategies for obtaining information that is accurate and interpretable. Thus, it is crucial for you to understand the implications of researchers' design decisions. Typically, developing a quantitative research design involves decisions with regard to the following aspects of the study:

▶ *Will there be an intervention?* In some studies, nurse researchers examine the effects of a new intervention (e.g., an innovative program to promote smoking cessation); in others, researchers gather information about existing phenomena. As noted in Chapter 2, this is a distinction between experimental and nonexperimental research. When there is an intervention, the research design specifies its features.

▶ *What types of comparison will be made?* Researchers usually design their studies to involve comparisons that enhance the interpretability of the results. Consider the example presented in Chapter 4 (Box 4.2), in which women who had an abortion were compared with women who delivered a baby in terms of emotional well-being. Without a comparison group, the researchers would not have known whether the abortion group members' emotional status was anomalous. Sometimes researchers use a before–after comparison (e.g., preoperative versus postoperative), and sometimes different groups are compared.

▶ *How will extraneous variables be controlled?* The complexity of relationships among variables makes it difficult to test hypotheses unambiguously unless efforts are made to control confounding factors (i.e., to control *extraneous variables*). This chapter discusses techniques for achieving such control.

▶ *When and how many times will data be collected?* In many studies, data are collected from participants at a single point in time, but some studies include multiple contacts with participants, for example, to determine how things have changed over time. The research design designates the frequency and timing of data collection.

▶ *In what setting will the study take place?* Data for quantitative studies sometimes are collected in real-world settings, such as in clinics or people's homes. Other studies are conducted in highly controlled environments established for research purposes (e.g., laboratories).

There is no single typology of research designs because they vary along a number of dimensions. The dimensions involve whether researchers control the independent variable, what type of comparison is made, how many times data are collected, and whether researchers look forward or backward in time for the occurrence of the independent and dependent variables (Table 9.1). Each dimension is, with a few exceptions, independent of the others. For example, an experimental design can be a between-subjects or within-subjects design; experiments can be cross-sectional or longitudinal, and so on (these terms are discussed later). The sections that follow describe different designs for quantitative nursing research. Qualitative research design is discussed in Chapter 10.

CONSUMER TIP

Research reports typically present information about the research design early in the method section. Complete information about the design is not always provided, however, and some researchers use terminology that is different from that used in this book. (Occasionally, researchers even misidentify the study design.) ■

TABLE 9.1	Dimensions of Quantitative Research Design	

DIMENSION	DESIGN	MAJOR FEATURES
Control over independent variable	Experimental	Manipulation of independent variable; control group; randomization
	Quasi-experimental	Manipulation of independent variable; no randomization and/or no comparison group; but efforts to compensate for this lack
	Preexperimental	Manipulation of independent variable; no randomization or no comparison group; limited control over extraneous variables
	Nonexperimental	No manipulation of independent variable
Type of group comparison	Between-subjects	Subjects in groups being compared are different people
	Within-subjects	Subjects in groups being compared are the same people at different times or in different conditions
Timeframes	Cross-sectional	Data are collected at a single point in time
	Longitudinal	Data are collected at two or more points in time over an extended period
Observance of independent and dependent variables	Retrospective	Study begins with dependent variable and looks backward for cause or influence
	Prospective	Study begins with independent variable and looks forward for the effect
Setting	Naturalistic setting	Data collected in real-world setting
	Laboratory	Data collected in contrived laboratory setting

EXPERIMENTAL, QUASI-EXPERIMENTAL, AND NONEXPERIMENTAL DESIGNS

This section describes designs that differ with regard to the amount of control the researcher has over the independent variable. We begin with research designs that offer the greatest amount of control: experimental designs.

Experiments

Experiments differ from nonexperimental studies in one key respect: researchers using an experimental design are active agents rather than passive observers. Early physical scientists found that, although observation of natural phenomena is valuable, the complexity of naturally occurring events often obscures relationships. This problem was addressed by isolating phenomena in laboratories and controlling the conditions under which they occurred. Procedures developed by physical scientists were adopted by biologists during the 19th century, resulting in many medical achievements. Researchers interested in human behaviour began using experimental methods in the 20th century.

CHARACTERISTICS OF EXPERIMENTS

To qualify as an experiment, a research design must have three properties:

1. *Manipulation*. Experimenters do something to participants in the study.
2. *Control*. Experimenters introduce controls, including the use of a control group.
3. *Randomization*. Experimenters assign participants to control or experimental groups randomly.

Using **manipulation**, experimenters consciously vary the independent variable and then observe its effect on the dependent variable. Researchers manipulate the independent variable by administering an experimental *treatment* (or *intervention*) to some subjects while withholding it from others. To illustrate, suppose we were investigating the effect of physical exertion on mood in healthy adults. One experimental design for this research problem is a **pretest–posttest design** (or *before–after design*). This design involves the observation of the dependent variable (mood) at two points in time: before and after the treatment. Participants in the experimental group are subjected to a demanding exercise routine, whereas those in the control group undertake a sedentary activity. This design permits us to examine what changes in mood were *caused* by the exertion because only some people were subjected to it, providing an important comparison. In this example, we met the first criterion of a true experiment by manipulating physical exertion, the independent variable.

This example also meets the second requirement for experiments, the use of a control group. Campbell and Stanley (1963), in a classic monograph on research design, noted that scientific evidence requires at least one comparison. But not all comparisons provide equally persuasive evidence. Let us look at an example. If we were to supplement the diet of a sample of premature neonates with special nutrients for 2 weeks, the infants' weight at the end of the 2-week period would give us no information about the treatment's effectiveness. At a minimum, we would need to compare posttreatment weight with pretreatment weight to determine whether, at least, their weights had increased. But suppose we find an average weight gain of 400 g. Does this finding indicate that there is a causal relationship between the nutritional supplements (the independent variable) and weight gain (the dependent variable)? No, it does not. Infants normally gain weight as they mature. Without a control group—a group that does not receive the supplements—it is impossible to separate the effects of maturation from those of the treatment. The term **control group** refers to a group of participants whose performance on a dependent variable is used to evaluate the performance of the **experimental group** (the group receiving the intervention) on the same dependent variable.

Experimental designs also involve placing subjects in groups at random. Through **randomization** (or *random assignment*), each participant has an equal chance of being in any group. If people are randomly assigned, there is no systematic bias in the groups with respect to attributes that may affect the dependent variable. *Randomly assigned groups are expected to be comparable, on average, with respect to an infinite number of biologic, psychological, and social traits at the outset of the study.* Group differences observed after random assignment can then be inferred as resulting from the treatment.

Random assignment can be accomplished by flipping a coin or pulling names from a hat. Researchers typically either use computers to perform the randomization or rely on a *table of random numbers*, a table displaying hundreds of digits arranged in a random order.

HOW-TO-TELL TIP

How can you tell if a study is experimental? Researchers usually indicate in their reports (in the method section) when they have used an experimental design, but they may also refer to the design as a *randomized design* or *clinical trial* (see Chapter 11). If such terms are missing, you can conclude that a study is experimental if the report says that a goal of the study was to "test," "evaluate," "assess," or "examine the effectiveness of" an "intervention," "treatment," or "innovation," *and* if individual participants were put into groups (or exposed to different conditions) at *random*. ▪

EXPERIMENTAL DESIGNS
Basic Designs

The most basic experimental design involves randomizing subjects to different groups and subsequently measuring the dependent variable. This design is a **posttest-only** (or *after-only*) **design.** A more widely used design, discussed previously, is the pretest–posttest design, which involves collecting **pretest data** (or **baseline data**) on the dependent variable before the intervention and **posttest data** (*outcome data*) after it.

Example of an after-only experimental design

Tranmer and Parry (2004) used an after-only design to test the effects of an advanced practice nursing intervention (telephone support for 4 weeks following hospital discharge) and patients' health-related quality of life, symptom distress, and satisfaction with care among cardiac surgery patients. The dependent variables were measured 5 weeks after hospital discharge.

Factorial Design

Researchers sometimes manipulate two or more variables simultaneously. Suppose we are interested in comparing two therapeutic strategies for premature infants: tactile stimulation versus auditory stimulation. We are also interested in learning whether the *amount* of stimulation affects infants' progress. Figure 9.1 illustrates the structure of this experiment. This **factorial design** allows us to address three questions: (1) Does auditory stimulation have a different effect on infant development than tactile stimulation? (2) Is the amount of stimulation (independent of modality) related to infant development? and (3) Is auditory stimulation most effective when linked to a certain dose and tactile stimulation most effective when coupled with a different dose?

TYPE OF STIMULATION

	Auditory A1	*Tactile* A2
15 min. B1	A1 B1	A2 B1
30 min. B2	A1 B2	A2 B2
45 min. B3	A1 B3	A2 B3

DAILY EXPOSURE

FIGURE 9.1 Schematic diagram of a factorial experiment.

The third question demonstrates a strength of factorial designs: they permit us to evaluate not only **main effects** (effects resulting from the manipulated variables, as in questions 1 and 2) but also **interaction effects** (effects resulting from combining the treatments). Our results may indicate, for example, that 15 minutes of tactile stimulation and 45 minutes of auditory stimulation are the most beneficial treatments. We could not have learned this by conducting two separate experiments that manipulated one independent variable at a time.

In factorial experiments, subjects are assigned at random to a combination of treatments. In our example, premature infants would be assigned randomly to one of the six cells. The term *cell* is used to refer to a treatment condition and is represented in a schematic diagram as a box. In a factorial design, the independent variables are referred to as *factors*. Type of stimulation is factor A, and amount of exposure is factor B. Each factor must have two or more *levels*. Level 1 of factor A is *auditory,* and level 2 of factor A is *tactile.* The research design in Figure 9.1 would be described as a 2 × 3 factorial design: two levels of factor A times three levels of factor B.

Example of a factorial design

McDonald, Wiczorek, and Walker (2004) used a 2 × 2 factorial design with a sample of college students to study the effect of background noise (noise versus no noise) and interruption (interruption versus no interruption) on learning health information.

Crossover Design

Thus far, we have described experiments in which subjects who are randomly assigned to treatments are different people. For instance, the infants given 15 minutes of auditory stimulation in the factorial experiment are not the same infants as those exposed to other treatment conditions. This broad class of designs is called **between-subjects designs** because the comparisons are *between* different people. When the same subjects are compared, the designs are **within-subjects designs.**

A crossover design (sometimes called a *repeated measures design*) involves exposing participants to more than one treatment. Such studies are true experiments only if participants are randomly assigned to different orderings of treatment. For example, if a crossover design were used to compare the effects of auditory and tactile stimulation on infants, some subjects would be randomly assigned to receive auditory stimulation first followed by tactile stimulation, and others would receive tactile stimulation first. In such a study, the three conditions for an experiment have been met: there is manipulation, randomization, and control—with *subjects serving as their own control group.*

A crossover design has the advantage of ensuring the highest possible equivalence between subjects exposed to different conditions. Such designs are inappropriate for certain research questions, however, because of possible *carryover effects*. When subjects are exposed to two different treatments, they may be influenced in the second condition by their experience in the first. Drug studies rarely use a crossover design because drug B administered after drug A is not necessarily the same treatment as drug B before drug A.

CONSUMER TIP

Research reports do not always identify the specific experimental design that was used; this may have to be inferred from information about the data collection plan (in the case of after-only and before–after designs) or from such statements as, "The subjects were used as their own controls" (in the case of a crossover design). Before–after and crossover designs are the most commonly used experimental designs in nursing research. ■

Example of a crossover design

Brooks, Sidani, Graydon, McBride, Hall, & Weinacht (2003) tested the effects of music on dyspnoea during exercise among patients with chronic obstructive pulmonary disease (COPD). Thirty patients walked for 10 minutes without music and for 10 minutes while listening to music; the ordering of the two sessions was determined at random.

EXPERIMENTAL AND CONTROL CONDITIONS

In designing experiments, researchers make many decisions about what the experimental and control conditions entail, and these decisions can affect the results.

To give an experimental intervention a fair test, researchers need to carefully design one that is appropriate and of sufficient intensity and duration that effects on the dependent variable might reasonably be expected. Researchers delineate the full nature of the intervention in formal *protocols* that stipulate exactly what the treatment is for those in the experimental group; research protocols usually are summarized in research reports.

The control group condition used as a basis of comparison is sometimes called the *counterfactual*. Researchers have choices about what to use as the counterfactual, and the decision has implications for interpreting the findings. Among the possibilities for the counterfactual are the following:

▶ No intervention—the control group gets no treatment at all
▶ An alternative treatment (e.g., auditory versus tactile stimulation)
▶ A **placebo** or pseudo-intervention presumed to have no therapeutic value
▶ Standard methods of care—normal procedures used to treat patients
▶ A lower dose or intensity of treatment, or only parts of the treatment
▶ Delayed treatment (i.e., exposure to the experimental treatment at a later point)

Example of a delayed treatment

Martens (2001) tested a school intervention in a Canadian Ojibwa community to provide adolescents with information about breastfeeding. The experimental group received the intervention, and the control group received it after the posttest data were collected.

Methodologically, the best possible test is between two conditions that are as different as possible, as when the experimental group gets a strong treatment and the control group gets no treatment. Ethically, however, the most appealing counterfactual is probably the delayed treatment approach, which may be difficult to do pragmatically. Testing two alternative interventions is also appealing ethically, but the risk is that the results will be inconclusive because it may be difficult to detect differential effects on the outcomes.

Ideally, participants should be *blinded* to which treatment group they are in, to avoid the risk that the outcomes would be affected by their *expectations* rather than by the actual intervention—although it is not always possible to mask the intervention.

Example of blinding

Davison and Degner (2002) used an experimental design to test the feasibility of using a computer-assisted intervention to enhance the way women with breast cancer communicate with their physicians. The women in the control and experimental groups signed different consent forms to conceal group assignment.

ADVANTAGES AND DISADVANTAGES OF EXPERIMENTS

Experiments are the most powerful designs for testing hypotheses of cause-and-effect relationships. Because of its special controlling properties, an experiment offers greater corroboration than other research designs that the independent variable (e.g., diet, drug dosage) affects the dependent variable (e.g., weight loss, blood pressure).

Lazarsfeld (1955) identified three criteria for causality. First, a cause must precede an effect in time. To test the hypothesis that saccharin causes bladder cancer, we would need to ensure that subjects had not developed cancer before exposure to saccharin. Second, there must be an empirical relationship between the presumed cause and the presumed effect. Thus, we would need to demonstrate an association between the ingestion of saccharin and the presence of cancer (i.e., that people who used saccharin experienced a higher incidence of cancer than those who did not). The final criterion for causality is that the relationship cannot be due to the influence of a third variable. Suppose that people who use saccharin tend also to drink more coffee than nonusers. Thus, a relationship between saccharin use and bladder cancer may reflect an underlying causal relationship between a substance in coffee and bladder cancer. It is particularly because of this third criterion that experimental designs are so strong. Through the controlling properties of manipulation, control groups, and randomization, alternative explanations to a causal interpretation can often be ruled out.

Experiments also have some limitations. First, not all interesting variables are amenable to manipulation. Many human characteristics, such as disease or health habits, cannot be randomly conferred on people. Second, there are many variables that could technically—but not ethically—be manipulated. For example, to date there have been no experiments to study the effect of cigarette smoking on lung cancer. Such an experiment would require us to assign people randomly to a smoking group (people forced to smoke) or a nonsmoking group (people prohibited from smoking).

In many health care settings, experimentation may not be feasible because it is impractical. It may, for instance, be impossible to secure the necessary cooperation from administrators or other key people to conduct an experiment.

Another potential problem is the **Hawthorne effect**, a term derived from a series of experiments conducted at the Hawthorne plant of the Western Electric Corporation in which various environmental conditions (e.g., light, working hours) were varied to determine their effect on worker productivity. Regardless of what change was introduced (i.e., whether the light was made better or worse), productivity increased. Thus, knowledge of being in a study may cause people to change their behaviour, thereby obscuring the effect of the research variables.

In health care settings, researchers sometimes contend with a double Hawthorne effect. For example, if an experiment investigating the effect of a new postoperative procedure were conducted, nurses as well as patients might be aware of participating in a study, and both groups could alter their actions accordingly. It is for this reason that **double-blind experiments**, in which neither the subjects nor those administering the treatment know who is in the experimental or control group, are so powerful. Unfortunately, the double-blind approach is not feasible in most nursing research because nursing interventions are often difficult to disguise.

In summary, experimental designs have some limitations that make them difficult to apply to real-world problems; nevertheless, experiments have a clearcut superiority to other designs for testing causal hypotheses.

Example of a double-blind study

Johnston, Filion, Snider, Majnemer, Limperopoulos, Walker, Veilleux, Pelausa, Cake, Stone, Sherrard, and Boyer (2002) used an experimental design to test the efficacy of sucrose analgesia for procedural pain during the first week of life in preterm neonates on enhancing later clinical outcomes (e.g., neurobehavioral development). Infants were randomized to a sucrose or sterile water condition. Both treating clinicians and the infants were blinded to group assignment.

Quasi-Experiments

Quasi-experiments look a lot like experiments because they also involve the manipulation of an independent variable (i.e., the institution of a treatment). Quasi-experiments, however, lack either the randomization or control-group features of true experiments—features whose absence weakens the ability to make causal inferences.

QUASI-EXPERIMENTAL DESIGNS
There are several quasi-experimental designs, but only the two most commonly used by nurse researchers are discussed here.

Nonequivalent Control Group Design
The most frequently used quasi-experimental design is the **nonequivalent control-group before–after design,** which involves two or more groups of subjects observed before and after the implementation of an intervention. As an example, suppose we wanted to study the effect of primary nursing on nursing staff morale in an urban hospital. The new system of nursing care is being implemented throughout the hospital, so randomization of nurses is not possible. Therefore, we decide to collect comparison data from nurses in a similar hospital that is not instituting primary nursing. We gather data on staff morale in both hospitals before implementing the primary nursing system (the pretest) and again after its implementation (the posttest).

This quasi-experimental research design is identical to the before–after experimental design discussed in the previous section, *except* subjects were not randomly assigned to the groups. The quasi-experimental design is weaker because, without randomization, *it cannot be assumed that the experimental and comparison groups are equivalent at the outset.* The design is, nevertheless, strong because the collection of pretest data allows us to determine whether the groups had similar morale initially. If the comparison and experimental groups were similar at the pretest, we could be relatively confident that posttest differences in self-reported morale resulted from the intervention. (Note that in quasi-experiments, the term **comparison group** is generally used in lieu of *control group* to refer to the group against which experimental group outcomes are evaluated.)

Now suppose we had been unable to collect pretest data before primary nursing care was introduced (i.e., only posttest data were collected). This design has a serious flaw because we have no basis for judging the initial equivalence of the two nursing staffs. If we found higher postintervention morale in the experimental group, could we conclude that primary nursing caused an improvement in staff morale? There could be several alternative explanations for such differences. Campbell and Stanley (1963), in fact, called this *nonequivalent control group after-only design* a **preexperimental design** rather than quasi-experimental because we would be constrained from making the desired inferences. Thus, even though quasi-experiments lack some of the controlling properties of experiments, the hallmark of quasi-experiments is the effort to introduce some controls.

Example of a nonequivalent control group before–after design

Gaudine and Saks (2004) used a strong quasi-experimental design to assess the effects of a training intervention on the self-efficacy and transfer of training performance of nurses receiving training on the McGill Model of Nursing. Although the random assignment of individual nurses was not possible, 12 training *groups* were randomly assigned to one of four treatments (cells) of a 2 × 2 factorial design (relapse prevention training crossed with transfer enhancement training). Data on the outcomes were collected before and after training.

Time-Series Design

In the designs just described, a control group was used, but randomization was not. The next design has neither a control group nor randomization. Suppose that a hospital was adopting a requirement that all its nurses accrue a certain number of continuing education credits before being eligible for a promotion. Administrators want to assess the effect of this mandate on turnover rate and number of promotions awarded. Let us assume there is no other hospital that can serve as a reasonable comparison for this study, so the only kind of comparison that can be made is a before–after contrast. If the requirement were inaugurated in January, one could compare the turnover rate, for example, for the 3-month period before the new rule with the turnover rate for the subsequent 3-month period.

This **one-group before–after design** seems logical, but it has a number of problems. What if one of the 3-month periods is atypical, apart from the mandate? What about the effect of any other rules instituted during the same period? What about the effects of external factors, like changes in the local economy? The design in question, which is preexperimental, offers no way of controlling any of these factors—although

Example of a preexperimental before–after design

Kirk-Gardner and Steven (2003) tested the effectiveness of a community-based educational intervention designed to promote cardiovascular health and reduce risk behaviours (e.g., smoking, high-risk eating habits). Risk behaviours were assessed before the intervention and again 3 months later.

the design can be profitably used in assessing the effectiveness of short-term educational interventions.

The inability to obtain a control group does not eliminate the possibility of conducting research with integrity. The previous design could be modified so that at least some of the alternative explanations for change in nurses' turnover rate could be ruled out. One such design is the **time-series design,** which involves collecting data over an extended time period, and introducing the treatment during that period. Our study could be designed with four observations before the new continuing education rule and four observations after it. For example, the first observation could be the number of resignations between January and March in the year before the new rule, the second observation could be the number of resignations between April and June, and so forth. After the rule is implemented, data on turnover would be collected for four consecutive 3-month periods, giving us observations 5 through 8.

Although the time-series design does not eliminate all the problems of interpreting changes in turnover rate, the extended time perspective strengthens our ability to attribute change to the intervention. This is because the time-series design rules out the possibility that changes in resignations represent a random fluctuation of turnover measured at only two points.

Example of a time-series design

Warren, Kerr, Smith, Godkin, and Schalm (2003) evaluated the effect of 14 adult day programs in Alberta on the perceived burden, quality of life, and health of family caregivers of elderly relatives. The outcomes were measured just before client admission into the program and then again 2 weeks, 2 months, and 6 months after admission.

ADVANTAGES AND DISADVANTAGES OF QUASI-EXPERIMENTS

Quasi-experiments are sometimes practical—it is not always feasible to conduct true experiments. In research in natural settings, it may be difficult to deliver an innovative treatment randomly to some people but not to others. Quasi-experimental designs introduce some research control when full experimental rigor is not possible.

The major disadvantage of quasi-experiments is that cause-and-effect inferences cannot be made as easily as with experiments. With quasi-experiments, there are alternative explanations for observed results. Suppose we wanted to evaluate the effect of a nursing intervention for infants of heroin-addicted mothers on infants' weight gain. If we use no comparison group or if we use a nonequivalent control group and then observe a weight gain, we must ask the following questions: Is it plausible that some other factor influenced the gain? Is it plausible that pretreatment group differences resulted in differential weight gains? Is it plausible that the changes would have occurred without an intervention? If the answer to any of these *rival hypotheses* is yes, inferences about treatment effectiveness are weakened. With quasi-experiments, there is almost always at least one plausible rival explanation.

HOW-TO-TELL TIP

How can you tell if a study is quasi-experimental? Researchers do not always identify their studies as quasi-experimental (or preexperimental). If a study involves an intervention (i.e., if the researcher has control over the independent variable) and if the report does not explicitly mention random assignment, it is probably safe to conclude that the design is quasi-experimental or preexperimental. Oddly, quite a few researchers *misidentify* true experimental designs as quasi-experimental. If individual subjects are randomized to groups or conditions, the design is *not* quasi-experimental. ▪

Nonexperimental Studies

Many research problems cannot be addressed with an experimental or quasi-experimental design. For example, suppose we were interested in studying the effect of widowhood on physical health. Our independent variable here is widowhood versus nonwidowhood. Clearly, we cannot manipulate widowhood; people lose their spouses by a process that is neither random nor subject to control. Thus, we would have to proceed by taking the two groups (widows and nonwidows) as they naturally occur and comparing their physical well-being. There are various reasons for doing a **nonexperimental study** (sometimes referred to as an *observational study* by medical researchers because the study involves making observations rather than intervening). Sometimes the independent variable inherently cannot be manipulated, and in other cases, it is unethical to manipulate the independent variable. Also, an experimental design is not appropriate if the study purpose is description.

TYPES OF NONEXPERIMENTAL STUDIES

One class of nonexperimental research is **correlational** (or *ex post facto*) **research**. The literal translation of the Latin term *ex post facto* is "from after the fact," indicating that the research has been conducted after variation in the independent variable has occurred.

The basic purpose of correlational research is the same as that of experimental research: to study relationships among variables. However, it is difficult to infer causal relationships in correlational studies. In experiments, investigators make a prediction that a deliberate variation in X, the independent variable, will result in changes to Y, the dependent variable. In correlational research, on the other hand, investigators do not control the independent variable—the presumed causative factor—because it has already occurred. It is risky to draw cause-and-effect conclusions in such a situation. A famous research dictum is relevant: *correlation does not prove causation.* That is, the mere existence of a relationship between variables does not warrant the conclusion that one variable caused the other, even if the relationship is strong.

Correlational studies that explore causal relationships can be classified as either retrospective or prospective. In correlational studies with a **retrospective design,** a phenomenon observed in the present is linked to phenomena occurring in the past: the researcher focuses on a presently occurring outcome and then tries to ascertain antecedent factors that have caused it. For example, in retrospective lung cancer research, the investigator begins with a sample of people who have lung cancer and those who do not. The researcher then looks for differences between the groups in antecedent behaviours or conditions, such as smoking habits.

Correlational studies with a **prospective design**, by contrast, start with a presumed cause and then go forward to the presumed effect. For example, in prospective lung cancer studies, researchers start with a sample of smokers and nonsmokers and later compare the two groups in terms of lung cancer incidence. Prospective studies are more costly than retrospective studies but are considerably stronger. For one thing, any ambiguity concerning the temporal sequence of phenomena is resolved in prospective research (i.e., the smoking is known to precede the lung cancer). In addition, samples are more likely to be representative of smokers and nonsmokers, and investigators may be in a position to rule out competing explanations for observed effects.

Example of a prospective nonexperimental study

Jensen, Rebeyka, Urquhart, and Roschkov (2004) studied the effect of presurgical anxiety on pain in adults after surgical repair for congenital heart defects. Preadmission anxiety was found to be predictive of pain on most days following surgery.

Researchers can sometimes strengthen a retrospective study, using a **case-control design**. This design involves comparing "cases" with a certain condition (e.g., breast cancer) with controls (women without breast cancer) who are selected to be similar to the cases with regard to background factors (e.g., family history of breast cancer) that could be linked to the condition. If researchers can demonstrate similarity between cases and controls with regard to extraneous traits, the inferences regarding the contribution of the independent variable (e.g., diet) to the disease are enhanced.

Example of a retrospective case-control study

Leslie, Derksen, Metge, Lix, Salamon, Steinman, and Roose (2005) studied demographic risk factors for fracture in First Nations people. More than 30,000 First Nations adults (cases) were matched by year of birth, gender, and area of residence to non–First Nations controls. Fracture rates were higher in the First Nations group, even after other potential determinants (e.g., income) were taken into consideration.

A second broad class of nonexperimental studies is **descriptive research**. The purpose of descriptive studies is to observe, describe, and document a phenomenon. For example, an investigator may wish to determine the percentage of teenaged mothers who receive adequate prenatal care. Sometimes, a report refers to the study design as **descriptive correlational**, meaning that researchers were interested in describing relationships among variables, without seeking to establish causal connections. For example, researchers might be interested in describing the relationship between fatigue and psychological distress in HIV patients. Because the intent in these situations is not specifically to explain or to understand the underlying causes of the variables of interest, a nonexperimental design is appropriate.

Example of a descriptive correlational study

Hall, Doran, and Pink (2004) conducted a study to describe relationships between nurse staffing models on the one hand and patient outcomes (e.g., falls, medication errors, wound infections) on the other, using data from 19 teaching hospitals in Ontario.

ADVANTAGES AND DISADVANTAGES OF NONEXPERIMENTAL RESEARCH

The major disadvantage of nonexperimental research is its inability to reveal causal relationships with assurance. Although this is not a problem when the aim is purely descriptive, correlational studies are often undertaken with an underlying desire to discover causes. Yet such studies are susceptible to faulty interpretation because researchers work with preexisting groups that have formed through **self-selection**. Kerlinger and Lee (2000) indicate that "self-selection occurs when the members of the groups being studied are in the groups, in part, because they differentially possess traits or characteristics extraneous to the research problem, characteristics that possibly influence or are otherwise related to the variables of the research problem" (p. 560). In other words, preexisting differences may be a plausible explanation for any observed group differences on the dependent variable.

As an example of such interpretive problems, suppose we studied differences in depression of patients with cancer who do or do not have adequate social support (i.e., emotional sustenance through a social network). The independent variable is social support, and the dependent variable is depression. Suppose we found that patients without social support were more depressed than patients with adequate support. We could interpret this to mean that people's emotional state is influenced by the adequacy of their social support,

CONSUMER TIP

Be prepared to think critically when a researcher claims to be studying the "effects" of an independent variable on a dependent variable in a nonexperimental study. For example, if a report is titled "The Effects of Dieting on Depression," the study is likely nonexperimental (i.e., subjects were not randomly assigned to dieting or not dieting). In such a situation, you might ask, Did dieting have an effect on depression—or did depression have an effect on dieting? or, Did a third variable (e.g., obesity) have an effect on both? ■

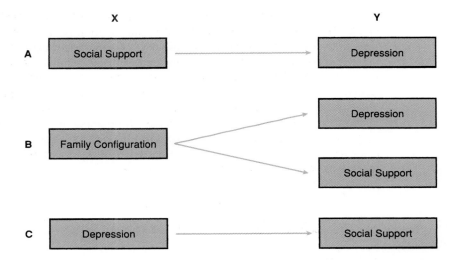

X   Y

FIGURE 9.2 Alternative explanations for relationship between depression and social support in cancer patients.

as diagrammed in Figure 9.2*A*. There are, however, other explanations for the findings. Perhaps a third variable influences *both* social support and depression, such as patients' family configuration. It may be that having family nearby affects how depressed cancer patients feel *and* the quality of their social support, as diagrammed in Figure 9.2*B*. A third possibility may be reversed causality, as shown in Figure 9.2*C*. Depressed cancer patients may find it more difficult to elicit social support than patients who are more cheerful. In this interpretation, it is the person's emotional state that causes the amount of received social support, and not the other way around. The point here is that correlational results should be interpreted cautiously, especially if the research has no theoretical basis.

Despite interpretive problems, correlational studies are important in nursing because many interesting problems cannot be studied experimentally. Correlational research is often an efficient means of collecting a large amount of data about a problem area. For example, it would be possible to collect extensive information about people's health problems and diet. Researchers could then study which health problems correlate with which nutritional patterns. By doing this, many relationships could be discovered in a short time. By contrast, an experimenter looks at only a few variables at a time. For example, one experiment might manipulate foods with different amounts of fat to observe the effects on physical outcomes, whereas another experiment might manipulate protein consumption, and so forth.

Quantitative Designs and Research Evidence

There is often a logical progression to knowledge expansion that begins with rich description, including description from qualitative research. Descriptive studies can be invaluable in documenting the prevalence, nature, and intensity of health-related conditions and behaviours and are critical in the conceptualization of effective interventions.

Correlational studies are often undertaken in the next phase of developing a knowledge base. Exploratory retrospective studies may pave the way for more rigorous case-control studies and prospective studies. As the evidence builds, conceptual models may be developed and tested using nonexperimental theory-testing strategies. These studies can provide hints about how to structure an intervention, who can most profit from it, and when it can best be instituted. Thus, the next important phase is to design interventions to improve health outcomes. Evidence regarding the effectiveness of interventions and health strategies is strongest when it comes from experiments. For this reason, experimental designs have earned the reputation among many of being the "gold standard" in an evidence-based practice environment. However, evidence for nursing practice depends on descriptive, correlational, and experimental research.

RESEARCH DESIGN AND THE TIME DIMENSION

The research design incorporates decisions about when and how often data will be collected in a study. In some studies, data are collected in a single time period, but others involve data collection on multiple occasions. Indeed, several designs involving multiple measurements have already been discussed, such as pretest–posttest designs, time-series designs, and prospective designs.

There are four situations in which it is appropriate to design a study with multiple points of data collection:

1. *Time-related processes.* Certain research problems involve phenomena that evolve over time. Examples include healing and recidivism.
2. *Time-sequenced phenomena.* It is sometimes important to ascertain the sequencing of phenomena. For example, if it is hypothesized that infertility contributes to depression, it would be important to determine that depression did not precede infertility.
3. *Comparative purposes.* Sometimes, multiple data points are used to compare phenomena over time. One example is a time-series study, in which the intent is to determine whether changes over time can be attributed to an intervention.
4. *Enhancement of research control.* Some designs collect data at multiple points to enhance interpretability of the results. For example, in nonequivalent control-group designs, the collection of preintervention data allows researchers to determine initial group differences.

Because of the importance of the time dimension in designing research, studies are sometimes categorized in terms of how they deal with time. The major distinction is between cross-sectional and longitudinal designs—terms that are most often (although not always) used to describe nonexperimental studies.

Cross-Sectional Designs

Cross-sectional designs involve the collection of data at one point in time (or multiple times in a short time period, such as 2 hours and 4 hours postoperatively). All phenomena under study are captured during one data collection period. Cross-sectional designs are appropriate for describing the status of phenomena or relationships among phenomena at a fixed point. For example, a researcher might study whether children's behaviour is correlated contemporaneously with their diet. Retrospective studies are almost always cross-sectional. Data with regard to the independent and dependent variables are collected concurrently (e.g., the lung cancer status of respondents and their smoking habits), but the independent variable usually captures events or behaviours occurring in the past.

When cross-sectional designs are used to study time-related phenomena, the designs are weaker than longitudinal ones. Suppose, for example, we were studying changes in children's health promotion activities between ages 7 and 10 years. One way to investigate this would be to interview the same children at age 7 and then 3 years later at age 10—a longitudinal design. On the other hand, we could use a cross-sectional design by interviewing different children ages 7 and 10 at one point in time and then comparing their responses. If 10-year-olds engaged in more health-promoting activities than the 7-year-olds, it might be inferred that children became more conscious of making good health choices as they age. To make this kind of inference, we would have to assume that the older children would have responded as the younger ones did had they been questioned 3 years earlier, or, conversely, that 7-year-olds would report more health-promoting activities if they were questioned again 3 years later.

The main advantage of cross-sectional designs is that they are economical and easy to manage. There are, however, problems in inferring changes over time using a cross-sectional design. The amount of social and technological change that characterizes our society makes it questionable to assume that differences in the behaviours or characteristics of different age groups are the result of the passage through time rather than cohort or generational differences. In the previous example, 7- and 10-year-old children may have different attitudes toward health and health promotion independent of maturational factors. In cross-sectional studies, there are often competing explanations for observed differences.

Example of a cross-sectional study

Using a cross-sectional design, Profetto-McGrath (2003) studied nursing students' critical thinking skills and critical thinking dispositions, using a sample of students from 4 years of a baccalaureate programme. Critical thinking skills among students in the 4 years of nursing school were compared and were generally found to increase from years 1 to 4.

Longitudinal Designs

Studies that collect data more than once over an extended period use a **longitudinal design**. Longitudinal designs are useful for examining changes over time and for ascertaining the temporal sequencing of phenomena.

Three types of longitudinal studies deserve special mention: trend, panel, and follow-up studies. **Trend studies** are investigations in which samples from a population are studied over time with respect to some phenomenon. Different samples are selected from the same population at repeated intervals. In trend studies, researchers can examine patterns of change and make predictions about future directions.

Example of a trend study

Keller, Hunter, and Shortt (2004) explored the effect of hospital restructuring on home care services by nurses by examining trends in the use of home care nursing services in Kingston, Ontario between 1996 and 2000.

In **panel studies**, the same people provide data at two or more points in time. The term *panel* refers to the sample of people in the study. Panel studies typically yield more information than trend studies because researchers can identify individuals who did and did not change and then explore characteristics that differentiate the two groups. Panel studies are appealing as a method of studying change but are difficult and expensive to manage. The most serious challenge is the loss of participants over time—a problem known as **attrition**. Subject attrition is problematic because those who drop out of the study may differ in important respects from those who continue to participate, resulting in potential biases and concerns about the generalizability of the findings.

Example of a panel study

Miller, Ratner, and Johnson (2003) used data from the Survey on Smoking in Canada, a national panel study with four rounds of data collection. In this study, all those who reported that they were former smokers in round 1 were divided into two groups: those who had a smoking relapse at some point during the next three rounds, and those who were continuously abstinent. The study focused on identifying predictors of smoking relapse prospectively.

Follow-up studies are undertaken to determine the subsequent status of subjects with a specified condition or who received a specified intervention. For example, patients who have received a smoking intervention may be followed up to ascertain its long-term effect. To take a nonexperimental example, samples of premature infants may be followed up to assess their later perceptual and motor development.

Example of a follow-up study

McCleary and Sanford (2002) undertook a longitudinal study of adolescents in Hamilton, Ontario who were diagnosed as having a major depressive disorder. Follow-up assessments of diagnosis and social functioning were completed 1 year after the initial screening.

In longitudinal studies, the number of data collection points and the time intervals between them depend on the nature of the study. When change or development is rapid, numerous data collection points at relatively short intervals may be required to document the pattern. By convention, however, the term *longitudinal* implies multiple data collection points over an extended period of time.

CONSUMER TIP

Not all longitudinal studies are prospective because sometimes the independent variable occurred well before the initial wave of data collection. And not all prospective studies are longitudinal in the classic sense. For example, an experimental study that collects data 2, 4, and 6 hours after a treatment would be prospective but not longitudinal (i.e., the independent variable occurred first, but outcome data are not collected over a long time period). ■

TECHNIQUES OF RESEARCH CONTROL

A major purpose of research design in quantitative studies is to maximize researchers' control over extraneous variables. There are two basic types of extraneous variables that need to be controlled—those that are intrinsic to study participants and those that are external, stemming from the research situation.

Controlling External Factors

Various external factors, such as the research environment, can affect study outcomes. In carefully controlled quantitative research, steps are taken to minimize situational contaminants (i.e., to achieve **constancy of conditions** for the collection of data) so that researchers can be confident that the conditions are not affecting the data.

The environment has been found to influence people's emotions and behaviour, and so, in designing quantitative studies, researchers strive to control the environmental context. Control over the environment is most easily achieved in laboratory experiments, in which all subjects are brought into an environment structured by the experimenter. Researchers have less control over the environment in studies that occur in natural settings, but some opportunities exist. For example, in interview studies, researchers can restrict data collection to one type of setting (e.g., respondents' homes).

A second external factor that may need to be controlled is time. Depending on the research topic, the dependent variable may be influenced by the time of day or the time of year in which data are collected. In these cases, researchers should ensure that constancy of time is maintained. If an investigator were studying fatigue, for example, it would matter whether the data were gathered in the morning, afternoon, or evening, and so data from all subjects should be collected at the same time of day.

Another issue concerns constancy of communications to subjects. Formal scripts are often prepared to inform subjects about the study purpose, the use that will be made of the data, and so forth. In research involving an intervention, formal research protocols are developed. For example, in an experiment to test the effectiveness of a new medication, care would be needed to ensure that subjects in the experimental group received the same chemical substance and the same dosage, that the substance was administered in the same way, and so forth.

Example of controlling external factors

Olson, Rennie, Hanson, Ryan, Gilpin, Falsetti, Heffner, and Gaudet (2004) took great care to ensure constancy of conditions in their experimental study, which tested whether central venous catheter-related sepsis could be reduced by removing (for half the subjects) a hypothesized reservoir for pathogens, gauze dressing at the exit site. All study participants received the same instructions regarding care on the day of insertion and the same information about whom to contact for assistance between appointments. All subjects were assessed for sepsis according to a well-defined protocol, and all microbiologic analyses were conducted at the same lab.

Controlling Intrinsic Factors

Control of study participants' extraneous characteristics is especially important. For example, suppose we were investigating the effects of an innovative physical training program on the cardiovascular functioning of nursing home residents. In this study, variables such as the subjects' age, gender, and smoking history would be extraneous variables; each is likely to be related to the outcome variable (cardiovascular functioning), independent of the physical training program. In other words, the effects that these variables have on the dependent variable are extraneous to the study. In this section, we review methods of controlling extraneous subject characteristics.

METHODS OF CONTROLLING SUBJECT CHARACTERISTICS
Randomization
We have already discussed the most effective method of controlling subject characteristics: randomization. The primary function of randomization is to secure comparable groups, that is, to equalize groups with respect to extraneous variables. A distinct advantage of randomization is that it controls all possible sources of extraneous variation, without any conscious decision by researchers about which variables need to be controlled. In our

Example of randomization with crossover

Watson, Moulin, Watt-Watson, Gordon, and Eisenhoffer (2003) compared the effects of controlled-release oxycodone versus a placebo on pain, disability, and quality of life among patients with diabetic neuropathy, using a random-ized crossover design.

example of the physical training intervention, random assignment of subjects to an experimental (intervention) group and control (no intervention) group would be an excellent control mechanism. Presumably, the two groups would be comparable in terms of age, gender, smoking history, and thousands of other preintervention characteristics. Randomization within a crossover design is especially powerful: participants serve as their own controls, thereby totally controlling all extraneous variables.

Homogeneity

When randomization is not feasible, other methods of controlling extraneous subject characteristics can be used. One alternative is **homogeneity,** in which only subjects who are homogeneous with respect to extraneous variables are included in the study. Extraneous variables, in this case, are not allowed to vary. In the physical training example, if gender were considered a confounding variable, we could recruit only men (or women) as participants. If we were concerned about the confounding effect of participants' age on physical fitness, participation could be limited to those within a specified age range. This strategy of using a homogeneous sample is easy, but its limitation is that the findings can be generalized only to the type of subjects who participated. If the physical training program were found to have beneficial effects on the cardiovascular functioning of men aged 65 to 75 years, its usefulness for improving the cardiovascular status of women in their 80s would need to be tested in a separate study.

Example of control through homogeneity

Boechler, Harrison, and Magill-Evans (2003) examined whether the amount of caregiving a father provided to his child was related to the quality of his teaching in structured interactions with his child. Because father–child interactions could be affected by other factors, the principle of homogeneity was used to restrict the sample. For example, the fathers could not be younger than 21, they could not be the primary caregiver to the child, and they had to be in a stable relationship with the child's mother.

Matching

A third method of dealing with extraneous variables is matching. **Matching** involves using information about subject characteristics to form comparison groups. For example, suppose we began with a sample of nursing home residents already set to participate in the physical training program. A comparison group of nonparticipating residents could be created by matching subjects, one by one, on the basis of important extraneous variables (e.g., age and gender). This procedure results in groups known to be comparable in terms of the extraneous variables of concern. Matching is the technique used to form comparable groups in case-control designs.

Matching has some drawbacks as a control method. To match effectively, researchers must know in advance what the relevant extraneous variables are. Also, after two or three variables, it becomes difficult to match. Suppose we wanted to control the age, gender, race, and length of nursing home stays of the participants. In this situation, if participant 1 in the physical training program were an African American woman, aged 80 years, whose length of stay was 5 years, we would have to seek another woman with these same or similar characteristics as a comparison group counterpart. With more than three variables, matching becomes cumbersome. Thus, matching as a control method is usually used only when more powerful procedures are not feasible.

Example of matching

Benzies, Harrison, and Magill-Evans (2004b) followed parents of preterm and full-term infants for 7 years to study the relationship between children's early characteristics and family environment and subsequent behavioural problems at age 7. At recruitment, the sample consisted of 56 families with a preterm infant and 58 families with a full-term infant. Participants in the two groups were matched in terms of hospital of birth and infant gender.

Statistical Control

Another method of controlling extraneous variables is through statistical analysis. You may be unfamiliar at this point with basic statistical procedures, let alone sophisticated ones such as those referred to here. Therefore, a detailed description of powerful statistical control mechanisms, such as **analysis of covariance,** will not be attempted. You should recognize, however, that nurse researchers are increasingly using powerful statistical techniques to control extraneous variables. A brief description of methods of statistical control is presented in Chapter 15.

Example of statistical control

Vissandjee, Desmeules, Cao, Abdool, and Kazanjian (2004) studied the relationship between a person's ethnicity and number of years since he or she immigrated to Canada on the one hand and health and chronic illness on the other. To rule out the effects of extraneous background characteristics, age, marital status, level of education, and income were statistically controlled.

EVALUATION OF CONTROL METHODS

Overall, random assignment is the most effective approach to controlling extraneous variables because randomization tends to cancel out individual variation on all possible extraneous variables. Crossover designs are especially powerful, but they cannot be applied to all nursing problems because of the possibility of carryover effects. The three remaining alternatives described here have two disadvantages in common. First, researchers must know which variables to control in advance. To select homogeneous samples, match, or perform an analysis of covariance, researchers must decide which variables to control. Second, these three methods control only for identified characteristics, possibly leaving others uncontrolled.

Although randomization is the best mechanism for controlling extraneous subject characteristics, randomization is not always possible. If the independent variable cannot be manipulated, other techniques should be used. It is far better to use matching or analysis of covariance than simply to ignore the problem of extraneous variables.

CHARACTERISTICS OF GOOD DESIGN

In evaluating the merits of a quantitative study, one overarching question is whether the research design did the best possible job of providing valid and reliable evidence. Cook and Campbell (1979), in their classic book on research design, describe four important considerations for evaluating quantitative research design. The questions that researchers must address (and consumers must evaluate) regarding research design are as follows:

1. What is the strength of the evidence that a relationship exists between two variables?
2. If a relationship exists, what is the strength of the evidence that the independent variable of interest (e.g., an intervention), rather than extraneous factors, caused the outcome?
3. What is the strength of evidence that observed relationships are generalizable across people, settings, and time?
4. What are the theoretical constructs underlying the related variables, and are those constructs adequately captured?

These questions, respectively, correspond to four aspects of a study's validity: (1) statistical conclusion validity; (2) internal validity; (3) external validity; and (4) construct validity. In this section we discuss aspects of the first three types of validity; construct validity, which concerns the measurement of variables, is discussed in Chapter 14.

Statistical Conclusion Validity

As noted earlier, the first criterion for establishing causality is demonstrating that there is, in fact, an empirical relationship between the independent and dependent variables. Statistical methods are used to determine whether such a relationship exists. Design decisions can influence whether statistical tests will actually detect true relationships, and so researchers need to make decisions that protect against reaching false statistical conclusions. Although we cannot at this point in the text discuss all aspects of **statistical conclusion validity**, we can describe a few design issues that can be threats to making valid statistical inferences.

One issue concerns **statistical power**, which is the ability of the design to detect true relationships among variables. Adequate statistical power can be achieved in various ways, the most straightforward of which is to use a sufficiently large sample. When small samples are used, statistical power tends to be low, and the analyses may fail to show that the independent and dependent variables are related—*even when they are*. Power and sample size are discussed in Chapter 12.

Another aspect of a powerful design concerns the construction or definition of the independent variable and the counterfactual. Both statistically and substantively, results are clearer when differences between the groups being compared are large. To enhance statistical conclusion validity, researchers should aim to maximize group differences on the independent variables so as to maximize differences on the dependent variable. If the groups or treatments are not very different, the statistical analysis might not be sufficiently sensitive to detect differences that actually exist.

A related issue is that the strength of an intervention (and hence statistical power) can be undermined if the intervention is not as powerful in reality as it is "on paper." An intervention can be weakened by a number of factors, such as lack of standardization, inadequate training, or premature withdrawal of subjects from the intervention. It is the researchers' responsibility to monitor the integrity of treatments in studies and to report deficiencies in achieving it.

Example of monitoring treatment integrity

Dennis (2002) conducted a randomized experimental study that evaluated the effects of a telephone-based peer support (mother-to-mother) intervention designed to support breastfeeding. A sample of 256 primiparous breastfeeding women were randomly assigned to either conventional care or conventional care plus peer support. Peer volunteers monitored and assessed the nature and intensity of the intervention by completing an activity log for each supported mother. The data from these logs revealed that contact was made between most sets of peers and experimental group participants—although different mothers did receive varying levels of treatment intensity.

Thus, if you are evaluating a study that indicates that groups being compared were not statistically different with respect to outcomes, one possibility is that the study had low statistical conclusion validity. The report might give clues about this possibility (e.g., too small a sample or substantial subject attrition) that should be taken into consideration in drawing conclusions about the study's evidence.

Internal Validity

Internal validity is the extent to which it is possible to make an inference that the independent variable is truly causing or influencing the dependent variable. Experiments possess a high degree of internal validity because randomization to different groups enables researchers to rule out competing explanations. With quasi-experiments and correlational studies, investigators must contend with rival hypotheses. There are various types of competing explanations, or *threats to internal validity*.

THREATS TO INTERNAL VALIDITY
History
The **history threat** is the occurrence of events concurrent with the independent variable that can affect the dependent variable. For example, suppose we were studying the effectiveness of an outreach program to encourage flu shots among community-dwelling elders using a time-series design. Now let us further suppose that, at about the same time the

outreach program was initiated, there was a national public media campaign focusing on the flu. Our dependent variable in this case, number of flu shots administered, is subject to the influence of at least two forces, and it would be difficult for us to disentangle the two effects. In experiments, history is not typically an issue because external events are as likely to affect one group as another. The designs most likely to be affected by the history threat are one-group before–after designs and time-series designs.

Selection

The **selection threat** encompasses biases resulting from preexisting differences between groups. When people are not assigned randomly to groups, the groups being compared may not be equivalent. In such a situation, researchers contend with the possibility that any group difference in the dependent variable is due to extraneous factors rather than to the independent variable. Selection biases are the most problematic threats to the internal validity of studies not using an experimental design (e.g., nonequivalent control group designs, case-control designs) but can be partially addressed using the control mechanisms described in the previous section.

Maturation

The **maturation threat** arises from processes occurring as a result of time (e.g., growth, fatigue) rather than the independent variable. For example, if we wanted to test the effect of a special sensorimotor development program for developmentally delayed children, we would have to contend with the fact that progress would occur even without the intervention. Remember that the term *maturation* here does not refer to developmental changes exclusively but rather to any kind of change that occurs as a function of time. Phenomena such as wound healing and postoperative recovery can occur with little nursing intervention, and thus maturation may be a rival explanation for positive posttreatment outcomes. One-group before–after designs are especially vulnerable to this threat.

Mortality

The **mortality threat** stems from differential attrition from groups. The loss of subjects during the study may differ among groups because of initial differences in interest or motivation. For example, suppose we used a nonequivalent control-group design to assess nurses' morale in two hospitals, only one of which initiated primary nursing. Nursing morale is measured before and after the intervention. The comparison group, which may have no particular commitment to the study, may be reluctant to complete a posttest questionnaire. Those who do fill it out may be unrepresentative of the group as a whole; they may be highly critical of their work environment, for example. Thus, on the average, it may appear that the morale of nurses in the comparison hospital declined, but this might only be an artefact of the *mortality* of a select segment of this group.

INTERNAL VALIDITY AND RESEARCH DESIGN

Quasi-experimental, preexperimental, and correlational studies are especially susceptible to threats to internal validity. These threats represent alternative explanations (rival hypotheses) that compete with the independent variable as a cause of the dependent variable. *The aim of a good quantitative research design is to rule out these competing explanations.* The control mechanisms previously reviewed are strategies for improving the internal validity of studies—and thus for strengthening the quality of evidence they yield.

An experimental design normally eliminates competing explanations, but this is not always the case. For example, if constancy of conditions is not maintained for experimental and control groups, history might be a rival explanation for obtained results. Experimental mortality is, in particular, a salient threat: because the experimenter does different things with the experimental and control groups, members of the two groups may drop out of the study differentially. This is particularly likely to happen if the experimental treatment is stressful or time-consuming or if the control condition is boring or aggravating. When this happens, participants remaining in the study may differ from those who left, thereby nullifying the initial equivalence of the groups.

You should pay careful attention to the possibility of competing explanations for reported results, especially in studies that do not use an experimental design. When the investigator does not have control over critical extraneous variables, caution in interpreting results and drawing conclusions about the evidence is appropriate.

External Validity

External validity is the generalizability of research findings to other settings or samples, an issue of great importance for those interested in an evidence-based practice. Quantitative studies are rarely conducted with the intention of discovering relationships among variables for a single group of people. If a nursing intervention is found to be effective—and if the study results are internally valid—then others will want to adopt it. Therefore, an important question is whether an intervention will work in another setting or with different patients.

One aspect of a study's external validity concerns the adequacy of the sampling design. If the characteristics of the sample are representative of those of the population, the generalizability of the results to the population is enhanced. Sampling designs are described in Chapter 12.

Various aspects of a research situation also affect the study's external validity. For example, when a treatment is new (e.g., a new protocol for pain management), participants and researchers alike might alter their behaviour. People may be either enthusiastic or sceptical about new methods of doing things. Thus, the results may reflect reactions to the novelty rather than to the intrinsic qualities of the treatment. Results may also reflect study participants' awareness of being in a study (the Hawthorne effect) or their expectations about benefits of an intervention, independent of the actual intervention (a **placebo effect**). It is because of these risks that blinding should be used whenever possible.

Example of a possible Hawthorne effect

Winterburn and Fraser (2000) used an experimental design to test the effect of long versus short postnatal stay on the decisions of first-time mothers to breastfeed. Length of hospital stay was unrelated to breastfeeding behaviours at 1 month, but in both groups, the breastfeeding rate was higher than city-wide rates. The researchers speculated that this could reflect a Hawthorne effect.

Sometimes, the demands for internal and external validity conflict. If a researcher exercises tight control in a study to maximize internal validity, the setting may become too artificial to generalize to a more naturalistic environment. Therefore, a compromise must sometimes be reached. The importance of replicating studies in different settings with new study participants cannot be overemphasized.

CRITIQUING QUANTITATIVE RESEARCH DESIGNS

The overriding consideration in evaluating a research design is whether the design enables the researcher to answer the research question conclusively. This must be determined in terms of both substantive and methodologic considerations.

Substantively, the issue is whether the researcher selected a design that matches the aims of the research. If the research purpose is descriptive or exploratory, an experimental design is not appropriate. If the researcher is searching to understand the full nature of a phenomenon about which little is known, a structured design that allows little flexibility might block insights (flexible designs are discussed in Chapter 10). We have discussed research control as a mechanism for reducing bias, but sometimes too much

BOX 9.1 Guidelines for Critiquing Research Designs in Quantitative Studies

1. Does the study involve an intervention? If yes, was an experimental, quasi-experimental, or preexperimental design used—and was this the most appropriate design?
2. If the study was experimental or quasi-experimental, was "blinding" used? Who was blinded?
3. If the study was nonexperimental, why didn't the researcher manipulate the independent variable? Was the decision regarding manipulation appropriate?
4. Was the study longitudinal or cross-sectional? Was the number of data collection points appropriate, given the research question?
5. What type of comparisons were called for in the research design (e.g., was the study design within-subjects or between-subjects)? Are the comparisons the most appropriate for illuminating the relationship between the independent and dependent variables?
6. What did the researcher do to control extraneous external factors and intrinsic subject characteristics? Were the procedures appropriate and adequate?
7. What steps did the researcher take in designing the study to enhance statistical conclusion validity? Were these steps adequate?
8. What steps did the researcher take to enhance the internal validity of the study? To what extent were those steps successful? What types of alternative explanations must be considered—what are the threats to internal validity? Does the design enable the researcher to draw causal inferences about the relationship between the independent and dependent variables?
9. To what extent is the study externally valid?
10. What are the major limitations of the design used? Are these limitations acknowledged by the researcher and taken into account in interpreting results?

control can introduce bias, for example, when the researcher tightly controls the ways in which the phenomena under study can be manifested and thereby obscures their true nature.

Methodologically, the main design issue in quantitative studies is whether the research design provides the most accurate, unbiased, interpretable, and replicable evidence possible. Indeed, there usually is no other aspect of a quantitative study that affects the quality of evidence as much as the research design. Box 9.1 provides questions to assist you in evaluating the methodologic aspects of quantitative research designs; these questions are key to a meaningful critique of a quantitative study.

RESEARCH EXAMPLES   Critical Thinking Activities

 EXAMPLE 1: Experimental Design

Aspects of an experimental nursing study, featuring terms and concepts discussed in this chapter, are presented below, followed by some questions to guide critical thinking.

Study
"Efficacy of a smoking-cessation intervention for elective-surgical patients" (Ratner, Johnson, Richardson, Bottorff, Moffat, Mackay, Fofonoff, Kingsbury, Miller, & Budz, 2004)

Statement of Purpose
The purpose of the study was to determine the effectiveness of a smoking-cessation intervention for presurgical patients.

Treatment Groups
The intervention consisted of three components: (1) a presurgical counselling session that recommended smoking cessation before surgery and provided nicotine replacement gum; (2) an in-hospital postoperative counselling session within 24 hours of surgery that reinforced smoking cessation messages; and (3) telephone counselling support (nine calls over a 4-month period). Subjects in a control group received standard care.

Design and Method
The intervention was implemented in a preadmission clinic in a large urban hospital in western Canada. A sample of 237 smokers scheduled for elective surgery were randomly assigned to the experimental or control group. Data were collected from all subjects before random assignment and then at three follow-up points: within 24 hours of surgery, and 6 and 12 months after surgery. Smoking status was measured by self-report and through biochemical measures (CO readings of expired air while in the hospital and urinary cotinine assays returned through the mail at the two follow-up points). In addition, the researchers gathered

(Research Examples continue on page 202)

Critical Thinking Activities (continued)

self-reported information about smoking cessation self-efficacy, anxiety, and depression, as well as background information such as smoking history. Nurses administered the baseline data collection instruments in a preadmission clinic before random assignment, which involved giving each subject a sealed envelope that contained a computer-generated, randomly determined group allocation. Assistants who gathered follow-up information by telephone were blinded to group assignment and hypotheses.

Key Findings

▶ The treatment and control groups did not differ significantly on any demographic or smoking-related characteristics at baseline.

▶ Subjects in the treatment group were more likely than those in the control group to fast before surgery and to be abstinent 6 months after surgery.

▶ The groups did not differ with regard to smoking abstinence 12 months after surgery.

Critical Thinking Suggestions*

*See the Student Resource CD-ROM for a discussion of these questions.

1. Answer questions 1, 2, and 4 through 9 from Box 9.1 regarding this study.

2. Also consider the following targeted questions, which may assist you in further assessing aspects of the study:

    a. What specific experimental design was used in this study? Was this appropriate?

    b. Could a crossover design have been used?

    c. Was randomization successful?

3. If the results of this study are valid and reliable, what are some of the uses to which the findings might be put in clinical practice?

 EXAMPLE 2: Quasi-Experimental Design

Aspects of a quasi-experimental nursing study, featuring terms and concepts discussed in this chapter, are presented below, followed by some questions to guide critical thinking.

Study

"Effects of a relationship-enhancing program of care on outcomes" (McGilton, O'Brien-Pallas, Darlington, Evans, Wynn, & Pringle, 2003)

Statement of Purpose

The purpose of the study was to test the effects of a relationship-enhancing program of care (REPC) for care providers in nursing homes on both resident and care provider outcomes. It was hypothesized that residents who received care from those trained in the REPC would perceive more empathic and reliable care, and that the care providers would exhibit more empathic and reliable behaviour, compared with those not getting the intervention.

Critical Thinking Activities (continued)

Treatment Conditions

The REPC intervention was an investigator-designed program based in part on a theory of relationships (Winnicott). The intervention began by providing participating supervisors a three-session educational program about the dynamics of providing support to care providers. Then a five-session program was offered directly to care providers (e.g., nurses, licensed practical nurses), focusing on skills needed to provide effective relational care. The program was not offered to care providers in a comparison group.

Design and Method

The study was conducted on two long-term care units in the nursing home section of a Canadian geriatric center. One unit received the intervention, and the other did not. A total of 90 residents and 32 care providers participated in the study. During the intervention, care providers in the intervention unit were asked not to discuss the program with, or distribute printed information to, colleagues from other units, to avoid contamination of treatment groups. Data were collected twice: once before program implementation and then 3 months after completion of the 7-month intervention. Some data were gathered by asking residents questions (e.g., about their perception of care providers' empathic care), and other data were gathered by observing care providers' behaviours with residents. The assistant who collected the observational data was blind to the study design.

Key Findings

▶ At baseline, the demographic characteristics of the care providers in the two units were comparable, but residents on the intervention unit were more physically and cognitively impaired than those on the comparison unit.

▶ Residents who were cared for by providers who received the special intervention showed increased perceptions of relational care from baseline to follow-up, whereas those receiving care from comparison group providers did not. Group differences of the measure of perceived close relationships with providers were not significant.

▶ Care providers who received the special training significantly improved their relational behaviours, whereas the empathic and reliable behaviours of providers in the comparison group declined somewhat from pretest to posttest.

Critical Thinking Suggestions

1. Answer questions 1, 2, and 4 through 9 from Box 9.1 regarding this study.
2. Also consider the following targeted questions, which may assist you in further assessing aspects of the study:
   a. What specific quasi-experimental design was used in this study? Was this appropriate?
   b. Comment on the researchers' decision to use two units from the same institution in their study.
3. If the results of this study are valid and reliable, what are some of the uses to which the findings might be put in clinical practice?

(Research Examples continue on page 204)

Critical Thinking Activities (continued)

 EXAMPLE 3: Nonexperimental Design

1. Read the method section from the study by Feeley and colleagues ("Mother–VLBW Infant Interaction") in Appendix A of this book, and then answer the relevant questions in Box 9.1.
2. Also consider the following targeted questions, which may further sharpen your critical thinking skills and assist you in assessing aspects of the study's merit:
   a. Was this study retrospective or prospective? Discuss the effect of the design on the researchers' ability to draw inferences about the direction of influence between the independent and dependent variables.
   b. In addition to the six independent variables used in this study, can you think of other possible predictors of the quality of mother–infant interactions? Can any of your suggested predictors be experimentally manipulated?

CHAPTER REVIEW

Summary Points

▶ The **research design** is the researcher's overall plan for answering research questions. In quantitative studies, the design indicates whether there is an intervention, the nature of any comparisons, the methods used to control extraneous variables, and the timing and location of data collection.

▶ **Experiments** involve **manipulation** (the researcher manipulates the independent variable by introducing a *treatment* or *intervention*), control (including the use of a **control group** that is compared to the **experimental group**), and **randomization** (wherein subjects are allocated to groups at random to make them comparable at the outset).

▶ **Posttest-only** (or *after-only*) designs involve collecting data only once—after random assignment and the introduction of the treatment; in **pretest–posttest** (or *before–after*) **designs,** data are collected both before and after the experimental manipulation.

▶ **Factorial designs**, in which two or more variables are manipulated simultaneously, allow researchers to test both **main effects** (effects from the experimentally manipulated variables) and **interaction effects** (effects resulting from combining the treatments).

▶ **Between-subjects designs**, in which different sets of people are compared, contrast with **within-subjects designs**, which involve comparisons of the same subjects.

▶ In a **crossover** (or *repeated-measures*) **design**, subjects are exposed to more than one experimental condition in random order and serve as their own controls.

▶ **Quasi-experiments** involve manipulation but lack a comparison group or randomization. Quasi-experimental designs introduce controls to compensate for these missing components. By contrast, **preexperimental designs** have no such safeguards.

▶ The **nonequivalent control-group before–after design** involves the use of a **comparison group** that was not created through random assignment and the collection of pretreatment data that permits an assessment of initial group equivalence.

▶ In a **time-series design,** there is no comparison group; information on the dependent variable is collected over a period of time before and after the treatment.

▶ **Nonexperimental research** includes **descriptive research**—studies that summarize the status of phenomena—and **correlational** (or *ex post facto*) **studies** that examine relationships among variables but involve no manipulation of the independent variable.

▶ Researchers use **retrospective** and **prospective** correlational designs to infer causality, but the findings from such studies are generally open to several interpretations.

▶ **Cross-sectional designs** involve the collection of data at one time period, whereas **longitudinal designs** involve data collection two or more times over an extended period. Three types of longitudinal studies, which are used to study changes or development over time, are **trend studies, panel studies,** and **follow-up studies.**

▶ Quantitative researchers strive to control external factors that could affect the study outcomes (e.g., the environment) and extraneous subject characteristics.

▶ Techniques for controlling subject characteristics include **homogeneity** (restricting the sample to eliminate variability on the extraneous variable); **matching** (matching subjects to make groups comparable); statistical procedures, such as **analysis of covariance**; and **randomization**—the most effective control procedure because it controls all possible extraneous variables without researchers having to identify or measure them.

▶ A well-designed study attends to statistical conclusion validity, internal validity, external validity, and construct validity.

▶ **Statistical conclusion validity** concerns the strength of evidence that a relationship exists between two variables. Threats to statistical conclusion validity include low **statistical power** (the ability to detect true relationships) and a weak treatment.

▶ **Internal validity** concerns the degree to which outcomes can be attributed to the independent variable. *Threats to internal validity* include **history, selection, maturation,** and **mortality** (caused by subject **attrition**).

▶ **External validity** refers to the generalizability of study findings to other samples and situations.

Additional Resources for Review

Chapter 9 of the *Study Guide to Accompany Essentials of Nursing Research,* 6th edition offers various exercises and study suggestions for reinforcing the concepts presented in this chapter. For additional review, see the Student Self-Study Review Questions section of the Student Resource CD-ROM provided with this book.

SUGGESTED READINGS

References for studies cited in the chapter appear at the end of the book.

Methodologic References

Campbell, D. T., & Stanley, J. C. (1963). *Experimental and quasi-experimental designs for research.* Chicago: Rand McNally.

Cook, T. D., & Campbell, D. T. (1979). *Quasi-experimental design and analysis issues for field settings.* Chicago: Rand McNally.

Ferguson, L. (2004). External validity, generalizability, and knowledge utilization. *Journal of Nursing Scholarship, 36,* 16–22.

Kerlinger, F. N., & Lee, H. B. (2000). *Foundations of behavioral research* (4th ed.). Orlando, FL: Harcourt College.

Lazarsfeld, P. (1955). Foreword. In H. Hyman (Ed.), *Survey design and analysis.* New York: The Free Press.

Understanding Qualitative Research Design

STUDENT OBJECTIVES

On completing this chapter, you will be able to:

▶ Discuss the rationale for emergent designs in qualitative research, and describe qualitative design features

▶ Identify the major research traditions for qualitative research and describe the domain of inquiry of each

▶ Describe the main features of ethnographic, phenomenological, and grounded theory studies

▶ Discuss the goals and methods of various types of research with an ideological perspective

▶ Define new terms in the chapter

THE DESIGN OF QUALITATIVE STUDIES

Quantitative researchers specify a research design before collecting their data and adhere to that design once the study is underway; they *design* and then they *do*. In qualitative research, by contrast, the research design typically evolves during the study; qualitative researchers *design* as they *do*. Decisions about how best to obtain data and from whom to obtain data are made in the field, as the study unfolds. Qualitative research design is an **emergent design**—a design that emerges as researchers make ongoing decisions reflecting what has already been learned. As noted by Lincoln and Guba (1985), an emergent design in qualitative studies is not the result of researchers' sloppiness or laziness, but rather of their desire to base the inquiry on the realities and viewpoints of those under study—realities and viewpoints that are not known at the outset.

CONSUMER TIP

Design decisions for a qualitative study are usually summarized in the method section of a report (e.g., a decision to interview a subset of study participants a second time), but the decision-making process for design decisions is rarely described. ■

Characteristics of Qualitative Research Design

Qualitative inquiry has been guided by a number of different disciplines, and each has developed methods best suited to address questions of interest. However, some general characteristics of qualitative research design apply across disciplines. Qualitative design:

▶ is flexible and elastic, capable of adjusting to what is being learned during the course of data collection;
▶ requires researchers to become intensely involved, often remaining in the field for lengthy periods of time;
▶ requires ongoing analysis of the data to formulate subsequent strategies and to determine when field work is done;
▶ tends to be holistic, striving for an understanding of the whole; and
▶ typically involves a merging together of various data collection strategies.

With regard to the last characteristic, qualitative researchers tend to put together a complex array of data from various sources. This tendency has been described as **bricolage**, and qualitative researchers have been referred to as bricoleurs, people who are "adept at performing a large number of diverse tasks, ranging from interviewing to observing, to interpreting personal and historical documents, to intensive reflection and introspection" (Denzin & Lincoln, 1994, p. 2).

Qualitative Design and Planning

Although design decisions are not made upfront, qualitative researchers typically do advance planning that supports their flexibility in developing an emergent design. In the absence of planning, design choices might actually be constrained. For example, a researcher initially might project a 6-month data collection period, but may need to be prepared to spend even longer in the field to pursue emerging opportunities. In other words, qualitative researchers plan for broad contingencies that may pose decision options in the field. Advance planning is usually important with regard to the following:

▶ Selection of the research tradition (described in the next section) that will guide certain design and analytic decisions
▶ Selection of a study site and identification of settings within the site that are likely to be especially fruitful for data collection

▶ Identification of the key "gatekeepers" who can provide (or deny) access to key data sources and can make arrangements for gaining entrée
▶ Determination of the maximum time available for the study
▶ Identification of all needed equipment for the collection and analysis of data in the field (e.g., audio and video recording equipment).

Thus, qualitative researchers plan for a variety of circumstances, but decisions about how they will deal with them must be resolved when the social context of time, place, and human interactions is better understood.

One further task that qualitative researchers typically undertake before (and during) data collection is an analysis of their own biases and ideology. Qualitative researchers tend to accept that research is subjective and may be ideologically driven. Decisions about research design are not value free. Qualitative researchers, then, often take on as an early research challenge the identification of their own biases. Such an activity is particularly important in qualitative inquiry because of the intensely personal nature of the data collection and analysis experience.

Example illustrating disclosure of possible bias

Rashid (2001) studied women's views about the use of the Norplant contraceptive implant in rural Bangladesh. She wrote: "My writing on this subject is influenced by my position as a native (born in Bangladesh) and as an outsider (I grew up overseas from 1979 to 1993). The kind of fieldwork I carried out was influenced by my cultural background, Muslim identity, status as an unmarried Bengali woman, and mixed cultural upbringing. . . ." (p. 89)

Phases in a Qualitative Study

Although the exact form of a qualitative study is not known in advance, Lincoln and Guba (1985) noted that a naturalistic inquiry typically progresses through three broad phases while in the field:

1. *Orientation and overview.* Quantitative researchers generally believe they know what they do not know (i.e., they know the type of knowledge they expect to obtain by doing a study and then strive to obtain it). A qualitative researcher, by contrast, enters the study "not knowing what is not known" (i.e., not knowing what it is about the phenomenon that will drive the inquiry forward). Therefore, the first phase of many qualitative studies is to get a handle on what is salient about the phenomenon of interest.
2. *Focused exploration.* The second phase is a more focused scrutiny and in-depth exploration of aspects of the phenomenon judged to be salient. The questions asked and the types of people invited to participate in the study are shaped by the understandings developed in the first phase.

3. *Confirmation and closure.* In the final phase, qualitative researchers make efforts to establish that their findings are trustworthy, often by going back and discussing their understanding with study participants. Phase 3 activities, which are crucial in the critique of a qualitative study, are described in Chapter 14.

The three phases are not discrete but overlap to a greater or lesser degree in different projects. For example, even the first few interviews or observations are typically used as a basis for selecting subsequent informants, even though the researcher is still striving to understand the scope of the phenomenon. The three phases might take only a few weeks to complete—or many months.

Janesick (2004), who also views qualitative design as having three phases, has likened it to choreography. The first phase is the warm-up or prechoreographic stage of design decisions. The second phase is the exploration or try-out and total work phase. Just as in choreography, qualitative design is viewed as a work in progress. The final stage is the cooling-down period, which Janesick calls illumination and formulation. The design decisions made toward the end of the study include deciding when to actually leave the field setting.

Qualitative Design Features

Some design features of quantitative studies also apply to qualitative studies, but they are often *post hoc* characterizations of what happened in the field rather than features specifically planned in advance. To further contrast qualitative and quantitative research design, we refer to the design elements identified in Table 9.1 in Chapter 9.

Experimental Versus Nonexperimental. Qualitative research is nonexperimental—although, as discussed in Chapter 11, a qualitative study sometimes is embedded within an experimental project. Qualitative researchers do not conceptualize their studies as having independent and dependent variables, and they do not manipulate any aspect of the people or environment under study. The goal of most qualitative studies is to develop a rich understanding of a phenomenon as it exists in the real world and as it is constructed by individuals within the context of that world.

Comparisons. Qualitative researchers typically do not plan in advance to make group comparisons because the intent is to thoroughly describe and explain a phenomenon. Nevertheless, patterns emerging in the data sometimes suggest that certain comparisons are relevant and illuminating.

Data Collection Points. Qualitative research, like quantitative research, can be cross-sectional, with one data collection point, or longitudinal, with multiple data collection points over an extended time period, to observe the evolution of a phenomenon. Qualitative researchers may plan in advance for multiple sessions, but in other cases, the decision to study a phenomenon longitudinally may be made in the field after preliminary data have been collected and analyzed.

Retrospective Versus Prospective. Qualitative researchers do not typically use the terms *retrospective* or *prospective.* Nevertheless, in trying to elucidate a phenomenon, they may look back retrospectively (with the help of study participants) for antecedent events leading to the occurrence of the phenomenon. Qualitative researchers may also study the evolution of a phenomenon prospectively.

Examples of the time dimension in qualitative studies

Cross-sectional: Dewar and Lee (2000) examined how people with a catastrophic illness or injury managed their circumstances. In one interview, the researchers asked participants (who had endured their condition for 3 to 25 years) to describe their coping processes over time.
 Longitudinal: Iwasiw, Goldenberg, Bol, and MacMaster (2003) conducted a longitudinal study of the first year in a long-term care facility for the residents and their relatives. Study participants were interviewed at 2 and 6 weeks, and at 3, 6, 8, and 12 months after admission.

Examples of exploring influences and causes in qualitative designs:

Retrospective exploration: Tarrant and Gregory (2003) studied First Nations parents' beliefs about childhood immunizations and retrospectively explored factors influencing immunization uptake.
 Prospective exploration: Olson, Tom, Hewitt, Whittingham, Buchanan, and Ganton (2002) conducted a prospective qualitative study to explore the evolution of routines among Canadian patients with cancer who were able to prevent fatigue; participants were interviewed before, during, and after treatment.

Research Setting. Qualitative researchers collect their data in real-world, naturalistic settings. And, whereas quantitative researchers usually strive to collect data in one type of setting to maintain constancy of conditions (e.g., conducting all interviews in study participants' homes), qualitative researchers may deliberately strive to study their phenomena in a variety of natural contexts.

Example of variation in settings

Woodgate, Degner, and Yanofsky (2003) conducted a longitudinal study to explore and describe the childhood cancer symptom course from the children's and their families' point of view. Data were collected in the children's homes and in inpatient and outpatient clinical settings.

QUALITATIVE RESEARCH TRADITIONS

Although qualitative research designs share some features, there is a wide variety of approaches. There is no readily agreed-on taxonomy, but one useful system is to describe qualitative research according to disciplinary traditions. As we have noted previously, these traditions vary in their view of what questions are important to ask in understanding human experiences. This section provides an overview of qualitative research traditions (some of which we have previously introduced), and subsequent sections describe ethnographies, phenomenological studies, and grounded theory studies in greater detail. In the discussion that follows, we describe "traditional" qualitative inquiry, but a later section examines qualitative studies that adopt a "critical" perspective.

Overview of Qualitative Research Traditions

The research traditions that have provided an underpinning for qualitative studies come primarily from anthropology, psychology, and sociology. As shown in Table 10.1, each discipline has tended to focus on one or two broad domains of inquiry.

The discipline of anthropology is concerned with human cultures. **Ethnography** is the primary research tradition within anthropology and provides a framework for studying the meanings, patterns, and experiences of a defined cultural group in a holistic fashion. **Ethnoscience** (or *cognitive anthropology*) focuses on the cognitive world of a culture, with particular emphasis on the semantic rules and the shared meanings that shape behaviour. Ethnoscientific studies may rely on quantitative as well as qualitative data.

TABLE 10.1   **Overview of Qualitative Research Traditions**

DISCIPLINE	DOMAIN	RESEARCH TRADITION	AREA OF INQUIRY
Anthropology	Culture	Ethnography	Holistic view of a culture
		Ethnoscience (cognitive anthropology)	Mapping of the cognitive world of a culture; a culture's shared meanings, semantic rules
Psychology/ philosophy	Lived experience	Phenomenology	Experiences of individuals within their lifeworld
		Hermeneutics	Interpretations and meanings of individuals' experiences
Psychology	Behaviour and events	Ethology	Behaviour observed over time in natural context
		Ecologic psychology	Behaviour as influenced by the environment
Sociology	Social settings	Grounded theory	Social structural processes within a social setting
		Ethnomethodology	Manner by which shared agreement is achieved in social settings
Sociolinguistics	Human communication	Discourse analysis	Forms and rules of conversation
History	Past behaviour, events, and conditions	Historical analysis	Description and interpretation of historical events

Example of an ethnoscientific study

Hirst (2002) used methods of ethnoscience to articulate a definition of resident abuse as perceived by nurses working in long-term care settings. She focused on the linguistic symbols and "folk terms" of the culture in long-term care institutions.

Phenomenology has its roots in both philosophy and psychology. As noted in Chapter 3, phenomenology is concerned with the lived experiences of humans. A closely related research tradition is **hermeneutics**, which uses the lived experiences of people as a tool to better understand the social, political, and historical context in which those experiences occur. Hermeneutic inquiry almost always focuses on meaning and interpretation—how socially and historically conditioned individuals interpret the world within their given context.

The discipline of psychology has several research traditions that focus on behaviour. Human **ethology**, which is sometimes described as the biology of human behaviour, studies behaviour as it evolves in its natural context. Human ethologists use observational methods to explore universal behavioural structures.

Example of an ethological study

Morse and Pooler (2002) used ethological methods to study the interactions of patients' family members with the patients and with nurses in the trauma-resuscitation room of an emergency department. The analysis was based on 193 videotapes of trauma room care.

Ecological psychology focuses on the environment's influence on human behaviour and attempts to identify principles that explain the interdependence of humans and the environment. Viewed from an ecological context, people are affected by (and affect) a multi-layered set of systems, including family, peer group, and neighbourhood, as well as the more indirect effects of health care and social services systems and the larger cultural belief and value systems of the society in which individuals live.

Example of an ecological study

Shamian, Kerr, Laschinger, and Thomson (2002) conducted an ecological analysis that explored the relationship between hospital-level indicators of the work environment and indicators of nurses' health and well-being among nurses working in acute care hospitals in Ontario.

Sociologists study the social world and have developed several research traditions of importance to qualitative researchers. The grounded theory tradition (described earlier and elaborated on in a later section of this chapter) seeks to understand the key social psychological and structural processes that occur in a social setting.

Ethnomethodology seeks to discover how people make sense of everyday activities and interpret their social world so as to behave in socially acceptable ways. Within this tradition, researchers attempt to understand a social group's norms and assumptions that are so deeply ingrained that members no longer think about the underlying reasons for their behaviours.

Example of an ethnomethodologic study

Montbriand (2004) explored the meaning that seniors from a Canadian prairie city ascribe to illness and healing. Seniors' analyses of their own lives revealed that their perceptions of having survived war and the Great Depression were related to their perceptions about current illnesses.

The domain of inquiry for sociolinguists is human communication. The tradition called discourse analysis seeks to understand the rules, mechanisms, and structure of conversations. The data for **discourse analysis** typically are transcripts from naturally occurring conversations, such as those between nurses and their patients.

Example of a discourse analysis

Espin and Lingard (2001) analyzed the communication patterns and discourse between nurses and surgeons in an Ontario teaching hospital and identified issues that are catalysts for tension.

Finally, **historical research**—the systematic collection and critical evaluation of data relating to past occurrences—also relies primarily on qualitative data. Historical research is undertaken to answer questions about phenomena or issues relating to past events that

Example of historical research

Grypma (2004) examined Canadian missionary nursing practice in China during the period of 1935 to 1947. Letters written by these missionary nurses and sent home to Canada were the main data source for this study. The letters portrayed the primary image of Canadian nurses as that of professional nurse as opposed to the media image of Angel of Mercy or Foreign Devil.

may shed light on present behaviours or practices. It is important not to confuse historical research with a review of the literature about historical events. Like other types of research, historical inquiry has as its goal the discovery of *new* knowledge.

It should be noted that some qualitative research reports do not identify a research tradition but simply say the study was qualitative. In some cases a research tradition can be inferred from information about the types of questions that were asked or the methods used to collect and analyze data. However, not all qualitative research *has* a link to one of the traditions we have discussed. Some *descriptive qualitative studies* simply focus on describing a phenomenon in a holistic fashion.

Example of a descriptive qualitative study

Mitchell (2004) conducted in-depth interviews with 42 Canadian women to describe how women perceive ultrasound when they receive unexpected abnormal ultrasound findings.

CONSUMER TIP

Research reports sometimes identify more than one tradition as having provided the framework for a qualitative inquiry (e.g., a phenomenological study using the grounded theory method). However, such "method slurring" (Baker, Wuest, & Stern, 1992) has been criticized because each research tradition has different intellectual assumptions and methodologic prescriptions. ■

Ethnography

Ethnographies are inquiries that involve the description and interpretation of cultural behaviour. Ethnographies are a blend of a process and a product: fieldwork and a written text. *Fieldwork* is the process by which ethnographers come to understand a culture; ethnographic texts are how that culture is communicated and portrayed. Because culture is, in itself, not visible or tangible, it must be constructed through ethnographic writing. Culture is inferred from the words, actions, and products of members of a group.

Ethnographic research is in some cases concerned with broadly defined cultures (e.g., a Haitian village culture), in a *macroethnography*. However, ethnographies some-

Example of a microethnography

Medves and Davies (2005) undertook an institutional ethnography of a rural Ontario hospital to study how nurses and physicians deliver maternity care to women in rural areas.

times focus on more narrowly defined cultures in a *microethnography*, which is an exhaustive, fine-grained study of a small unit within a group or culture (e.g., the culture of homeless shelters). An underlying assumption of ethnographers is that every human group eventually evolves a culture that guides the members' view of the world and the way they structure their experiences.

Ethnographers seek to learn from (rather than to study) members of a cultural group. Ethnographers sometimes refer to emic and etic perspectives. An **emic perspective** is the way members of the culture envision their world—the insiders' view. The emic is the local concepts or means of expression used by the members of the group under study to characterize their experiences. The **etic perspective**, by contrast, is the outsiders' interpretation of the culture's experiences; it is the language used by those doing the research to refer to the same phenomena. Ethnographers strive to acquire an emic perspective of a culture. Moreover, they strive to reveal **tacit knowledge**, information about the culture that is so deeply embedded in cultural experiences that members do not talk about it or may not even be consciously aware of it.

Ethnographic research is a labour-intensive and time-consuming endeavour—months and even years of fieldwork may be required to learn about a cultural group. The study of a culture requires a certain level of intimacy with members of the cultural group, and such intimacy can only be developed over time and by working directly with those members as active participants. The concept of *researcher as instrument* is used by anthropologists to describe the significant role ethnographers play in analyzing and interpreting a culture.

Three broad types of information are usually sought by ethnographers: cultural behaviour (what members of the culture do); cultural artefacts (what members of the culture make and use); and cultural speech (what people say). This implies that ethnographers rely on various data sources, including observations, in-depth interviews, and other types of physical evidence (photographs, diaries, letters, and so on). Ethnographers typically conduct in-depth interviews with about 25 to 50 informants. They also typically use a strategy known as **participant observation** in which they make observations of a community or group while participating in its activities (see Chapter 13).

The products of ethnographic research are rich, holistic descriptions of a culture. Ethnographers also make cultural interpretations, describing normative behavioural and social patterns. Among health care researchers, ethnography provides information about the health beliefs and health-related practices of a culture or subculture. Ethnographic inquiry can thus facilitate understanding of behaviours affecting health and illness. Many nurse researchers have undertaken ethnographic studies, and Madeleine Leininger has coined the phrase **ethnonursing research**, which she defines as "the study and analysis of the local or indigenous people's viewpoints, beliefs, and practices about nursing care behavior and processes of designated cultures" (1985, p. 38).

Ethnographers are often, but not always, "outsiders" to the culture under study. If nurse researchers studied, for example, the culture of an intensive care unit, however, this would be called **insider research** (or *peer research* or *auto-ethnography*). There are practical and substantive advantages to such a study, including ease of entry into the culture, access to information and informants that might not otherwise be available, and an abundance of prior knowledge. The drawback is that an "insider" may have developed biases about certain issues or may be so entrenched in the culture that valuable pieces of data get overlooked. Insider research demands that researchers maintain a high level of consciousness about their role and monitor their beliefs and their interactions with others.

Example of insider research

Lipson (2001) conducted an ethnographic study about the experiences of people with multiple chemical sensitivity (MCS). She gathered her data over a 2-year period through in-depth interviews and observations in two U.S. and two Canadian settings, and through participation in a weekly MCS chat room. Lipson, who herself suffers from MCS, included a valuable discussion of issues relating to the conduct of insider research.

Phenomenology

Phenomenology, rooted in a philosophical tradition developed by Husserl and Heidegger, is an approach to thinking about people's life experiences. Phenomenological researchers ask: What is the *essence* of this phenomenon as experienced by these people, and what does it *mean?* Phenomenologists assume there is an essence—an essential invariant structure—that can be understood, in much the same way that ethnographers assume that cultures exist. Phenomenologists investigate subjective phenomena in the belief that key *truths* about reality are grounded in people's lived experiences. The phenomenological approach is especially useful when a phenomenon has been poorly understood. The topics appropriate to phenomenology are ones that are fundamental to the life experiences of humans; for health researchers, these include such topics as the meaning of stress or the experience of bereavement.

Phenomenologists believe that lived experience gives meaning to each person's perception of a particular phenomenon. The goal of phenomenological inquiry is to understand fully lived experience and the perceptions to which it gives rise. Four aspects of lived experience that are of interest are *lived space*, or spatiality; *lived body*, or corporeality; *lived time*, or temporality; and *lived human relation*, or relationality.

Phenomenologists view human existence as meaningful and interesting because of people's consciousness of that existence. The phrase **being-in-the-world** (or *embodiment*) is a concept that acknowledges people's physical ties to their world—they think, see, hear, feel, and are conscious through their bodies' interaction with the world.

In phenomenological studies, the main data source is in-depth conversations, with researchers and informants as co-participants. Through in-depth conversations, researchers strive to gain entrance into the informants' world, to have full access to their experiences as lived. Two or more separate interviews are sometimes needed. Typically, phenomenological studies involve a small number of study participants—often 10 or fewer. For some phenomenological researchers, the inquiry includes not only gathering information from informants but also efforts to experience the phenomenon in the same way, typically through participation, observation, and introspective reflection.

There are a number of variants and methodologic interpretations of phenomenology. The two main schools of thought are descriptive phenomenology and interpretive phenomenology (hermeneutics).

Example of a phenomenological study

O'Brien and Fothergill-Bourbonnais (2004) conducted a phenomenological study of patients' experience of trauma resuscitation in the emergency department. In-depth interviews were conducted with seven patients 2 to 7 days after trauma resuscitation in a trauma hospital in Ontario.

DESCRIPTIVE PHENOMENOLOGY

Descriptive phenomenology was developed first by Husserl (1962), who was interested in the question: What do we know as persons? His philosophy emphasized descriptions of human experience. Descriptive phenomenologists insist on the careful description of ordinary conscious experience of everyday life—a description of "things" as people experience them. These "things" include hearing, seeing, believing, feeling, remembering, deciding, evaluating, acting, and so forth.

Descriptive phenomenological studies often involve four steps: bracketing, intuiting, analyzing, and describing. **Bracketing** refers to the process of identifying and holding in abeyance preconceived beliefs about the phenomenon under study. Although bracketing can never be achieved totally, researchers strive to bracket out the world and any presuppositions in an effort to confront the data in pure form. Phenomenological researchers (as well as other qualitative researchers) often maintain a **reflexive journal** in their efforts to bracket.

Intuiting occurs when researchers remain open to the meanings attributed to the phenomenon by those who have experienced it. Phenomenological researchers then proceed to the analysis phase (i.e., extracting significant statements, categorizing, and making sense of the essential meanings of the phenomenon). Chapter 16 provides further information regarding data analysis in phenomenological studies. Finally, the descriptive phase occurs when researchers come to understand and define the phenomenon.

Example of a descriptive phenomenological study

Perreault, Fothergill-Bourbonnais, and Fiset (2004) did a phenomenological study designed to describe the experience of family members caring for a dying loved one. They elicited richly detailed narrative descriptions of the experience in interviews with family caregivers.

INTERPRETIVE PHENOMENOLOGY

Heidegger, a student of Husserl, moved away from his professor's philosophy into **interpretive phenomenology,** or hermeneutics. To Heidegger (1962), the critical question is: What is Being? He stressed interpreting and understanding—not just describing—human experience. Heidegger argued that hermeneutics ("understanding") is a basic characteristic of human existence. Indeed, the term hermeneutics refers to the art and philosophy of interpreting the meaning of an object (such as a *text*, work of art, and so on). The goals of interpretive phenomenological research are to enter another's world and to discover the practical wisdom, possibilities, and understandings found there.

It should be noted that an important distinction between descriptive and interpretive phenomenology is that in an interpretive phenomenological study, bracketing does not occur. For Heidegger, it was not possible to bracket one's being-in-the-world. Hermeneutics presupposes prior understanding on the part of the researcher.

Example of an interpretive phenomenological study

Sinding, Gray, Fitch, and Greenberg (2002) used a hermeneutic approach to explore the meanings of living with metastatic breast cancer. The research team, a theatre troupe, and women with breast cancer who were interviewed as part of the study co-created a performance ("Handle With Care"); the performance context allowed certain illness meanings to emerge and intensify.

Interpretive phenomenologists, like descriptive phenomenologists, rely primarily on in-depth interviews with individuals who have experienced the phenomenon of interest, but, as in the above example, they may go beyond a traditional approach to gathering and analyzing data. For example, interpretive phenomenologists sometimes augment their understandings of the phenomenon through an analysis of supplementary texts, such as novels, poetry, or other artistic expressions—or they use such materials in their conversations with study participants.

Example of a hermeneutic study using artistic expression

Lauterbach (2001) studied the phenomenon of maternal mourning over the death of a wished-for-baby. She increased her "attentive listening" to this phenomenon by turning to examples of infant death experiences illustrated in the arts, literature, and poetry. For example, she included a poem written by Shakespeare as he mourned his son's death. She also described the painting "Rachel Weeping" by Charles Wilson Peale, which depicts the artist's daughter, who had died of smallpox, laid out in her burial dress. Lauterbach also visited cemeteries to discover memorial art in babies' grave stones. She used the examples of memorial art and of literature to validate the themes of mothers' experiences in her research.

Grounded Theory

Grounded theory has become an important method for the study of nursing problems and has contributed to the development of many middle-range theories of phenomena of relevance to nurses. Grounded theory began more as a systematic method of qualitative research than as a philosophy. It was developed in the 1960s by two sociologists, Glaser

HOW-TO-TELL TIP

How can you tell if a phenomenological study is descriptive or interpretive? Phenomenologists often use key terms in their report that can help you make a determination. In a descriptive phenomenological study, such terms may be bracketing, description, essence, Husserl, and phenomenological reduction. The names of Colaizzi, Van Kaam, and Giorgi may be found in the method section. In an interpretive phenomenological study, key terms can include being-in-the-world, shared interpretations, hermeneutics, understanding, and Heidegger. The names van Manen, Benner, and Diekelmann may appear in the method section. These names will be discussed in Chapter 16. ■

and Strauss (1967), whose theoretical roots were in *symbolic interactionism*, which focuses on the manner in which people make sense of social interactions and the interpretations they attach to social symbols (e.g., language).

As noted in Chapter 3, grounded theory comprises methods for studying social processes and social structures. The focus of most grounded theory studies is on the discovery of a basic social psychological problem that a group of people experience and on the social psychological stages or phases that characterize the process used to cope with or resolve this basic problem. The primary purpose is to generate a theory that explains a pattern of behaviour that is problematic and relevant to study participants.

Grounded theory methods constitute an entire approach to the conduct of field research. For example, a study that truly follows Glaser and Strauss' precepts does not begin with the identification of a specific research problem. In grounded theory, both the research problem and the process used to resolve it are discovered during the study. A fundamental feature of grounded theory research is that data collection, data analysis, and sampling of participants occur simultaneously. The grounded theory process is recursive: researchers collect data, categorize them, describe the emerging central phenomenon, and then recycle earlier steps.

A procedure called **constant comparison** is used to identify the basic problem and to develop and refine theoretically relevant categories. The categories elicited from the data are constantly compared with data obtained earlier so that commonalities and variations can be determined, and categories can be condensed and collapsed. As data collection proceeds, the inquiry becomes focused on emerging theoretical concerns and core processes. Data analysis in grounded theory studies is described in Chapter 16.

Example of a grounded theory study

Jack, DiCenso, and Lohfield (2005) conducted a grounded theory study of the process by which mothers of children at risk for developmental delays engage with public health nurses and family visitors in a home visiting program. Data were collected through in-depth interviews with 20 mothers and through review of client records.

In-depth interviews are the most common data source in grounded theory studies, but observation (including participant observation) and existing documents may also be used. Typically, a grounded theory study involves interviews with a sample of about 25 to 50 informants.

HOW-TO-TELL TIP

Grounded theory studies often use gerunds in their titles, which suggest action and change. A gerund is a part of speech ending in "ing." It is part verb (signifying action) and part noun. An example is the title of one of Beck's studies, "Teetering on the Edge: A Substantive Theory of Postpartum Depression." ■

ALTERNATIVE VIEWS OF GROUNDED THEORY

In 1990, Strauss and Corbin published what became a controversial book, *Basics of Qualitative Research: Grounded Theory Procedures and Techniques*. Strauss and Corbin stated that the purpose of the book was to provide beginning grounded theory students with a more concrete description of the procedures involved in building theory at the substantive level.

Glaser, however, disagreed with some of the procedures advocated by Strauss (his original co-author) and Corbin (a nurse researcher). Glaser published a rebuttal in 1992, *Emergence Versus Forcing: Basics of Grounded Theory Analysis.* Glaser believed that Strauss and Corbin developed a method that is not grounded theory but rather what he calls "full conceptual description." According to Glaser, the purpose of grounded theory is to generate concepts and theories about their relationships that explain and interpret variation in behaviour in the substantive area under study. *Conceptual description*, in contrast, is aimed at describing the full range of behaviour of what is occurring in the substantive area, "irrespective of relevance and accounting for variation in behavior" (Glaser, 1992, p. 19).

Nurse researchers have conducted grounded theory studies using both the original Glaser and Strauss and the Strauss and Corbin approaches. We discuss aspects of the two approaches in more detail in the chapter on data analysis (see Chapter 16).

FORMAL GROUNDED THEORY

Glaser and Strauss (1967) distinguished two types of grounded theory: substantive and formal. **Substantive theory** is grounded in data on a specific substantive area, such as postpartum depression. It can serve as a springboard for **formal grounded theory**, which involves developing a higher, more abstract level of theory from a compilation of substantive grounded theory studies regarding a particular phenomenon. Glaser and Strauss' (1971) theory of status passage is an example of a formal grounded theory.

Kearney (1998) used an interesting analogy to differentiate substantive theories (custom-tailored clothing) and formal theory (ready-to-wear clothing). Formal grounded theories were likened to clothing sold in department stores that can fit a wider variety of users. Formal grounded theory is not personally tailored like substantive theory, but rather provides a conceptualization that applies to a broader population experiencing a common phenomenon. Formal grounded theories are not situation specific. The best data for constructing grounded formal theories are substantive grounded theories.

Example of a formal grounded theory

Kearney and O'Sullivan (2003) used a formal grounded theory approach to synthesize the findings of 14 studies, with the goal of identifying common elements of individuals' efforts to change a variety of unhealthy behaviours. The concept of *identity shift* was discovered as a core process.

CONSUMER TIP

Avoid jumping to conclusions about the research tradition of a study based on the report's title. For example, the study "The Personal Significance of Home: Habitus and the Experience of Receiving Long-Term Home Care" (Angus, Kontos, Dyck, McKeever, & Poland, 2005) is not a phenomenological study but rather an ethnographic study of home care in 16 homes in Ontario—even though the word "experience" in the title might suggest otherwise. As another example, despite the title's suggestion of a focus on cultural issues, "Giving Birth: The Voices of Orthodox Jewish Women Living in Canada" (Semenic, Callister, & Feldman, 2004) is a phenomenological study, not an ethnographic one. ■

RESEARCH WITH IDEOLOGICAL PERSPECTIVES

An emerging trend in nursing research is to conduct inquiries within ideological frameworks, typically to draw attention to certain social problems or the needs of certain groups. These approaches, which represent important investigative avenues, usually rely primarily on qualitative data and interpretive methods of analysis.

Critical Theory

Critical theory originated within a group of Marxist-oriented German scholars in the 1920s, collectively referred to as the Frankfurt School. Essentially, critical researchers are concerned with a critique of society and with envisioning new possibilities.

Critical research is typically action oriented. Its broad aim is to integrate theory and practice so that people become aware of contradictions and disparities in their beliefs and social practices, and become inspired to change them. Critical researchers reject the idea of an objective, disinterested inquirer and are oriented toward a transformation process. Critical theory calls for inquiries that foster enlightened self-knowledge and sociopolitical action. Moreover, critical theory involves a self-reflexive aspect. To prevent a critical theory of society from becoming yet another self-serving ideology, critical theorists must account for their own transformative effects.

The design of research within critical theory often begins with a thorough analysis of certain aspects of a problem. For example, critical researchers might analyze and critique taken-for-granted assumptions that underlie a problem, the language used to depict the

TABLE 10.2	Comparison of Traditional Qualitative Research and Critical Research	
ISSUE	**TRADITIONAL QUALITATIVE RESEARCH**	**CRITICAL RESEARCH**
Research aims	Understanding; reconstruction of multiple constructions	Critique; transformation; consciousness raising; advocacy
View of knowledge	Transactional/subjective; knowledge is created in interaction between investigator and participants	Transactional/subjective; value mediated and value dependent; importance of historical insights
Method	Dialectic: truth arrived at logically through conversations	Dialectic and didactic: dialogue designed to transform naivety and misinformation
Evaluative criteria for inquiry quality	Authenticity; trustworthiness	Historical situatedness of the inquiry; erosion of ignorance; stimulus for change
Researcher's role	Facilitator of multivoice reconstruction	Transformative agent; advocate; activist

situation, and the biases of prior researchers investigating the problem. Critical researchers often triangulate multiple methodologies and emphasize multiple perspectives (e.g., alternative racial or social class perspectives) on problems. Critical researchers interact with study participants in ways that emphasize participants' expertise. Some of the features that distinguish more traditional qualitative research and critical research are summarized in Table 10.2.

Critical theory has played an especially important role in ethnography. **Critical ethnography** focuses on raising consciousness and aiding emancipatory goals in the hope of effecting social change. Critical ethnographers address the social, political, and economic dimensions of cultures and their value-laden agendas. An assumption in critical ethnographic research is that actions and thoughts are mediated by power relationships. Critical ethnographers attempt to increase the political dimensions of cultural research and undermine oppressive systems.

Example of a critical ethnography

Kushner (2005) undertook a critical ethnographic study to explicate ways that health decision making among Canadian working mothers was socially organized through the institutions of motherhood, the family, the workplace, and broader health and social systems. Twenty mothers took part in the study over a 2-year period.

Feminist Research

Feminist research uses approaches that are similar to those of critical theory research, but it focuses sharply on gender domination and discrimination within patriarchal societies.

Like critical researchers, feminist researchers seek to establish collaborative, nonexploitive relationships with their informants, to avoid objectification, and to conduct research that is transformative. Feminist researchers stress *intersubjectivity* between researchers and participants and the mutual creation of knowledge.

Gender is the organizing principle in feminist research, and investigators seek to understand how gender and a gendered social order have shaped women's lives. The aim is to alter the "invisibility and distortion of female experience in ways relevant to ending women's unequal social position" (Lather, 1991, p. 71). The purpose of feminist research is to provide information *for* women, not just *about* women.

The scope of feminist research ranges from studies of the particular and subjective views of individual women, to studies of social movements and broad policies that affect (and often exclude) women. Olesen (1994), a sociologist who studied nurses' career patterns and definitions of success, has noted that some of the best feminist research on women's subjective experiences has been done in the area of women's health.

Feminist research methods generally include in-depth, collaborative individual interviews or group interviews that offer the possibility of reciprocally educational encounters. Feminists generally seek to negotiate the meanings of the results with those participating in the study, and to be self-reflexive about what they themselves are experiencing and learning. In feminist research, the researcher's history, assumptions, interests, motives, and interpretations are explicitly scrutinized in the process of the study.

Feminist research, like other research with an ideological perspective, has raised the bar for the conduct of ethical research. With the emphasis on trust, empathy, and nonexploitive relationship, proponents of these newer modes of inquiry view any type of deception or manipulation as abhorrent. As Punch (1994) has noted in speaking about ethics and feminist research, "you do not rip off your sisters" (p. 89).

Example of a feminist research

Wuest, Merritt-Gray, and Ford-Gilboe (2004) conducted a feminist grounded theory study of family health promotion in the aftermath of intimate family violence. The researchers found, through interviews with 40 women in two Canadian provinces over a 3-year period, that families strengthened their emotional health by replacing previously destructive patterns of interaction with supportive ways of getting along through a process called *regenerating family.*

Participatory Action Research

Participatory action research (PAR) is closely allied to both critical research and feminist research. PAR, one of several types of *action research* that originated in the 1940s with social psychologist Kurt Lewin, is based on a recognition that the use and production of knowledge can be political and can be used to exert power. PAR researchers typically work with groups or communities that are vulnerable to the control or oppression of a dominant group or culture.

PAR is, as the name implies, participatory. There is collaboration between researchers and study participants in the definition of the problem, the selection of an approach and research methods, the analysis of the data, and the use to which findings are put. The aim of PAR is to produce not only knowledge but also action and consciousness-raising. Researchers specifically seek to empower people through the process of constructing knowledge. The PAR tradition has as its starting point a concern for the powerlessness of the group under study. Thus, a key objective is to produce action that is directly used to make improvements through education and sociopolitical action.

In PAR, the research methods take second place to emergent processes of collaboration and dialogue that can motivate, increase self-esteem, and generate solidarity. Thus, data-gathering strategies are not only the traditional methods of interview and observation (including both qualitative and quantitative approaches) but also may include storytelling, sociodrama, drawing and painting, and other activities designed to encourage people to find creative ways to explore their lives and recognize their own strengths.

Example of participatory action research

Mill (2003) used PAR to study the experience of HIV-positive Ghanaian women and to identify factors that influenced their vulnerability to infection. Over a period of several months, Mill conducted individual and group interviews with HIV-positive women, HIV-positive men, nurses, other health care professionals, and traditional healers.

CRITIQUING QUALITATIVE DESIGNS

Evaluating a qualitative design is often difficult. Qualitative researchers do not always document design decisions and are even less likely to describe the process by which such decisions were made. Researchers often do, however, indicate whether the study was conducted within a specific qualitative tradition. This information can be used to come to some conclusions about the study design. For example, if a report indicated that the researcher conducted 1 month of fieldwork for an ethnographic study, there would be reason to suspect that insufficient time had been spent in the field to obtain a true emic perspective of the culture under study. Ethnographic studies may also be critiqued if their only source of information was from interviews, rather than from a broader range of data sources including observations.

In a grounded theory study, you might also be concerned if the researcher relied exclusively on data from interviews; a stronger design might have been obtained by including participant observations. Also, look for evidence about when the data were collected and analyzed. If the researcher collected all the data before analyzing any of it, you might question whether the constant comparative method was used correctly.

In critiquing a phenomenological study, you should first determine whether the study is descriptive or interpretive. This will help you to assess how closely the researcher kept to the basic tenets of that qualitative research tradition. For example, in a descriptive phenomenological study, did the researcher bracket?

No matter what qualitative design is identified in a study, look to see if the researchers stayed true to a single qualitative tradition throughout the study or if they mixed qualitative traditions, possibly weakening the rigour of the study. For example, did the researcher state that a grounded theory design was used, but then present results that described *themes* instead of generating a substantive theory?

The guidelines in Box 10.1 are intended to assist you in critiquing the designs of qualitative studies.

BOX 10.1   Guidelines for Critiquing Qualitative Designs

1. Is the research tradition for the qualitative study identified? If none was identified, can one be inferred? If more than one was identified, is this justifiable or does it suggest "method slurring"?
2. Is the research question congruent with a qualitative approach and with the specific research tradition (i.e., is the domain of inquiry for the study congruent with the domain encompassed by the tradition)? Are the data sources, research methods, and analytic approach congruent with the research tradition?
3. How well is the research design described? Are design decisions explained and justified? Does it appear that the researcher made all design decisions up-front, or did the design emerge during data collection, allowing researchers to capitalize on early information?
4. Is the design appropriate, given the research question? Does the design lend itself to a thorough, in-depth, intensive examination of the phenomenon of interest? What design elements might have strengthened the study (e.g., a longitudinal perspective rather than a cross-sectional one)?
5. Was there appropriate evidence of reflexivity in the design?
6. Was the study undertaken with an ideological perspective? If so, is there evidence that ideological methods and goals were achieved? (e.g., Was there evidence of full collaboration between researchers and participants? Did the research have the power to be transformative, or is there evidence that a transformative process occurred?)

CONSUMER TIP

In this age of the Internet, students and researchers have access to information on qualitative design at their fingertips. Two important websites are:
www.phenomenologyonline.com
www.groundedtheory.com

RESEARCH EXAMPLES   **Critical Thinking Activities**

 EXAMPLE 1: Critical/Feminist Ethnography

Aspects of an ethnographic nursing study, featuring terms and concepts discussed in this chapter, are presented here, followed by some questions to guide critical thinking.

(Research Examples continue on page 226)

Critical Thinking Activities (continued)

Study

"First Nations women's encounters with mainstream health services" (Browne & Fiske, 2001)

Statement of Purpose

The purpose of the study was to address two key questions: How do First Nations women describe their encounters with local mainstream health care services? and How are these encounters shaped by social, political, and economic factors?

Community Setting and Sociopolitical Context

The research was conducted in partnership with a First Nations reserve community with a population of 600 in rural northwest Canada. The community believed it would benefit from a thorough description of women's encounters as it developed plans to improve health and health care for its members. Women from the community (including one of the researchers) were renowned locally as leaders in health, and yet First Nations people were rarely invited to join nearby mainstream health boards or decision-making bodies.

Theoretical Perspectives

The construct of *cultural safety*, originally developed by indigenous nurses in New Zealand to address the health concerns of the Maori, informed this research. The emphasis of cultural safety is on transforming attitudes and practices by gaining an awareness of the forces shaping the health and status of indigenous people.

Method

The study was a critical ethnography drawing on feminist perspectives. The researchers made efforts to "equalize power within the research team and between the participants and researchers" (p. 132). This was accomplished in a variety of ways, including the adoption of a "critically reflective research process." Using input from community leaders and elders, the researchers selected 10 women to participate in two rounds of interviews. Each woman was interviewed separately for 1 to 2 hours. The second interviews were used to clarify and verify information from the first interviews. Participants were asked to describe both positive encounters (model cases) and negative encounters (contrary cases) with health care services. An interpretive thematic analysis was conducted with transcripts from these interviews. The initial analysis was subjected to critical questioning, reflection, and discussions with participants.

Key Findings

▶ The narratives revealed that the "women's encounters were shaped by racism, discrimination, and structural inequalities that continue to marginalize and disadvantage First Nations women" (p. 126).

▶ Participants described situations in which their health concerns or reported symptoms were not taken seriously. Encounters that revealed health care workers' discriminatory attitudes and behaviours were found to be pervasive.

Critical Thinking Activities (continued)

*Critical Thinking Suggestions**

*See the Student Resource CD-ROM for a discussion of these questions.

1. Answer questions 1 through 6 from Box 10.1 regarding this study.

2. Also consider the following targeted questions, which may assist you in further assessing aspects of the study:

    a. Would you consider this an example of insider research? If yes, explain some of the issues the researchers faced.

    b. The report did not indicate over how long a period the researchers conducted their fieldwork. Comment on the fieldwork for this ethnographic study.

    c. Could this study have been conducted as a phenomenological study? As a grounded theory study? Why or why not?

3. If the results of this study are trustworthy, what are some of the uses to which the findings might be put in clinical practice?

 EXAMPLE 2: Grounded Theory Study

Aspects of a grounded theory study, featuring terms and concepts discussed in this chapter, are presented below, followed by some questions to guide critical thinking.

Study

"Struggling to understand: The experience of nonsmoking parents with adolescents who smoke" (Small, Brennan-Hunter, Best, & Solberg, 2002)

Statement of Purpose

The purpose of this grounded theory study was to understand what nonsmoking parents experience as a result of their adolescent children's smoking. The aim was to develop a theory to explain the process nonsmoking parents go through in dealing with their children's risk-taking behaviour.

Context

The researchers noted that there has been little research on the experience of parenting adolescents. Research has tended to be unidirectional—the effect that parents have on children has been extensively studied, but there has been little research on the effects that children's actions have on parents.

Method

Small and her colleagues chose a grounded theory approach "because of the scarcity of knowledge in the area of parenting adolescents who smoke and the need to develop an explanatory model of the process nonsmoking parents experience in their interactions with adolescents who smoke" (p. 1203). They recruited 25 nonsmoking parents with children who smoked through schools in a Canadian city. Participants were asked to talk about their experience during in-depth interviews, which were audiotaped and transcribed. The early interviews asked broad and exploratory questions, but in later interviews the researchers asked more

(Research Examples continue on page 228)

Critical Thinking Activities (continued)

focused and direct questions when they "required information that was more specific to expand on certain aspects of the parents' experiences" (p. 1204). Data collection and analysis occurred simultaneously in an interactive process. Data analysis began when the first interview transcript was completed, and emergent findings increasingly guided subsequent data collection. Data were analyzed using the constant comparison method, using the Strauss and Corbin approach. The researchers validated their model by discussing it with 8 additional parents.

Key Findings

The researchers used their interview data to generate a schematic model they called "Struggling to Understand." In this model, parents' attempt to understand and cope was reflected by their passage through four stages: discovering the smoking, facing the problem, reflecting, and waiting it out. Each of these stages consisted of several activities in which the parents engaged. For example, during Stage 1 (discovering the smoking), the parents' actions included (1) seeing the evidence, (2) putting the pieces together, and (3) confirming the behaviour.

Critical Thinking Suggestions

1. Answer questions 1 through 6 from Box 10.1 regarding this study.
2. Also consider the following targeted questions, which may assist you in further assessing aspects of the study:
   a. Did the researchers develop a substantive theory or a formal theory?
   b. Was this study longitudinal or cross-sectional?
   c. Could this study have been conducted as a phenomenological study? As an ethnographic study? Why or why not?
3. If the results of this study are trustworthy, what are some of the uses to which the findings might be put in clinical practice?

 EXAMPLE 3: Phenomenological Study

1. Read the Method section from the Beck's phenomenological study ("Birth Trauma") in Appendix B of this book, and then answer the relevant questions in Box 10.1.
2. Also consider the following targeted questions, which may further sharpen your critical thinking skills and assist you in assessing aspects of the study's merit:
   a. Was this study a descriptive or interpretive phenomenology?
   b. Could this study have been conducted as a grounded theory study? As an ethnographic study? Why or why not?
   c. Could this study have been conducted as a feminist inquiry? If yes, what might Beck have done differently?

CHAPTER REVIEW
Summary Points

▶ Qualitative research typically involves an **emergent design**—a design that emerges as the study unfolds.

▶ As **bricoleurs**, qualitative researchers are creative and intuitive, putting together data drawn from many sources to arrive at a holistic understanding of a phenomenon.

▶ Although qualitative design is flexible, qualitative researchers nevertheless plan for broad contingencies that are expected to pose decision opportunities for design decisions in the field.

▶ A naturalistic inquiry typically progresses through three broad phases in the field: an orientation phase to determine what it is about the key phenomenon that is salient; a focused exploration phase that closely examines important aspects of the phenomenon; and a confirmation and closure phase to confirm findings.

▶ Qualitative research traditions have their roots in anthropology (e.g., *ethnography* and **ethnoscience**); philosophy (*phenomenology* and **hermeneutics**); psychology (**ethology, ecological psychology**); sociology (**grounded theory, ethnomethodology**); sociolinguistics (**discourse analysis**); and history (**historical research**).

▶ Some *descriptive qualitative* studies are not linked to any research tradition and are designed to describe some phenomenon in an in-depth, holistic fashion.

▶ Ethnography focuses on the culture of a group of people and relies on extensive field work. The ethnographer strives to acquire an **emic**, or insider's, **perspective** of the culture under study and to discover deeply embedded **tacit knowledge**; the outsider's perspective is known as **etic**.

▶ Phenomenology seeks to determine the essence and meaning of a phenomenon as it is experienced by people.

▶ In **descriptive phenomenology**, researchers describe lived experiences by **bracketing out** any preconceived views and **intuiting** the essence of the phenomenon by remaining open to the meanings attributed to it by those who have experienced it.

▶ Bracketing is not a feature of **interpretive phenomenology** (**hermeneutics**), which focuses on interpreting the meaning of experiences.

▶ *Grounded theory* is an approach to generating a theory to explain a pattern of behaviour that is problematic and relevant to participants. This approach uses **constant comparison:** categories elicited from the data are constantly compared with data obtained earlier so that shared patterns and variations can be determined.

▶ There are two types of grounded theory: **substantive theory**, which is grounded in data on a specific substantive area, and **formal grounded theory** (often using data from substantive theory studies) that is at a higher level of abstraction.

▶ Research is sometimes conducted within an ideological perspective, and such research tends to rely primarily on qualitative research.

▶ **Critical theory** is concerned with a critique of existing social structures; critical researchers conduct inquiries that involve collaboration with participants and foster enlightened transformation. *Critical ethnography* uses the principles of critical theory in the study of cultures.

▶ **Feminist research**, like critical research, is designed to be transformative, but the focus is sharply on how gender domination and discrimination shape women's lives.

▶ **Participatory action research** (PAR) produces knowledge through close collaboration with groups or communities that are vulnerable to control or oppression by a dominant culture; in PAR, research methods take second place to emergent processes that can motivate people and generate community solidarity.

Additional Resources for Review

Chapter 10 of the *Study Guide to Accompany Essentials of Nursing Research,* 6th edition offers various exercises and study suggestions for reinforcing the concepts presented in this chapter. For additional review, see the Student Self-Study Review Questions section of the Student Resource CD-ROM provided with this book.

SUGGESTED READINGS

References for studies cited in the chapter appear at the end of the book.

Methodologic References

Baker, C., Wuest, J., & Stern, P. N. (1992). Method slurring: The grounded theory/phenomenology example. *Journal of Advanced Nursing, 17,* 1355–1360.

Creswell, J. W. (1998). Qualitative inquiry and research design: Choosing among five traditions. Thousand Oaks, CA: Sage Publications.

Denzin, N. K., & Lincoln, Y. S. (Eds.). (2000). *Handbook of qualitative research* (2nd ed.). Thousand Oaks, CA: Sage Publications.

Glaser, B. G. (1992). *Emergence versus forcing: Basics of grounded theory analysis.* Mill Valley, CA: Sociology Press.

Glaser, B. G., & Strauss, A. L. (1967). The discovery of grounded theory: Strategies for qualitative research. Chicago: Aldine.

Glaser, B., & Strauss, A. (1971). *Status passage: A formal theory.* Mill Valley, CA: Sociology Press.

Heidegger, M. (1962). *Being and time.* New York: Harper & Row.

Husserl, E. (1962). Ideas: General introduction to pure phenomenology. New York: MacMillan.

Janesick, V. J. (2004). *Stretching exercises for qualitative researchers.* Thousand Oaks, CA: Sage Publications.

Kearney, M. H. (1998). Ready-to-wear: Discovering grounded formal theory. *Research in Nursing & Health, 21,* 179–186.

Leininger, M. M. (Ed.). (1985). *Qualitative research methods in nursing.* New York: Grune & Stratton.

Lincoln, Y. S., & Guba, E. G. (1985). *Naturalistic inquiry.* Newbury Park, CA: Sage Publications.

Morse, J. M. (1991). Qualitative nursing research: A contemporary dialogue. Newbury Park, CA: Sage Publications.

Morse, J. M. (1999). Qualitative methods: The state of the art. *Qualitative Health Research, 9,* 393–406.

Morse, J. M., & Field, P. A. (1995). *Qualitative research methods for health professionals* (2nd ed.). Thousand Oaks, CA: Sage Publications.

Lather, P. (1991). Getting smart: Feminist research and pedagogy within the postmodern. New York: Routledge.

Olesen, V. (1994). Feminism and models of qualitative research. In N. K. Denzin & Y. S. Lincoln (Eds.), *Handbook of qualitative research.* Thousand Oaks, CA: Sage Publications.

Punch, M. (1994). Politics and ethics in qualitative research. In N. K. Denzin & Y .S. Lincoln (Eds.), *Handbook of qualitative research.* Thousand Oaks, CA: Sage Publications.

Strauss, A. L., & Corbin, J. M. (1990). *Basics of qualitative research: Grounded theory procedures and techniques.* Newbury Park, CA: Sage Publications.

11

Examining Specific Types of Research

STUDENT OBJECTIVES

On completing this chapter, you will be able to:

▶ Identify the purposes and some of the distinguishing features of specific types of research (e.g., clinical trials, surveys)
▶ Determine whether researchers' primary approach (qualitative versus quantitative) and design were appropriate for the type of research
▶ Identify several advantages of mixed method research and describe specific applications
▶ Define new terms in the chapter

A ll quantitative studies can be categorized as either experimental, quasi-experimental/preexperimental, or nonexperimental, as discussed in Chapter 9. And, most qualitative studies lie within one of the research traditions described in Chapter 10. This chapter describes types of qualitative and quantitative research that vary according to study purpose rather than according to research design or tradition. The chapter also describes mixed method research that combines qualitative and quantitative approaches in a single project.

STUDIES THAT ARE TYPICALLY QUANTITATIVE

The research described in this section usually uses quantitative approaches, but it is important to note that for certain types of research (e.g., evaluation research), qualitative methods may also be added as a component in a mixed method strategy.

Clinical Trials

Clinical trials are studies designed to assess the effectiveness of clinical interventions. Methods associated with clinical trials have been developed for medical and epidemiological research, but nurse researchers are increasingly adopting these methods to test nursing interventions.

Clinical trials undertaken to test innovative therapies often are designed in a series of phases.

▶ *Phase I* of the trial occurs after the initial development of the drug or therapy and is designed primarily to determine things like drug dose (or strength of the therapy), safety, and patient tolerance. This phase typically uses preexperimental designs (e.g., before–after designs without a control group). The focus is not on efficacy, but on developing the best possible treatment.

▶ *Phase II* of the trial involves seeking preliminary evidence of the effectiveness of the treatment as it has been designed in Phase I, typically using a preexperimental or quasi-experimental design, but sometimes an experimental design with a small sample. During this phase, researchers assess the feasibility of launching a larger, more rigourous test, seek evidence that the treatment holds promise, and look for possible side effects. This phase is considered a *pilot test* of the treatment. There have been clinical trials of drug therapies that have shown such powerful effects during this phase that further phases were considered unnecessary and even unethical, but this would rarely be true in nursing studies.

Example of a Phase II clinical trial

Olson, Hanson, and Michaud (2003) conducted a Phase II trial that compared pain levels, quality of life, and analgesic use with a sample of 24 Canadian patients with cancer who received either standard opioid pain management plus Reiki or standard pain opioid management plus rest.

▶ *Phase III* is a full experimental test of the treatment, involving random assignment to groups or to orderings of treatment conditions. The objective of this phase is to determine the efficacy of the innovation compared with the standard treatment or an alternative counterfactual. When the term *clinical trial* is used in the nursing literature, it usually is referring to a Phase III trial, which may also be called a **randomized clinical trial** (RCT). Phase III clinical trials usually involve the use of a large and heterogeneous sample of subjects, frequently selected from multiple, geographically dispersed sites to ensure that findings are not unique to a single setting.

▶ *Phase IV* of a trial occurs after the decision to adopt an innovation has been made. In this phase, researchers monitor the long-term consequences of the intervention as it is used in actual practice, including both benefits and side effects. This phase might use a nonexperimental, preexperimental, or quasi-experimental design.

Example of a multisite randomized clinical trial

Hodnett, Lowe, Hannah, Willan, Stevens, Weston, Ohlsson, Gafni, Muir, Myhr, Stremler, and the Nursing Supportive Care in Labor Trial Group (2002) undertook a large-scale clinical trial that assessed the effectiveness of nurses as providers of labour support. Nearly 7000 women in 13 Canadian and U.S. hospitals were randomly assigned to receive either usual care or continuous labour support by a specially trained nurse during labour.

Evaluations

Evaluations are used to find out how well a program, treatment, or policy works. Clinical nurses, nurse administrators, and nursing educators often need to pose such questions as the following: How are current practices working? Should a new practice be adopted? Which approach is most effective? In this era of accountability, evaluations of the effectiveness of nursing actions are common. Evaluations can employ experimental, quasi-experimental, or nonexperimental designs and can be either cross-sectional or longitudinal. Although most evaluations are quantitative, certain aspects of programs are often evaluated using qualitative methods.

Clinical trials are sometimes evaluations. As an example, Steel-O'Connor, Mowat, Scott, Carr, Dorland, and Young-Tai (2003) evaluated the effectiveness of two public health nurse follow-up programs (home visits and telephone follow-up) in terms of infant health problems, breastfeeding rates, and use of postpartum health services. Their program evaluation involved a multisite clinical trial in Ontario. Generally, the term *evaluation research* is used when researchers are trying to determine the effectiveness of a rather complex program, rather than when they are testing a specific entity (e.g., alternative drugs or sterilizing solutions). Thus, not all clinical trials would be called evaluations, and not all evaluations use methods associated with clinical trials. Moreover, evaluations often try to answer broader questions than simply whether an intervention is more effective clinically than care as usual. Evaluations may involve determining how the intervention was actually put into place, for example.

There are various types of evaluations. A **process analysis** (or an **implementation analysis**) obtains descriptive information about the process of implementing a new program or procedure and about its functioning in actual operation. Process evaluations, which often rely on both qualitative and quantitative data, are designed to address such questions as the following: What are the strongest and weakest aspects of the program?

What exactly *is* the treatment, and how does it differ from traditional practices? What were the barriers to implementing the program successfully?

Example of a process analysis

A team of researchers in Canada (Chalmers, Gupton, Katz, Hack, Hildes-Ripstein, Brown, McMillan, Labossiere, Mackay, Pickerl, Savard-Preston, Vincent, Morris, and Cann, 2004) used a participatory process to develop a community-based smoking cessation intervention for perinatal women. Their report summarized descriptive information about the development and implementation of the intervention and participants' reactions to its various components.

An **outcome analysis** documents the extent to which the goals of a program are attained, to obtain preliminary evidence about program success (e.g., the extent to which positive outcomes are in line with the original intent). Outcome analyses are descriptive and do not use experimental designs; before–after designs without a comparison group are common.

Example of an outcome analysis

Lavorato, Grypma, Spenceley, Hagen, and Nowatzki (2003) studied the outcomes of a cardiac rehabilitation program. Health-related quality of life and health outcomes were studied before and after program participation for 64 clients in the program.

An **impact analysis** attempts to identify the *impacts* or *net effects* of an intervention (i.e., the effects over and above what would have occurred in its absence). Impact analyses use an experimental or quasi-experimental design because their goal is to attribute a causal connection between outcomes and the intervention. Many nursing evaluations are impact analyses, although they are not necessarily labelled as such.

Example of an impact analysis

Harkness, Morrow, Smith, Kiczula, and Arthur (2003) evaluated the impact of a psychoeducational nursing intervention on the anxiety levels of patients during the waiting period for elective cardiac catheterization. Intervention patients received a detailed, nurse-delivered information session within 2 weeks of being placed on the waiting list, whereas those not in the intervention group received usual care. A before–after experimental design was used.

Finally, evaluations sometimes include a **cost–benefit analysis** to determine whether the monetary benefits of a program outweigh the costs. Administrators make decisions about resource allocations for health services not only on the basis of whether something "works" but also on the basis of whether it is economically viable. Cost–benefit analyses are typically done in connection with impact analyses and Phase III clinical trials, that is, when researchers establish solid evidence regarding program effectiveness.

Example of a cost analysis

In their evaluation of the effects of public health nurse follow-up programs, described earlier, Steel-O'Connor and colleagues (2003) studied the costs associated with the two alternative programs. Direct costs, indirect costs (i.e., overhead), and total costs of health services per 100 infants were greater for the home visit group than for the telephone screen group in both research sites.

Outcomes Research

Outcomes research, designed to document the effectiveness of health care services, is gaining momentum in nursing and health care fields. Outcomes research overlaps with evaluation research, but evaluations typically appraise a specific new intervention, whereas outcomes research is a more global assessment of health care services. The impetus for outcomes research comes from the quality assessment and quality assurance functions that grew out of the professional standards review organizations (PSROs) in the 1970s. Outcomes research represents a response to the increasing demand from policy makers, insurers, and the public to justify care practices in terms of improved patient outcomes and costs.

Although many nursing studies are concerned with examining patient outcomes and patient satisfaction, specific efforts to appraise and document the quality of nursing care—as distinct from the care provided by the overall health care system—are not numerous. A major obstacle is attribution—that is, linking patient outcomes to specific nursing actions, distinct from the actions of other members of the health care team. It is also difficult in some cases to determine a causal connection between outcomes and health care interventions because factors outside the health care system (e.g., patient characteristics) affect outcomes in complex ways.

Nevertheless, outcomes research continues to expand. There is increasing interest, for example, in describing the work that nurses do in terms of established classification, and there is also interest in maintaining complete and accurate records of nursing actions in computerized datasets (referred to as *nursing minimal data sets* or *NMDS*). A number of research-based classification systems of nursing interventions are being developed, refined, and tested, including the Nursing Diagnoses Taxonomy of the North American Nursing Diagnosis Association (NANDA) and the Nursing Intervention Classification (NIC) developed at the University of Iowa. Studies with these classification systems have thus far focused on descriptions of patient problems and nursing interventions, and assessments of the utility of these systems.

Example of a study using the NIC system

Within the context of an RCT that evaluated postdischarge nursing interventions for stroke survivors, two nurse case managers provided care to 90 community-dwelling patients in the intervention group. Nursing documentation was analyzed, using the NIC system, to identify and quantify the interventions that were provided. (McBride, White, Sourial, & Mayo, 2004)

Just as there have been efforts to develop classifications of nursing interventions, work has been undertaken to develop outcome classification systems. Of particular note is the Nursing Outcomes Classification (NOC) developed by nurses at the University of Iowa College of Nursing to complement the NIC (Johnson & Maas, 1998). The NOC system was designed to measure patient outcomes that are sensitive to nursing care and to help standardize these outcomes. The NOC includes 260 patient outcomes categorized into seven domains: functional health, physiologic health, psychosocial health, health knowledge and behaviour, perceived health, family health, and community health.

Sidani, Doran, and Mitchell (2004) recently advocated a theory-driven approach to evaluating the quality of nursing care. Their approach focuses on the identification of patient, professional, and setting characteristics that affect processes of health care and that, in turn, affect patient outcomes.

Example of outcomes research

Linda McGillis Hall and Diane Doran are leading Canadian nurse researchers involved in outcomes research. For example, Hall and Doran (2004) explored whether nurse staffing models and nurse characteristics were related to differences in quality outcomes (e.g., unit communication, perceived quality of care) in 77 patient care units in 19 hospitals. As another example, Hall, Doran, Baker, Pink, Sidani, O'Brien-Pallas, and Donner (2003) examined the relationship between different nurse staffing models on the one hand and patient outcomes (e.g., functional status, pain control, patient satisfaction with nursing care) on the other.

Surveys

A **survey** obtains information regarding the prevalence, distribution, and interrelationships of variables within a population. Political opinion polls are examples of surveys. Surveys collect information on people's actions, knowledge, intentions, opinions, and attitudes.

Survey data are based on **self-reports**—respondents answer questions posed by researchers. Survey data can be collected in a number of ways, but the most respected method is through **personal interviews** (or *face-to-face interviews*), in which interviewers meet with respondents to ask them questions. Personal interviews are usually costly because they tend to involve a lot of personnel time. Nevertheless, personal interviews are considered the best means of collecting survey data because the quality of data they yield is higher than other methods and because relatively few people refuse to be interviewed in person. **Telephone interviews** are a less costly, but often less effective, method of gathering survey data. When the interviewer is unknown, respondents may be uncooperative on the telephone. Telephoning can, however, be a convenient method of collecting information if the interview is short and not too personal. Telephone interviews may be difficult for certain groups of respondents, including low-income people (who do not always have a telephone) and the elderly (who may have hearing problems).

Survey researchers can also distribute **questionnaires**, which are self-administered. Because respondents differ in their reading levels and in their ability to communicate in writing, questionnaires are *not* merely a printed form of an interview. Self-administered questionnaires are economical but are not appropriate for surveying certain populations (e.g., the elderly, children). Survey questionnaires are generally distributed through the mail but may also be distributed in other ways (e.g., through the Internet).

Survey research is highly flexible: it can be applied to many populations, and it can focus on a wide range of topics. Survey data tend, however, to be relatively superficial. Survey research is better suited to extensive rather than intensive analysis. Although surveys can be done within the context of experiments, surveys are usually nonexperimental.

Example of a survey

Robinson, Clements, and Land (2003) studied the prevalence, distribution, correlates, and predictors of vicarious trauma and burnout among registered psychiatric nurses in Canada. Questionnaires were distributed to more than 1000 nurses in Manitoba.

STUDIES THAT CAN BE QUALITATIVE OR QUANTITATIVE

The studies described in the previous section are typically conducted with formal instruments designed to yield quantitative data. The types of studies described in this section can be either qualitative or quantitative.

Case Studies

Case studies are in-depth investigations of a single entity or a small number of entities. The entity may be an individual, family, group, community, or other social unit. In a case study, researchers obtain a wealth of descriptive information and may examine relationships among different phenomena. Case study researchers attempt to analyze and understand issues that are important to the history, development, or circumstances of the person or entity under study.

One way to think of a case study is to consider what is center stage. In most studies, whether qualitative or quantitative, a certain phenomenon or variable (or set of variables) is the core of the inquiry. In a case study, the *case* itself is central. As befits an intensive analysis, the focus of case studies is typically on determining the dynamics of *why* an individual thinks, behaves, or develops in a particular manner rather than on *what* his or her status or actions are. It is not unusual for probing research of this type to require detailed study over a considerable period. Data are often collected that relate not only to the person's present state but also to past experiences and situational factors relevant to the problem being examined.

The greatest strength of case studies is the depth that is possible when a limited number of individuals or groups are being investigated. On the other hand, this same strength is a potential weakness because researchers' familiarity with the person or group may make objectivity more difficult. The biggest criticism of case studies concerns generalizability: if researchers discover important relationships, it is difficult to know whether the same relationships would occur with others. However, case studies can often play a critical role in challenging generalizations based on other types of research.

It is important to recognize that case study research is not simply anecdotal descriptions of a particular incident or patient. Case study research is a disciplined process and typically requires an extended period of systematic data collection.

Example of a quantitative case study

Kolanowski, Litaker, and Catalano (2002) studied the self-reported mood and affective pattern of an older man with severe cognitive impairments. Data were collected through observation of the man and through his self-reports of mood collected three times a day over a 35-day period.

Example of a qualitative case study

Graham, Logan, Davies, and Nimrod (2004) conducted a case study of factors influencing the successful and unsuccessful introduction of an evidence-based foetal health surveillance guideline in two tertiary and one community hospital.

Secondary Analysis

Secondary analysis involves the use of data gathered in a previous study to test new hypotheses or explore new phenomena. In a typical study, researchers collect far more data than can be analyzed. Secondary analysis of existing data is efficient because data collection is typically the most time-consuming and expensive part of a study. Nurse researchers have done secondary analyses with both large national data sets and smaller, localized sets, and with both qualitative and quantitative data.

A number of avenues are available for making use of an existing set of quantitative data. For example, variables and relationships among variables that were previously unanalyzed can be examined (e.g., a dependent variable in the original study could become the independent variable in the secondary analysis). Or, the secondary analysis can focus on a particular subgroup rather than on the full original sample (e.g., survey data about health habits from a national sample could be analyzed to study smoking among urban teenagers). As another example, the unit of analysis can be changed. A **unit of analysis** is the basic unit that yields data for an analysis; in nursing studies, each individual subject is typically the unit of analysis. However, data are sometimes aggregated to yield information about larger units (e.g., a study of individual nurses from 25 hospitals could be converted to aggregated data about the hospitals). In qualitative studies, wider theories can be generated by using data from several different datasets. Or, a qualitative researcher could scrutinize an existing data set for particular themes or content coverage that was previously unexplored.

The use of available data makes it possible to bypass time-consuming steps in a study, but there are some noteworthy disadvantages in working with existing data. In particular, if researchers do not play a role in collecting the data, the chances are pretty high that the data set will be deficient in one or more ways, such as in the sample used, the variables measured, and so forth. Researchers may continuously face "if only" problems: if only they had asked questions on a certain topic or had measured a particular variable differently. Nevertheless, existing data sets present exciting opportunities for exploring phenomena of importance to nurses.

Example of a secondary analysis of quantitative data

Forbes, Stewart, Morgan, Anderson, Parent, and Janzen (2003) used data from three cross-sectional waves of Statistics Canada's National Population Health Surveys. The purpose was to identify individual factors (e.g., age, gender, income) that predicted the use of publicly funded home care nursing and housework assistance in Canadian adults.

Example of a secondary analysis of qualitative data

Thorne, Con, McGuinness, McPherson, and Harris (2004) analyzed previously collected qualitative data from a larger study that explored patterns in health care communication across several chronic diseases. The new study involved an analysis of people with multiple sclerosis and their perceptions of helpful and unhelpful communication in their health care.

Methodologic Research

Methodologic research examines methods of obtaining and analyzing research data and addresses the development, validation, and evaluation of instruments or methods. Nurse researchers have become increasingly interested in methodologic research; this is not surprising in light of growing demands for sound and reliable outcome measures and for sophisticated procedures for obtaining and analyzing qualitative and quantitative data.

Quantitative methodologic studies often focus on instrument development and testing. For example, suppose we developed and evaluated an instrument to measure patients' satisfaction with nursing care. In such a study, we would not examine levels of patient satisfaction, nor how satisfaction relates to characteristics of nurses or patients. Our goal would be to develop an effective, trustworthy instrument that could be used by others, and to determine our success.

Most methodologic studies are descriptive and nonexperimental, but occasionally quantitative researchers use an experimental or quasi-experimental design to test competing methodologic strategies. For example, a researcher might test whether a financial incentive increases the number of volunteers willing to participate in a study. Potential participants could be randomly assigned to an incentive or no-incentive condition. The dependent variable in this case is whether people agree to participate.

In qualitative research, methodologic issues often arise within the context of a substantive study, rather than having a study originate as a purely methodologic endeavour. In such instances, however, the researcher typically performs separate analyses designed to highlight a methodologic issue and to generate strategies for solving a methodologic problem.

Methodologic research may appear less provocative than substantive research, but it is virtually impossible to produce high-quality research evidence on a substantive topic with inadequate research methods.

Example of a quantitative methodologic study

Bottorff, Ratner, Richardson, Balneaves, McCullum, Hack, Chalmers, and Buxton (2003) undertook a methodologic study by means of a telephone survey to evaluate alternative ways of asking women about their interest in genetic testing for breast cancer risk.

Example of a qualitative methodologic study

Miranda (2004) was involved in a study in which prospective study participants were asked about their willingness to be randomly assigned to alternative interventions to address their insomnia. The majority of study participants were unwilling to be randomized, and Miranda analyzed the qualitative data regarding the underlying reasons for their treatment allocation preferences. The study offers useful information for the conduct of experimental studies in this area.

MIXED METHOD STUDIES

An emerging trend, and one that we believe will gain momentum, is the planned integration of qualitative and quantitative data within single studies or coordinated clusters of studies. This section discusses the rationale for such **mixed method** (or **multimethod**) studies and presents a few applications.

Rationale for Mixed Method Studies

The dichotomy between quantitative and qualitative data represents a key methodologic distinction in the social, behavioural, and health sciences. Some argue that the paradigms that underpin qualitative and quantitative research are fundamentally incompatible. Others, however, believe that many areas of inquiry can be enriched and the evidence base enhanced through the judicious blending of qualitative and quantitative data. The advantages of such a triangulated design include the following:

▶ *Complementarity.* Qualitative and quantitative data represent words and numbers, the two fundamental languages of human communication. The strengths and weaknesses of these two types of data and associated methods are complementary. By using multiple methods, researchers can allow each method to do what it does best, possibly avoiding the limitations of a single approach.

▶ *Incrementality.* Progress on a topic tends to be incremental, relying on multiple feedback loops. Qualitative findings can generate hypotheses to be tested, and quantitative findings can be clarified through in-depth probing. It can be productive to build such a loop into the design of a single study.

▶ *Enhanced validity.* When a hypothesis or model is supported by multiple and complementary types of data, researchers can be more confident about the validity of their results.

▶ *Creating new frontiers.* Sometimes qualitative and quantitative findings are inconsistent with each other. This lack of congruity—when it happens in a single study—can lead to insights that can push a line of inquiry further. Inconsistencies in separate studies may reflect differences in study participants and circumstances rather than theoretically meaningful distinctions. In a single study, discrepancies can be used as a springboard for further exploration.

CONSUMER TIP

Mixed method studies rarely combine qualitative and quantitative findings in a single report. Typically, the quantitative findings are reported in one journal article, and the qualitative findings appear in a separate article in a different journal. This sometimes makes it difficult for readers to grasp the contributions of all the components. ▬

Applications of Mixed Method Research

The integration of qualitative and quantitative data can be used to address various research goals.

1. *Instrumentation.* Researchers sometimes collect qualitative data for the development and validation of formal instruments used in research or clinical applications. The questions for such an instrument are sometimes derived from clinical experience or prior research, but when a construct is new, these sources may be inadequate to capture its full complexity. Qualitative data can be used to generate questions for instruments that are subsequently subjected to rigorous testing in methodologic studies.

Example of instrumentation

Joy Johnson and her colleagues (Johnson, Bottorff, Moffat, Ratner, Shoveller, & Lovato, 2003; Johnson, Tucker, Ratner, Bottorff, Prkachin, Shoveller, & Zumbo, 2004) developed and refined a measure of tobacco dependence in adolescence, the Dimensions of Tobacco Dependence Scale. The instrument's five dimensions (social, pleasurable, empowering, emotional, and physical dependence) were identified in a thematic analysis of in-depth interviews with 72 youths. The purpose of the qualitative study was to identify the patterns of language that young people use to describe tobacco dependence and the meaning that tobacco dependence holds for them. Using the language of the adolescents, the researchers developed a 54-item scale representing these five dimensions. For example, "Smoking helps me fit in at school" is a scale item for the social dimension. The researchers rigorously tested their scale with 513 students from high schools in British Columbia.

2. *Hypothesis Generation and Testing.* In-depth qualitative studies are often fertile with insights about constructs or relationships among them. These insights then can be tested and confirmed in quantitative studies, and the generalizability of the insights can be assessed. This most often happens in the context of discrete investigations. One problem, however, is that it usually takes years to do a study and publish the results, which means that considerable time may elapse between qualitative insights and formal quantitative testing of hypotheses based on those insights. A research team interested in a phenomenon might wish to collaborate in a research program that has hypothesis generation and testing as an explicit goal.

Example of hypothesis generation

McClement, Chochinov, Hack, Kristjanson, and Harlos (2004) used qualitative and quantitative methods to develop a comprehensive understanding of the concept of *dignity* in terminally ill patients. Analysis of data from in-depth interviews with 50 palliative cancer patients resulted in a model of dignity and the generation of hypotheses about factors influencing patients' perceptions of dignity. The quantitative data were used to examine how disease-specific variables were related to dignity.

3. *Illustration.* Qualitative data are sometimes used to illustrate the meaning of quantitative descriptions or relationships. Such illustrations help to clarify important concepts, to corroborate the findings from the statistical analysis, and to guide the interpretation of results. Qualitative materials can be used to illustrate specific statistical findings and to provide more global and dynamic views of the phenomena under study, sometimes in the form of illustrative case studies.

4. *Understanding relationships and causal processes.* Quantitative methods can demonstrate that variables are systematically related but may fail to provide insights about *why* they are related. Interpretations are often speculative, representing hypotheses that

Example of illustrating with qualitative data

Polit, London, and Martinez (2000, 2001) used data from the ethnographic component of a study of poor urban families to illustrate how food insecurity and hunger—reported by more than half of the sample from the survey component—were actually experienced and managed. The following excerpt illustrates the sustenance problems some women had: "*It was hard, especially when you got kids at home saying, 'I'm hungry.' . . . I started working at the church as a babysitter. I was getting paid $20 a week and a bag of food every Thursday. . . . Then I was doing very odd jobs that most people would not dare to do. I was making deliveries on pizza in bad neighborhoods where most people wouldn't go. I mean, I literally took my life in my own hands*" (2001, p. 58).

could be tested in another study. When a study integrates qualitative and quantitative data, however, the researcher may be in a stronger position to derive meaning immediately from the statistical findings.

Example of illuminating with qualitative data

Benzies, Harrison, and Magill-Evans (2004a, 2004b) collected both qualitative and quantitative data about child behaviour problems. The longitudinal study of preterm and full-term infants, with follow-up when the children were 7 years old, included quantitative measures that allowed the researchers to examine factors predictive of the behaviour problems—including parental stress during infancy. The qualitative data, based on an intensive study of four families, allowed the researchers to more fully explore the interaction of parental stress and stressful life circumstances on the one hand and children's problem behaviours on the other.

5. *Theory building, testing, and refinement.* The most ambitious application of mixed method research is in the area of theory development. A theory gains acceptance as it escapes disconfirmation, and the use of multiple methods provides great opportunity for potential disconfirmation of a theory. If the theory can survive these assaults, it can provide a stronger context for the organization of clinical and intellectual work.

Example of theory building

Morgan and Stewart (2002) conducted a mixed-method evaluation of a dementia special care unit in a midwestern Canadian city that involved a quasi-experimental component and a grounded theory component. The study led to a better understanding of how the nursing home environment affects residents with dementia, which in turn helped to advance theory development in person–environment interaction.

Mixed Method Strategies

The ways in which researchers can design studies to integrate qualitative and quantitative methods are almost limitless. The three following scenarios are especially common:

1. *Adding qualitative methods to a survey.* Once researchers have gained the cooperation of survey respondents, they may be in a good position to collect more in-depth data from them. If in-depth interviews can be postponed until after the analysis of quantitative data, researchers can probe into the reasons for any obtained results. The second-stage respondents, in other words, can be used as informants to help researchers interpret outcomes.

Example of a qualitative component within a survey

Degner, Hack, O'Neil, and Kristjanson (2003) conducted a survey of more than 1000 women at various points after diagnosis of breast cancer. The survey obtained extensive data (e.g., demographic, disease, and treatment information). At the end of the interview, the women were asked to describe the meaning that breast cancer had for them. The women's detailed statements were recorded and transcribed for qualitative analysis.

2. *Embedding quantitative measures into an ethnography.* Although qualitative data prevail in ethnographic field studies, ethnographers can often profit from the collection of structured information, either from the study participants or from a larger or more representative sample. Having already gained entrée into the community and the cooperation of its members, ethnographers may be in an ideal position to pursue a survey or a record-extraction activity. For example, if a researcher's in-depth fieldwork focused on family violence, community-wide police and hospital records could be used to gather systematic data amenable to statistical analysis.

Example of a multimethod ethnography

Lipson and colleagues (Lipson, Weinstein, Gladstone, & Sarnoff, 2003; Weinstein, Sarnoff, Gladstone, & Lipson, 2000) did a mixed method study of the health and health care needs of refugees in Santa Clara County, California after resettlement in the United States. The study had three parts. The first was a secondary analysis of a data set containing health records from 2361 refugees who sought services from county health facilities. The second part involved an analysis of 187 randomly selected medical records from the County Refugee Clinic with regard to diagnosis, use of services, and quality of care. The third component involved ethnographies of the Bosnian and former Soviet Union refugee communities. In the ethnographies, the researchers observed community events, interviewed refugees in their homes, and interviewed health care providers. Data from the ethnographic component, which indicated that certain health problems were especially common in the refugee population, helped to focus certain aspects of the medical records component.

3. *Embedding qualitative approaches into experimental research.* Qualitative data can often enrich clinical trials and evaluations that rely on experimental designs. Through in-depth approaches, researchers can, for example, better understand qualitative differences between groups, including differences in the experiences and processes underlying experimental effects. Qualitative data may be especially useful when researchers are evaluating complex interventions. When an experimental treatment is straightforward (e.g., a new drug), it might be easy to interpret the results. However, many nursing interventions are more complicated; they may involve new ways of interacting with patients or new approaches to organizing the delivery of care. At the end of the experiment, even when hypothesized results are obtained, people may ask, What was it that really caused the group differences? In-depth qualitative data may help researchers to address the **black box** question—understanding what it is about the intervention that is driving observed effects. Also, mixed method approaches are sometimes useful in the early stages of an experiment or clinical trial. For example, through in-depth questioning, researchers can gather information about the feasibility and acceptability of an intervention, or about how best to promote it.

Example of qualitative data collection in a clinical trial

Majumdar, Browne, Roberts, and Carpio (2004) conducted a randomized clinical trial to determine the effectiveness of cultural sensitivity training on health care providers' knowledge and attitudes, and on patient satisfaction and outcomes among minority patients cared for by those with the training. The quantitative results indicated that there were several improvements for patients in the experimental group (e.g., enhanced overall functional capacity). During the study, participating nurses kept personal journals that were analyzed qualitatively. These data suggested that the training was successful in increasing cultural awareness.

CRITIQUING STUDIES DESCRIBED IN THIS CHAPTER

It is somewhat difficult to provide guidance on critiquing the types of studies described in this chapter because they are so diverse and because many of the fundamental methodologic issues that would be critiqued concern the overall design. Table 11.1 provides a very crude guide to the types of quantitative research designs that are usually considered appropriate for the various types of studies described in this chapter. Note that qualitative approaches could be integrated as an adjunct in *any* of these types in a mixed method study, and in some cases (e.g., a process analysis), qualitative data could be collected exclusively in lieu of quantitative data. Despite the limitations of the table, you can see, for example, that an impact analysis or Phase III clinical trial that used a preexperimental design would be problematic.

TABLE 11.1	Guide to Study Types and Quantitative Research Designs
TYPE OF STUDY	**USUAL TYPE OF QUANTITATIVE DESIGN**
Clinical trial	
Phase I	Preexperimental, nonexperimental*
Phase II	Small-scale experimental, quasi-experimental
Phase III	Experimental
Phase IV	Nonexperimental, preexperimental, quasi-experimental
Evaluation	
Process analysis	Nonexperimental*
Outcome analysis	Preexperimental
Impact analysis	Experimental, quasi-experimental
Cost–benefit analysis	Experimental, quasi-experimental
Outcomes research	Nonexperimental,* preexperimental, quasi-experimental, experimental
Survey	Nonexperimental
Case study	Nonexperimental*
Secondary analysis	Nonexperimental*
Methodologic	Nonexperimental, preexperimental, quasi-experimental, experimental*

*Information collected could be qualitative data rather than quantitative data. In deliberately mixed method studies, both qualitative and quantitative data could be gathered for *any* of these types of study.

You should also consider whether researchers took appropriate advantage of the possibilities of a mixed method design. Collecting both qualitative and quantitative data is not always necessary or practical, but in critiquing studies, you can consider whether the study would have been strengthened by triangulating different types of data. In studies in which mixed methods were used, you should carefully consider whether the inclusion of both types of data was justified and whether the researcher really made use of both types of data to enhance knowledge on the research topic.

Box 11.1 offers a few specific questions for critiquing the types of studies included in this chapter.

 BOX 11.1   **Guidelines for Critiquing Studies Described in This Chapter**

1. Does the study purpose match the study design? Was the best possible design (or research tradition) used to address the study purpose?
2. Is the study exclusively qualitative or exclusively quantitative? If so, could the study have been strengthened by including both types of data?
3. If both qualitative and quantitative data were collected, was the use of both types justified? How (if at all) did the inclusion of both types of data strengthen the study and further the aims of the research?

RESEARCH EXAMPLES Critical Thinking Activities

 EXAMPLE 1: Mixed Method Research—Survey and Qualitative Inquiry

Aspects of a coordinated series of studies on ovarian cancer using qualitative and quantitative approaches by a team of nurse researchers from Toronto are presented below, followed by some questions to guide critical thinking.

Studies
Qualitative: "Women's experience with recurrent ovarian cancer" (Howell, Fitch, & Deane, 2003a); "Impact of ovarian cancer perceived by women" (Howell, Fitch, & Deane, 2003b); "Living with ovarian cancer: Women's perspectives on treatment and treatment decision-making" (Fitch, Deane, & Howell, 2003)
 Quantitative: "Canadian women's perspectives on ovarian cancer" (Fitch, Gray, DePetrillo, Franssen, & Howell, 1999); "Women's perspectives regarding the impact of ovarian cancer: Implications for nursing" (Fitch, Gray, & Franssen, 2000)

Statement of Purpose
The overall project involved gathering information about the experiences of women with a diagnosis of ovarian cancer.

Method
The researchers began by gathering qualitative data through face-to-face interviews with women with ovarian cancer. The 18 study participants were recruited through nurses and gynaecologists at two cancer centres and through an ovarian cancer support group. The in-depth interviews included questions about the women's experiences with diagnosis and treatment, therapy choice decisions, changes in lifestyle, and the acquisition of information and supportive care. The qualitative findings provided the basis for developing a cross-sectional survey of the ovarian cancer experience. In this part of the project, 26 cancer programs throughout Canada agreed to distribute questionnaire packets to women with ovarian cancer who could speak either English or French. Questionnaires were returned in the mail by 315 women, who represented all Canadian provinces and territories. The structured questions in the survey concerned many of the same issues covered in the in-depth interviews.

Key Findings
The research team's reports based on these studies lay the foundation for improved care and support for women with ovarian cancer. The survey data were used to describe problems the women experienced (Fitch et al., 1999) and to compare the experiences of women who had versus those who did not have recurrent disease (Fitch et al., 2000). One qualitative report probed more deeply into the experiences of women with recurrent ovarian cancer (Howell et al., 2003a), whereas another focused on the women's treatment decision making (Fitch et al., 2003). A few highlights of the findings are presented on the next page.

(Research Examples continue on page 248)

Critical Thinking Activities (continued)

▶ In the survey, the majority of women reported that their lifestyles had changed as a result of the disease; nearly half reported sleeping difficulties, and 58% reported treatment side effects.

▶ One of the themes in the qualitative analysis was that the women, who were aware of the risk of recurrence, went through a frightening stage of waiting for the recurrence; follow-up medical visits were seen as a fearful experience.

▶ In the paper on treatment decision making, women described how personal involvement with treatment decisions tended to be minimal, and that initial treatment plans were overwhelming.

*Critical Thinking Suggestions**
*See the Student Resource CD-ROM for a discussion of these questions.

1. Answer the questions from Box 11.1 regarding this study.

2. Also consider the following targeted questions, which may assist you in further assessing aspects of the study:

  a. Comment on the researchers' decision to collect survey data by a self-administered questionnaire distributed through the mail.

  b. Comment on the sequencing of the survey and the in-depth interviews.

3. If the results of this study are valid and trustworthy, what are some of the uses to which the findings might be put in clinical practice?

 EXAMPLE 2: Mixed Method Study: Randomized Clinical Trial and In-Depth Interviews

Aspects of a mixed method nursing study, featuring terms and concepts discussed in this chapter, are presented below, followed by some questions to guide critical thinking. (The research report is included in an appendix of the associated *Study Guide to Accompany Essentials of Nursing Research,* 6th edition.)

Study
"A randomized control trial of nursing-based case management for patients with chronic obstructive pulmonary disease" (Egan, Clavarino, Burridge, Teuwen, & White, 2002)

Statement of Purpose
The main purpose of the study was to test the effectiveness of nursing-based case management for patients with chronic obstructive pulmonary disease (COPD). The study also investigated issues relating to the implementation of the intervention and satisfaction with it among patients, caregivers, and health care staff.

Method
A sample of 66 hospitalized patients with COPD in Brisbane, Australia were randomly assigned to either an intervention group (which received individualized nursing-based case management during and after hospitalization over a 6-week period) or a control group (which received normal care). The following outcomes

Critical Thinking Activities (continued)

were measured upon admission and then 1 and 3 months after discharge: health-related quality of life, including frequency and severity of respiratory symptoms; social support availability; anxiety; depression; and subjective well-being. Nurses in the hospital were surveyed to determine their perceptions about the case management intervention. Additionally, 2 physicians, 10 patients, and 8 caregivers of the patients were interviewed in depth regarding their experiences during the study period.

Key Findings

▶ The experimental and control groups did not differ significantly in terms of unplanned readmissions, depression, symptoms, support, and subjective well-being.
▶ The in-depth interviews indicated that intervention group patients placed a high value on case management, recognizing that they had gained access to resources they otherwise would not have had.
▶ Most nursing and medical staff found case management beneficial to patients.

Critical Thinking Suggestions

1. Answer the questions from Box 11.1 regarding this study.
2. Also consider the following targeted questions, which may assist you in further assessing aspects of the study:
    a. What phase of a clinical trial would you consider this research?
    b. Would you consider this study an evaluation? Why or why not? If yes, what type of evaluation would this be?
    c. The results of the qualitative and quantitative portions of the study are not totally congruent. Why do you think that might be the case?
3. If the results of this study are valid and trustworthy, what are some of the uses to which the findings might be put in clinical practice?

CHAPTER REVIEW
Summary Points

▶ Quantitative and qualitative studies vary according to purpose as well as design and tradition. Several specific types of study are described in this chapter.
▶ **Clinical trials**—studies designed to assess the effectiveness of clinical interventions—are often designed in a series of phases. *Phase I* is designed to finalize the features of the intervention; *Phase II* involves seeking preliminary evidence of treatment effectiveness; *Phase III* is a full experimental test of the treatment, often called a **randomized clinical trial** (RCT); and *Phase IV* monitors generalizability and long-term consequences.
▶ **Evaluations,** which assess the effectiveness of a program, policy, or procedure, can answer a variety of questions. **Process** or **implementation analyses** describe the process by which a program gets implemented and how it functions in practice. **Outcome analyses** describe the status of some condition after the introduction of an intervention. **Impact analyses** test whether an intervention caused any *net effects* relative to a counterfactual. **Cost–benefit analyses** examine whether the monetary costs of a program are outweighed by benefits.

▶ **Outcomes research** is undertaken to document the quality and effectiveness of health care and nursing services. Classification systems that help to standardize descriptions of nursing actions and outcomes sensitive to nursing care can contribute to outcomes research.

▶ **Surveys** examine people's characteristics, attitudes, and intentions by asking them questions. The preferred survey method is through **personal interviews**, in which interviewers meet respondents face-to-face and question them. **Telephone interviews** are more economical, but are not suitable for lengthy surveys or for ones with sensitive questions. **Questionnaires** are self-administered; that is, questions are read by respondents, who then give written responses.

▶ **Case studies** are intensive investigations of a single entity or small number of entities (e.g., people, organizations). Such studies, which can be qualitative or quantitative, typically involve data collection over an extended period.

▶ **Secondary analysis** refers to studies in which researchers analyze previously collected data—either qualitative or quantitative. Secondary analysts may examine unanalyzed concepts, focus on a particular subsample, or change the **unit of analysis**.

▶ In **methodologic research**, investigators are concerned with the development and assessment of methodologic tools or strategies.

▶ **Mixed method** (or **multimethod**) **research,** the blending of qualitative and quantitative data in a single project, can be advantageous in developing an evidence base for nursing practice. Qualitative and quantitative methods have complementary strengths and weaknesses, and an integrated approach can lead to theoretical and substantive insights.

▶ In nursing, one of the most frequent uses of multimethod research has been in the area of instrument development and refinement. Qualitative data are also used to illustrate, clarify, or amplify the meaning of quantified descriptions or relationships. Multimethod studies can help to interpret relationships and can also be used to generate and test hypotheses.

▶ Researchers can implement a multimethod study in a variety of ways, including the use of qualitative data as an adjunct in clinical trials, experimental evaluations, and surveys. The collection of quantitative data within the context of a primarily qualitative study is somewhat less common, but is most likely to happen in ethnographies.

Additional Resources for Review

Chapter 11 of the *Study Guide to Accompany Essentials of Nursing Research,* 6th edition offers various exercises and study suggestions for reinforcing the concepts presented in this chapter. For additional review, see the Student Self-Study Review Questions section of the Student Resource CD-ROM provided with this book.

SUGGESTED READINGS

*References for studies cited in the chapter appear at the end of the book.

Methodologic References

Johnson, M., & Maas, M. (1998). The nursing outcomes classification. *Journal of Nursing Care Quality, 12,* 9–20.

Morse, J. M. (1991). Approaches to qualitative-quantitative methodological triangulation. *Nursing Research, 40,* 120–122.

Sandelowski, M. (2000). Combining qualitative and quantitative sampling, data collection, and analysis techniques in mixed-method studies. *Research in Nursing & Health, 23,* 246–255.

Sidani, S., Doran, D. M., & Mitchell, P. H. (2004). A theory-driven approach to evaluating quality of nursing care. *Journal of Nursing Scholarship, 36,* 60–65.

Sidani, S., & Epstein, D. R. (2003). Enhancing the evaluation of nursing care effectiveness. *Canadian Journal of Nursing Research, 35*(3), 26–38.

Examining Sampling Plans

STUDENT OBJECTIVES

On completing this chapter, you will be able to:

▶ Describe the rationale for sampling in research
▶ Identify differences in the logic and evaluation criteria used in sampling for quantitative versus qualitative studies
▶ Distinguish between nonprobability and probability samples and compare their advantages and disadvantages
▶ Identify several types of sampling in qualitative and quantitative studies and describe their main characteristics
▶ Evaluate the appropriateness of the sampling method and sample size used in a study
▶ Define new terms in the chapter

Sampling is a process familiar to all of us—we gather information, make decisions, and formulate predictions about phenomena based on contact with a limited portion of them. Researchers, too, draw conclusions from samples. In testing the efficacy of a nursing intervention for patients with cancer, nurse researchers reach conclusions without testing the intervention with every victim of the disease. However, researchers cannot afford to draw conclusions about nursing interventions and health-related phenomena based on flawed samples. The consequences of faulty inferences are more vital in professional decisions than in private ones.

BASIC SAMPLING CONCEPTS

Sampling is an important step in the research process. In quantitative studies in particular, the findings can be seriously compromised by sampling inadequacies. Let us first consider some terms associated with sampling—terms that are used primarily (but not exclusively) in connection with quantitative studies.

Populations

A **population** is the entire aggregation of cases that meet specified criteria. For instance, if a researcher were studying Canadian nurses with doctoral degrees, the population could be defined as all Canadian citizens who are RNs and who have acquired a DNSc, PhD, or other doctoral-level degree. Other possible populations might be all cardiac patients hospitalized in University of Alberta Hospital in 2004; all individuals diagnosed with schizophrenia in Calgary; or all children in New Brunswick with leukemia. Thus, a population may be broadly defined, involving millions of people, or narrowly specified to include a few hundred people.

Populations are not restricted to human subjects. A population might consist of all the shift reports from the Shriners Hospital from 2001 to 2004, or all the Canadian high schools with a clinic that dispenses contraceptives. Whatever the basic unit, the population comprises the aggregate of entities in which a researcher is interested.

Quantitative researchers (and sometimes qualitative researchers) specify the characteristics that delimit the study population through the **eligibility criteria** (or *inclusion criteria*). For example, consider the population of Canadian nursing students.

Example of eligibility criteria in a quantitative study

Momtahan, Berkman, Sellick, Kearns, and Lauzon (2004) studied cardiac patients' understanding of cardiac risk factors. Patients who were hospitalized at the University of Ottawa Heart Institute were invited to participate in the study, unless they were deemed ineligible according to the following exclusion criteria: (1) not literate in French or English; (2) too confused or too ill to participate; and (3) too close in time to a procedure or operation.

Example of eligibility criteria in a qualitative study

Doiron-Maillet and Meagher-Stewart (2003) conducted a qualitative study of women's experiences following a myocardial infarction (MI). The eligibility criteria for the study included (1) female, less than 61 years of age; (2) experienced a complicated or uncomplicated MI; (3) functioning at cardiac activity level IV or V; (4) resident of New Brunswick; and (5) able to give informed consent.

Would this population include part-time students? Would RNs returning to school for a bachelor's degree be included? Researchers establish these criteria to determine whether a person qualifies as a member of the population. Readers of research reports need to know the eligibility criteria to understand the population to which the findings apply. Sometimes a population is defined in terms of traits that people must *not* possess through *exclusion criteria* (e.g., the population may be defined to exclude people who do not speak English).

Quantitative researchers sample from an accessible population in the hope of generalizing to a target population. The **target population** is the entire population in which a researcher is interested. The **accessible population** comprises cases from the target population that are accessible to the researcher as a pool of subjects. For example, the researcher's target population might consist of all patients with diabetes in Canada, but, in reality, the population that is accessible to him or her might consist of patients with diabetes who receive health care at a particular clinic.

CONSUMER TIP

The development of an evidence-based practice is dependent on good information about the population about whom research has been conducted. Many quantitative researchers fail to identify their target populations, or to discuss the issue of the generalizability of their findings. Researchers should clearly identify their populations so that users will know whether the findings have external validity and are relevant to groups with whom they work. ▬

Samples and Sampling

Sampling is the process of selecting a portion of the population to represent the entire population. A **sample,** then, is a subset of the population. The entities that make up the samples and populations are *elements*. In nursing research, the elements are usually humans.

Researchers work with samples rather than with populations because it is more practical to do so. Researchers have neither the time nor the resources to study all members of a population. Furthermore, it is unnecessary to study everyone because it is usually possible to obtain reasonably good information from a sample.

Still, information from samples can lead to erroneous conclusions. In quantitative studies, *the overriding criterion of adequacy is a sample's representativeness*—the extent to which the sample is similar to the population. Unfortunately, there is no method for ensuring that a sample is representative. Certain sampling plans are less likely to result in biased samples than others, but there is never a guarantee of a representative sample. Researchers operate under conditions in which error is possible, but quantitative researchers strive to minimize or control those errors. Consumers must assess their success in having done so—their success in minimizing sampling bias.

Sampling bias is the systematic overrepresentation or underrepresentation of some segment of the population in terms of a characteristic relevant to the research question. Sampling bias is affected by many things, including the homogeneity of the population. If the elements in a population were all identical on the critical attribute, any sample would be as good as any other. Indeed, if the population exhibited no variability at all, a single element would be a sufficient sample for drawing conclusions about the population. For many physical or physiologic attributes, it may be safe to assume a reasonable degree of homogeneity. For example, the blood in a person's veins is relatively homogeneous; hence, a single blood sample chosen haphazardly from a patient is adequate for clinical purposes. Most human attributes, however, are not homogeneous. Variables, after all, derive their name from the fact that traits vary from one person to the next. Age, blood pressure, and stress level, for example, are all attributes that reflect human heterogeneity.

Strata

Populations consist of subpopulations, or **strata.** Strata are mutually exclusive segments of a population based on a specific trait. For instance, a population consisting of all RNs in Ontario could be divided into two strata based on gender. Strata are used in the sample selection process in quantitative studies to enhance the sample's representativeness.

CONSUMER TIP

The sampling plan is usually discussed in a report's method section, sometimes in a subsection called "Sample," "Subjects," or "Participants." A description of sample characteristics, however, may be reported in the results section. If researchers have undertaken analyses to detect sample biases, these may be described in either the method or results section (e.g., researchers might compare the characteristics of patients who were invited to participate in the study but who declined to do so with those of patients who actually became subjects).

SAMPLING DESIGNS IN QUANTITATIVE STUDIES

Quantitative and qualitative researchers have different approaches to sampling. Quantitative researchers develop a sampling plan before data collection begins, with the goals of achieving statistical conclusion validity and generalizing their results to a population. Qualitative researchers, by contrast, focus on achieving an in-depth, holistic understanding of the phenomenon of interest. They allow sampling decisions to emerge during the course of data collection based on informational needs. This section discusses sampling strategies used by quantitative researchers, and the next section focuses on sampling in qualitative investigations.

The two main sampling design issues in quantitative studies are how the sample is selected and how many elements are included. There are two broad types of sampling designs in quantitative research: probability sampling and nonprobability sampling.

Nonprobability Sampling

In **nonprobability sampling**, researchers select elements by nonrandom methods. There is no way to estimate the probability of including each element in a nonprobability sample, and every element does *not* have a chance for inclusion. Three methods of nonprobability sampling used in quantitative studies are convenience, quota, and purposive sampling.

CONVENIENCE AND SNOWBALL SAMPLING

Convenience sampling (or *accidental sampling*) entails using the most conveniently available people as participants. A nurse who distributes questionnaires about vitamin use to the first 100 available community-dwelling elders is using a convenience sample. The problem with convenience sampling is that available subjects might be atypical of the population; therefore, the price of convenience is the risk of bias.

Another type of convenience sampling is **snowball sampling** (or *network sampling* or *chain sampling*). With this approach, early sample members are asked to refer others who meet the eligibility criteria. This method of sampling is often used when the population consists of people with specific traits who might be difficult to identify by ordinary means (e.g., people who are afraid of hospitals).

Convenience sampling is the weakest (but most widely used) form of sampling for quantitative studies. In heterogeneous populations, there is no other sampling method in which the risk of bias is greater—and there is no way to evaluate the biases. Caution is needed in interpreting findings and generalizing results from quantitative studies based on convenience samples.

Example of a convenience sample

Roshkov and Jensen (2004) studied the intensity and quality of pain experienced during the removal of temporary epicardial pacing wires in coronary artery bypass graft (CABG) patients. Their study was done with a convenience sample of 100 CABG patients.

QUOTA SAMPLING

In **quota sampling,** researchers identify strata of the population and then determine how many participants are needed from each stratum to meet a quota. By using information about population characteristics, researchers can ensure that diverse segments are represented.

As an example, suppose we were interested in studying the attitudes of undergraduate nursing students toward working on an AIDS unit. The accessible population is a nursing school with an enrolment of 500 undergraduates; a sample size of 100 students is desired. With a convenience sample, we could distribute questionnaires to 100 students as they entered the nursing school library. Suppose, however, that we suspect that male and female students have different attitudes toward working with AIDS victims. A convenience sample might result in too many men, or too few. Table 12.1 presents some fictitious data showing the gender distribution for the population and for a convenience sample (second and third columns). In this example, the convenience sample seriously overrepresents

TABLE 12.1	Numbers and Percentages of Students in Strata of a Population, Convenience Sample, and Quota Sample		
STRATA	**POPULATION**	**CONVENIENCE SAMPLE**	**QUOTA SAMPLE**
Male	100 (20%)	5 (5%)	20 (20%)
Female	400 (80%)	95 (95%)	80 (80%)
Total	500 (100%)	100 (100%)	100 (100%)

women and underrepresents men. In a quota sample, researchers can guide the selection of subjects so that the sample includes an appropriate number of cases from both strata. The far-right panel of Table 12.1 shows the number of men and women required for a quota sample for this example.

If we pursue this example a bit further, you may better appreciate the dangers of a biased sample. Suppose a key question in this study was: Would you be willing to work on a unit that cared exclusively for patients with AIDS? The percentage of students in the population who would respond "yes" to this question is shown in the first column of Table 12.2. Of course, these values would not be known; they are displayed to illustrate a point. Within the population, males are more likely than females to express willingness to work on an AIDS unit, yet men were underrepresented in the convenience sample. As a result, there is a notable discrepancy between the population and sample values: nearly twice as many students in the population are favourable toward working with AIDS victims (20%) than in the convenience sample (11%). The quota sample, on the other hand, does a reasonably good job of reflecting the population's views.

Except for identifying key strata, quota sampling is similar to convenience sampling: subjects are a convenience sample from each population stratum. Because of this fact, quota sampling shares many of the weaknesses of convenience sampling. For instance, if we were required by the quota sampling plan to interview 20 male nursing students, a trip to the dormitories might be a convenient method of recruiting those subjects. Yet this approach would fail to give any representation to male students living off campus, who may have distinctive views about working with patients with AIDS. Despite its problems, however,

TABLE 12.2	Students Willing to Work on AIDS Unit: Population, Convenience Sample, and Quota Sample		
	NUMBER IN POPULATION	**NUMBER IN CONVENIENCE SAMPLE**	**NUMBER IN QUOTA SAMPLE**
Willing males	28 (out of 100)	2 (out of 5)	6 (out of 20)
Willing females	72 (out of 400)	9 (out of 95)	13 (out of 80)
Total number of willing students	100 (out of 500)	11 (out of 100)	19 (out of 100)
Percentage willing	20%	11%	19%

quota sampling is an important improvement over convenience sampling. Quota sampling is a relatively easy way to enhance the representativeness of a nonprobability sample, and does not require sophisticated skills. Surprisingly, few researchers use this strategy.

Example of a quota sample

Kaasalainen and Crook (2004) conducted a study to evaluate the ability of elderly residents of a long-term care facility to report pain. Their sample of 130 residents was stratified according to their level of cognitive impairment (cognitively intact, mild impairment, moderate impairment, and extreme impairment).

PURPOSIVE SAMPLING

Purposive sampling (or *judgmental sampling*) is based on the belief that researchers' knowledge about the population can be used to hand pick the cases (or types of cases) to be included in the sample. Researchers might decide purposely to select the widest possible variety of respondents or might choose subjects who are judged to be typical of the population in question or knowledgeable about the issues under study. Sampling in this subjective manner, however, provides no external, objective method for assessing the typicality of the selected subjects. Nevertheless, this method can be used to advantage in certain instances. For example, sometimes researchers want to ask questions of a group of experts. Also, as discussed in a later section, purposive sampling is often used productively by qualitative researchers.

Example of a purposive sample

Gagnon and Grenier (2004) conducted a study to identify, validate, and rank order quality care indicators relating to empowerment for patients with a chronic complex illness. One phase of their study involved gathering quantitative information from a purposive sample of nurses and other health care professionals selected for their expertise—at least 5 years' experience working with patients with chronic illness.

EVALUATION OF NONPROBABILITY SAMPLING

Nonprobability samples are rarely representative of the target population—some segment of the population is likely to be systematically underrepresented. And, when there is sampling bias, there is a good chance that the results will be misleading. Why, then, are nonprobability samples used at all in quantitative research? Clearly, the advantage of these designs lies in their convenience and economy. Probability sampling requires resources and time. There may be no option but to use a nonprobability sampling plan. Researchers using a nonprobability sample out of necessity should be cautious about their conclusions, and you as reader should be alert to the possibility of sampling bias.

HOW-TO-TELL TIP

How can you tell what type of sampling design was used in a quantitative study? Researchers who have made explicit efforts to achieve a representative sample usually indicate the type of sampling design used. If the sampling design is not specified, it is probably safe to assume that a sample of convenience was used.　■

Probability Sampling

Probability sampling involves the random selection of elements from the population. *Random selection* should not be confused with *random assignment*, which was described in Chapter 9. Random assignment is the process of allocating subjects to different treatments on a random basis in experimental designs. Random assignment has no bearing on how subjects in the experiment were selected in the first place. A **random selection** process is one in which each element in the population has an equal, independent chance of being selected. Because probability samples involve selecting units at random, some confidence can be placed in their representativeness. The four most commonly used probability sampling designs are simple random, stratified random, cluster, and systematic sampling.

SIMPLE RANDOM SAMPLING

Simple random sampling is the most basic probability sampling design. Because more complex probability sampling designs incorporate features of simple random sampling, the procedures are briefly described so that you can understand what is involved.

After defining the population, researchers establish a *sampling frame*, the technical name for the actual list of population elements. If nursing students at McGill University were the accessible population, then a student roster would be the sampling frame. If the population were 300-bed or larger hospitals in Ontario, then a list of all those hospitals would be the sampling frame. Populations are sometimes defined in terms of an existing sampling frame. For example, a researcher might use a telephone directory as a sampling frame. In such a case, the population would be defined as the residents of a certain community who have listed telephone numbers. After a list of population elements has been developed, the elements are numbered consecutively. A table of random numbers or a computer program is then used to draw, at random, a sample of the desired size.

Samples selected randomly in such a fashion are not subject to researcher biases. There is no *guarantee* that the sample will be representative of the population, but random selection does guarantee that differences between the sample and the population are purely a function of chance. The probability of selecting a deviant sample through random sampling is low, and this probability decreases as the sample size increases.

Simple random sampling is a laborious process. The development of the sampling frame, enumeration of the elements, and selection of the sample are time-consuming chores, particularly with a large population. Moreover, it is rarely possible to get a complete listing of population elements; hence, other methods are often used.

Example of a random sample

Patterson, Kaczorowski, Arthur, Smith, and Mills (2003) conducted a study to identify the clinical role functions of advanced practice nurses (ANPs) with respect to complementary therapies. Questionnaires were mailed to a random sample of 389 ANPs registered with the College of Nurses of Ontario.

STRATIFIED RANDOM SAMPLING

In **stratified random sampling,** the population is divided into homogeneous subsets from which elements are selected at random. As in quota sampling, the aim of stratified sampling is to enhance the sample's representativeness. The most common procedure for drawing a stratified random sample is to group together those elements that belong to a stratum and to randomly select the desired number of elements.

Researchers may sample either proportionately (in relation to the size of the stratum) or disproportionately. If a population of students in a nursing school in Canada consisted of 10% Asian, 5% Aboriginals, and 85% whites, a **proportionate sample** of 100 students, stratified on race/ethnicity, would consist of 10, 5, and 85 students from the respective strata. Researchers often use a **disproportionate sample** whenever comparisons between strata of unequal size are desired. In our example, the researcher might select 20 Asian, 20 Aboriginal, and 60 whites to ensure a more adequate representation of the viewpoints of the two racial minorities. (When disproportionate sampling is used, however, it is necessary to make a mathematic adjustment—**weighting**—to arrive at the best estimate of overall population values.)

By using stratified random sampling, researchers can sharpen the representativeness of their samples. Stratified sampling may, however, be impossible if information on the stratifying variables is unavailable (e.g., a student roster might not include information on race and ethnicity). Furthermore, a stratified sample requires even more labour than simple random sampling because the sample must be drawn from multiple enumerated listings.

Example of a stratified random sample

Minore, Boone, and Hill (2004) conducted a survey of nurses to explore the viability of establishing a relief pool of nurses to serve the aboriginal communities of northwestern Ontario. A stratified random sample was drawn from 1126 registrants of the College of Nurses of Ontario who lived in the targeted communities. A proportionate sample of 622 nurses from the population, with nursing preparation as the stratifying variable, was drawn: 170 BScN nurses and 452 diploma RNs.

CLUSTER SAMPLING

For many populations, it is impossible to obtain a listing of all elements. For example, there is no listing of all full-time nursing students in Canada. Large-scale studies rarely use simple or stratified random sampling. The most common procedure for national surveys is cluster sampling.

In **cluster sampling,** there is a successive random sampling of units. The first unit to be sampled is large groupings, or clusters. For example, in drawing a sample of nursing students, researchers might first draw a random sample of nursing schools and then sample students from the selected schools. The usual procedure for selecting samples from a general population is to sample such administrative units as provinces, cities, census tracts, and then households, successively. Because of the successive stages of sampling, this approach is sometimes referred to as *multistage sampling.*

For a specified number of cases, cluster sampling tends to contain more sampling error than simple or stratified random sampling. Nevertheless, cluster sampling is more economical and practical when the population is large and widely dispersed.

Example of a cluster/multistage sample

Durbin, Goering, Streiner, and Pink (2004) studied continuity of mental health care through a survey of users of community and outpatient mental health programs. To select a sample, they first drew a random sample of clients, stratified by program, from staff assessments (2293 assessments). From the staff assessment sample, they randomly sampled 432 clients for a self-report survey.

SYSTEMATIC SAMPLING

Systematic sampling involves the selection of every kth case from a list or group, such as every 10th person on a patient list. Systematic sampling can be applied in such a way that an essentially random sample is drawn. First, the size of the population is divided by the size of the desired sample to obtain the sampling interval width. The *sampling interval* is the standard distance between the selected elements. For instance, if we wanted a sample of 50 from a population of 5000, our sampling interval would be 100 (5000/50 = 100). In other words, every 100th case would be sampled. Next, the first case would be selected randomly (e.g., by using a table of random numbers). If the random number chosen were 73, the people corresponding to numbers 73, 173, 273, and so forth would be included in the sample. Systematic sampling conducted this way is essentially identical to simple random sampling and is often preferable because of its convenience.

Example of a systematic random sample

Then, Rankin, and Fofonoff (2001) compared the clinical manifestations of first-time myocardial infarction in three groups of men and women who presented to the emergency departments of three acute tertiary care hospitals. Phase I of the study involved a retrospective review of a systematic random sample of 153 patient charts.

EVALUATION OF PROBABILITY SAMPLING

Probability sampling is the only reliable method of obtaining representativeness because it avoids the risk of conscious or unconscious biases. If all the elements in the population have an equal probability of being selected, there is a high likelihood that the sample will represent the population adequately. Probability sampling also allows researchers to estimate the magnitude of sampling error. **Sampling error** is the difference between population values (e.g., the average heart rate of the population) and sample values (e.g., the average heart rate of the sample). It is rare that a sample is perfectly representative of a population and contains no sampling error; however, probability sampling permits estimates of the degree of expected error. On the other hand, probability sampling is expensive and demanding. Unless the population is narrowly defined, it is beyond the scope of most researchers to draw a probability sample.

CONSUMER TIP

The quality of the sampling plan is of particular importance in survey research because the purpose of surveys is to obtain descriptive information about the prevalence or average values for a population. All national surveys, such as the National Population Health Survey in Canada, use probability samples (usually multistage samples). Probability samples are rarely used in experimental and quasi-experimental studies, in part because the main focus of such inquiries is on between-group differences rather than absolute values for a population. ■

Sample Size in Quantitative Studies

Sample size—the number of subjects in a sample—is a major issue in quantitative research. There is no simple equation to determine how large a sample is needed, but quantitative researchers are generally advised to use the largest sample possible. The larger the sample, the more representative it is likely to be. Every time researchers calculate a percentage or an average based on sample data, the purpose is to estimate a population value. The larger the sample, the smaller the sampling error.

Let us illustrate this with an example of estimating monthly aspirin consumption in a nursing home. The population is 15 nursing home residents whose aspirin consumption averages 16 per month. Two simple random samples with sample sizes of 2, 3, 5, and 10 were drawn from this population (Table 12.3). Each sample average on the right represents an estimate of the population average, which we know is 16. (Under ordinary circumstances, the population value would be unknown, and we would draw only one sample.) With a sample size of 2, our estimate might have been wrong by as many as 8 aspirins (sample 1B). As the sample size increases, the average gets closer to the population value, *and* differences in the estimates between samples A and B get smaller. As the sample size increases, the probability of getting a deviant sample diminishes because large samples provide the opportunity to counterbalance atypical values.

Sophisticated researchers estimate how large their samples should be to test their research hypotheses adequately through **power analysis** (Cohen, 1988). A simple example can illustrate basic principles of power analysis. Suppose we were testing an intervention to

TABLE 12.3	Comparison of Population and Sample Values and Averages in Nursing Home Aspirin Consumption Example		

NUMBER IN GROUP	GROUP	VALUES (MONTHLY NUMBER OF ASPIRINS CONSUMED)	AVERAGE
15	Population	2, 4, 6, 8, 10, 12, 14, 16, 18, 20, 22, 24 26, 28, 30	16.0
2	Sample 1A	6, 14	10.0
2	Sample 1B	20, 28	24.0
3	Sample 2A	16, 18, 8	14.0
3	Sample 2B	20, 14, 26	20.0
5	Sample 3A	26, 14, 18, 2, 28	17.6
5	Sample 3B	30, 2, 26, 10, 4	14.4
10	Sample 4A	18, 16, 24, 22, 8, 14, 28, 20, 2, 6	15.8
10	Sample 4B	14, 18, 12, 20, 6, 14, 28, 12, 24, 16	16.4

help people quit smoking; we assign smokers randomly to either an experimental or a control group. How many subjects should we use in this study? When using power analysis, researchers estimate how big group differences will be on the outcomes (e.g., the difference in the average number of cigarettes smoked a week after the intervention). The estimate might be based on previous research, on our personal experience, or on other factors. When expected differences are large, it does not take a large sample to ensure that the differences will be revealed in a statistical analysis; but when small differences are predicted, large samples are needed. Cohen (1988) claimed that, for new areas of research, group differences are likely to be small. In our example, if we expected a small group difference in postintervention smoking, the sample size needed to test the effectiveness of the new program, assuming standard statistical criteria, would be about 800 smokers (400 per group). If a medium-sized difference were expected, the total sample size would still need to be several hundred smokers.

When samples are too small, researchers run the risk of gathering data that will not support their hypotheses—even when those hypotheses are correct. This poses a potential threat to the study's statistical conclusion validity. Large samples are no assurance of accuracy, however. With nonprobability sampling, even a large sample can harbour extensive bias. The famous example from the United States illustrating this point is the 1936 U.S. presidential poll conducted by the magazine *Literary Digest,* which predicted that Alfred M. Landon would defeat Franklin D. Roosevelt by a landslide. An extremely large sample—about 2.5 million people—participated in this poll, but biases arose because the sample was drawn from telephone directories and automobile registrations during a Depression year when only the well-to-do (who favoured Landon) had a car or telephone.

A large sample cannot correct for a faulty sampling design; nevertheless, a large nonprobability sample is preferable to a small one. When critiquing quantitative studies, you must assess both the sample size and the sample selection method to judge how representative the sample likely was.

CONSUMER TIP

The sampling plan is often one of the weakest aspects of quantitative research. Most nursing studies use samples of convenience, and many are based on samples that are too small to provide an adequate test of the hypotheses. Most quantitative studies are based on samples of fewer than 200 participants, and a great many studies have fewer than 100 participants. Power analysis is not used by many nurse researchers, and research reports typically offer no justification for the size of the study sample. Small samples run a high risk of leading researchers to erroneously reject their research hypotheses. Therefore, you should be especially prepared to critique the sampling plan of studies that fail to support research hypotheses.

SAMPLING IN QUALITATIVE RESEARCH

Qualitative studies typically use small, nonrandom samples. This does not mean that qualitative researchers are unconcerned with the quality of their samples, but rather that they use different criteria for selecting participants. This section examines sampling considerations in qualitative studies.

The Logic of Qualitative Sampling

Quantitative research is concerned with measuring attributes and relationships in a population, and therefore a representative sample is needed to ensure that the measurements accurately reflect and can be generalized to the population. The aim of most qualitative studies is to discover meaning and to uncover multiple realities; therefore, generalizability, as quantitative researchers use this term, is not a guiding criterion.

Qualitative researchers ask such sampling questions as: Who would be an information-rich data source for my study? Whom should I talk to, or what should I observe, to maximize my understanding of the phenomenon? A critical first step in qualitative sampling is selecting settings with high potential for "information richness."

As the study progresses, new sampling questions emerge, such as the following: Whom can I talk to or observe to confirm my understandings? To challenge, modify, or enrich my understandings? Thus, as with the overall design in qualitative studies, sampling design is an emergent one that capitalizes on early learning to guide subsequent direction.

Types of Qualitative Sampling

Qualitative researchers usually eschew probability samples. A random sample is not the best method of selecting people who will make good informants—people who are knowledgeable, articulate, reflective, and willing to talk at length with a researcher.

CONVENIENCE AND SNOWBALL SAMPLING

Qualitative researchers sometimes begin with a convenience sample, which is sometimes referred to as a **volunteer sample**. Volunteer samples are especially useful when researchers need participants to come forward to identify themselves (*e.g.*, by placing notices in newspapers for people with certain experiences) or when they need to rely on referrals from others.

Sampling by convenience is efficient, but it is not usually a preferred sampling approach, even in qualitative studies. The key aim in qualitative studies is to extract the greatest possible information from the small number of informants in the sample, and a convenience sample may not provide the most information-rich sources. Convenience sampling is frequently used as a way to begin the sampling process.

Qualitative researchers also use snowball sampling (or *nominated sampling*), asking early informants to make referrals for other study participants. Researchers may use this method to gain access to people who are difficult to identify. A weakness of this approach is that the eventual sample might be restricted to a rather small network of acquaintances. Moreover, the quality of the referrals may be affected by whether the referring sample member trusted the researcher and truly wanted to cooperate.

Example of a snowball sample

Hall and Callery (2003) conducted an international study (in Canada and the United Kingdom) of the manner in which dual-earner couples with preschool children manage work and family life. In Canada, the researchers first recruited couples through a hospital and municipal employers and then got additional couples through referrals from participants who had volunteered.

PURPOSIVE SAMPLING

Qualitative sampling may begin with volunteer informants and may be supplemented with new participants through snowballing, but many qualitative studies eventually evolve to a purposive (or *purposeful*) sampling strategy—a strategy in which researchers hand pick the cases or types of cases that will best contribute to the information needs of the study. Qualitative researchers often strive to select sample members purposefully based on the information needs emerging from the early findings: whom to sample next depends on who has been sampled already.

Example of a purposive sample

Tweedell, Forchuk, Jewell, and Steinnagel (2004) explored families' experiences relating to a family member's recovery or nonrecovery from psychosis. Their sample included nine families, many of whom had relatives whose mental illness had endured for more than a decade. The last four families were purposively chosen to include families with briefer experience (3 years or less).

Within purposive sampling, several strategies have been identified (Patton, 2002), only some of which are mentioned here. Note that researchers themselves do not necessarily refer to their sampling plans with Patton's labels; his classification shows the kind of diverse strategies qualitative researchers have adopted to meet the conceptual needs of their research:

▶ **Maximum variation sampling** involves purposefully selecting cases with a range of variation on dimensions of interest

▶ **Homogeneous sampling** involves a deliberate reduction of variation to permit a more focused inquiry

▶ **Extreme/deviant case sampling** provides opportunities for learning from the most unusual and extreme informants (e.g., outstanding successes and notable failures)

▶ **Typical case sampling** involves selecting participants who will illustrate or highlight what is typical or average

▶ **Criterion sampling** involves studying cases that meet a predetermined criterion of importance

Example of maximum variation sampling

Chouinard, Ntetu, Lapierre, Gagnon, and Hudon (2004) studied patients' perceptions of the nursing services they received in a cardiovascular disease prevention clinics network. Their multimethod studied involved a phenomenological component in which 19 patients were interviewed in depth. Patients were selected to ensure variation in diagnosis, gender, and length of program participation.

Maximum variation sampling is often the sampling mode of choice in qualitative research because it is useful in documenting the scope of a phenomenon and in identifying important patterns that cut across variations. Other strategies can also be used advantageously, however, depending on the nature of the research question.

CONSUMER TIP

A qualitative research report will not necessarily use such terms as "maximum variation sampling" but may describe the researcher's selection of a diverse sample of participants. ■

A strategy of sampling confirming and disconfirming cases is another purposive strategy that is used toward the end of data collection in qualitative studies. As researchers note trends and patterns in the data, emerging conceptualizations may need to be checked. **Confirming cases** are additional cases that fit researchers' conceptualizations and offer enhanced credibility. **Disconfirming cases** are new cases that do not fit and serve to challenge researchers' interpretations. These "negative" cases may offer new insights about how the original conceptualization needs to be revised or expanded.

CONSUMER TIP

Some qualitative researchers appear to call their sample purposive simply because they "purposely" selected people who experienced the phenomenon of interest. However, experience with the phenomenon is actually an eligibility criterion—the population of interest comprises people with that experience. If the researcher then recruits *any* person with that experience, the sample is selected by convenience, not purposively. Purposive sampling implies an intent to carefully choose *particular* exemplars or *types* of people who can best enhance the researcher's understanding of the phenomenon. ■

THEORETICAL SAMPLING

Theoretical sampling is a method of sampling used in grounded theory studies. Glaser (1978) defined this sampling approach as "the process of data collection for generating theory whereby the analyst jointly collects, codes, and analyzes his data and decides what data to collect next and where to find them, in order to develop his theory as it emerges" (p. 36). This complex sampling technique requires researchers to be involved with multiple lines and directions as they go back and forth between data and categories as the theory emerges.

Theoretical sampling is not the same as purposeful sampling. The purpose of theoretical sampling is to discover categories and their properties and to offer interrelationships that occur in the substantive theory. Glaser noted that the basic question in theoretical sampling is: what groups or subgroups should the researcher turn to next? The groups are chosen as they are needed for their theoretical relevance in furthering the emerging conceptualization.

Example of a theoretical sample

Beck (2002) used theoretical sampling in her grounded theory study of mothering twins during the first year of life, in which 16 mothers of twins were interviewed. An example of theoretical sampling concerned what the mothers kept referring to as the "blur period"—the first few months of caring for the twins. Initially, Beck interviewed mothers whose twins were about 1 year old. Her rationale was that these mothers would be able to reflect back over the entire first year of parenting. When these mothers referred to the "blur period," Beck asked them to describe this period more fully, but they could not provide many details because the period was "such a blur!" Beck then chose to interview mothers whose twins were 3 months old or younger, to ensure that mothers still immersed in the "blur period" would be able to provide rich detail about what this phase of mothering twins was like.

Sample Size in Qualitative Studies

There are no rules for sample size in qualitative research. Sample size is largely a function of the purpose of the inquiry, the quality of the informants, and the type of sampling strategy used. For example, a larger sample is likely to be needed with maximum variation sampling than with typical case sampling. Patton argues that purposive sample sizes should "be judged on the basis of the purpose and rationale of each study. . . . The sample, like all other aspects of qualitative inquiry, must be judged in context . . ." (2002, p. 245).

A guiding principle in qualitative sampling is **data saturation** (i.e., sampling to the point at which no new information is obtained). Information redundancy can typically be achieved with a fairly small number of cases, if the information from each is of sufficient depth. Morse (2000) noted that the number of participants needed to reach saturation depends on a number of factors. For example, the broader the scope of the research question, the more participants will likely be needed. Data quality can also affect sample size. If participants are good informants who are able to reflect on their experiences and communicate effectively, saturation can be achieved with relatively few informants. Also, if longitudinal data are collected, fewer participants may be needed because each will provide a greater amount of information. As discussed in the next section, sample size is also partly a function of the type of qualitative inquiry that is undertaken.

CONSUMER TIP

The sample size adequacy for quantitative studies can be estimated by consumers after the fact through power analysis. However, sample size adequacy in a qualitative study is more difficult to critique because redundancy of information is difficult for consumers to judge. Some qualitative reports explicitly state that data saturation was achieved. ■

Sampling in the Three Main Qualitative Traditions

There are similarities among the various qualitative traditions with regard to sampling: samples are generally small, probability sampling is almost never used, and final sampling decisions generally take place during data collection. However, there are some differences as well.

SAMPLING IN ETHNOGRAPHIC STUDIES

Ethnographers often begin by adopting a "big net" approach—that is, mingling with and having conversations with as many members of the culture under study as possible. Starting with this wide-angle lens of the culture provides ethnographers with the "lay of the land."

Although they may converse with many people (usually 25 to 50), ethnographers often rely on a smaller number of **key informants**, who are highly knowledgeable about the culture and who develop special, ongoing relationships with them. These key informants are ethnographers' main link to the "inside."

Key informants usually are chosen purposively, guided by ethnographers' informed judgments (although sampling may become more theoretical as the study progresses). Developing a pool of potential key informants often depends on ethnographers' prior knowledge to construct a relevant framework. For example, an ethnographer might make decisions about different types of key informants to seek out based on roles (e.g., physicians, nurse practitioners) or on some other theoretically meaningful distinction. Once a pool of potential key informants is developed, the main considerations for final selection are their level of knowledge about the culture and how willing they are to collaborate with the ethnographer in revealing and interpreting the culture. Ethnographers typically attempt to develop relationships with as diverse a group of informants as possible.

Sampling in ethnography typically involves more than selecting informants because observation and other data sources play a big role in helping researchers understand a culture. Ethnographers have to decide not only *whom* to sample but also *what* to sample. For example, ethnographers have to make decisions about observing *events* and *activities*, about examining *records* and *artefacts*, and about exploring *places* that provide clues about the culture. Key informants can help ethnographers decide what to sample.

Example of an ethnographic sample

Kirkham (2003) conducted an institutional ethnography, informed by feminist and cultural theories, to examine the theme of "belonging" within the social context of intercultural health care in Canada. Fieldwork was undertaken in three medical-surgical units in two hospitals. Kirkham began with a core of 11 nurses in one of the units. She then "buddied" with 20 nurses during the course of several shifts and had formal and informal interviews with them. Sampling was purposive: she sought to represent a range of nursing experiences and ethnocultural backgrounds. Kirkham also interviewed administrators and patients, as well as policy makers and educators from outside the settings.

SAMPLING IN PHENOMENOLOGICAL STUDIES

Phenomenologists tend to rely on very small samples of participants—typically 10 or fewer. There is one guiding principle in selecting the sample for a phenomenological study: all participants must have experienced the phenomenon under study and must be able to articulate what it is like to have lived that experience. Although phenomenological researchers seek participants who have had the targeted experiences, they also want to explore diversity of individual experiences. Thus, as described by Porter (1999), they may specifically look for people with demographic or other differences who have shared a common experience. To study a phenomenon of interest in depth, phenomenologists may also

Example of a sample in a phenomenological study

Struthers (2003) conducted a phenomenological study of the experience of being a traditional healer with a purposive sample of six Ojibwa and Cree indigenous women healers from Canada and the United States.

sample experiences of place and of events in time because a person's experience of the phenomenon under study is situated in a specific place and time.

Interpretive phenomenologists may, in addition to sampling people, sample artistic or literary sources. Experiential descriptions of the phenomenon may be selected from a wide array of literature, such as poetry, novels, biographies, diaries, and journals. These sources can help increase phenomenologists' insights into the phenomena under study. Art—including paintings, film, photographs, and music—is viewed as another source of lived experience by interpretive phenomenologists. Each artistic medium is viewed as having its own specific language or way of expressing the experience of the phenomenon.

SAMPLING IN GROUNDED THEORY STUDIES

Grounded theory research is typically done with samples of about 20 to 30 people, using theoretical sampling. The goal in a grounded theory study is to select informants who can best contribute to the evolving theory. Sampling, data collection, data analysis, and theory construction occur concurrently, and so study participants are selected serially and contingently—that is, contingent on the emerging conceptualization. Theoretical sampling is used to develop and refine categories. As grounded theorists identify gaps or holes in their emerging theory, they go back to the field and sample data to fill in thin areas. At this point in their research, grounded theorists become very selective in their sampling: participants are sampled only in regard to specific issues. Theoretical sampling is used not to increase the sample size but to refine the developing theory and to gain more insight into the properties of the categories. Sampling might evolve as follows:

1. The researcher begins with a general notion of where and with whom to start. The first few cases may be solicited purposively, by convenience, or through snowballing.
2. In the early part of the study, a strategy such as maximum variation sampling might be used to gain insights into the range and complexity of the phenomenon under study.
3. The sample is adjusted in an ongoing fashion. Emerging conceptualizations help to focus the sampling process to maximize understanding of the categories.
4. Sampling continues until saturation is achieved.
5. Final sampling often includes a search for confirming and disconfirming cases to test, refine, and strengthen the theory.

Example of a sample in a grounded theory study

In her grounded theory study of the evolving process of women caring for husbands with Alzheimer's disease, Perry (2002) recruited sample members from a support group, a day care centre, and diagnostic and outreach clinics. Although initial sampling was by convenience, emerging themes provided direction for theoretical sampling. For example, to better understand the evolution of what Perry called "interpretive caring" as the disease progressed, participants were sought whose husbands were in the middle or advanced stages of Alzheimer's disease.

CRITIQUING THE SAMPLING PLAN

The sampling plan of a study—particularly a quantitative study—merits particular scrutiny because, if the sample is seriously biased or too small, the findings may be misleading or just plain wrong. In critiquing a sampling plan, you should consider two issues. The first is whether the researcher has adequately described the sampling strategy. Ideally, research reports should include a description of the following aspects of the sample:

▶ The type of sampling approach used (e.g., convenience, snowball, purposive, simple random)
▶ The population under study and the eligibility criteria for sample selection in quantitative studies; the nature of the setting and study group in qualitative ones (qualitative studies may also articulate eligibility criteria)
▶ The number of participants in the study and a rationale for the sample size
▶ A description of the main characteristics of participants (e.g., age, gender, medical condition, race/ethnicity, and so forth) and, in a quantitative study, of the population
▶ In quantitative studies, the number and characteristics of potential subjects who declined to participate in the study

If the description of the sample is inadequate, you may not be in a position to deal with the second and principal issue, which is whether the researcher made good sampling decisions.

Critiquing Quantitative Sampling Plans

We have stressed that the main criterion for assessing a sampling plan in quantitative research is whether the sample is representative of the population. You will never be able to know for sure, of course, but if the sampling strategy is weak or if the sample size is small, there is reason to suspect some bias. When researchers have adopted a sampling plan in which the risk for bias is high, they should take steps to estimate the direction and degree of this bias so that readers can draw some informed conclusions.

Even with a rigourous sampling strategy, the sample may contain some bias if not all people invited to participate in a study agree to do so. If certain segments of the population refuse to participate, then a biased sample can result, even when probability sampling is used. The research report ideally should provide information about **response rates** (i.e., the number of people participating in a study relative to the number of people sampled) and about possible **nonresponse bias**—differences between participants and those who declined to participate (also sometimes referred to as *response bias*).

In developing the sampling plan, quantitative researchers make decisions about the specification of the population as well as the selection of the sample. If the target population is defined broadly, researchers may have missed opportunities to control extraneous variables, and the gap between the accessible and the target population may be too great. Your job as reviewer is to come to conclusions about the reasonableness of generalizing the findings from the researcher's sample to the accessible population and from the accessible population to a broader target population. If the sampling plan is seriously flawed, it may be risky to generalize the findings at all.

BOX 12.1   Guidelines for Critiquing Quantitative Sampling Designs

1. Is the population under study identified and described? Are eligibility criteria specified? Are the sample selection procedures clearly delineated?
2. What type of sampling plan was used? Would an alternative sampling plan have been preferable? Was the sampling plan one that could be expected to yield a representative sample?
3. How were participants recruited into the sample? Does the method suggest potential biases?
4. Did some factor other than the sampling plan (e.g., a low response rate) affect the representativeness of the sample?
5. Are possible sample biases or weaknesses identified?
6. Are key characteristics of the sample described (e.g., mean age, percent female)?
7. Is the sample size sufficiently large? Was the sample size justified on the basis of a power analysis or other rationale?
8. To whom can the study results reasonably be generalized?

Box 12.1 presents some guiding questions for critiquing the sampling plan of a quantitative research report.

Evaluating Qualitative Sampling Plans

In a qualitative study, sampling can be evaluated in terms of adequacy and appropriateness (Morse, 1991). *Adequacy* refers to the sufficiency and quality of the data the sample yielded. An adequate sample provides data without any "thin" spots. When the researcher has truly obtained saturation with a sample, informational adequacy has been achieved, and the resulting description or theory is richly textured and complete.

Appropriateness concerns the methods used to select a sample. An appropriate sample is one resulting from the identification and use of study participants who can best

BOX 12.2   Guidelines for Critiquing Qualitative Sampling Designs

1. Is the setting or context adequately described? Is the setting appropriate for the research question?
2. Are the sample selection procedures clearly delineated? What type of sampling strategy was used?
3. Were the eligibility criteria for the study specified? How were participants recruited into the study? Did the recruitment strategy yield information-rich participants?
4. Given the information needs of the study—and, if applicable, its qualitative tradition— was the sampling approach appropriate? Are dimensions of the phenomenon under study adequately represented?
5. Is the sample size adequate and appropriate for the qualitative tradition of the study? Did the researcher indicate that information redundancy had been achieved? Do the findings suggest a richly textured and comprehensive set of data without any apparent "holes" or thin areas?
6. Are key characteristics of the sample described (e.g., age, gender)? Is a rich description of participants provided, allowing for an assessment of the transferability of the findings?

supply information according to the conceptual requirements of the study. Researchers must use a strategy that will yield the fullest possible understanding of the phenomenon of interest. A sampling approach that excludes negative cases or that fails to include participants with unusual experiences may not meet the information needs of the study.

Another important issue concerns the potential for transferability of the findings. The degree of transferability of study findings is a function of the similarity between the study sample and the people at another site to which the findings might be applied. **Fittingness** is the degree of congruence between these two groups. Thus, in critiquing a report, you should see whether the researcher provided an adequately thick description of the sample, setting, and context so that someone interested in transferring the findings could make an informed decision.

Further guidance to critiquing sampling in a qualitative study is presented in Box 12.2 on page 271.

RESEARCH EXAMPLES   **Critical Thinking Activities**

 **EXAMPLE 1: Quantitative Research**

Aspects of a quantitative nursing study, featuring terms and concepts discussed in this chapter, are presented below, followed by some questions to guide critical thinking.

Study
"Level of RN educational preparation: Its impact on collaboration and the relationship between collaboration and professional identity" (Miller, 2004)

Purpose
Miller's study had two purposes: (1) to determine whether educational preparation affects nurses' perceptions of their interprofessional collaboration; and (2) to explore the relationship between such collaboration and nurses' professional identity.

Design
The researcher conducted a cross-sectional mailed survey that assessed professional identity and four dimensions of collaboration (mutual safeguarding of concerns, power/control, clarity of patient care goals, and practice spheres).

Sampling Plan
Miller drew a stratified random sample of nurses from the membership of a provincial nursing association. Using information available in the listing, she first removed association members who were deemed unlikely to interact with professionals from other disciplines in matters related to patient care (e.g., nursing education administrators, those not in the labour market). The resulting sampling frame was then stratified by highest level of nursing preparation: those with a diploma or baccalaureate degree were in one stratum, and those with a master's or doctoral degree were in another. Before randomly selecting names, Miller

Critical Thinking Activities (continued)

determined how many nurses should be included in the sample by performing a power analysis. The power analysis assumed a modest effect size and took into account the likelihood that many people would not complete a mailed survey. The sample size for each stratum was set at 400. Of the 800 surveys mailed, 379 (47%) usable questionnaires were received: 174 from the diploma/baccalaureate stratum and 205 from the master's/doctoral stratum.

Key Findings
▶ For the first three of the four dimensions of collaboration, both groups reported reasonably effective collaboration with other health professionals.
▶ Higher level of education was positively related to interprofessional collaboration.
▶ The relationship between collaboration and professional identity scores tended to be modest and mostly nonsignificant.

Critical Thinking Suggestions*
*See the Student Resource CD-ROM for a discussion of these questions.
1. Answer questions 1 through 5, 7, and 8 from Box 12.1 regarding this study.
2. Also consider the following targeted questions, which may assist you in further assessing aspects of the study:
   a. Was the sampling likely to be proportionate or disproportionate?
   b. Comment on Miller's decision to stratify the sample.
   c. Identify some of the major potential sources of bias in the final sample of 379 participants.
3. If the results of this study are valid and reliable, what are some of the uses to which the findings might be put in clinical practice?

 EXAMPLE 2: Qualitative Research

Aspects of a qualitative nursing study, featuring terms and concepts discussed in this chapter, are presented below, followed by some questions to guide critical thinking.

Study
"Precarious ordering: Toward a formal theory of women's caring" (Wuest, 2001)

Research Purpose
Wuest undertook a grounded theory study to develop a middle-range theory that captures the common processes of women's caring in a wide array of circumstances.

Method
Wuest noted that there are social and political trends that place increasing demands on women to provide care. She argued that a conceptualization of caring that

(Research Examples continue on page 274)

Critical Thinking Activities (continued)

captures the full range of women's caring experiences could have consequences for health and social policy. She undertook a feminist grounded theory study that combined new data with data she had gathered in earlier studies.

Sampling Plan

Wuest recruited participants by distributing letters to potential respondents through community contacts. As data collection progressed, she relied on theoretical sampling. This approach was particularly important in Wuest's study because she sought to develop an explanatory theory that reflected the complex reality and diversity of women's caring experiences. She used theoretical sampling not only to guide her selection of new participants but also to "sample" from other data sources: "Theoretical sampling took many forms: choosing new participants on the basis of what they could contribute, looking for comparisons in data already collected, returning to participants to ask new questions, observing participants, and looking at literature and other written data" (p. 172). As an example of her approach to sampling participants, Wuest began by interviewing women who were raising children and discovered such issues as the competing demands of caring for spouse versus caring for children, and caring for parents versus caring for their own family. This led her to ask, "Are there other problematic properties of *demands*?" and subsequently to seek as study participants women who had greater demands (e.g., mothers of physically disabled children) and fewer demands (e.g., widows with adult children). Wuest sampled women until she achieved saturation and had a sufficiently large sample to conduct a detailed analysis. She conducted 32 new interviews with 21 women who had diverse characteristics and caring responsibilities, and also drew on 43 previously completed interviews.

Key Findings

Wuest's grounded theory provided insight into the process she called *precarious ordering*, which accounts for the complex strategies that women use to manage the dissonance created by the competing and changing caring demands in their lives. The theory demonstrates the power and resilience in women's management through the interrelated processes of *setting boundaries*, *negotiating*, and *repatterning care*.

Critical Thinking Suggestions

1. Answer questions 1 through 6 from Box 12.2 regarding this study.
2. Also consider the following targeted questions, which may assist you in further assessing aspects of the study:
   a. Comment on the characteristics of the participants, given the researcher's aims.
   b. Could Wuest have achieved her goal by using a random sample?
3. If the results of this study are trustworthy, what are some of the uses to which the findings might be put in clinical practice?

Critical Thinking Activities (continued)

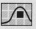 **EXAMPLE 3: Quantitative Research**

1. Read the Method section from the study by Feeley and colleagues
   ("Mother–VLBW Infant Interaction") in Appendix A of this book and then
   answer the relevant questions in Box 12.1.
2. Also consider the following targeted questions, which may further sharpen your
   critical thinking skills and assist you in assessing aspects of the study:
   a. What type of sampling plan might have improved the representativeness of
      the sample?
   b. The report indicates that participants and nonparticipants (those declining to
      participate in the study) differed in some respects. Discuss the nature of the
      differences and what effect this might have had on the study findings.

 EXAMPLE 4: Qualitative Research

1. Read the Method section from Beck's study ("Birth Trauma") in Appendix B of
   this book, and then answer the relevant questions in Box 12.2.
2. Also consider the following targeted questions, which may further sharpen your
   critical thinking skills and assist you in assessing aspects of the study.
   a. Comment on the characteristics of the participants, given the purpose of this
      study.
   b. Do you think that Beck should have limited her sample to women from one
      country only? Provide a rationale for your answer.

CHAPTER REVIEW
Summary Points

▶ **Sampling** is the process of selecting a portion of the **population**, which is an entire
aggregate of cases.

▶ An *element* (the basic unit about which information is collected) must meet the **eligibility criteria** to be included in the sample.

▶ The main consideration in assessing a sample in a quantitative study is its *representativeness*—the extent to which the sample is similar to the population and avoids bias.
Sampling bias refers to the systematic overrepresentation or underrepresentation of
some segment of the population.

▶ Quantitative researchers usually sample from an **accessible population** but typically
want to generalize to a larger **target population**.

▶ **Nonprobability sampling** (wherein elements are selected by nonrandom methods)
includes convenience, quota, and purposive sampling. Nonprobability sampling designs
are convenient and economical; a major disadvantage is their potential for bias.

▶ **Convenience sampling** (or *accidental sampling*) uses the most readily available or
most convenient group of people for the sample. **Snowball sampling** is a type of

convenience sampling in which referrals for potential participants are made by those already in the sample.

▶ **Quota sampling** divides the population into homogeneous **strata** (subgroups) to ensure representation of those subgroups in the sample; within each stratum, researchers select participants by convenience sampling.

▶ In **purposive** (or *judgmental*) **sampling**, participants or types of participants are hand picked based on the researcher's knowledge about the population.

▶ **Probability sampling** designs, which involve the **random selection** of elements from the population, yield more representative samples than nonprobability designs and permit estimates of the magnitude of **sampling error**. Probability samples, however, are expensive and demanding.

▶ **Simple random sampling** involves the selection of elements on a random basis from a *sampling frame* that enumerates all the elements.

▶ **Stratified random sampling** divides the population into homogeneous subgroups from which elements are selected at random.

▶ **Cluster sampling** (or *multistage sampling*) involves the successive selection of random samples from larger to smaller units by either simple random or stratified random methods.

▶ **Systematic sampling** is the selection of every *k*th case from a list. By dividing the population size by the desired sample size, the researcher establishes the *sampling interval*, which is the standard distance between the selected elements.

▶ In addition to representativeness, **sample size** is another important concern in quantitative studies, especially with regard to a study's statistical conclusion validity.

▶ Advanced researchers use **power analysis** to estimate sample size needs. Large samples are preferable to small ones in quantitative studies because larger samples tend to be more representative, but even large samples do not guarantee representativeness.

▶ Qualitative researchers use the theoretical demands of the study to select articulate and reflective informants with certain types of experience in an emergent way, capitalizing on early learning to guide subsequent sampling decisions.

▶ Qualitative researchers most often use purposive or, in grounded theory studies, **theoretical sampling** to guide them in selecting data sources that maximize information richness.

▶ Various purposive sampling strategies have been used by qualitative researchers. One strategy is **maximum variation sampling**, which entails purposely selecting cases with a wide range of variation. Other strategies include **homogeneous sampling** (deliberately reducing variation); **extreme case sampling** (selecting the most unusual or extreme cases); and **criterion sampling** (studying cases that meet a predetermined criterion of importance).

▶ Another strategy in qualitative research is **sampling confirming and disconfirming cases**, that is, selecting cases that enrich and challenge the researchers' conceptualizations.

▶ Samples in qualitative studies are typically small and based on information needs. A guiding principle is **data saturation**, which involves sampling to the point at which no new information is obtained and redundancy is achieved.

▶ Ethnographers make numerous sampling decisions, including not only *whom* to sample but also *what* to sample (e.g., activities, events, documents, artefacts); these decisions are often aided by **key informants** who serve as guides and interpreters of the culture.

▶ Phenomenologists typically work with a small sample of people (10 or fewer) who meet the criterion of having lived the experience under study.

▶ Grounded theory researchers typically use theoretical sampling and work with samples of about 20 to 30 people.

▶ Criteria for evaluating qualitative sampling are informational adequacy and appropriateness; potential for transferability is another issue of concern.

Additional Resources for Review

Chapter 12 of the *Study Guide to Accompany Essentials of Nursing Research,* 6th edition offers various exercises and study suggestions for reinforcing the concepts presented in this chapter. For additional review, see the Student Self-Study Review Questions section of the Student Resource CD-ROM provided with this book.

SUGGESTED READINGS

References for studies cited in the chapter appear at the end of the book.

Methodologic References

Cohen, J. (1988). *Statistical power analysis for the behavioral sciences* (2nd. ed.). Mahwah, NJ: Erlbaum.

Glaser, B. (1978). *Theoretical sensitivity.* Mill Valley, CA: Sociology Press.

Morse, J. M. (1991). Strategies for sampling. In J. M. Morse (Ed.), *Qualitative nursing research: A contemporary dialogue.* Newbury Park, CA: Sage Publications.

Morse, J. M. (2000). Determining sample size. *Qualitative Health Research, 10,* 3–5.

Patton, M. Q. (2002). *Qualitative evaluation and research methods* (3rd ed.). Newbury Park, CA: Sage Publications.

Polit, D. F., & Beck, C. T. (2004). *Nursing research: Principles and methods* (7th ed.). Philadelphia: Lippincott Williams & Wilkins.

Porter, E. J. (1999). Defining the eligible, accessible population for a phenomenological study. *Western Journal of Nursing Research, 21,* 796–804.

Data Collection

Scrutinizing Data Collection Methods

STUDENT OBJECTIVES

On completing this chapter, you will be able to:

▶ Identify phenomena that lend themselves to self-reports, observation, and physiologic measurement
▶ Distinguish between and evaluate structured and unstructured self-reports; open-ended and closed-ended questions; and interviews and questionnaires
▶ Distinguish between and evaluate structured and unstructured observations and describe various methods of collecting, sampling, and recording observational data
▶ Describe the major features of biophysiologic measures
▶ Critique a researcher's decisions regarding the data collection plan (degree of structure, general method, mode of administration) and its implementation
▶ Define new terms in the chapter

The concepts in which researchers are interested must be measured, observed, or recorded. The task of selecting or developing methods for gathering data is among the most challenging in the research process.

OVERVIEW OF DATA COLLECTION AND DATA SOURCES

There are many alternative approaches to data collection, and these approaches vary along several dimensions. This section provides an overview of some important dimensions.

Existing Data Versus New Data

One of the first data decisions an investigator makes concerns the use of existing data versus new data gathered specifically for the study. Most of this chapter is devoted to methods researchers use to generate new data, but they sometimes can take advantage of existing information.

We have already discussed several types of studies that rely on existing data. Meta-analyses and meta-syntheses (see Chapter 7) are examples of studies that involve analyses of available data—that is, data from research reports. Historical research (see Chapter 10) typically relies on available data in the form of written, narrative records of the past: diaries, letters, newspapers, minutes of meetings, and so forth. As we discussed in Chapter 11, researchers sometimes perform a secondary analysis, which is the use of data gathered in a previous study to test new hypotheses or address new research questions.

An important existing data source for nurse researchers is **records**. Hospital records, nursing charts, physicians' order sheets, and care plan statements all constitute rich data sources. Records are an economical and convenient source of information. Because the researchers were not responsible for collecting and recording information, however, they may be unaware of the records' limitations, biases, or incompleteness. If the records available for use are not the entire set of all possible records, investigators must consider the records' representativeness. Existing records have been used in both qualitative and quantitative nursing studies.

Example of a study using records

Gélinas, Fortier, Viens, Fillion, and Puntillo (2004) extracted data from the medical records of two health care centres in Québec to describe approaches to pain assessment and pain management in critically ill intubated patients.

CONSUMER TIP

Researchers describe their data collection plan in the methods section of a research report. In a report for a quantitative study, the specific data collection methods are often described in a subsection labelled "Measures" or "Instruments." The actual steps taken to collect the data are sometimes described in a separate subsection with the heading "Procedures." ■

Major Types of Data for Nursing Studies

If existing data are unavailable or unsuitable for a research question, researchers must collect new data. In developing their data collection plan, researchers make many decisions, including the decision about the basic type of data to gather. Three types have been used most frequently by nurse researchers: self-reports, observations, and biophysiologic measures. **Self-reports** are participants' responses to questions posed by the researcher, as in an interview. Direct **observation** of people's behaviours or characteristics is an alternative to self-reports for certain research questions. Nurses also use **biophysiologic measures** to assess important clinical variables. Sections of this chapter are devoted to these three major types of data collection.

In quantitative studies, researchers decide up front how to operationalize their variables and how best to gather their data. Their data collection plans are almost always "cast in stone" before a single piece of data is collected. Self-reports are the most common data collection approach in quantitative nursing studies

Qualitative researchers typically go into the field knowing the most likely sources of data, but they do not rule out other possible data sources that might come to light as data collection progresses. As in quantitative studies, the primary method of collecting qualitative data is through self-report, that is, through interviews with study participants. Observation is often a part of many qualitative studies as well. Physiologic data are rarely collected in a naturalistic inquiry.

Table 13.1 compares the types of data used by researchers in the three main qualitative traditions, as well as other aspects of the data collection process for each tradition. Ethnographers almost always triangulate data from various sources, with observation and interviews being the most important methods. Ethnographers also gather or examine products of the culture under study, such as documents, records, artefacts, photographs, and so on. Phenomenologists and grounded theory researchers rely primarily on in-depth interviews with individual participants, although observation also plays a role in some grounded theory studies.

Key Dimensions of Data Collection Methods

Regardless of the type of data collected in a study, data collection methods vary along several important dimensions:

▶ *Structure.* Research data can be collected in a highly structured manner: the same information is gathered from all participants in a comparable, prespecified way. Sometimes, however, it is more appropriate to be flexible and to allow participants to reveal relevant information in a naturalistic way.

▶ *Quantifiability.* Data that will be analyzed statistically must be gathered in such a way that they can be quantified. On the other hand, data that are to be analyzed qualitatively are collected in narrative form. Structured data collection approaches tend to yield data that are more easily quantified.

▶ *Obtrusiveness.* Data collection methods differ in terms of the degree to which people are aware of their status as study participants. If participants are fully aware of their role in a study, their behaviour and responses might not be normal. When data are collected unobtrusively, however, ethical problems may emerge.

TABLE 13.1	Data Collection in the Three Main Qualitative Traditions		
ISSUE	**ETHNOGRAPHY**	**PHENOMENOLOGY**	**GROUNDED THEORY**
Type of data	Primarily participant observation and interviews, plus documents, artefacts, maps, photographs, social network diagrams, genealogies	Primarily in-depth interviews, sometimes diaries, artwork, or other materials	Primarily individual interviews, sometimes group interviews, participant observations, journals
Unit of data collection	Cultural systems	Individuals	Individuals
Period of data collection	Extended period, many months or years	Typically moderate	Typically moderate
Salient field issues	Gaining entrée, determining a role, learning how to participate, encouraging candor, identification with group, premature exit	Bracketing one's views, building rapport, encouraging candor, listening intently while preparing next question, keeping "on track," handling personal emotions	Building rapport, encouraging candor, keeping "on track," listening intently while preparing next question, handling personal emotions

▶ *Objectivity.* Some data collection approaches require more subjective judgment than others. Quantitative researchers generally strive for methods that are as objective as possible. In qualitative research, however, the researcher's subjective judgment is considered a valuable tool.

Research questions may dictate where on these four dimensions the data collection method will lie. For example, questions that are best suited for a phenomenological study tend to use methods that are low on structure, quantifiability, and objectivity, whereas research questions appropriate for a survey tend to require methods that are high on all four dimensions. However, researchers often have latitude in selecting or designing appropriate data collection plans.

CONSUMER TIP

Most data that are analyzed quantitatively actually begin as qualitative data. If a researcher asked respondents if they have been severely depressed, moderately depressed, somewhat depressed, or not at all depressed in the past week, they answer in words, not numbers. The words are transformed, through a coding process, into quantitative categories. ■

SELF-REPORT METHODS

A good deal of information can be gathered by directly questioning people. If, for example, we were interested in learning about patients' perceptions of hospital care, their preoperative fears, or their health-promoting activities, we would likely talk to them and ask them questions. For some research variables, alternatives to direct questioning exist, but the unique ability of humans to communicate verbally on a sophisticated level ensures that self-reports will always be a fundamental tool in nurse researchers' repertoire of data collection techniques.

Self-report techniques can vary in structure. At one extreme are loosely organized methods that do not involve a formal set of questions. At the other extreme are tightly structured methods involving the use of forms such as questionnaires. Some characteristics of different self-report approaches are discussed next.

Qualitative Self-Report Techniques

Self-report methods used in qualitative studies offer flexibility. When these unstructured methods are used, researchers do not have a set of questions that must be asked in a specific order and worded in a given way. Instead, they start with some general questions and allow respondents to tell their stories in a naturalistic, narrative fashion. In other words, unstructured or semi-structured interviews are conversational in nature.

Unstructured interviews, which are used by researchers in all qualitative research traditions, encourage respondents to define the important dimensions of a phenomenon and to elaborate on what is relevant to them, rather than being guided by investigators' *a priori* notions of relevance. Unstructured interviews are the mode of choice when researchers do not have a clear idea of what it is they do not know.

TYPES OF QUALITATIVE SELF-REPORTS

There are several approaches to collecting qualitative self-report data. **Completely unstructured interviews** are used when researchers have no preconceived view of the content or flow of information to be gathered. Their aim is to elucidate respondents' perceptions of the world without imposing the researchers' views. Typically, researchers begin by asking a broad **grand tour question** such as, "What happened when you first learned that you had AIDS?" Subsequent questions usually are more focused and are guided by initial responses. Ethnographic and phenomenological studies sometimes use completely unstructured interviews.

Semi-structured (or *focused*) **interviews**, which are used more frequently than totally unstructured interviews, are used when researchers have a list of topics or broad questions that must be addressed in an interview. Interviewers use a written **topic guide** (or *interview guide*) to ensure that all question areas are covered. The interviewer's function is to encourage participants to talk freely about all the topics on the guide.

Focus group interviews are interviews with groups of about 5 to 10 people whose opinions and experiences are solicited simultaneously. The interviewer (or *moderator*) guides the discussion according to a topic guide or set of questions. The advantages of a group format are that it is efficient and can generate a lot of dialogue. Some people,

Example of semi-structured interviews

Coulson and Doran (2003) conducted a phenomenological study to explore how nurses integrate outcomes assessment data into their practice. Their semi-structured interviews were guided by three broad questions. For example, one question was, "How relevant and useful are the outcomes data in supporting your clinical decision-making?"

however, are uncomfortable expressing their views or describing their experiences in front of a group. Focus groups have been used by researchers in many qualitative research traditions and can play a particularly important role in feminist, critical theory, and participatory action research.

Example of focus group interviews

Clark, Barbour, White, and MacIntyre (2004) studied patients' beliefs and decision making about participation in a cardiac rehabilitation program. Some 44 patients who were eligible for cardiac rehabilitation took part in eight focus groups. There were four groups of high attendees, two groups with people who attended irregularly, and two groups of nonattendees.

Life histories are narrative self-disclosures about individual life experiences. With this approach, researchers ask respondents to describe, often in chronologic sequence, their experiences regarding a specified theme, either orally or in writing. Some researchers have used this approach to obtain a total life health history.

The **think aloud method** is a qualitative method that has been used to collect data about cognitive processes, such as thinking, problem solving, and decision making. This method involves having people use audio-recording devices to talk about decisions as they are being made or while problems are being solved, over an extended period (e.g., throughout a shift). The method produces an inventory of decisions and underlying processes as they occur in a naturalistic context.

Example of the think aloud method

Neufeld, Harrison, Rempel, Larocque, Dublin, Stewart, and Hughes (2004) studied appraisals of nonsupport among female family caregivers. One part of the study involved card-sorting exercises in which participants sorted statements relating to family caregiving. For example, one exercise involved sorting statements into two piles—helpful or unhelpful. The researchers used the think aloud method to capture participants' decision making during the card-sorting task.

Personal **diaries** have long been used as a source of data in historical research. It is also possible to generate new data for a nonhistorical study by asking participants to maintain a diary or journal over a specified period. Diaries can be useful in providing an intimate description of a person's everyday life. The diaries may be completely unstructured; for example, individuals who have undergone organ transplantation could be asked simply to spend 10 to 15 minutes a day jotting down their thoughts and feelings. Frequently, however, participants are requested to make entries into a diary regarding some specific aspect of their experience (e.g., about fatigue).

The **critical incidents technique** is a method of gathering information about people's behaviours by examining specific incidents relating to the behaviour under study. The technique focuses on a factual *incident*—an integral episode of human behaviour; *critical* means that the incident must have had a discernible impact on some outcome. The technique differs from other self-report approaches in that it focuses on something specific about which respondents can be expected to testify as expert witnesses.

Example of the critical incident technique

Care and Udod (2003) used the critical incidents technique in their study of the competencies nurse managers need to fulfill their roles. They asked participants to elaborate on a specific incident in their practice when they "performed at their best" as a manager.

GATHERING QUALITATIVE SELF-REPORT DATA

Researchers gather narrative self-report data to develop a construction of a phenomenon that is consistent with that of participants. This goal requires researchers to take steps to overcome communication barriers and to enhance the flow of meaning. For example, researchers should strive to learn if a group under study uses any special terms or jargon.

Although qualitative interviews are conversational, this does not mean that researchers engage in them casually. The conversations are purposeful and require advance thought and preparation. For example, the wording of questions should make sense to respondents and reflect their world view. In addition to being good questioners, researchers must be good listeners. Only by attending carefully to what respondents are saying can in-depth interviewers develop appropriate follow-up questions.

Unstructured interviews are typically long—sometimes lasting several hours. The issue of how best to record such abundant information is a difficult one. Some researchers take sketchy notes as the interview progresses, filling in the details after the interview is completed—but this method is risky in terms of data accuracy. Most prefer tape recording the interviews for later transcription. Although some respondents are self-conscious when their conversation is recorded, they typically forget about the presence of recording equipment after a few minutes.

Quantitative Self-Report Techniques

Structured approaches to collecting self-report data are appropriate when researchers know in advance exactly what they need to know and can, therefore, frame appropriate questions to obtain the needed information. Structured self-report data are usually collected by means of a formal, written document—an **instrument.** The instrument is an **interview schedule** when the questions are asked orally in either a face-to-face or telephone format and is a **questionnaire** when respondents complete the instrument themselves.

QUESTION FORM

In a structured instrument, respondents are asked to respond to the same questions in the same order, and they are given the same set of response options. **Closed-ended questions** (also called **fixed-alternative questions**) are ones in which the **response alternatives** are prespecified by the researcher. The alternatives may range from a simple yes or no to complex expressions of opinion. The purpose of using questions with fixed alternatives is to ensure comparability of responses and to facilitate analysis.

Many structured instruments also include some **open-ended questions,** which allow participants to respond to questions in their own words. In questionnaires, respondents must write out their responses to open-ended questions. In interviews, the interviewer writes down responses verbatim. Some examples of open-ended and closed-ended questions are presented in Box 13.1.

Both open-ended and closed-ended questions have strengths and weaknesses. Closed-ended questions are more difficult to construct than open-ended ones but easier to administer and, especially, to analyze. Closed-ended questions are more efficient: people can complete more closed-ended questions than open-ended ones in a given amount of time. Also, respondents may be unwilling to compose lengthy written responses to open-ended questions in questionnaires.

The major drawback of closed-ended questions is that researchers might overlook some potentially important responses. Another concern is that closed-ended questions can be superficial; open-ended questions allow for richer and fuller information if the respondents are verbally expressive and cooperative. Finally, some respondents object to choosing from alternatives that do not reflect their opinions precisely.

INSTRUMENT CONSTRUCTION

In drafting questions for a structured instrument, researchers must carefully monitor the wording of each question for clarity, sensitivity to respondents' psychological state, absence of bias, and (in questionnaires) reading level. Questions must be sequenced in a psychologically meaningful order that encourages cooperation and candour.

Draft instruments are usually critically reviewed by colleagues and then pretested with a small sample of respondents. A *pretest* is a trial run to determine whether the instrument is useful in generating desired information. In large studies, the development and pretesting of self-report instruments may take many months.

INTERVIEWS VERSUS QUESTIONNAIRES

Researchers using structured self-reports must decide whether to use interviews or questionnaires. You should be aware of the limitations and strengths of these alternatives because the decision may affect the findings and the quality of the evidence. Questionnaires, relative to interviews, have the following advantages:

▶ Questionnaires are less costly and require less time and effort to administer; this is a particular advantage if the sample is geographically dispersed. Web-based questionnaires are especially economical.

BOX 13.1   **Examples of Question Types**

Open-Ended

- What led to your decision to stop smoking?
- What did you do when you discovered you had AIDS?

Closed-Ended

1. Dichotomous Question

Have you ever been hospitalized?
- ❏ 1. Yes
- ❏ 2. No

2. Multiple-Choice Question

How important is it to you to avoid a pregnancy at this time?
- ❏ 1. Extremely important
- ❏ 2. Very important
- ❏ 3. Somewhat important
- ❏ 4. Not at all important

3. "Cafeteria" Question

People have different opinions about the use of hormone-replacement therapy for women in menopause. Which of the following statements best represents your point of view?
- ❏ 1. Hormone replacement is dangerous and should be totally banned.
- ❏ 2. Hormone replacement may have some undesirable side effects that suggests the need for caution in its use.
- ❏ 3. I am undecided about my views on hormone-replacement therapy.
- ❏ 4. Hormone replacement has many beneficial effects that merit its promotion.
- ❏ 5. Hormone replacement is a wonder cure that should be administered widely to menopausal women.

4. Rank-Order Question

People value different things about life. Below is a list of principles or ideals that are often cited when people are asked to name things they value most. Please indicate the order of importance of these values to you by placing a 1 beside the most important, 2 beside the next most important, and so forth.
- ❏ Career achievement/work
- ❏ Family relationships
- ❏ Friendships and social interaction
- ❏ Health
- ❏ Money
- ❏ Religion

5. Forced-Choice Question

Which statement most closely represents your point of view?
- ❏ 1. What happens to me is my own doing.
- ❏ 2. Sometimes I feel I don't have enough control over my life.

6. Rating Question

On a scale from 0 to 10, where 0 means extremely dissatisfied and 10 means extremely satisfied, how satisfied are you with the nursing care you received during your hospitalization?

Extremely dissatisfied   Extremely satisfied

0 1 2 3 4 5 6 7 8 9 10

▶ Questionnaires offer the possibility of complete anonymity, which may be crucial in obtaining information about illegal or deviant behaviours or about embarrassing traits.

Example of mailed questionnaires

Adlaf, Glikdman, Demers, and Newton-Taylor (2003) studied rates and patterns of illicit drug use among undergraduates in Canadian universities. Questionnaires were mailed to 16,000 students from 16 universities.

The strengths of interviews far outweigh those of questionnaires. These strengths include the following:

▶ Response rates tend to be high in face-to-face interviews. Respondents are less likely to refuse to talk to an interviewer than to ignore a questionnaire, especially a mailed questionnaire. Low response rates can lead to bias because respondents are rarely a random subset of those sampled. In the mailed questionnaire study described earlier (Adlaf et al., 2003), the response rate was 51%, despite fairly elaborate efforts to encourage student participation in the survey.
▶ Many people simply cannot fill out a questionnaire; examples include young children, the blind, and the very elderly. Interviews are feasible with most people.
▶ Interviewers can produce additional information through observation of respondents' living situation, level of understanding, degree of cooperativeness, and so on—all of which can be useful in interpreting responses.

Most advantages of face-to-face interviews also apply to telephone interviews. Complicated or detailed instruments are not well suited to telephone interviewing, but for relatively brief instruments, the telephone interview combines relatively low costs with high response rates.

Example of in-person interviews

Ing and Reutter (2003) studied the relationships among socioeconomic status, sense of coherence, and health in Canadian women. The data were collected in personal interviews with a national sample of more than 25,000 households, from which 6748 women were selected for this secondary analysis. The response rate was 88.7% of eligible households.

Scales and Other Special Forms of Structured Self-Reports

Several special types of structured self-reports are used by nurse researchers. These include composite social-psychological scales, vignettes, and Q sorts.

SCALES

Social-psychological scales are often incorporated into a questionnaire or interview schedule. A **scale** is a device designed to assign a numeric score to people to place them on a continuum with respect to attributes being measured, like a scale for measuring weight. Social-psychological scales quantitatively discriminate among people with different attitudes, motives, perceptions, and needs.

The most common scaling technique is the **Likert scale**, which consists of several declarative statements (or *items*) that express a viewpoint on a topic. Respondents are asked to indicate how much they agree or disagree with the statement. Table 13.2 presents an illustrative, five-point Likert scale for measuring attitudes toward condom use. In this example, agreement with positively worded statements and disagreement with negatively worded statements are assigned higher scores. The first statement is positively phrased;

TABLE 13.2   Example of a Likert Scale to Measure Attitudes Toward Condoms

DIRECTION OF SCORING*	ITEM	RESPONSES† SA	A	?	D	SD	SCORE PERSON 1 (✔)	PERSON 2 (✗)
+	1. Using a condom shows you care about your partner.		✔			✗	4	1
−	2. My partner would be angry if I talked about using condoms.			✗	✔		5	3
−	3. I wouldn't enjoy sex as much if my partner and I used condoms.		✗	✔			4	2
+	4. Condoms are a good protection against AIDS and other sexually transmitted diseases.			✔	✗		3	2
+	5. My partner would respect me if I insisted on using condoms.	✔				✗	5	1
−	6. I would be too embarrassed to ask my partner about using a condom.		✗		✔		5	2
	Total score						26	11

* Researchers would not indicate the direction of scoring on a Likert scale administered to subjects. The scoring direction is indicated in this table for illustrative purposes only.
† SA, strongly agree; A, agree; ?, uncertain; D, disagree; SD, strongly disagree.

agreement indicates a favourable attitude toward condom use. Because the item has five response alternatives, a score of 5 would be given to someone strongly agreeing, 4 to someone agreeing, and so forth. The responses of two hypothetical respondents are shown by a check or an X, and their item scores are shown in the right-hand columns. Person 1, who agreed with the first statement, has a score of 4, whereas person 2, who strongly disagreed, has a score of 1. The second statement is negatively worded, and so the scoring is reversed—a 1 is assigned to those who strongly agree, and so forth. This reversal is necessary so that a high score consistently reflects positive attitudes toward condom use. A person's total score is determined by summing item scores; hence, these scales are sometimes called **summated rating scales.** The total scores of the two respondents reflect a considerably more positive attitude toward condoms on the part of person 1 (score = 26) than person 2 (score = 11). Summing item scores makes it possible to make fine discriminations among people with different points of view. A six-item scale, such as the one in Table 13.2, could yield a range of possible scores, from a minimum of 6 (6 × 1) to a maximum of 30 (6 × 5).

Example of a Likert scale

Lobchuk and Vorauer (2003) studied family caregivers' accuracy in estimating symptom experiences of patients with cancer. A sample of 98 dyads (patients with advanced-stage cancer and their caregivers) completed the Memorial Symptom Assessment Scale, a 32-item Likert-type scale for assessing the frequency and severity of symptoms.

Another technique for measuring attitudes is the **semantic differential** (SD). With the SD, respondents rate concepts (e.g., primary nursing, team nursing) on a series of *bipolar adjectives*, such as good/bad, strong/weak, important/unimportant. Respondents are asked to place a check at the appropriate point on a seven-point scale that extends from one extreme of the dimension to the other. An example of an SD format is shown in Figure 13.1. The SD method is flexible and easy to construct. The concept being rated can be virtually anything—a person, concept, issue, and so on. Scoring is similar to that for Likert scales. Scores from 1 to 7 are assigned to each bipolar scale response, and responses are then summed across the scales to yield a total score.

Another type of psychosocial measure is the **visual analog scale** (VAS), which can be used to measure subjective experiences, such as pain, fatigue, and dyspnoea. The VAS is a straight line, the end anchors of which are labelled as the extreme limits of a sensation. Participants mark a point on the line corresponding to the amount of sensation experienced. Traditionally, a VAS line is 100 mm in length, which makes it easy to derive a score from 0 to 100 by simply measuring the distance from one end of the scale to the mark on the line. An example of a VAS is presented in Figure 13.2.

Scales permit researchers to efficiently quantify subtle gradations in the strength or intensity of individual characteristics. Scales can be administered either verbally or in writing and thus are suitable for use with most people. Scales are susceptible to several

NURSE PRACTITIONERS

competent	7*	6	5	4	3	2	1	incompetent
worthless	1	2	3	4	5	6	7	valuable
important								unimportant
pleasant								unpleasant
bad								good
cold								warm
responsible								irresponsible
successful								unsuccessful

*The score values would not be printed on the form administered to actual subjects. The numbers are presented here solely for the purpose of illustrating how semantic differentials are scored.

FIGURE 13.1 Example of a semantic differential.

Example of a visual analog scale

Nemeth, Harrison, Graham, and Burke (2003) studied the prevalence of venous leg ulcer pain over three seasons (autumn, winter, and spring). A VAS was used to measure pain.

common problems, however, the most troublesome of which are referred to as **response set biases.** The most important biases include the following:

▶ *Social desirability response set bias*—a tendency to misrepresent attitudes or traits by giving answers that are consistent with prevailing social views

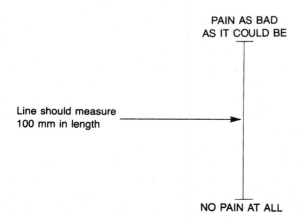

PAIN AS BAD
AS IT COULD BE

Line should measure
100 mm in length

NO PAIN AT ALL

FIGURE 13.2 Example of a visual analog scale.

▶ *Extreme response set bias*—a tendency to consistently express attitudes or feelings in extreme responses (e.g., strongly agree), leading to distortions because extreme responses may not necessarily signify the greatest intensity of the trait being measured

▶ *Acquiescence response set bias*—a tendency to agree with statements regardless of their content by people who are referred to as *yea-sayers*. Other people (*nay-sayers*) disagree with statements independently of the question content.

These biases can be reduced through such strategies as *counterbalancing* positively and negatively worded statements, developing sensitively worded questions, creating a nonjudgmental atmosphere, and guaranteeing the confidentiality of responses.

CONSUMER TIP

Most studies that collect self-report data involve one or more social-psychological scale. Typically, the scales are ones that were developed previously by other researchers. ■

VIGNETTES

Vignettes are brief descriptions of situations to which respondents are asked to react. The descriptions are structured to elicit information about respondents' perceptions, opinions, or knowledge about a phenomenon. Questions about the vignettes can be open ended (e.g., How would you recommend handling this situation?) or closed ended (e.g., On the 7-point scale below, rate how well you think the nurse handled the situation).

Vignettes are an economical means of eliciting information about how people might behave in situations that would be difficult to observe in daily life. For example, we might want to assess how patients would react to or feel about nurses with different cultural backgrounds. The principal problem with vignettes concerns response validity. If respondents describe how they would react in a situation portrayed in the vignette, how accurate is that description of their actual behaviour? Thus, although the use of vignettes can be profitable, the possibility of response biases should be recognized.

Example of vignettes

Valente and Saunders (2004) studied nurses' experiences in the detection, assessment, and intervention of patients who are suicidal. Their questionnaires, which were sent to more than 1000 members of the Oncology Nursing Society from Canada and the United States, included a vignette of a suicidal patient.

Q SORTS

In a **Q sort,** participants are presented with a set of cards on which statements or phrases are written. Participants are asked to sort the cards along a specified bipolar dimension, such as agree/disagree. Typically, there are between 60 and 100 cards to be sorted into 9 or 11 piles, with the number of cards to be placed in each pile predetermined by the researcher.

The sorting instructions in a Q sort can vary. For example, personality can be studied by writing descriptions of personality traits on the cards; participants can then be asked to sort items on a continuum from "exactly like me" to "not at all like me." Or, patients could be asked to rate various aspects of their treatment on a most distressing to least distressing continuum.

Q sorts can be useful, but they also have drawbacks. On the positive side, Q sorts are versatile and can be applied to a wide variety of problems. Requiring people to place a predetermined number of cards in each pile eliminates many response biases. On the other hand, it is time-consuming to administer Q sorts to a large sample of people. Some critics argue that the forced distribution of cards according to researchers' specifications is artificial and excludes information about how participants would ordinarily distribute their responses.

Example of a Q sort

Ryan and Zerwic (2004) used Q sorts as an approach to studying the cluster of symptoms that individuals at high risk for acute myocardial infarction (AMI) believe to be associated with AMI. A sample of patients with known coronary artery disease sorted 49 statements about symptoms of AMI from "most like a heart attack" to "most unlike a heart attack."

Evaluation of Self-Report Methods

Self-report techniques—the most common method of data collection in nursing studies—are strong with respect to their directness. If researchers want to know how people feel or what they believe, the most direct approach is to ask them. Moreover, self-reports frequently yield information that would be impossible to gather by other means. Behaviours can be directly *observed*, but only if people are willing to engage in them publicly. It is usually impossible for researchers to observe such behaviours as contraceptive practices or drug use. Furthermore, observers can only observe behaviours occurring at the time of the study; self-report instruments can gather retrospective data about activities occurring in the past or about behaviours in which participants plan to engage in the future. Information about feelings, values, opinions, and motives can sometimes be inferred through observation, but people's actions do not always indicate their state of mind. Self-report instruments can be used to measure psychological characteristics through direct communication with participants.

Despite these advantages, self-report methods have some weaknesses. The most serious issue concerns the validity and accuracy of self-reports: How can we be sure that respondents feel or act the way they say they do? How can we trust the information that respondents provide, particularly if the questions ask them to admit to potentially undesirable traits? Investigators often have no alternative but to assume that most respondents have been frank. Yet, we all have a tendency to present ourselves in the best light, and this may conflict with the truth. When reading research reports, you should be alert to potential biases in self-reported data, particularly with respect to behaviours or feelings that society judges to be controversial or wrong.

You should also be familiar with the merits of unstructured and structured self-reports. In general, unstructured (qualitative) interviews are of greatest utility when a new area of research is being explored. A qualitative approach allows researchers to ascertain what the basic issues are, how individuals conceptualize and talk about a phenomenon, and what the range is of opinions or behaviours that are relevant to the topic. Qualitative methods may also help elucidate the underlying meaning of a pattern or relationship repeatedly observed in quantitative research.

Qualitative methods, however, are extremely time-consuming and demanding and are not appropriate for capturing the measurable aspects of a phenomenon, such as incidence (e.g., the percentage of women who experience postpartum depression, or PPD), frequency (how often symptoms of PPD are experienced); duration (e.g., average time period during which PPD is present), or magnitude (e.g., degree of severity of PPD). Structured self-reports are also appropriate when researchers want to test hypotheses concerning relationships.

Critiquing Self-Reports

One of the first questions you should ask is whether the researcher made the right decision in obtaining the data by self-report rather than by an alternative method. Attention then should be paid to the adequacy of the actual methods used. Box 13.2 presents some guiding questions for critiquing self-reports.

It may be difficult to perform a thorough critique of self-report methods in studies reported in journals because researchers seldom include detailed descriptions of the data collection methods. What you can expect is information about the following aspects of the self-report data collection:

▶ The degree of structure used in the questioning
▶ Whether interviews or questionnaires (or variants such as a Q sort) were used
▶ How the instruments were administered (e.g., by telephone, in person, by mail, over the Internet)
▶ Where the interviews (if relevant) took place

BOX 13.2   Guidelines for Critiquing Self-Reports

1. Does the research question lend itself to a self-report method of data collection? Would an alternative method have been more appropriate?
2. Is the degree of structure consistent with the nature of the research question?
3. Given the research question and respondent characteristics, did the researcher use the best possible mode for collecting the data (i.e., personal interviews, telephone interviews, or self-administered questionnaires)?
4. Do the questions included in the instrument or topic guide adequately cover the complexities of the problem under investigation?
5. If a composite scale was used, does its use seem appropriate? Does the scale adequately capture the target research variable?
6. If a vignette or Q sort was used, does its use seem appropriate?

Degree of structure is especially important in your assessment of a data collection plan. The decision about an instrument's structure should be based on considerations that you can often evaluate. For example, respondents who are not very articulate are more receptive to instruments with many closed-ended questions than to questioning that forces them to compose lengthy answers. Other considerations include the amount of time available (structured instruments are more efficient); the expected sample size (open-ended questions and qualitative interviews are difficult to analyze with large samples); the status of existing information on the topic (in a new area of inquiry, a quantitative approach may not be warranted); and, most important, the nature of the research question.

CONSUMER TIP

In research reports, descriptions of data collection instruments are often quite brief. For example, if a study involved the use of a depression scale (e.g., the Center for Epidemiological Studies Depression Scale, or CES-D), the research report most likely would not describe individual items on this scale—although the report should provide an appropriate reference. Moreover, there is typically insufficient space in journals for detailed rationales (e.g., a rationale for choosing the CES-D instead of the Beck Depression Scale). It may thus be hard for you to undertake a thorough critique of the data collection plan.   ■

OBSERVATIONAL METHODS

For some research questions, direct observation of people's behaviour is an alternative to self-reports. Within nursing research, observational methods have broad applicability, particularly for clinical inquiries. Nurses are in an advantageous position to observe, relatively unobtrusively, the behaviours and activities of patients, their families, and health care staff. Observational methods can be used to gather such information as the characteristics and conditions of individuals (e.g., patients' sleep–wake state); verbal communication (e.g., exchange of information at change-of-shift); nonverbal communication (e.g., body language); activities (e.g., patients' self-grooming activities); and environmental conditions (e.g., noise levels in nursing homes).

In observational studies, researchers have flexibility with regard to several issues:

▶ *The focus of the observation.* The focus can be broadly defined events (e.g., patient mood swings), or small, specific behaviours (e.g., facial expressions).

▶ *Concealment.* As discussed in Chapter 5, awareness of being observed may cause people to behave abnormally, thereby jeopardizing the validity of the observations. The problem of behavioural distortions due to the known presence of an observer is called **reactivity.**

▶ *Duration of observation.* Some observations can be made in a short period of time, but others, particularly those in ethnographic and other field studies, may require months or years in the field.

▶ *Method of recording observations.* Observations can be made through the human senses and then recorded by paper-and-pencil methods, but they can also be done with sophisticated technical equipment (e.g., video equipment, audio-recording equipment).

In summary, observational techniques can be used to measure a broad range of phenomena and are versatile. Like self-report techniques, an important dimension for observational methods is degree of structure—that is, whether the observational data are amenable to qualitative or quantitative analysis.

Qualitative Observational Methods

Qualitative researchers collect observational data with a minimum of structure and researcher-imposed constraints. Skilful unstructured observation permits researchers to see the world as the study participants see it, to develop a rich understanding and appreciation of key phenomena, to extract meaning from events and situations, and to grasp the subtleties of cultural variation.

Naturalistic observations often are made in field settings through a technique called **participant observation**. A participant observer participates in the functioning of the group or institution under study and strives to observe and record information within the contexts, experiences, and symbols that are relevant to the participants. By assuming a participating role, observers may have insights that would have eluded more passive observers. Of course, not all qualitative observational studies use *participant* observation; some unstructured observations involve watching and recording unfolding behaviours without the observers' participation in activities. The great majority of qualitative observations, however, do involve some participation, particularly in ethnographic and grounded theory research.

Example of qualitative nonparticipant observation

Moules, Simonson, Prins, Angus, and Bell (2004) conducted a hermeneutic study of the experience of grief, based on a qualitative analysis of videotaped clinical interviews with families seen in the Family Nursing Unit at the University of Calgary.

THE OBSERVER-PARTICIPANT ROLE IN PARTICIPANT OBSERVATION

In participant observation, the role observers play in the social group under study is important because their social position determines what they are likely to see. That is, the behaviours that are likely to be available for observation depend on the observers' position in a network of relations.

The extent of the observers' actual participation in a group is best thought of as a continuum. At one extreme of the continuum is complete immersion in the setting, with researchers assuming full participant status; at the other extreme is complete separation, with researchers assuming an onlooker status. Researchers may in some cases assume a fixed position on this continuum throughout the study.

On the other hand, researchers' role as participants may evolve over the course of the field work. A researcher may begin primarily as a bystander, with participation in group activities increasing over time. In other cases, it might be profitable to become immersed in a social setting quickly, with participation diminishing to allow more time for pure observation.

CONSUMER TIP

It is not unusual to find research reports that state that participant observation was used when in fact the description of the method suggests that observation, but not participation, was involved. Some researchers appear to use the term "participant observation" to refer generally to unstructured observations conducted in the field. ▬

Observers must overcome at least two major hurdles in assuming a satisfactory role vis-à-vis participants. The first is to gain entrée into the social group under study; the second is to establish rapport and develop trust within that group. Without gaining entrée, the study cannot proceed; but without the trust of the group, the researcher will typically be restricted to "front stage" knowledge—that is, information distorted by the group's protective facades (Leininger, 1985). The goal of participant observers is to "get back stage"—to learn about the true realities of the group's experiences and behaviours. On the other hand, being a fully participating member does not *necessarily* offer the best perspective for studying a phenomenon—just as being an actor in a play does not offer the most advantageous view of the performance.

Example of participant observation

A team of researchers (Estabrooks, Rutakumwa, O'Leary, Profetto-McGrath, Milner, Levers, & Scott-Finlay, 2005) conducted an ethnographic study of nurses' research utilization behaviour and the sources of nurses' practice knowledge. The study took place in seven patient care units in four Canadian hospitals. Participant observation fieldwork was performed over a 6-month period in each unit by nurses trained for the study.

GATHERING PARTICIPANT OBSERVATION DATA

Participant observers typically place few restrictions on the nature of the data collected, in keeping with the goal of minimizing observer-imposed meanings and structure. Nevertheless, participant observers often do have a broad plan for the types of information to be gathered. Among the aspects of an observed activity likely to be considered relevant are the following:

1. *The physical setting—"where" questions.* Where is the activity happening? What are the main features of the physical setting?
2. *The participants—"who" questions.* Who is present? What are their characteristics and roles? Who is given free access to the setting—who "belongs"?

3. *Activities*—*"what"* *questions.* What is going on? What are participants doing? How do participants interact with one another?
4. *Frequency and duration*—*"when"* *questions.* When did the activity begin and end? How regularly does the activity recur?
5. *Process*—*"how"* *questions.* How is the activity organized? How does the event unfold?
6. *Outcomes*—*"why"* *questions.* Why is the activity happening, or why is it happening in this manner? What did *not* happen—and why?

The next decision is to identify a way to sample observations and to select observational locations. Researchers generally use a combination of positioning approaches. *Single positioning* means staying in a single location for a period to observe transactions. *Multiple positioning* involves moving around the site to observe behaviours from different locations. *Mobile positioning* involves following a person throughout a given activity or period.

Because participant observers cannot spend a lifetime in one site and cannot be in more than one place at a time, observation is usually supplemented with information from unstructured interviews or conversations. For example, informants may be asked to describe what went on in a meeting the observer was unable to attend, or to describe an event that occurred before the observer entered the field. In such cases, the informant functions as the observer's observer.

RECORDING OBSERVATIONS

The most common forms of record keeping in participant observation studies are logs and field notes, but photographs and videotapes may also be used. A **log** (or *field diary*) is a daily record of events and conversations. **Field notes** are broader, more analytic, and more interpretive. Field notes represent the observer's efforts to record information, synthesize, and understand the data.

Field notes can be descriptive or reflective. *Descriptive notes* (or *observational notes*) are objective, *thick* descriptions of events and conversations. Descriptions of what has transpired must include contextual information about time, place, and actors to fully portray the situation. *Reflective notes* document researchers' personal experiences and reflections while in the field. Reflective notes can serve various purposes. *Theoretical notes* are interpretive attempts to attach meaning to observations. *Methodologic notes* are instructions or reminders about how subsequent observations will be made. *Personal notes* are comments about the researcher's own feelings during the research process. Box 13.3 presents examples of various types of field notes from Beck's (2002) study of mothering twins.

The success of any participant observation study depends on the quality of the logs and field notes. Observers must develop the skill of making detailed mental notes that can later be written or tape-recorded. The use of laptop computers can greatly facilitate the recording and organization of notes in the field.

Quantitative Observational Methods

Structured observation differs from unstructured techniques in the specificity of what will be observed and in the advance preparation of forms. The creativity of structured

> ### BOX 13.3   Example of Field Notes: Mothering Multiples Grounded Theory Study
>
> **Observational Notes:** O.L. attended the mothers of multiples support group again this month but she looked worn out today. She wasn't as bubbly as she had been at the March meeting. She explained why she wasn't doing as well this month. She and her husband had just found out that their house has lead-based paint in it. Both twins do have increased lead levels. She and her husband are in the process of buying a new home.
>
> **Theoretical Notes:** So far all the mothers have stressed the need for routine in order to survive the first year of caring for twins. Mothers, however, have varying definitions of routine. I.R. had the firmest routine with her twins. B.L. is more flexible with her routine, i.e., the twins are always fed at the same time but aren't put down for naps or bed at night at the same time. Whenever one of the twins wants to go to sleep is fine with her. B.L. does have a daily routine in regards to housework. For example, when the twins are down in the morning for a nap, she makes their bottles up for the day (14 bottles total).
>
> **Methodologic Notes:** The first sign-up sheet I passed around at the Mothers of Multiples Support Group for women to sign up to participate in interviews for my grounded theory study only consisted of two columns: one for the mother's name and one for her telephone number. I need to revise this sign-up sheet to include extra columns for the age of the multiples, the town where the mother lives, and older siblings and their ages. My plan is to start interviewing mothers with multiples around 1 year of age so that the moms can reflect back over the process of mothering their infants for the first 12 months of their lives.
>
> Right now I have no idea of the ages of the infants of the mothers who signed up to be interviewed. I will need to call the nurse in charge of this support group to find out the ages.
>
> **Personal Notes:** Today was an especially challenging interview. The mom had picked the early afternoon for me to come to her home to interview her because that is the time her 2-year-old son would be napping. When I arrived at her house her 2-year-old ran up to me and said hi. The mom explained that he had taken an earlier nap that day and that he would be up during the interview. So in the living room with us during our interview were her two twin daughters (3 months old) swinging in the swings and her 2-year-old son. One of the twins was quite cranky for the first half hour of the interview. During the interview the 2-year-old sat on my lap and looked at the two books I had brought as a little present. If I didn't keep him occupied with the books, he would keep trying to reach for the microphone of the tape recorder.

From Beck, C. T. (2002). Releasing the pause button: Mothering twins during the first year of life. *Qualitative Health Research*, 12, 593–608.

observation lies not in the observation itself but rather in the development of a system for accurately categorizing, recording, and encoding the observations and sampling the phenomena of interest.

CATEGORIES AND CHECKLISTS

The most common approach to making structured observations is to use a category system for classifying observed phenomena. A **category system** represents a method of recording in a systematic fashion the behaviours and events of interest that transpire in a setting.

Some category systems are constructed so that *all* observed behaviours within a specified domain (e.g., all body positions and movements) can be classified into one and only one category. A contrasting technique is to develop a system in which only particular types of behaviour (which may or may not be manifested) are categorized. For example, if we were studying autistic children's aggressive behaviour, we might develop such categories as "strikes another child," or "throws objects around the room." In this category system, many behaviours—all that are nonaggressive—would not be classified, and some children may exhibit *no* aggressive actions. Nonexhaustive systems are adequate for many purposes, but one risk is that resulting data might be difficult to interpret. When a large number of behaviours are not categorized, the investigator may have difficulty placing categorized behaviour into perspective.

Example of a nonexhaustive observational checklist

Harrison, Magill-Evans, and Sadoway (2001) examined interactions between fathers and their 13- to 24-month-old infants. The researchers used an instrument called the Nursing Child Assessment Teaching Scale (NCATS), an observational checklist that taps 50 parent behaviours and 23 infant behaviours during a teaching task. Specific behaviours are recorded as being observed or not. In this study, the fathers' scores on the NCATS scale were compared with scores for mothers of similar ethnicity and marital status.

One of the most important requirements of a category system is the careful and explicit operational definition of the behaviours and characteristics to be observed. Each category must be carefully explained, giving observers clearcut criteria for assessing the occurrence of the phenomenon. Even with detailed definitions of categories, observers often are faced with making numerous on-the-spot inferences. Virtually all category systems require observer inference, to a greater or lesser degree.

Example of moderate observer inference

Drummond, Fleming, McDonald, & Kysela (2005) studied the effect of a family problem-solving intervention on group problem solving and cooperative parenting communication, which were measured using observational instruments that required moderate inference. For example, parents were videotaped playing with their child, and an instrument called the Interactive Language Assessment Device was used to measure parent initiations and parent responses. Examples of types of parent responses that needed to be coded are "repeating," "expansion," "seeking clarification," and "negative feedback."

After a category system has been developed, researchers typically construct a **checklist,** which is the instrument used to record observations. The checklist is generally formatted with the list of behaviours from the category system on the left and space for tallying their frequency or duration on the right. The task of the observer using an exhaustive category system is to place *all* observed behaviours in one category for each integral unit of behaviour (e.g., a sentence in a conversation, a time interval). Checklists based on

Example of low observer inference

Walker, Kudreikis, Sherrard, and Johnston (2003) studied the effect of repeated neonatal pain on maternal behaviour in rats. The mother rats were observed (by videotape) after their pups were separated from them and then reunited after receiving a painful procedure. Various maternal behaviours were coded, including nesting, defined as "the time when the mother was over her pups in the crouching position . . . and more than 3 pups were attached to the nipples." (p. 255)

exhaustive category systems tend to be demanding because the recording task is continuous. With nonexhaustive category systems, categories of behaviours that may or may not be manifested by participants are listed. The observer's tasks are to watch for instances of these behaviours and to record their occurrence.

RATING SCALES

Another approach to structured observations is to use a **rating scale**, which requires observers to rate some phenomena along a descriptive continuum. Observers may be required to make ratings of behaviour at intervals throughout the observation or to summarize an entire event or transaction after observation is completed.

Rating scales can be used as an extension of checklists, in which the observer records not only the occurrence of some behaviour but also some qualitative aspect of it, such as its magnitude or intensity. When rating scales are coupled with a category scheme in this fashion, considerably more information about the phenomena under study can be obtained, but this approach places an immense burden on observers.

Example of observational ratings

A team of nurses at the University of Alberta (Morse, Beres, Spiers, Mayan, and Olson, 2003) studied emotional suffering among people who had experienced a life-threatening illness or had cared for a significant other with a terminal illness. In-depth interviews with 19 participants were videotaped, and facial expressions were coded to link verbal and behavioural expressions of suffering. The researchers used an observational system that involved rating facial muscle movements for intensity (from 1 to 5) at 1-second intervals.

OBSERVATIONAL SAMPLING

Researchers must decide when structured observational systems will be applied. Observational sampling methods provide a mechanism for obtaining representative examples of the behaviours being observed. One system is **time sampling,** which involves the selection of time periods during which observations will occur. Time frames may be systematically selected (e.g., every 30 seconds at 2-minute intervals) or selected at random.

Example of time sampling

Billinghurst, Morgan, and Arthur (2003) conducted a study to determine the frequency of rhythm disturbance events among patients on remote cardiac telemetry and to identify how many of the events were detected by telemetry nurses. Observational data were collected in a coronary respiratory care unit over a 9-day period. Two-hour blocks of time were randomly selected within 8-hour time periods.

Event sampling selects integral behaviours or events for observation. Event sampling requires researchers to either have knowledge about the occurrence of events or be in a position to wait for or precipitate their occurrence. Examples of integral events that may be suitable for event sampling include shift changes of nurses in a hospital or cast removals of paediatric patients. This sampling approach is preferable to time sampling when the events of interest are infrequent and may be missed if time sampling is used. When behaviours and events are relatively frequent, however, time sampling enhances the representativeness of the observed behaviours.

Evaluation of Observational Methods

The field of nursing is particularly well suited to observational research. Nurses are often in a position to watch people's behaviours and may, by training, be especially sensitive observers. Moreover, certain research questions are better suited to observation than to self-reports, such as when people cannot adequately describe their own behaviours. This may be the case when people are unaware of their own behaviour (e.g., stress-induced behaviour), when people are embarrassed to report their activities (e.g., aggressive actions), when behaviours are emotionally laden (e.g., grieving behaviour), or when people are not capable of articulating their actions (e.g., young children or the mentally ill). Observational methods have an intrinsic appeal for directly capturing behaviours and events. Furthermore, observational methods can provide information of great depth and variety. With this approach, humans—the observers—are used as measuring instruments and provide a uniquely sensitive (if fallible) tool.

Several of the shortcomings of the observational approach have already been mentioned. These include possible ethical difficulties and reactivity of the observed when the observer is conspicuous. However, one of the most pervasive problems is the vulnerability of observations to bias. A number of factors interfere with objective observations, including the following:

▶ Emotions, prejudices, and values of the observer may result in faulty inference.
▶ Personal interest and commitment may colour what is seen in the direction of what the observer wants to see.
▶ Anticipation of what is to be observed may affect what is perceived.
▶ Hasty decisions may result in erroneous conclusions or classifications.

Observational biases probably cannot be eliminated, but they can be minimized through careful observer training.

Both unstructured and structured observational methods have pros and cons. Qualitative observational methods potentially yield a richer understanding of human behaviours and social situations than is possible with structured procedures. Skilful participant observers can "get inside" a situation and lead to a solid understanding of its complexities. Furthermore, qualitative observational approaches are flexible and give observers freedom to reconceptualize the problem after becoming familiar with the situation. On the other hand, observer bias may pose a threat: once researchers begin to participate in a group's activities, the possibility of emotional involvement becomes a salient issue. Participant observers may develop a myopic view on issues of importance to the group. Another issue is that qualitative observational methods are highly dependent on the observational and interpersonal skills of the observer.

Researchers generally choose an approach that matches the research problem—and their paradigmatic orientation. Qualitative observational methods are especially profitable for in-depth research in which the investigator wishes to establish an adequate conceptualization of the important issues in a social setting or to develop hypotheses. Structured observation is better suited to formal hypothesis testing regarding measurable human behaviours.

Critiquing Observational Methods

As in the case of self-reports, the first question you should ask when critiquing an observational study is whether the data should have been collected by some other approach. The advantages and disadvantages of observational methods, discussed previously, should be helpful in considering the appropriateness of using observation.

Some additional guidelines for critiquing observational studies are presented in Box 13.4. A research report should usually document the following aspects of the observational plan:

▶ The degree of structure in the observations
▶ The focus of the observations

BOX 13.4   Guidelines for Critiquing Observational Methods

1. Does the research question lend itself to an observational approach? Would an alternative method have been more appropriate?
2. Is the degree of structure consistent with the nature of the research question?
3. To what degree were observers concealed during data collection? If there was no concealment, what effect might the observers' presence have had on the behaviours being observed?
4. To what degree did the observer participate in activities with those being observed, and was this appropriate?
5. Where did the observations take place? To what extent did the setting influence the naturalness of the behaviours observed?
6. How were data actually recorded (e.g., on field notes, checklists)? Did the recording procedure appear appropriate?
7. What was the plan by which events or behaviours were sampled? Did this plan appear appropriate?
8. What steps were taken to minimize observer biases?

▶ The degree to which the observer was concealed
▶ For qualitative studies, how entry into the observed group was gained, the relationship between the observer and those observed, the time period over which data were collected, and the method of recording data
▶ For quantitative studies, a description of the category system or rating scales and the settings in which observations took place
▶ The plan for sampling events and behaviours to observe

BIOPHYSIOLOGIC MEASURES

One result of the trend toward clinical, patient-centred studies is greater use of biophysiologic and physical variables. Clinical nursing studies involve biophysiologic instruments both for creating independent variables (e.g., an intervention using biofeedback equipment) and for measuring dependent variables. For the most part, our discussion focuses on the use of biophysiologic measures as dependent (outcome) variables.

Nurse researchers have used biophysiologic measures in a variety of ways. Some have studied basic biophysiologic processes that have relevance for nursing care, using healthy participants or an animal species. Some have evaluated specific nursing interventions or products to enhance patient health or comfort. Yet others have examined the correlates of physiologic functioning in patients with health problems. Studies have also been undertaken to evaluate the measurement of biophysiologic information gathered by nurses, with an eye toward improving clinical measurements.

Example of evaluating clinical measurements

Chin-Peuckert, Rennick, Jednak, Capolicchio, and Salle (2004) hypothesized that warm infusion solution should be used for urodynamic evaluations of children. They used a crossover design comparing outcomes for room temperature and body temperature cystometrograms with 91 hospitalized children. Outcome measures included maximum cystometric bladder capacity, maximum flow rate, and pressure at maximum flow.

Types of Biophysiologic Measures

Biophysiologic measures include both *in vivo* and *in vitro* measures. *In vivo* measures are performed directly within or on living organisms. Examples of *in vivo* measures include blood pressure and vital capacity measurement. *In vivo* instruments are available to measure all bodily functions, and technologic advances continue to improve the ability to measure biophysiologic phenomena more accurately and conveniently.

With *in vitro* measures, data are gathered from participants by extracting some biophysiologic material from them and subjecting it to laboratory analysis. The analysis is normally done by specialized laboratory technicians. *In vitro* measures include chemical

Example of a study with *in vivo* measures

Using an experimental design, Gibbins, Stevens, Hodnett, Pinelli, Ohlsson, and Darlington (2002) compared the efficacy and safety of three interventions for relieving pain from heel lances in neonates. Physiologic indicators (heart rate, oxygen saturation) were incorporated into their measure of infant pain. (Note that this study appears in its entirety in Appendix A of the *Study Guide to Accompany Essentials of Nursing Research*, 6th edition).

measures (e.g., the measurement of hormone, sugar, or potassium levels); microbiologic measures (e.g., bacterial counts and identification); and cytologic or histologic measures (e.g., tissue biopsies).

Example of a study with *in vitro* measures

Olson, Rennie, Hanson, Ryan, Gilpin, Falsetti, Heffner, and Gaudet (2004) hypothesized that sepsis could be reduced through a no-dressing intervention for tunnelled central venous catheter exit sites. Skin swabs collected from the catheter exit sites and blood cultures were submitted for laboratory analysis.

Evaluation of Biophysiologic Measures

Biophysiologic measures offer a number of advantages to nurse researchers. First, biophysiologic measures are relatively accurate and precise, especially when compared with psychological measures, such as self-report measures of anxiety, pain, and so forth. Biophysiologic measures are also objective. Two nurses reading from the same spirometer output are likely to record identical tidal volume measurements, and two different spirometers are likely to produce the same readouts. Patients cannot easily distort measurements of biophysiologic functioning deliberately. Finally, biophysiologic instrumentation provides valid measures of the targeted variables: thermometers can be depended on to measure temperature and not blood volume, and so forth. For nonbiophysiologic measures, there are typically concerns about whether an instrument is really measuring the target concept.

In short, biophysiologic measures are plentiful, tend to be accurate and valid, and are extremely useful in clinical nursing studies. However, care must be exercised in using them with regard to practical, ethical, medical, and technical considerations.

Critiquing Biophysiologic Measures

As always, the most important consideration in evaluating a data collection strategy is the appropriateness of the measures for the research question. The objectivity, accuracy, and availability of biophysiologic measures are of little significance if an alternative method

> ### BOX 13.5   Guidelines for Critiquing Biophysiologic Methods
>
> 1. Does the research question lend itself to a biophysiologic approach? Would an alternative method have been theoretically more appropriate?
> 2. Was the proper instrumentation used to obtain the biophysiologic measurements? Would an alternative instrument or method have been more appropriate?
> 3. Does the researcher appear to have the skills necessary for proper interpretation of the biophysiologic measures?

would have resulted in a better measurement of the key concepts. Stress, for example, could be measured in various ways: through self-report (e.g., through the use of a scale such as the State-Trait Anxiety Inventory); through direct observation of participants' behaviour during exposure to stressful stimuli; or by measuring heart rate, blood pressure, or levels of adrenocorticotropic hormone in urine samples. The choice of which measure to use must be linked to the way that stress is conceptualized in the research problem.

Additional criteria for assessing the use of biophysiologic measures are presented in Box 13.5. The general questions to consider are these: Did the researcher select the correct biophysiologic measure? Was care taken in the collection of the data? Did the researcher competently interpret the data?

 CONSUMER TIP

Many nursing studies—especially qualitative ones—integrate a variety of data collection approaches. Qualitative studies are especially likely to combine unstructured observations and self-reports. If multiple approaches are used in a quantitative study, structured self-reports combined with biophysiologic measures are most common. ■

IMPLEMENTING THE DATA COLLECTION PLAN

In addition to selecting methods for collecting data, researchers must develop and implement a plan for gathering their data. This involves decisions that could affect the quality of the data being collected.

One important decision concerns who will collect the data. Researchers often hire assistants to collect data rather than doing it personally. This is especially likely to be the case in large-scale quantitative studies. In other studies, nurses or other health care staff are asked to assist in the collection of data. From your perspective as a consumer, the critical issue is whether the people collecting data were able to produce valid and accurate data. In any research endeavour, adequate training of data collectors is essential.

Another issue concerns the circumstances under which data were gathered. For example, it may be essential to ensure total privacy to participants. In most cases, it is important for researchers to create a nonjudgmental atmosphere in which participants are encouraged to be candid or behave naturally. Again, you as a consumer must ask whether

BOX 13.6   Guidelines for Critiquing Data Collection Procedures

1. Who collected the research data? Were the data collectors qualified for their role, or is there something about them (e.g., their professional role, their relationship with study participants) that could undermine the collection of unbiased, high-quality data?
2. How were data collectors trained? Does the training appear adequate?
3. Where and under what circumstances were the data gathered? Were other people present during that data collection? Could the presence of others have created any distortions?
4. Did the collection of data place any undue burdens (in terms of time or stress) on participants? How might this have affected data quality?

there is anything about the way in which the data were collected that could have created bias or otherwise affected data quality.

In evaluating the data collection plan of a study, then, you should critically appraise not only the actual methods chosen but also the procedures used to collect the data. Box 13.6 provides some specific guidelines for critiquing the procedures used to collect research data.

RESEARCH EXAMPLES   Critical Thinking Activities

 EXAMPLE 1: Unstructured Observation and Interviews

Aspects of a qualitative study, featuring terms and concepts discussed in this chapter, are presented below, followed by some questions to guide critical thinking.

Study
"Daughters of cardiac patients: The process of caregiving" (Gage-Rancoeur & Purden, 2003)

Statement of Purpose
The purpose of this study was to explore the caregiving role that adult daughters play when a parent is hospitalized for a cardiac condition and to examine how the role develops and changes during the recovery period.

Method
Gage-Rancoeur and Purden collected self-report and observational data from daughters of parents hospitalized with cardiac illness. A sample of nine daughters, all of whom were identified as actively involved in their parents' care, participated in the study. After a daughter agreed to participate, the researchers began to observe her interactions with her parent, and field notes were maintained. The daughters were also interviewed in-depth to explore their thoughts and feelings, using a semi-structured approach. Interviewing began with such broad questions as, "In every family, children help out in different ways; could you tell me about

(Research Examples continue on page 310)

Critical Thinking Activities (continued)

your experience?" For logistical reasons, the interviews were not audiotaped, but the conversations were recorded immediately following the interaction, and detailed field notes were completed the same day. Additional data were collected through interviews and conversations with the patients themselves and with other family members. Follow-up interviews were conducted by telephone with some of the daughters after discharge. The number of contacts per family ranged from one to seven, with variation related to the patients' length of stay in hospital.

Key Findings
▶ The daughters were engaged in a dynamic process of "knowing" in order to care for their ill parent.
▶ The daughters' caregiving was characterized by a nonlinear process of knowing that included "caring to know" (knowledge seeking), "coming to know" (knowledge consolidation), and "knowing to care" (actions based on knowledge).
▶ The daughters' level of involvement was defined by four different caregiving modes (*we all support each other; my siblings help out in different ways; the chosen one;* and *I am the only one left*).

Critical Thinking Suggestions*
*See the Student Resource CD-ROM for a discussion of these questions.
1. Answer the following questions, many of which are adapted from the critiquing guidelines presented in this chapter:
   a. How much structure did the researchers use in their data collection? Is the degree of structure used appropriate for the study purpose?
   b. Some of the researchers' data were gathered through observation; does the research question lend itself to an observational approach? If the researchers had not done observations, would the findings likely be affected?
   c. The report indicated that *participant* observation had been used. Describe how this might have been accomplished.
   d. Much of the data for this study were gathered through self-report; does the research question lend itself to a self-report approach? If the researchers had not gathered self-report data, would their findings likely have been affected?
   e. Comment on the fact that the interviews were not audiotaped.
   f. Comment on the researchers' strategy to gather additional data by interviewing the patients and other family members.
2. If the results of this study are trustworthy, what are some of the uses to which the findings might be put in clinical practice?

 EXAMPLE 2: Physiologic, Self-Report, and Observational Measures

Aspects of a quantitative nursing study, featuring terms and concepts discussed in this chapter, are presented below, followed by some questions to guide critical thinking.

Critical Thinking Activities (continued)

Study
"Tub bathing versus traditional sponge bathing for the newborn" (Bryanton, Walsh, Barrett, & Gaudet, 2004)

Statement of Purpose
The study was designed to compare the effects of tub bathing versus traditional sponge bathing in healthy, term infants on newborn outcomes and maternal confidence.

Method
A true experimental design was used in which 102 mother–infant pairs were randomly assigned to the experimental tub bath or to a sponge bath (usual care) control group. A wide range of data was gathered at the baby's initial and one additional bath, including data from records (demographic information), physiologic measures, observations, and self-reports. The main physiologic variable was infant temperature, measured using the axillary route, within 10 minutes before and after bathing. Structured observations were used to measure umbilical cord healing and infant contentment. Nurses on the night shift rated the infant cords using the Cord Rating Scale, which encompassed observational ratings of redness, discharge, odour, and dryness. The nurse bathing the infant assessed contentment using a scale from a formal observational instrument known as the Brazelton Neonatal Behavioral Assessment Scale. Newborn state of consciousness was also rated on a 6-point scale from State 1 (quiet sleep) to State 6 (crying). Finally, mothers completed a brief self-report instrument in which they were asked to rate, on a 5-point scale, their degree of pleasure with the bathing procedure (which they observed) and their level of confidence with bathing.

Key Findings
▶ Tub-bathed infants had significantly less temperature loss than sponge-bathed infants.
▶ Tub-bathed infants were significantly more content than infants in the control group, and mothers of tub-bathed infants also had higher ratings of pleasure.
▶ Cord healing did not differ in the two groups.

Critical Thinking Suggestions
1. Answer the following questions, many of which are adapted from the critiquing guidelines presented in this chapter:
  a. How much structure did the researchers use in their data collection? Is the degree of structure appropriate for the research question?
  b. Some of the researchers' outcome data were gathered through self-report; does the research question lend itself to a self-report approach? If they had not gathered self-report data, would their findings likely have been affected?
  c. How do you think the self-report data were gathered (by interview or questionnaire)?

(Research Examples continue on page 312)

Critical Thinking Activities (continued)

d. Some of the outcome data were gathered through observation; does the research question lend itself to an observational approach? If the researchers had not undertaken observational work, would the findings likely be affected?

e. To what extent do you think the behaviours of those being observed were affected by the presence of observers? Do you think that the risk of observational bias was high?

f. Some of the researchers' outcome data were biophysiologic measures; is this compatible with the research question? Was this the best method to use?

2. If the results of this study are valid and reliable, what are some of the uses to which the findings might be put in clinical practice?

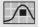 **EXAMPLE 3: Structured Self-Reports and Physiologic Measures**

1. Read the Method section from the study by Feeley and colleagues ("Mother–VLBW Infant Interaction") in Appendix A of this book, and then answer questions 1 through 4 in Box 13.2.

2. Also consider the following targeted questions, which may further sharpen your critical thinking skills and assist you in assessing aspects of the study's merit:

a. Comment on the researchers' decision to use a structured observational measure for the dependent variable.

b. Why do you think the researchers videotaped the mother–infant interaction? What are the advantages and disadvantages of such an approach?

c. What steps were taken to minimize observer bias?

 EXAMPLE 4: Unstructured Self-Reports

1. Read the Procedure section from Beck's study ("Birth Trauma") in Appendix B of this book, and then answer questions 1 through 3 in Box 13.2.

2. Also consider the following targeted questions, which may further sharpen your critical thinking skills and assist you in assessing aspects of the study:

a. Comment on the potential added value of having some of the respondents' journals as a data source.

b. Comment on Beck's procedure of following up with further questions after she received the respondents' birth trauma stories.

C H A P T E R   R E V I E W
S u m m a r y   P o i n t s

▶ Some researchers use existing data in their studies—for example, those doing historical research, meta-analyses, secondary analyses, or analyses of available **records**.

▶ Data collection methods vary along four dimensions: structure, quantifiability, researcher obtrusiveness, and objectivity.

▶ The three principal data collection methods for nurse researchers are self-reports, observations, and biophysiologic measures.

▶ Self-reports are the most widely used method of collecting data for nursing studies. Qualitative studies—especially ethnographies—are more likely than quantitative studies to triangulate data from different sources.

▶ **Self-report** data are collected by means of an oral interview or written questionnaire. Self-report methods are an indispensable means of collecting data but are susceptible to errors of reporting.

▶ Unstructured self-reports, used in qualitative studies, include **completely unstructured interviews**, which are conversational discussions on the topic of interest; **semi-structured** (or *focused*) **interviews**, using a broad **topic guide**; **focus group interviews**, which involve discussions with small groups; **life histories**, which encourage respondents to narrate their life experiences about a theme; the **think aloud method,** which involves having people talk about decisions as they are making them; **diaries**, in which respondents are asked to maintain daily records about some aspects of their lives; and the **critical incidents technique**, which involves probes about the circumstances surrounding an incident that is critical to an outcome of interest.

▶ Structured self-reports used in quantitative studies employ a formal **instrument**—a **questionnaire** or **interview schedule**—that may contain a combination of **open-ended questions** (which permit respondents to respond in their own words) and **closed-ended questions** (which offer respondents fixed alternatives from which to choose).

▶ Questionnaires are less costly than interviews, offer the possibility of anonymity, and run no risk of interviewer bias; however, interviews yield higher response rates, are suitable for a wider variety of people, and provide richer data than questionnaires.

▶ Social-psychological **scales** are self-report tools for quantitatively measuring the intensity of such characteristics as attitudes, needs, and perceptions.

▶ **Likert scales** (or **summated rating scales**) present respondents with a series of *items* worded favourably or unfavourably toward some phenomenon; responses indicating level of agreement or disagreement with each statement are scored and summed into a composite score.

▶ The **semantic differential** (SD) technique consists of a series of scales with bipolar adjectives (e.g., good/bad) along which respondents rate their reactions toward phenomena.

▶ A **visual analog scale** (VAS) is used to measure subjective experiences (e.g., pain, fatigue) along a line designating a bipolar continuum.

▶ Scales are versatile and powerful but are susceptible to **response set biases**—the tendency of some people to respond to items in characteristic ways, independently of item content.

▶ **Vignettes** are brief descriptions of some person or situation to which respondents are asked to react.

▶ With a **Q sort**, respondents sort a set of statements into piles according to specified criteria.

▶ Direct **observation** of phenomena, which includes both structured and unstructured procedures, is a technique for gathering data about behaviours and events.

▶ One type of unstructured observation is **participant observation**, in which the researcher gains entrée into the social group of interest and participates to varying degrees in its functioning while making in-depth observations of activities and events.

> **Logs** of daily events and **field notes** of the observer's experiences and interpretations constitute the major data collection instruments in unstructured observation.

▶ Structured observations, which dictate what the observer should observe, often involve **checklists**—tools based on **category systems** for recording the appearance, frequency, or duration of prespecified behaviours or events. Alternatively, the observer may use **rating scales** to rate phenomena along a dimension of interest (e.g., energetic/lethargic).

▶ Structured observations often use a sampling plan (such as **time sampling** or **event sampling**) for selecting the behaviours or events to be observed.

▶ Observational techniques are a versatile and important alternative to self-reports, but observational biases can pose a threat to the validity and accuracy of observational data.

▶ Data may also be derived from **biophysiologic measures**, which can be classified as either *in vivo* measurements (those performed within or on living organisms) or *in vitro* measurements (those performed outside the organism's body, such as blood tests). Biophysiologic measures have the advantage of being objective, accurate, and precise.

▶ In developing a data collection plan, the researcher must decide who will collect the data, how the data collectors will be trained, and what the circumstances for data collection will be.

Additional Resources for Review

Chapter 13 of the *Study Guide to Accompany Essentials of Nursing Research,* 6th edition offers various exercises and study suggestions for reinforcing the concepts presented in this chapter. For additional review, see the Student Self-Study Review Questions section of the Student Resource CD-ROM provided with this book.

SUGGESTED READINGS

*References for studies cited in the chapter appear at the end of the book.

Methodologic References

Frank-Stromberg, M., & Olsen, S. J. (Eds.). (2004). *Instruments for clinical health care.* Sudbury, MA: Jones & Bartlett.

Kerlinger, F. N., & Lee, H. B. (2000). *Foundations of behavioral research* (4th ed.). Orlando, FL: Harcourt College.

Leininger, M. M. (Ed.). (1985). *Qualitative research methods in nursing.* New York: Grune & Stratton.

Polit, D. F., & Beck, C. T. (2004). *Nursing research: Principles and methods* (7th ed.). Philadelphia: Lippincott Williams & Wilkins.

Rew, L., Bechtel, D., & Sapp, A. (1993). Self-as-instrument in qualitative research. *Nursing Research, 42,* 300–301.

Waltz, C. F., Strickland, O. L., & Lenz, E. R. (1991). *Measurement in nursing research* (2nd ed.). Philadelphia: F. A. Davis.

Evaluating Measurements and Data Quality

STUDENT OBJECTIVES

On completing this chapter, you will be able to:

◗ Describe the major characteristics of measurement and identify major sources of measurement error
◗ Describe aspects of reliability and validity, and specify how each aspect can be assessed
◗ Interpret the meaning of reliability and validity coefficients
◗ Describe the four dimensions used in establishing the trustworthiness of qualitative data and identify methods of enhancing data quality in qualitative studies
◗ Evaluate the overall quality of a measuring tool or data collection approach used in a study
◗ Define new terms in the chapter

An ideal data collection procedure is one that captures a phenomenon or concept in a way that is relevant, accurate, truthful, and sensitive. For most concepts of interest to nurse researchers, few, if any, data collection procedures match this ideal. In this chapter, we discuss criteria for evaluating the quality of data obtained in both quantitative and qualitative studies.

MEASUREMENT AND THE ASSESSMENT OF QUANTITATIVE DATA

Quantitative studies derive data through the measurement of variables. Before discussing the assessment of quantitative measures, we briefly discuss the concept of measurement.

Measurement

Measurement involves rules for assigning numeric values to *qualities* of objects to designate the *quantity* of the attribute. No attribute inherently has a numeric value; human beings invent rules to measure concepts. An often-quoted statement by an American psychologist, L. L. Thurstone, summarizes a position assumed by many quantitative researchers: "Whatever exists, exists in some amount and can be measured." The notion here is that attributes are not constant: they vary from day to day or from one person to another. This variability is capable of a numeric expression that signifies *how much* of an attribute is present. Quantification is used to communicate that amount. The purpose of assigning numbers is to differentiate among people who possess varying degrees of the critical attribute.

Measurement requires numbers to be assigned to objects according to rules rather than haphazardly. The rules for measuring temperature, weight, and other physical attributes are widely known and accepted. Rules for measuring many variables, however, have to be invented. What are the rules for measuring patient satisfaction? Pain? Depression? Whether the data are collected through observation, self-report, or some other method, researchers must specify how numeric values are to be assigned.

ADVANTAGES OF MEASUREMENT

A major strength of measurement is that it removes guesswork in gathering information. Consider how handicapped nurses and doctors would be in the absence of measures of body temperature, blood pressure, and so on. Because measurement is based on explicit rules, the information tends to be objective: two people measuring a person's weight using the same scale would likely get identical results. Two people scoring responses to a self-report stress scale would likely arrive at identical scores. Not all quantitative measures are completely objective, but most incorporate rules for minimizing subjectivity.

Measurement also makes it possible to obtain reasonably precise information. Instead of describing Nathan as "rather tall," for example, we can depict him as a man who is 1.9 meters tall. If it were necessary, we could obtain even more precise height measurements. Such precision allows researchers to differentiate among people who possess different amounts of an attribute.

Finally, measurement is a language of communication. Numbers are less vague than words and can thus communicate information broadly. If a researcher reported that the average oral temperature of a sample of patients was "somewhat high," different readers might develop different ideas about the sample's physiologic state. If the researcher reported an average temperature of 37.6°C, however, there is no ambiguity.

ERRORS OF MEASUREMENT

Researchers work with fallible measures. Values and scores from even the best instruments have a certain amount of error. We can think of every piece of quantitative data as consisting of two parts: a true component and an error component. This can be written as an equation, as follows:

Obtained score = True score ± Error

The **obtained** (or observed) **score** could be, for example, a patient's heart rate or score on an anxiety scale. The **true score** is the true value that would be obtained if it were possible to have an infallible measure of the target attribute. The true score is hypothetical; it can never be known because measures are not infallible. The **error of measurement**—the difference between true and obtained scores—reflects extraneous factors that affect the measurement and distort the results. Many factors contribute to errors of measurement. Among the most common are the following:

▶ *Situational contaminants.* Measurements can be affected by the conditions under which they are produced (e.g., people's awareness of an observer can affect their behaviour; environmental factors such as temperature or time of day can be sources of measurement error).
▶ *Response set biases.* A number of relatively enduring characteristics of respondents can interfere with accurate measures of an attribute (see Chapter 13).
▶ *Transitory personal factors.* Temporary personal factors (e.g., fatigue) can influence people's motivation or ability to cooperate, act naturally, or do their best.
▶ *Administration variations.* Alterations in the methods of collecting data from one person to the next can affect obtained scores (e.g., if some biophysiologic measures are taken before a feeding and others are taken postprandially).
▶ *Item sampling.* Errors can be introduced as a result of the sampling of items used to measure an attribute. For example, a student's score on a 100-item research methods test will be influenced to a certain extent by *which* 100 questions are included.

This list is not exhaustive, but it illustrates that data are susceptible to measurement error from a variety of sources.

Reliability

The reliability of a quantitative measure is a major criterion for assessing its quality. **Reliability** is the consistency with which an instrument measures the attribute. If a spring scale gave a reading of 50 kg for a person's weight one minute and a reading of 60 kg the next minute, we would naturally be wary of using such an unreliable scale. The less variation an instrument produces in repeated measurements, the higher is its reliability.

Another way to define reliability is in terms of accuracy. An instrument is reliable if its measures accurately reflect true scores. A reliable measure is one that maximizes the true score component and minimizes the error component of an obtained score.

Three aspects of reliability are of interest to quantitative researchers: stability, internal consistency, and equivalence.

STABILITY

The *stability* of a measure is the extent to which the same scores are obtained when the instrument is used with the same people on separate occasions. Assessments of stability are derived through **test–retest reliability** procedures. The researcher administers the same measure to a sample of people on two occasions, and then compares the scores.

CONSUMER TIP

Many psychosocial scales contain two or more **subscales**, each of which tap distinct, but related, concepts (e.g., a measure of independent functioning might include subscales for motor activities, communication, and socializing). The reliability of each subscale is typically assessed and, if subscale scores are summed for an overall score, the scale's overall reliability would also be assessed. ■

Suppose, for example, we were interested in the stability of a self-report scale that measured self-esteem in adolescents. Because self-esteem is a fairly stable attribute that would not change markedly from one day to the next, we would expect a reliable measure of it to yield consistent scores on two separate tests. As a check on the instrument's stability, we arrange to administer the scale 3 weeks apart to a sample of teenagers. Fictitious data for this example are presented in Table 14.1. On the whole, differences on the two tests are not large. Researchers compute a **reliability coefficient,** a numeric index of a measure's reliability, to objectively determine exactly how small the differences are. Reliability coefficients (designated as r) range from .00 to 1.00.* The higher the value, the IQ1 more reliable (stable) is the measuring instrument. In the example shown in Table 14.1, the reliability coefficient is .95, which is quite high.

CONSUMER TIP

For most purposes, reliability coefficients higher than .70 are satisfactory, but coefficients in the .85 to .95 range are far preferable. ■

TABLE 14.1	**Fictitious Data for Test–Retest Reliability of Self-Esteem Scale**	
SUBJECT NUMBER	**TIME 1**	**TIME 2**
1	55	57
2	49	46
3	78	74
4	37	35
5	44	46
6	50	56
7	58	55
8	62	66
9	48	50
10	67	63

$r = .95$

*Computation procedures for reliability coefficients are not presented in this textbook, but formulas can be found in the references cited at the end of this chapter. Although reliability coefficients can technically be less than .00 (i.e., a negative value), they are almost invariably a number between .00 and 1.00).

The test–retest approach to estimating reliability has certain disadvantages. The major problem is that many traits do change over time, independently of the instrument's stability. Attitudes, knowledge, and so forth can be modified by experiences between two measurements. Thus, stability indexes are most appropriate for relatively enduring characteristics, such as personality and abilities. Even with such traits, test–retest reliability tends to decline as the interval between the two administrations increases.

Example of test–retest reliability

Fillion, Gélinas, Simard, Savard, & Gagnon (2003) evaluated the French Canadian adaptation of the Multidimensional Fatigue Inventory among patients with cancer. Some study participants completed the scale twice—at weeks 2 and 4 of radiation treatment. The test–retest reliability for the total scale was .83, whereas that for subscales ranged from .51 (mental fatigue) to .78 (physical fatigue).

INTERNAL CONSISTENCY

Scales that involve summing items usually are evaluated for their internal consistency. Ideally, scales are composed of items that all measure the same critical attribute and nothing else. On a scale to measure nurses' empathy, it would be inappropriate to include an item that is a better measure of spirituality than empathy. An instrument has **internal consistency** reliability to the extent that all its subparts measure the same characteristic. This approach to reliability assesses an important source of measurement error in multi-item measures: the sampling of items.

One of the oldest methods for assessing internal consistency is the *split-half technique*. In this approach, the items comprising a scale are split into two groups (usually, odd versus even items) and scored, and then scores on the two half-tests are used to compute a reliability coefficient. If the two half-tests are really measuring the same attribute, the correlation between the two and hence the reliability coefficient will be high. More sophisticated and accurate methods of computing internal consistency are now in use, most notably, **Cronbach's alpha** (or **coefficient alpha**). This method gives an estimate of the split-half correlation for all possible ways of dividing the measure into two halves, not just odd versus even items. As with test–retest reliability coefficients, indexes of internal consistency range in value between .00 and 1.00. The higher the reliability coefficient, the more accurate (internally consistent) the measure.

Example of internal consistency reliability

Durbin, Goering, Streiner, and Pink (2004) refined and evaluated the Alberta Continuity of Services Scale—Mental Health, a measure of continuity of care for individuals with persistent mental illness. The overall scale had an alpha of .88, and the alphas for the three subscales ranged from .74 to .80.

EQUIVALENCE

The *equivalence* approach to estimating reliability—used primarily with observational instruments—determines the consistency or equivalence of the instrument by different observers or raters. As noted in Chapter 13, a potential weakness of direct observation is the risk for observer error. The degree of error can be assessed through **interrater** (or **interobserver**) **reliability**, which is estimated by having two or more trained observers make simultaneous, independent observations. The resulting data can then be used to calculate an index of equivalence or agreement. That is, a reliability coefficient can be computed to demonstrate the strength of the relationship between the observers' ratings. When two independent observers score some phenomenon congruently, the scores are likely to be accurate and reliable.

Example of interrater reliability

Olson, Hanson, Hamilton, Stacey, Eades, Gue, Plummer, Janes, Fitch, Bakker, Baker, and Oliver (2004) assessed the reliability of a scale (the Western Consortium for Cancer Nursing Research scale) for staging the severity of chemotherapy-induced stomatitis. Pairs of raters used the instrument with 207 patients from 10 Canadian cancer centres. Interrater agreement between the raters was good in five sites, but agreement was lower in the remaining sites.

INTERPRETATION OF RELIABILITY COEFFICIENTS

Reliability coefficients are an important indicator of an instrument's quality. A measure with low reliability prevents an adequate testing of research hypotheses. If data fail to confirm a hypothesis, one possibility is that the measuring tool was unreliable—not necessarily that the expected relationships do not exist. Knowledge about an instrument's reliability thus is critical in interpreting research results, especially if research hypotheses are not supported.

Reliability estimates vary according to the procedure used to obtain them. Estimates of reliability computed by different procedures for the same instrument are not identical.

Example of different forms of reliability

Davies and Hodnett (2002) developed and evaluated a scale to measure nurses' perceived self-efficacy for providing support to women in labour, the Self-Efficacy Labor Support Scale. The test–retest reliability for the 14-item scale over a 1-week period was .93; the internal consistency reliability was .98.

In addition, reliability of an instrument is related to sample heterogeneity. The more homogeneous the sample (i.e., the more similar the scores), the lower the reliability coefficient will be. This is because instruments are designed to measure differences, and if sample members are similar to one another, it is more difficult for the instrument to discriminate reliably among those who possess varying degrees of the attribute. Finally, longer instruments (i.e., those with more items) tend to have higher reliability than shorter ones.

CONSUMER TIP

If a research report provides information on the reliability of a quantitative scale without specifying the type of reliability measure used, it is probably safe to assume that internal consistency reliability was assessed by the Cronbach alpha method. ■

Validity

The second important criterion for evaluating a quantitative instrument is its validity. **Validity** is the degree to which an instrument measures what it is supposed to be measuring. If a researcher develops an instrument to measure patients' stress, he or she should take steps to ensure that the resulting scores validly reflect this variable and not some other concept.

The reliability and validity of an instrument are not totally independent. A measuring device that is not reliable cannot be valid. An instrument cannot validly be measuring the attribute of interest if it is erratic or inaccurate. An instrument can be reliable, however, without being valid. Suppose we had the idea to measure patients' anxiety by measuring the circumference of their wrists. We could obtain highly accurate, consistent, and precise measurements of wrist circumferences, but they would not be valid indicators of anxiety. Thus, the high reliability of an instrument provides no evidence of its validity; the low reliability of a measure *is* evidence of low validity.

CONSUMER TIP

Some methodologic studies are designed to determine the quality of instruments used by clinicians or researchers. In these **psychometric assessments,** information about the instrument's reliability and validity is carefully documented. ■

Like reliability, validity has a number of aspects and assessment approaches. One aspect is known as face validity. **Face validity** refers to whether the instrument *looks* as though it is measuring the appropriate construct. Although it is often useful for an instrument to have face validity, three other types of validity are of greater importance in assessing an instrument: content validity, criterion-related validity, and construct validity.

CONTENT VALIDITY

Content validity is concerned with adequacy of coverage of the content area being measured. Content validity is crucial for tests of knowledge. In such a context, the validity question is: How representative are the questions on this test of the universe of all questions that might be asked on this topic?

Content validity is also relevant in measures of complex psychosocial traits. A person who wanted to create a new instrument would begin by developing a thorough conceptualization of the construct of interest so that the measure would adequately capture the whole domain. Such a conceptualization might come from first-hand knowledge but is more likely to come from qualitative studies or from a literature review.

The content validity of an instrument is necessarily based on judgment. There are no totally objective methods for ensuring the adequate content coverage of an instrument. Experts in the content area are often called on to analyze the items' adequacy in representing the hypothetical content universe in the correct proportions. It is also possible to calculate a **content validity index** (CVI) that indicates the extent of expert agreement, but ultimately the experts' subjective judgments must be relied on.

Example of content validity

McGilton (2003) developed and evaluated scales to measure supportive leadership (effective support for nursing staff) in long-term care settings. After an initial review of items on one scale by five experts, the CVI score was calculated at 83.5% (usually a minimally acceptable CVI score is 80%). After revisions, the panel re-evaluated the items, and the CVI score improved to 100%.

CRITERION-RELATED VALIDITY

In **criterion-related validity** assessments, researchers seek to establish a relationship between scores on an instrument and some external criterion. The instrument, whatever attribute it is measuring, is said to be valid if its scores correspond strongly with scores on some criterion. (One difficulty of criterion-related validation, however, is finding a criterion that is, in itself, reliable and valid.) After a criterion is established, validity can be estimated easily. A **validity coefficient** is computed by using a mathematic formula that correlates scores on the instrument with scores on the criterion variable. The magnitude of the coefficient indicates how valid the instrument is. These coefficients (r) range between .00 and 1.00, with higher values indicating greater criterion-related validity. Coefficients of .70 or higher are desirable.

Sometimes, a distinction is made between two types of criterion-related validity. **Predictive validity** is an instrument's ability to differentiate between people's performances or behaviours on some future criterion. When a school of nursing correlates students' incoming high school grades with their subsequent grade-point averages, the predictive validity of the high school grades for nursing school performance is being evaluated. **Concurrent validity** refers to an instrument's ability to distinguish among people who differ in their present status on some criterion. For example, a psychological test to differentiate between patients in a mental institution who could and could not be released could be correlated with current ratings by nurses. The difference between predictive and concurrent validity, then, is the difference in the timing of obtaining measurements on a criterion.

Example of predictive validity

Dennis (2003) developed a short form of the Breastfeeding Self-Efficacy Scale (BSES-SF), a scale to measure breastfeeding confidence. She determined the predictive validity of the scale by correlating mothers' scale scores with their method of infant feeding at 4 and 8 weeks postpartum—a strong and objective criterion.

CONSTRUCT VALIDITY

Validating an instrument in terms of **construct validity** is challenging. Construct validity is concerned with the following question: What construct is the instrument actually measuring? The more abstract the concept, the more difficult it is to establish the construct validity of the measure; at the same time, the more abstract the concept, the less suitable it is to use a criterion-related validation approach. What objective criterion is there for concepts such as empathy and separation anxiety? Construct validation is addressed in several ways, but there is always an emphasis on testing relationships predicted on the basis of theoretical considerations. Researchers make predictions about the manner in which the construct will function in relation to other constructs.

One approach to construct validation is the **known-groups technique.** In this procedure, groups that are expected to differ on the critical attribute are administered the instrument, and group scores are compared. For instance, in validating a measure of fear of the labour experience, the scores of primiparas and multiparas could be contrasted. Women who had never given birth would likely experience more anxiety than women who had already had children; one might question the validity of the instrument if such differences did not emerge.

Another method of construct validation involves an examination of relationships based on theoretical predictions. Researchers might reason as follows: According to theory, construct X is related to construct Y; instrument A is a measure of construct X, and instrument B is a measure of construct Y; scores on A and B are related to each other, as predicted by the theory; therefore, it is inferred that A and B are valid measures of X and Y. This logical analysis is fallible, but it does offer supporting evidence.

Another approach to construct validation employs a statistical procedure known as **factor analysis**, which is a method for identifying clusters of related items on a scale. The procedure is used to identify and group together different measures of some underlying attribute and to distinguish them from measures of different attributes.

In summary, construct validation employs both logical and empirical procedures. Like content validity, construct validity requires a judgment pertaining to what the instrument is measuring. Construct validity and criterion-related validity share an empirical component, but, in the latter case, there is a pragmatic, objective criterion with which to compare a measure rather than a second measure of an abstract theoretical construct.

INTERPRETATION OF VALIDITY

Like reliability, validity is not an all-or-nothing characteristic of an instrument. An instrument cannot really be said to possess or lack validity; it is a question of degree. The testing of an instrument's validity is not proved but rather is supported by an accumulation of evidence.

Example of construct validity

Tourangeau and McGilton (2004) evaluated the Leadership Practice Inventory in applications designed to measure leadership practices of nurses. They used various techniques to assess the scale's construct validity, including a factor analysis and the known-groups technique (comparing aspiring and established nurse leaders). They also correlated scale scores with scores on an observational measure of the nurses' organizational effectiveness.

Strictly speaking, researchers do not validate an instrument *per se* but rather some application of the instrument. A measure of anxiety may be valid for presurgical patients but may not be valid for nursing students before a final examination. Validation is a never-ending process: the more evidence that can be gathered that an instrument is measuring what it is supposed to be measuring, the greater the confidence researchers have in its validity.

CONSUMER TIP

In quantitative studies involving self-report or observational instruments, the research report usually provides validity and reliability information from an earlier study—often a study conducted by the person who developed the instrument. If the sample characteristics in the original study and the new study are similar, the citation provides valuable information about data quality in the new study. Ideally, researchers should also compute new reliability coefficients for the actual research sample. ■

Sensitivity and Specificity

Reliability and validity are the two most important criteria for evaluating quantitative instruments, but researchers sometimes need to consider other qualities. In particular, for screening and diagnostic instruments, sensitivity and specificity need to be evaluated.

Sensitivity is the ability of an instrument to correctly identify a "case," that is, to correctly screen in or diagnose a condition. An instrument's sensitivity is its rate of yielding "true positives." **Specificity** is the instrument's ability to correctly identify noncases, that is, to correctly screen *out* those without the condition. Specificity is an instrument's rate of yielding "true negatives." To determine an instrument's sensitivity and specificity, researchers need a reliable and valid criterion of "caseness" against which scores on the instrument can be assessed.

There is, unfortunately, a tradeoff between the sensitivity and specificity of an instrument. When sensitivity is increased to include more true positives, the number of true negatives declines. Therefore, a critical task is to develop the appropriate *cut-off point*, that is, the score value used to distinguish cases and noncases. Instrument developers use sophisticated procedures to make such a determination.

THE ASSESSMENT OF QUALITATIVE DATA

The assessment procedures described thus far cannot be meaningfully applied to such qualitative materials as narrative responses in interviews or participant observers' field notes. This does not imply, however, that qualitative researchers are unconcerned with data quality. The central question underlying the concepts of validity and reliability is: Do the data reflect the truth? Certainly, qualitative researchers are as eager as quantitative researchers to have data reflecting the true state of human experience.

Nevertheless, there has been considerable controversy about the criteria to use for assessing the "truth value" of qualitative research. Whittemore, Chase, and Mandle (2001), who listed different criteria recommended by ten influential authorities, noted that the difficulty in achieving universally accepted criteria (or even universally accepted labels for those criteria) stems in part from various tensions, such as the tension between the desire for rigour and the desire for creativity.

The criteria currently thought of as the "gold standard" for qualitative researchers are those outlined by Lincoln and Guba (1985). As noted in Chapter 2, these researchers have suggested four criteria for establishing the **trustworthiness** of qualitative data: credibility, dependability, confirmability, and transferability. It should be noted that these criteria go beyond an assessment of qualitative *data* alone, but rather are concerned with evaluations of interpretations and conclusions as well. These standards are often used by researchers in all major qualitative research traditions.

CONSUMER TIP

Qualitative research reports are uneven in the amount of information they provide about data quality. Some do not address data quality issues at all, whereas others elaborate on the steps taken to assess trustworthiness. The absence of information undermines consumers' ability to draw conclusions about the believability of qualitative findings. ■

Credibility

Careful qualitative researchers take steps to improve and evaluate data **credibility,** which refers to confidence in the truth of the data and interpretations of them. Lincoln and Guba note that the credibility of an inquiry involves two aspects: first, carrying out the investigation in a way that believability is enhanced; and second, taking steps to *demonstrate* credibility. Lincoln and Guba suggest various techniques for improving and documenting the credibility of qualitative data. A few that are especially relevant to the evaluation of qualitative studies are mentioned here.

PROLONGED ENGAGEMENT AND PERSISTENT OBSERVATION
Lincoln and Guba recommend activities that increase the likelihood of producing credible data and interpretations. A first and very important step is **prolonged engagement**—the investment of sufficient time in data collection activities to have an in-depth understanding of the culture, language, or views of the group under study and to test for misinformation. Prolonged engagement may also be essential for building trust and rapport with informants.

Credible data collection also involves **persistent observation,** which refers to the researcher's focus on the aspects of a situation that are relevant to the phenomena being studied. As Lincoln and Guba note, "If prolonged engagement provides scope, persistent observation provides depth" (1985, p. 304).

Example of prolonged engagement and persistent observation

Schafer and Peternelj-Taylor (2003) explored therapeutic relationships from the perspectives of forensic patients enrolled in a treatment program for violent offenders. They interviewed 12 informants three or four times, with some interviews lasting more than 2 hours, over a 6-month period. At each interview, participants were given the opportunity to confirm, correct, or extend transcripts of prior interviews. The researchers maintained field notes and reflective journals throughout data collection.

TRIANGULATION

Triangulation can also enhance credibility. As previously noted, triangulation refers to the use of multiple referents to draw conclusions about what constitutes truth. The aim of triangulation is to "overcome the intrinsic bias that comes from single-method, single-observer, and single-theory studies" (Denzin, 1989, p. 313). It has also been argued that triangulation helps to capture a more complete and contextualized portrait of the phenomenon under study—a goal shared by researchers in all qualitative traditions. Denzin (1989) identified four types of triangulation:

1. *Data source triangulation*: using multiple data sources in a study (e.g., interviewing diverse key informants such as nurses and patients about the same topic)
2. *Investigator triangulation*: using more than one person to collect, analyze, or interpret a set of data
3. *Theory triangulation:* using multiple perspectives to interpret a set of data
4. *Method triangulation*: using multiple methods to address a research problem (e.g., observations plus interviews)

Triangulation provides a basis for convergence on the truth. By using multiple methods and perspectives, researchers strive to distinguish true information from information with errors.

Example of data source and investigator triangulation

Rempel, Cender, Lynam, Sandor, and Farquharson (2004) studied parents' decision-making processes after learning antenatally of their baby's congenital heart disease. Interviews were conducted with both mothers and fathers (some separately and some conjointly). Most parents were interviewed three times, both during pregnancy and after delivery. Two members of the research team coded each interview.

EXTERNAL CHECKS: PEER DEBRIEFING AND MEMBER CHECKS

Two other techniques for establishing credibility involve external checks on the inquiry. **Peer debriefing** is a session held with objective peers to review and explore various aspects of the inquiry. Peer debriefing exposes investigators to the searching questions of others who are experienced in either qualitative research or in the phenomenon being studied, or both. Peer review can also be useful to researchers interested in testing some working hypotheses or in exploring new interpretive avenues.

Member checks involve soliciting study participants' reactions to preliminary findings and interpretations. Member checking can be carried out both informally in an ongoing way as data are being collected and more formally after data have been collected and analyzed. Lincoln and Guba (1985) consider member checking the most important technique for establishing the credibility of qualitative data. However, not all qualitative researchers use member checking to ensure credibility. For example, member checking is not a component of Giorgi's method of descriptive phenomenology. Giorgi (1989) argued that asking participants to evaluate the researchers' interpretation of their own descriptions exceeds the role of participants.

Example of peer debriefing and member checking

Brathwaite and Williams (2004) studied the childbirth experiences of professional Chinese Canadian women. Their qualitative study was based on in-depth interviews with six women. The researchers asked study participants to review their findings and confirm or refute them. They also validated emerging themes by consulting with three colleagues who were members of the Chinese Canadian community.

SEARCHING FOR DISCONFIRMING EVIDENCE

Data credibility can be enhanced by researchers' systematic search for data that challenge an emerging conceptualization or descriptive theory. The search for **disconfirming evidence** occurs through purposive sampling but is facilitated through other processes already described, such as prolonged engagement and peer debriefings. The sampling of individuals who can offer conflicting viewpoints can greatly strengthen a comprehensive description of a phenomenon.

Lincoln and Guba (1985) refer to a similar activity of **negative case analysis**—a process by which researchers revise their hypotheses through the inclusion of cases that appear to disconfirm earlier hypotheses. The goal of this procedure is to refine a hypothesis or theory continuously until it accounts for all cases.

Example of negative case analysis

Sinding, Barnoff, and Grassau (2004) studied the experiences of lesbians with cancer to explore their perceptions of homophobia and discrimination during their treatment. The authors specifically noted that they "deliberately read for and coded negative cases (instances where participants' experiences of commentary departed from or challenged an emerging theme)." (p. 175)

RESEARCHER CREDIBILITY
Another aspect of credibility discussed by Patton (2002) is **researcher credibility,** the faith that can be put in the researcher. In qualitative studies, researchers *are* the data collecting instruments—as well as creators of the analytic process—and, therefore, the researchers' training, qualifications, and experience are important in establishing confidence in the data.

Research reports ideally should contain information about the researchers, including information about credentials and about any personal connections the researchers had to the people, topic, or community under study. For example, it is relevant for a reader of a report on AIDS patients' coping mechanisms to know that the researcher is HIV positive. Patton argues that the researcher should report "any personal and professional information that may have affected data collection, analysis and interpretation—negatively or positively..." (2002, p. 566).

Dependability

The **dependability** of qualitative data refers to data stability over time and over conditions. It might be said that credibility (in qualitative studies) is to validity (in quantitative studies) what dependability is to reliability. Like the reliability–validity relationship in quantitative research, there can be no credibility in the absence of dependability.

One approach to assessing data dependability is to undertake a **stepwise replication.** This approach, which is conceptually similar to a split-half technique, involves having several researchers who can be divided into two teams. These teams deal with data sources separately and conduct, essentially, two independent inquiries through which data and conclusions can be compared.

Another technique relating to dependability is the **inquiry audit.** An inquiry audit involves a scrutiny of the data and relevant supporting documents by an external reviewer, an approach that also has a bearing on data confirmability, as we discuss next.

Example of dependability

Gaudine and Beaton (2002) studied nurse managers' accounts of ethical conflicts within their places of work. Fifteen nurse managers from an eastern province were interviewed in depth, and the taped interviews were transcribed verbatim. Stepwise replication was used; the two researchers separately analyzed the data, then cross-checked each other's categories, themes, and interpretations. The minimal differences in the two analyses were resolved.

Confirmability

Confirmability refers to the objectivity or neutrality of the data, that is, the potential for congruence between two or more independent people about the data's accuracy, relevance, or meaning. Bracketing (in phenomenological studies) and maintaining a reflexive journal are methods that can enhance confirmability, although these strategies do not actually document that it has been achieved.

Inquiry audits can be used to establish both the dependability and confirmability of the data. In an inquiry audit, the investigator develops an **audit trail,** which is a systematic collection of documentation that allows an independent auditor to come to conclusions about the data. After the audit trail materials are assembled, the inquiry auditor proceeds to audit, in a fashion analogous to a financial audit, the trustworthiness of the data and the meanings attached to them. Examples of the classes of records that are important in creating an adequate audit trail include the raw data (e.g., field notes, interview transcripts), analytic products (e.g., documentation on working hypotheses, notes from member check sessions); and materials relating to intentions and dispositions (e.g., reflective notes).

Researchers can also enhance the **auditability** of their inquiry (i.e., the degree to which an outside person can follow the researchers' methods, decisions, and conclusions) by maintaining an adequate **decision trail.** A decision trail articulates the researchers' decision rules for categorizing data and making inferences in the analysis. When researchers share decision trail information in their research report, readers are in a better position to evaluate the soundness of the decisions and to draw conclusions about the trustworthiness of the study.

Example of confirmability

In their in-depth study of Chinese Canadians' beliefs toward organ donation, Molzahn, Starzomski, McDonald, and O'Loughlin (2005) enhanced the trustworthiness of their inquiry by maintaining an audit trail that documented all methodologic decisions, the evolution of the findings, and the researchers' orientation to the problem.

Transferability

In Lincoln and Guba's (1985) framework, **transferability** refers to the extent to which the findings from the data can be transferred to other settings and is thus similar to the concept of generalizability. This is, to some extent, an issue relating to sampling and design rather than to the soundness of the data *per se.* As Lincoln and Guba note, however, a researcher's responsibility is to provide sufficient descriptive data in the research report for consumers to evaluate the applicability of the data to other contexts: "Thus the naturalist cannot specify the external validity of an inquiry; he or she can provide only the thick description necessary to enable someone interested in making a transfer to reach a conclusion about whether transfer can be contemplated as a possibility" (1985, p. 316). **Thick description** refers to a rich, thorough description of the research setting and of the transactions and processes observed during the inquiry. Thus, if there is to be transferability, the burden rests with researchers to provide sufficient information to permit judgments about contextual similarity.

Example of transferability

In their ethnographic study, Banister, Jakubec, and Stern (2003) explored Canadian adolescent girls' health concerns in their dating relationships. Focus group sessions were held with four groups of young women. To achieve diversity and enhance transferability, five sites were used to recruit participants. To assess the transferability of their results, the researchers showed the findings "to a number of practitioners at various sites in the community, who perceived them as congruent with their practice experiences." (p. 22)

CONSUMER TIP

Because the process of assessing data quality in qualitative studies may be inextricably linked to data analysis, discussions of data quality are sometimes included in the results section rather than the method section of the report. In some cases, the text will not explicitly point out that data quality issues are being discussed. Readers may have to be alert to evidence of triangulation or other verification techniques in such statements as, "Informants' reports of experiences of serious illness were supported by discussions with three public health nurses." ■

CRITIQUING DATA QUALITY

If data are seriously flawed, the study cannot contribute useful evidence. Therefore, it is important for you as a consumer to consider whether researchers have taken appropriate steps to collect data that accurately reflect reality. In both qualitative and quantitative studies, you have the right—indeed, the obligation—to ask: Can I trust the data? Do the data accurately reflect the true state of the phenomenon under study?

In quantitative studies, you should expect some discussion of the reliability and validity of the measures—preferably, information collected directly with the sample under study (rather than evidence from other studies). You should be wary about the results of quantitative studies when the report provides no information about data quality or when it suggests unfavourable reliability or validity. Also, data quality deserves special scrutiny when the research hypotheses are not confirmed. There may be many reasons that hypotheses are not supported by data (e.g., too small a sample or a faulty theory), but the quality of the measures is an important area of concern. When hypotheses are not supported, one possibility is that the instruments were not good measures of the research constructs. Box 14.1 provides some guidelines for critiquing data quality in quantitative studies.

Information about data quality is equally important in qualitative studies. You should be particularly alert to information on data quality when a single researcher has been responsible for collecting, analyzing, and interpreting all the data, as is frequently the case. Some guidelines for critiquing the trustworthiness of data in qualitative studies are presented in Box 14.2.

CONSUMER TIP

The amount of detail about data quality in a research report varies considerably. Some articles have virtually no information. Sometimes such information is not needed (e.g., when biophysiologic instrumentation with a proven and widely known record for accuracy is used). Most research reports, however, should provide some evidence that data quality was sufficiently high to answer the research questions. Information about data quality normally is presented in the method section of the report. ■

BOX 14.1   Guidelines for Evaluating Data Quality in Quantitative Studies

1. Is there congruence between the research variables as conceptualized (i.e., as discussed in the introduction of the report) and as operationalized (i.e., as described in the method section)?
2. If operational definitions (or scoring procedures) are specified, do they clearly indicate the rules of measurement? Do the rules seem sensible? Were data collected in such a way that measurement errors were minimized?
3. Does the report offer evidence of the reliability of measures? Does the evidence come from the research sample itself, or is it based on other studies? If the latter, is it reasonable to conclude that data quality would be similar for the research sample as for the reliability sample (e.g., are sample characteristics similar)?
4. If reliability is reported, which estimation method was used? Was this method appropriate? Should an alternative or additional method of reliability appraisal have been used? Is the reliability sufficiently high?
5. Does the report offer evidence of the validity of the measures? Does the evidence come from the research sample itself, or is it based on other studies? If the latter, is it reasonable to believe that data quality would be similar for the research sample as for the validity sample (e.g., are the sample characteristics similar)?
6. If validity information is reported, which validity approach was used? Was this method appropriate? Does the validity of the instrument appear to be adequate?
7. If there is no reliability or validity information, what conclusion can you reach about the quality of the data in the study?
8. If a diagnostic or screening tool was used, is information provided about its sensitivity and specificity, and were these qualities adequate?
9. Were the research hypotheses supported? If not, might data quality play a role in the failure to confirm the hypotheses?

BOX 14.2   Guidelines for Evaluating Data Quality in Qualitative Studies

1. Does the report discuss efforts to enhance or evaluate the trustworthiness of the data? If so, is the description sufficiently detailed and clear? If not, is there other information that allows you to conclude that data are of high quality?
2. Which techniques (if any) did the researcher use to enhance and appraise the credibility of the data? Was the investigator in the field for an adequate amount of time? Was triangulation used, and if so, of what type? Did the researcher search for disconfirming evidence? Were there peer debriefings and/or member checks? Do the researcher's qualifications enhance the credibility of the data?
3. Which techniques (if any) did the researcher use to enhance and appraise the dependability, confirmability, and transferability of the data?
4. Given the efforts to enhance data quality, what can you conclude about the trustworthiness of the data? In light of this assessment, how much faith can be placed in the results of the study?

RESEARCH EXAMPLES | **Critical Thinking Activities**

EXAMPLE 1: Quantitative Research

Aspects of two related psychometric assessments by one of the authors of this book, featuring terms and concepts discussed in this chapter, are presented below, followed by some questions to guide critical thinking.

Studies
"Postpartum Depression Screening Scale: Development and psychometric testing" (Beck & Gable, 2000); and "Further validation of the Postpartum Depression Screening Scale" (Beck & Gable, 2001)

Statement of Purpose
The two methodologic studies involved developing and testing the quality of a new scale to screen women for postpartum depression (PPD).

Background
Beck had studied PPD in a series of qualitative studies, using both a phenomenological approach (1992, 1996) and a grounded theory approach (1993). Based on her in-depth understanding of PPD, she began in the late 1990s to develop a scale that could be used to screen for PPD, the Postpartum Depression Screening Scale (PDSS). Working with Gable, an expert psychometrician, Beck refined and evaluated the PDSS. (Psychometric testing of the Spanish version of the PDSS was reported in Beck and Gable, 2003.)

Content Validity
Content validity was enhanced by using direct quotes from the qualitative studies as items on the Likert-type scale (e.g., "I felt like I was losing my mind"). A pilot version of the PDSS was subjected to ratings by a panel of five content experts. This content validity effort led to some modifications.

Construct Validity
The PDSS was administered to a sample of 525 new mothers in six states (Beck & Gable, 2000). Preliminary analyses resulted in the deletion of several items. The PDSS was finalized as a 35-item scale with seven subscales, each with 5 items. This version of the PDSS was subjected to factor analyses, which indicated that the items mapped well onto underlying constructs. In their subsequent study, Beck and Gable (2001) administered the PDSS and other scales to 150 new mothers. To further validate their scale, they tested theoretically driven hypotheses about how scores on the PDSS would correlate with scores on other scales.

Criterion-Related Validity
In the second study, Beck and Gable correlated scores on the PDSS with an expert clinician's diagnosis of PPD for each woman. The validity coefficient was .70.

Critical Thinking Activities (continued)

Internal Consistency Reliability

In both studies, Beck and Gable evaluated the internal consistency reliability of the PDSS and its subscales. Reliability for the subscales ranged from .83 to .94 in the first study and from .80 to .91 in the second study.

Sensitivity and Specificity

In the second study, Beck and Gable used the expert diagnosis of PPD to establish a cut-off score and evaluate the scale's sensitivity and specificity. Based on their analyses, Beck and Gable recommended a cut-off score of 80 for major postpartum depression. This cut-off accurately screened in 94% of true PPD cases and mistakenly screened in 2% who did not have the mood disorder.

Critical Thinking Suggestions*

*See the Student Resource CD-ROM for a discussion of these questions.

1. Answer questions 3 through 6 and 8 from Box 14.1 regarding this study.

2. Also consider the following targeted questions, which may assist you in further assessing aspects of the study:

   a. Was the criterion-related validity effort an example of concurrent or predictive validity?

   b. The researchers determined that there should be seven subscales to the PDSS. Why do you think this might be the case?

   c. Each item on the PDSS is scored on a 5-point scale from 1 to 5. What is the range of possible scores on the scale (and what is the range of scores on each subscale)? Comment on where the cut-off score of 80 falls on the total scale.

   d. Comment on the researchers credentials for undertaking this study together, and on the appropriateness of their overall effort.

3. What are some of the uses to which the scale might be put in clinical practice?

 EXAMPLE 2: Qualitative Research

Aspects of a qualitative nursing study, featuring terms and concepts discussed in this chapter, are presented below, followed by some questions to guide critical thinking.

Study

"The structure of everyday self-care decision making in chronic illness" (Thorne, Paterson, & Russell, 2003)

Statement of Purpose

The overall purpose of this study (a secondary analysis of two qualitative data sets) was to explore self-care decision making of individuals with chronic illness.

Method

The study involved the collection and analysis of multiple forms of data from 43 individuals with type 1 or type 2 diabetes, HIV/AIDS, or multiple sclerosis. Study

(Research Examples continue on page 334)

Critical Thinking Activities (continued)

participants were interviewed at the outset of the study, and the audiotaped interviews were transcribed and checked for accuracy against the tapes. Initial interviews were followed by 2 or 3 think aloud sessions lasting 1 week each, in which participants audiotaped their thoughts about self-care decisions. The think aloud sessions were followed by in-depth interviews to probe into the underlying logic of the decisions. Toward the end of the study, participants were invited to focus group sessions to review preliminary analyses.

Credibility

In addition to method triangulation, the researchers enhanced credibility through prolonged engagement and persistent observation: the researchers were in contact with the participants on multiple occasions over a 12-month period. Member checks were done by reviewing preliminary themes with participants in focus group sessions. The entire research team also held regular meetings for the purposes of peer debriefing. The report also indicates that the researchers identified and explored cases that contradicted their hypotheses.

Dependability and Confirmability

The researchers maintained a research audit trail, consisting of a written record of their methodologic and theoretic decisions during data collection and data analysis.

Transferability

Transferability was facilitated through rich description of the participants' decision making processes. Also, the sample was selected to reflect various types of chronic illness. With data collected over a 12-month period, the researchers ensured that they captured seasonal variation and some life cycle events. The report included information about the demographic characteristics of the participants, which could be used to determine transferability of the study findings.

Key Findings

For participants representing three chronic disease categories, self-care decision making reflected the outcome of a conscious decision to gain control of the management of their disease. Within each disease category, the specific nature of decisions was distinct, yet common patterns and processes clearly emerged.

Critical Thinking Suggestions

1. Answer the questions from Box 14.2 regarding this study.
2. Also consider the following targeted questions, which may assist you in further assessing aspects of the study:
   a. Can you think of other types of triangulation that the researchers could have used?
   b. Explain how investigator triangulation and peer debriefings could affect confirmability as well as credibility in this study.
   c. How did audiotaping and transcription enhance the trustworthiness of the data?

Critical Thinking Activities (continued)

3. If the results of this study are trustworthy, what are some of the uses to which the findings might be put in clinical practice?

 EXAMPLE 3: Quantitative Research

1. Read the Method section from the study by Feeley and colleagues ("Mother–VLBW Infant Interaction") in Appendix A of this book, and then answer questions 1 through 6 and 9 in Box 14.1.

2. Also consider the following targeted questions, which may further sharpen your critical thinking skills and assist you in assessing aspects of the study:

    a. Suggest some "known groups" that might be used to assess the construct validity of the NCAST scale that was used in this study.

    b. The maternal State Anxiety scale was administered at 3 and 9 months postpartum. Would it make sense for the researchers to use these scores to assess the scale's test–retest reliability? Why or why not?

 EXAMPLE 4: Qualitative Research

1. Read the Method section from Beck's (2002) study in Appendix B of this book ("Birth Trauma"), and then answer the relevant questions in Box 14.2.

2. Also consider the following targeted questions, which may assist you in assessing aspects of the study's merit:

    a. Beck is a mother of two children. She herself has not experienced birth trauma, but she has interacted with pregnant women and new mothers extensively both clinically and in her research. Discuss how Beck's background has relevance for this study.

    b. Give one or two examples of additional (or alternative) steps Beck could have taken to address issues of trustworthiness in her study.

C H A P T E R   R E V I E W

S u m m a r y   P o i n t s

▶ **Measurement** involves a set of rules according to which numeric values are assigned to objects to represent varying degrees of an attribute.

▶ Few quantitative measuring instruments are infallible. Sources of measurement error include situational contaminants, response biases, and transitory personal factors (e.g., fatigue).

▶ **Obtained scores** from an instrument consist of a **true score** component—the value that would be obtained if it were possible to have a perfect measure of the attribute—and an error component, or **error of measurement**, that represents measurement inaccuracies.

▶ **Reliability** is the degree of consistency or accuracy with which an instrument measures an attribute. The higher the reliability of an instrument, the lower the amount of error in the obtained scores.

▶ There are different methods for assessing reliability and computing a **reliability coefficient**. The *stability* aspect, which concerns the extent to which an instrument yields the same results on repeated administrations, is evaluated by **test–retest procedures**.

▶ The **internal consistency** aspect of reliability, which refers to the extent to which all the instrument's items are measuring the same attribute, is assessed using either the *split-half reliability technique* or, more likely, **Cronbach's alpha method**.

▶ When the focus of a reliability assessment is on establishing *equivalence* between observers in rating or coding behaviours, estimates of **interrater** (or **interobserver**) **reliability** are obtained.

▶ **Validity** is the degree to which an instrument measures what it is supposed to be measuring.

▶ **Face validity** refers to whether an instrument appears, on the face of it, to be measuring the appropriate construct.

▶ **Content validity** is concerned with the sampling adequacy of the content of a measure.

▶ **Criterion-related validity** focuses on the correlation between the instrument and an outside criterion.

▶ **Construct validity** refers to the adequacy of an instrument in measuring the construct of interest. One construct validation method is the **known-groups technique**, which contrasts the scores of groups that are presumed to differ on the attribute; another is **factor analysis**, a statistical procedure for identifying unitary clusters of items or measures.

▶ Sensitivity and specificity are criteria for evaluating screening or diagnostic instruments. **Sensitivity** is the instrument's ability to correctly identify a case, that is, its rate of true positives. **Specificity** is the instrument's ability to correctly identify a noncase, that is, its rate of true negatives.

▶ Qualitative researchers evaluate the **trustworthiness** of their data using the criteria of credibility, dependability, confirmability, and transferability.

▶ **Credibility**, roughly analogous to validity in a quantitative study, refers to the believability of the data. Techniques to improve the credibility of qualitative data include **prolonged engagement**, which strives for adequate scope of data, and **persistent observation**, which is aimed at achieving adequate depth.

▶ **Triangulation** is the process of using multiple referents to draw conclusions about what constitutes the truth. The four major forms are *data source triangulation, investigator triangulation, theoretical triangulation,* and *method triangulation.*

▶ Two important tools for establishing credibility are **peer debriefings**, wherein the researcher obtains feedback about data quality and interpretation from peers, and **member checks**, wherein informants are asked to comment on the researcher's conclusions and interpretations.

▶ **Dependability** of qualitative data refers to the stability of data over time and over conditions and is somewhat analogous to the concept of reliability in quantitative studies.

▶ **Confirmability** refers to the objectivity or neutrality of the data. Independent **inquiry audits** by external auditors can be used to assess and document dependability and confirmability.

▶ The **auditability** of a study is enhanced when researchers maintain and share portions of an **audit trail** and **decision trail** in their reports.

▶ **Transferability** is the extent to which findings from the data can be transferred to other settings or groups. Transferability can be enhanced through **thick descriptions** of the context of the data collection.

Additional Resources for Review

Chapter 14 of the *Study Guide to Accompany Essentials of Nursing Research,* 6th edition offers various exercises and study suggestions for reinforcing the concepts presented in this chapter. For additional review, see the Student Self-Study Review Questions section of the Student Resource CD-ROM provided with this book.

SUGGESTED READINGS

*References for studies cited in the chapter appear at the end of the book.

Methodologic References

Denzin, N. K. (1989). *The research act* (3rd ed.). New York: McGraw-Hill.

Chiovitti, R. F., & Piran, N. (2003). Rigour and grounded theory research. *Journal of Advanced Nursing, 44,* 427–435.

Giorgi, A. (1989). Some theoretical and practical issues regarding the psychological and phenomenological method. *Saybrook Review, 7,* 71–85.

Hall, J. M., & Stevens, P. E. (1991). Rigor in feminist research. *Advances in Nursing Science, 13,* 16–29.

Kerlinger, F. N. (1986). *Foundations of behavioral research* (3rd ed.). New York: Holt, Rinehart & Winston.

Lincoln, Y. S., & Guba, E. G. (1985). *Naturalistic inquiry.* Newbury Park, CA: Sage Publications.

Morse, J. M. (1999). Myth # 93: Reliability and validity are not relevant to qualitative inquiry. *Qualitative Health Research, 9,* 717–718.

Nunnally, J., & Bernstein, I. H. (1994). *Psychometric theory* (3rd ed.). New York: McGraw-Hill.

Patton, M. Q. (2002). *Qualitative evaluation and research methods* (3rd ed.). Thousand Oaks, CA: Sage Publications.

Whittemore, R., Chase, S. K., & Mandle, C. L. (2001). Validity in qualitative research. *Qualitative Health Research, 11,* 522–537.

Data Analysis

Analyzing Quantitative Data

STUDENT OBJECTIVES

On completing this chapter, you will be able to:

▶ Identify the four levels of measurement and compare their characteristics
▶ Identify and interpret various descriptive statistics
▶ Describe the logic and purpose of tests of statistical significance and describe hypothesis testing procedures
▶ Specify the appropriate applications for *t*-tests, analysis of variance, chi-squared tests, correlation coefficients, multiple regression, and analysis of covariance
▶ Understand the results of simple statistical procedures described in a research report
▶ Define new terms in the chapter

T he data collected in a study do not by themselves answer research questions or test hypotheses. Data need to be systematically analyzed so that patterns can be detected. This chapter describes procedures for analyzing quantitative data, and Chapter 16 discusses the analysis of qualitative data.

LEVELS OF MEASUREMENT

A quantitative measure can be classified according to its **level of measurement.** This classification is important because the analyses that can be performed on data depend on their measurement level. There are four major levels of measurement:

1. **Nominal measurement,** the lowest level, involves using numbers simply to categorize attributes. Examples of variables that are nominally measured include gender and blood type. The numbers assigned in nominal measurement do not have quantitative meaning. If we code males as 1 and females as 2, the number 2 does not mean "more than" 1. Nominal measurement provides information only about categorical equivalence and nonequivalence; the numbers cannot be treated mathematically. It is nonsensical, for example, to compute the sample's average gender by adding the values of the codes and dividing by the number of subjects.

Example of nominal measurement

King, Ghali, Faris, Curtis, Galbraith, Graham, and Knudtson (2004) studied gender differences in outcomes after cardiac catheterization using data from a clinical database in Alberta. The independent variable (gender) was a nominal-level variable, and a key outcome variable (mortality) was also nominal.

2. **Ordinal measurement** ranks objects based on their relative standing on an attribute. If a researcher rank-orders people from heaviest to lightest, this is ordinal measurement. As another example, consider this ordinal coding scheme for measuring ability to perform activities of daily living: 1 = completely dependent; 2 = needs another person's assistance; 3 = needs mechanical assistance; and 4 = completely independent. The numbers signify incremental ability to perform activities of daily living independently. Ordinal measurement does not, however, tell us how much greater one level is than another. For example, we do not know if being completely independent is twice as good as needing mechanical assistance. As with nominal measures, the mathematic operations permissible with ordinal-level data are restricted.

Example of ordinal measurement

Coulson, Strang, Mariño, and Minichiello (2004) studied lifestyle behaviours in healthy older adults related to preventing vascular dementia. Several variables were measured on an ordinal scale. For example, participants rated their level of stress as follows: no stress, mild stress, moderate stress, severe stress, and severe stress treated by a doctor.

3. **Interval measurement** occurs when researchers can specify the ranking of objects on an attribute *and* the distance between those objects. Most psychological tests are based on interval scales. For example, the Stanford-Binet Intelligence Scale—a standardized intelligence quotient (IQ) test used in many countries—is an interval measure. A score of 140 on the Stanford-Binet is higher than a score of 120, which, in turn, is higher than 100. Moreover, the difference between 140 and 120 is presumed to be equivalent to the difference between 120 and 100. Interval scales expand analytic possibilities: interval-level data can be averaged meaningfully, for example. Many statistical procedures require interval measurements.

Example of interval measurement

Lebel, Jakubovits, Rosberger, Loiselle, Seguin, Cornaz, Ingram, August, and Lisbona (2003) examined the emotional distress and coping strategies of women waiting for a breast biopsy. Several variables were measured on an interval scale. For example, anxiety was measured with the State Anxiety Scale, a 20-item scale whose scores could range from 20 to 80.

4. **Ratio measurement** is the highest level of measurement. Ratio scales, unlike interval scales, have a meaningful zero and therefore provide information about the absolute magnitude of the attribute. The Centigrade scale for measuring temperature (interval measurement) has an arbitrary zero point. Zero on the thermometer does not signify the absence of heat; it would not be appropriate to say that 30°C is twice as hot as 15°C. Many physical measures, however, are ratio measures with a real zero. A person's weight, for example, is a ratio measure. It is acceptable to say that someone who weighs 120 kg is twice as heavy as someone who weighs 60 kg. Statistical procedures suitable for interval data are also appropriate for ratio-level data.

Example of ratio measurement

Cesario (2004) surveyed maternity care agencies in Canada, Mexico, and the United States to re-evaluate the average length of each phase of labour for women in North America. Several variables in the study were ratio-level measures, including descriptors of the agencies (number of births per year, number of full-time nurses on staff) and the main outcome variables, number of minutes in the first and second stages of labour.

Researchers usually strive to use the highest levels of measurement possible—especially for their dependent variables—because higher levels yield more information and are amenable to more powerful analysis than lower levels.

HOW-TO-TELL TIP

How can you tell the measurement level of a variable? A variable is *nominal* if the values could be interchanged (e.g., 1 = male, 2 = female, OR 1 = female, 2 = male—the codes are arbitrary). A variable is usually *ordinal* if there is a quantitative ordering of values AND if there are only a small number of values (e.g., very important, important, not too important, unimportant). A variable is usually considered *interval* if it is measured with a composite scale or psychological test. A variable is *ratio* level if it makes sense to say that one value is twice as much as another (e.g., 100 mg is twice as much as 50 mg). ■

DESCRIPTIVE STATISTICS

Statistical procedures enable researchers to organize, interpret, and communicate numeric information. Statistics are either descriptive or inferential. **Descriptive** statistics, such as averages and percentages, are used to synthesize and describe data. When such indexes are calculated on data from a population, they are called **parameters.** A descriptive index from a sample is a **statistic.** Most scientific questions are about parameters; researchers calculate statistics to estimate them.

Frequency Distributions

Data that are not analyzed or organized are overwhelming. It is not even possible to discern general trends without some structure. Consider the 60 numbers in Table 15.1. Let us assume that these numbers are the scores of 60 preoperative patients on a six-item measure of anxiety—scores that we will consider to be on an interval scale. Visual inspection of the numbers in this table provides little insight on patients' anxiety levels.

Frequency distributions are a method of imposing order on numeric data. A **frequency distribution** is a systematic arrangement of numeric values from lowest to highest, together with a count (or percentage) of the number of times each value was obtained. The 60 anxiety scores are presented as a frequency distribution in Table 15.2. This arrangement makes it convenient to see at a glance the highest and lowest scores, the most common scores, and how many patients were in the sample (total sample size is typically designated as *N* in research reports). None of this was easily discernible before the data were organized.

TABLE 15.1		Patients' Anxiety Scores							
22	27	25	19	24	25	23	29	24	20
26	16	20	26	17	22	24	18	26	28
15	24	23	22	21	24	20	25	18	27
24	23	16	25	30	29	27	21	23	24
26	18	30	21	17	25	22	24	29	28
20	25	26	24	23	19	27	28	25	26

TABLE 15.2	Frequency Distribution of Patients' Anxiety Scores	
SCORE	FREQUENCY	PERCENTAGE
15	1	1.7
16	2	3.3
17	2	3.3
18	3	5.0
19	2	3.3
20	4	6.7
21	3	5.0
22	4	6.7
23	5	8.3
24	9	15.0
25	7	11.7
26	6	10.0
27	4	6.7
28	3	5.0
29	3	5.0
30	2	3.3
	$N = 60$	100.0

Some researchers display frequency data graphically in a *frequency polygon* (Figure 15.1). In such graphs, scores are on the horizontal line, with the lowest value on the left, and frequency counts or percentages are on the vertical line. Distributions can be described by their shapes. **Symmetric distribution** occurs if, when folded over, the two halves of a frequency polygon would be superimposed (Figure 15.2). In an asymmetric or **skewed distribution,** the peak is off centre, and one tail is longer than the other. When the longer tail is pointed toward the right, the distribution has a **positive skew,** as in the first graph of Figure 15.3. Personal income is an example of a positively skewed attribute. Most people have moderate incomes, with few high-income people at the right end of the distribution. If the longer tail points to the left, the distribution has a **negative skew,** as in the second graph in Figure 15.3. Age at death is an example: here, the bulk of people are at the far right end of the distribution, with relatively few people dying at an early age.

Another aspect of a distribution's shape concerns how many peaks or high points it has. A *unimodal distribution* has one peak (graph A, Figure 15.2), whereas a *multimodal distribution* has two or more peaks—that is, two or more values of high frequency. A multimodal distribution with two peaks is a *bimodal distribution,* illustrated in graph B of Figure 15.2.

A distribution of particular interest is the **normal distribution** (sometimes called *a bell-shaped curve*). A normal distribution is symmetric, unimodal, and not very peaked, as illustrated in graph A of Figure 15.2. Many human attributes (e.g., height, intelligence) approximate a normal distribution.

Frequency distributions can be constructed with data for variables measured on any of the four measurement scales.

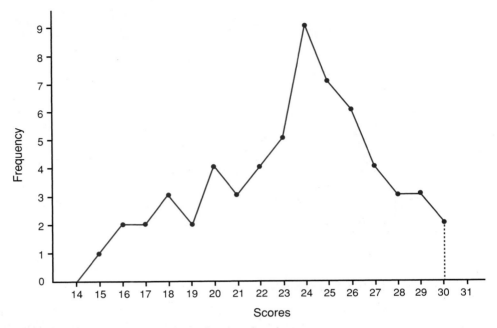

FIGURE 15.1 Frequency polygon of patients' anxiety scores.

Example of frequency information

Table 15.3 presents distribution information on sample characteristics from a study of clients of adult day programs in Alberta (Ross-Kerr, Warren, Schalm, Smith, & Godkin, 2003). This table shows, for selected background characteristics, both the frequency and percentage of participants in various categories. For example, 179 of the 477 clients (37.5%) were men, and 298 (62.5%) were women. Most subjects were either married (41.5%) or widowed (46.1%).

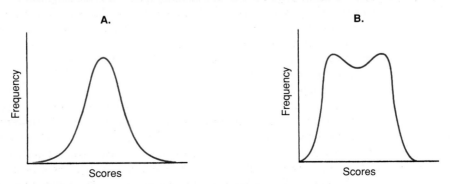

FIGURE 15.2 Examples of symmetric distributions.

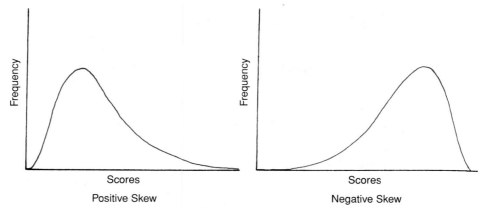

FIGURE 15.3 Examples of skewed distributions.

Central Tendency

For variables on an interval or ratio scale, a distribution of values is usually of less inter-est than an overall summary. Researchers ask such questions as: What was the patients' average blood pressure? How depressed was the typical mother postpartum? These ques-tions seek a single number that best represents the whole distribution. Such indexes are measures of **central tendency.** To lay people, the term *average* is normally used to desig-nate central tendency. There are three commonly used kinds of averages, or measures of central tendency: the mode, the median, and the mean.

▶ **Mode**: The mode is the number that occurs most frequently in a distribution. In the fol-lowing distribution, the mode is 53:

  50 51 51 52 53 53 53 53 54 55 56

  The value of 53 occurred four times, a higher frequency than for other numbers. The mode of the patients' anxiety scores in Table 15.2 is 24. The mode, in other words, identifies the most popular value. The mode is used most often to describe typical or high-frequency values for nominal measures. For example, in the study by Ross-Kerr and co-researchers (see Table 15.3), we could make the following statement: The typi-cal (modal) client was a widowed female.

▶ **Median**: The median is the point in a distribution that divides scores in half. Consider the following set of values:

  2 2 3 3 4 5 6 7 8 9

  The value that divides the cases in half is midway between 4 and 5, and thus 4.5 is the median. For the patient anxiety scores, the median is 24, the same as the mode. An important characteristic of the median is that it does not take into account individ-ual values and is thus insensitive to extremes. In the above set of numbers, if the value of 9 were changed to 99, the median would remain 4.5. Because of this property, the median is the preferred index of central tendency to describe a highly skewed distribu-tion. The median may be abbreviated as *Md* or *Mdn*.

TABLE 15.3	Example of Table With Frequency Information: Selected Characteristics of Clients Attending Adult Day Programs	
CLIENT CHARACTERISTIC	**NUMBER (N = 477)**	**PERCENTAGE**
Type of Program		
Adult day support program	234	49.1
Adult day hospital program	243	50.9
Gender		
Male	179	37.5
Female	298	62.5
Marital Status		
Widowed	220	46.1
Married	198	41.5
Separated/divorced	30	6.3
Never married	29	6.1

Adapted from Rose-Kerr, J. C., Warren, S., Schalm, C., Smith, D., & Godkin, M. D. (2003). Adult day programs: Are they needed? *Journal of Gerontological Nursing, 29*(12), 1–7.

▶ **Mean**: The mean equals the sum of all values divided by the number of participants—what people refer to as the average. The mean of the patients' anxiety scores is 23.4 (1405 + 60). As another example, here are the weights of eight people:

50 55 61 66 72 78 86 92

In this example, the mean is 70. Unlike the median, the mean is affected by every score. If we were to exchange the 92-kg person for one weighing 132 kg, the mean weight would increase from 70 to 75 kg. A substitution of this kind would leave the median unchanged. The mean is often symbolized as M or $\bar{X}$ (e.g., $\bar{X} = 145$).

For interval-level or ratio-level measurements, the mean, rather than the median or mode, is usually the statistic reported. The mean is the most stable of these indexes: if repeated samples were drawn from a population, the means would fluctuate less than the modes or medians. Because of its stability, the mean usually is the best estimate of a population central tendency. When a distribution is highly skewed, however, the mean does not characterize the centre of the distribution; in such situations, the median is preferred. For example, the median is a better central tendency measure of family income than the mean because income is positively skewed.

Variability

Two sets of data with identical means could be quite different with respect to **variability**, that is, how different people are from one another. Consider the distributions in Figure 15.4, which represent hypothetical scores of students from two schools on the Stanford-Binet IQ test. Both distributions have an average score of 100, but the two groups are very different. In school A, there is a wide range of scores—from scores below 70 to above 130. In school B, by contrast, there are few low scorers but also few outstanding performers. School A is more heterogeneous (i.e., more variable) than school B; school B is more homogeneous than school A.

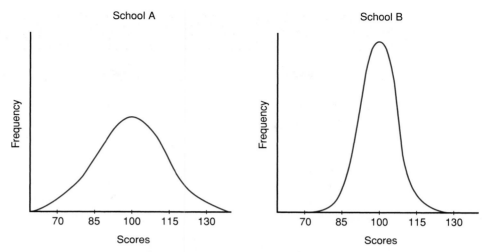

FIGURE 15.4 Two distributions of different variability.

Researchers compute an index of variability to summarize the extent to which scores in a distribution differ from one another. Several such indexes have been developed, the most important of which are the range and the standard deviation.

▶ **Range:** The range is the highest score minus the lowest score in a distribution. In the example of the patients' anxiety scores, the range is 15 (30 − 15). In the distributions in Figure 15.4, the range for school A is about 80 (140 − 60), whereas the range for school B is about 50 (125 − 75). The chief virtue of the range is ease of computation. Because it is based on only two scores, however, the range is unstable: from sample to sample drawn from the same population, the range tends to fluctuate widely. Moreover, the range ignores variations between the two extremes. In school B of Figure 15.4, if a single student obtained a score of 60 and another obtained a score of 140, the range of both schools would then be 80—despite clear differences in heterogeneity. For these reasons, the range is used largely as a gross descriptive index.

▶ **Standard deviation:** The most widely used variability index is the standard deviation. Like the mean, the standard deviation is calculated based on every value in a distribution. The standard deviation summarizes the *average* amount of deviation of values from the mean. In the anxiety scale example, the standard deviation is 3.725.* In research reports, the standard deviation is often abbreviated as *s* or *SD*. Occasionally, the standard deviation is simply shown in relation to the mean without a formal label, such as M = 4.0 (1.5) or M = 4.0 ± 1.5, where 4.0 is the mean and 1.5 is the standard deviation. †

---

*Formulas for computing the standard deviation, as well as other statistics discussed in this chapter, are not shown in this textbook. The emphasis here is on helping you to understand statistical applications. References at the end of the chapter can be consulted for computation formulas.

†Research reports occasionally refer to an index of variability known as the **variance**. The variance is simply the value of the standard deviation squared. In the example of the patients' anxiety scores, the variance is 3.725^2, or 13.88.

A standard deviation is more difficult to interpret than the range. With regard to the SD of the anxiety scores, you might ask, 3.725 *what?* What does the number mean? We can answer these questions from several angles. First, as discussed, the SD is an index of how variable scores in a distribution are. If male and female nursing students had means of 23 on the anxiety scale, but females had an SD of 7 and males had an SD of 3, we would immediately know that the males were more homogeneous (i.e., their scores were more similar to one another).

The SD represents the *average* of deviations from the mean. The mean tells us the single best point for summarizing an entire distribution, and an SD tells us how much, on average, the scores deviate from that mean. In the anxiety scale example, they deviated by an average of just under 4 points. A standard deviation might thus be interpreted as an indication of our degree of error when we use a mean to describe an entire sample.

In normal and near-normal distributions, there are roughly three standard deviations above and below the mean. Suppose we had a normal distribution with a mean of 50 and an SD of 10 (Figure 15.5). In such a distribution, a fixed percentage of cases fall within certain distances from the mean. Sixty-eight percent of all cases fall within 1 SD above and below the mean. Thus, in this example, nearly 7 of 10 scores are between 40 and 60. In a normal distribution, 95% of the scores fall within 2 SDs from the mean. Only a handful of cases—about 2% at each extreme—lie more than 2 SDs from the mean. Using this figure, we can see that a person with a score of 70 had a higher score than about 98% of the sample.

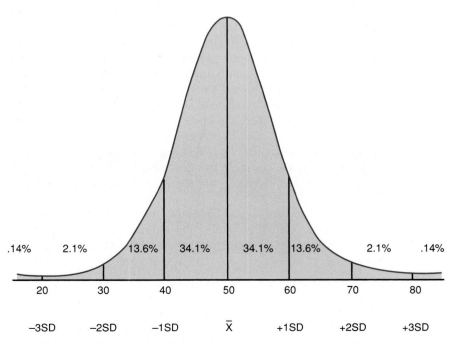

FIGURE 15.5 Standard deviations in a normal distribution.

Example of means and SDs

Table 15.4 presents descriptive statistics from a clinical trial designed to assess the effect of alternative modes of early labour support for pregnant women (Janssen, Iker, & Carty, 2003). The table shows the means and SDs of selected background characteristics for the two research groups (women getting support through a home visit or through telephone triage). According to these data, the two groups had similar means with regard to age, weight, weight gain, and gestational age at delivery. The telephone triage group, however, tended to be slightly more heterogeneous. For example, the SD for gestational age was much larger in the telephone triage group than in the home visit group, even though the means were identical.

Bivariate Descriptive Statistics

So far, our discussion has focused on *univariate* (one-variable) *descriptive statistics*. The mean, mode, standard deviation, and so forth are used to describe one variable at a time. *Bivariate* (two-variable) *descriptive statistics* describe relationships between two variables.

CONTINGENCY TABLES

A **contingency table** is a two-dimensional frequency distribution in which the frequencies of two variables are **cross-tabulated.** Suppose we had data on patients' gender and whether they were nonsmokers, light smokers (<1 pack of cigarettes a day), or heavy smokers (≥1 pack a day). The question is whether there is a tendency for the men to smoke more heavily than the women or *vice versa*. Some fictitious data on these two variables are shown in a contingency in Table 15.5. Six cells are created by using one variable (gender) for columns and the other variable (smoking status) for rows. After all subjects are allocated to the appropriate cells, percentages can be computed. This simple procedure allows us to see at a glance that, in this sample, women were more likely than men to be

TABLE 15.4	Example of Table With Descriptive Statistics: Characteristics of Women in Two Research Groups				
	HOME VISIT GROUP (n = 117)			TELEPHONE TRIAGE GROUP (n = 120)	
CHARACTERISTIC	Mean	SD		Mean	SD
Age	31.3	4.7		30.4	5.6
Prepregnancy weight (kg)	60.7	11.3		60.7	11.8
Weight gain during pregnancy (kg)	15.0	15.9		14.0	15.7
Gestational age at delivery (wk)	39.5	1.42		39.5	2.92

Adapted from Janssen, P. A., Iker, C. E., & Carty, E. A. (2003). Early labour assessment and support at home: A randomized controlled trial. *Journal of Obstetrics and Gynaecology Canada, 25,* 734–741.

TABLE 15.5	Contingency Table for Gender and Smoking Status Relationship					
	GENDER					
	Female		**Male**		**Total**	
SMOKING STATUS	*n*	%	*n*	%	*n*	%
Nonsmoker	10	45.4	6	27.3	16	36.4
Light smoker	8	36.4	8	36.4	16	36.4
Heavy smoker	4	18.2	8	36.4	12	27.3
TOTAL	22	50.0	22	50.0	44	100.0

nonsmokers (45.4% versus 27.3%) and less likely to be heavy smokers (18.2% versus 36.4%). Contingency tables usually are used with nominal data or ordinal data that have few levels or ranks. In the present example, gender is a nominal measure, and smoking status is an ordinal measure.

Example of a contingency table

Table 15.6 presents a contingency table from an actual study that examined the relationship between degree of psychological distress and the use of psychotropic drugs in a sample of elders from Québec (Voyer, McCubbin, Preville, & Boyer, 2003). Overall, 15.3% of the sample of more than 3000 elders reported using an anxiolytic, sedative, or hypnotic (ASH) drug; 5.9% reported being in high psychological distress. About one third (33.4%) of those in high distress reported using an ASH drug, compared with only 8.9% of those in low distress.

A comparison of Tables 15.5 and 15.6 illustrates that cross-tabulated data can be presented two ways: within each cell, percentages can be computed based on either row totals or column totals. In Table 15.5, the number 10 in the first cell (female nonsmokers) was divided by the column total (i.e., by the total number of females—22) to arrive at the percentage (45%) of females who were nonsmokers. The table could have shown 63% in this cell (10 + 16)—the percentage of nonsmokers who were female. In Table 15.6, the number 81 in the first cell was divided by the row total of 915 (i.e., the number of elders in low distress) to yield 8.9%—the percentage of those in low distress who are ASH users. Computed the other way, the researchers would have gotten 17.6% (81 + 461)—the percentage of ASH users who were in low distress. Either approach is acceptable, although the former is often preferred because then the percentages in a column add up to 100%.

TABLE 15.6	Example of a Contingency Table: Psychological Distress and Consumption of Anxiolytic, Sedative, and Hypnotic (ASH) Drug Use in the Elderly					
PSYCHOLOGICAL DISTRESS	**ASH CONSUMPTION**					
	Yes		**No**		**Total**	
	n	%	*n*	%	*n*	%
Low	81	8.9	834	91.1	915	30.4
Intermediate	320	16.7	1599	83.3	1919	63.7
High	60	33.6	118	66.5	178	5.9
Total	461	15.3	2551	84.7	3012	100.0

Calculations and adaptations from Voyer, P., McCubbin, M., Preville, M., & Boyer, R. (2003). Factors in duration of anxiolytic, sedative, and hypnotic drug use in the elderly. *Canadian Journal of Nursing Research, 35*(4), 126–149.

CONSUMER TIP

You may need to spend an extra minute inspecting contingency tables to determine which total—row or column—was used as the basis for calculating percentages. ■

CORRELATION

Relationships between two variables are usually described through **correlation** procedures. The correlation question is: To what extent are two variables related to each other? For example, to what degree are anxiety scores and blood pressure measures related? This question can be answered quantitatively by calculating a **correlation coefficient,** which describes the *intensity* and *direction* of a relationship.

Two variables that are related are height and weight: tall people tend to weigh more than short people. The relationship between height and weight would be a *perfect relationship* if the tallest person in a population was the heaviest, the second tallest person was the second heaviest, and so on. The correlation coefficient summarizes how "perfect" a relationship is. The possible values for a correlation coefficient range from −1.00 through .00 to +1.00. If height and weight were perfectly correlated, the correlation coefficient expressing this would be 1.00 (the actual correlation coefficient is in the vicinity of .50 to .60 for a general population). Height and weight have a **positive relationship** because greater height tends to be associated with greater weight.

When two variables are unrelated, the correlation coefficient is zero. One might expect that women's shoe size is unrelated to their intelligence. Women with large feet are as likely to perform well on IQ tests as those with small feet. The correlation coefficient summarizing such a relationship would presumably be near .00.

Correlation coefficients running between .00 and –1.00 express a **negative,** or *inverse*, **relationship.** When two variables are inversely related, increments in one variable are associated with decrements in the second. For example, there is a negative correlation between depression and self-esteem: on average, people with *high* self-esteem tend to be *low* on depression. If the relationship were perfect (i.e., if the person with the highest self-esteem score had the lowest depression score and so on), then the correlation coefficient would be −1.00. In actuality, the relationship between depression and self-esteem is moderate—usually in the vicinity of −.40 or −.50. Note that the higher the *absolute value* of the coefficient (i.e., the value disregarding the sign), the stronger the relationship. A correlation of −.80, for instance, is much stronger than a correlation of +.20.

The most commonly used correlation index is the **product–moment correlation coefficient** (also called **Pearson's** *r*), which is computed with interval or ratio measures. One correlation index for ordinal measures is **Spearman's rank-order correlation** (r_s), sometimes referred to as **Spearman's rho.**

It is difficult to offer guidelines on what should be interpreted as strong or weak relationships because it depends on the nature of the variables. If we were to measure patients' body temperature both orally and rectally, a correlation (*r*) of .70 between the two measurements would be low. For most psychosocial variables (e.g., stress and severity of illness), however, an *r* of .70 would be rather high. Perfect correlations (+1.00 and −1.00) are extremely rare.

Correlation coefficients are often reported in tables displaying a two-dimensional **correlation matrix,** in which variables are displayed in both rows and columns. To read a correlation matrix, one finds the row for one variable and reads across until the row intersects with the column for another variable, and the intersection gives the corresponding value for *r*.

Example of a correlation matrix

Table 15.7 presents an abridged correlation matrix from a study that examined factors associated with psychological distress in family caregivers of persons with psychiatric disabilities (Provencher, Perreault, St.-Onge, & Rousseau, 2003). The table lists, on the left, four possible predictors of distress (the caregivers' age, caregivers' perceptions of the family members' problematic behaviours, the number of caregiving tasks the caregiver had assumed, and self-reported subjective burden), and then the outcome variable, psychological distress. The numbers in the top row, from 1 to 5, correspond to the 5 variables: 1 is caregiver's age, 2 is problematic behaviours, and so on. At the intersection of row 1 and column 1, we find the value 1.00, which simply indicates that the variable "age of caregiver" is perfectly correlated with itself. The next entry represents the correlation between age and problematic behaviours. The value of −.11 (i.e., *r* = −.11) indicates a weak negative relationship between these variables: As caregivers' age increased, there was a very slight tendency for them to list fewer problematic behaviours on the part of their relatives; there was also a tendency for older caregivers to report less psychological distress than younger ones (−.22). On the other hand, caregivers' psychological distress was positively correlated with family members' problematic behaviours (.40). The strongest correlation in this matrix is between psychological distress and subjective burden (.70), and the weakest correlation is between caregivers' age and the number of caregiving tasks (−.08).

TABLE 15.7	Example of a Correlation Matrix: Psychological Distress in Family Caregivers of Persons With Psychiatric Disabilities				
	1	**2**	**3**	**4**	**5**
1. Age of caregiver	1.00				
2. Problematic behaviours of family member	−.11	1.00			
3. Number of caregiving tasks in prior month	−.08	.54	1.00		
4. Subjective burden (e.g., guilt, embarrassment)	−.16	.51	.43	1.00	
5. Caregivers' psychological distress	−.22	.40	.33	.70	1.00

Adapted from Provencher, H.L., Perreault, M., St. Onge, M., & Rousseau, M. (2003). Predictors of psychological distress in family caregivers of persons with psychiatric disabilities. *Journal of Psychiatric and Mental Health Nursing, 10,* 592–607.

INTRODUCTION TO INFERENTIAL STATISTICS

Descriptive statistics are useful for summarizing data, but researchers usually do more than simply describe. **Inferential statistics,** which are based on the *laws of probability*, provide a means for drawing conclusions about a population, given data from a sample.

Sampling Distributions

When using a sample to estimate population characteristics, it is important to obtain a sample that is representative, and random sampling is the best means of securing such samples. Inferential statistics are based on the assumption of random sampling from populations—although this assumption is widely violated.

Even with random sampling, however, sample characteristics are seldom identical to those of the population. Suppose we had a population of 30,000 nursing school applicants whose mean score on a standardized entrance exam was 500 with a standard deviation of 100. Suppose that we do not know these parameters but that we must estimate them based on scores from a random sample of 25 applicants. Should we expect a sample mean of exactly 500 and a standard deviation of 100? It would be improbable to obtain identical values. Suppose that the sample mean was 505. If a completely new random sample of 25 students were drawn, the mean might be 497. Sample statistics fluctuate and are unequal to the population parameter because of sampling error. Researchers need a way to determine whether sample statistics are good estimates of population parameters.

To understand the logic of inferential statistics, we must perform a mental exercise. Consider drawing a sample of 25 students from the population of all applicants, calculating a mean test score, replacing the students, and drawing a new sample. Each mean is considered one datum. If we drew 10,000 samples of 25 applicants, we would have 10,000 means (data points) that could be used to construct a frequency polygon (Figure 15.6). This distribution is called a **sampling distribution of the mean**, which is a theoretical rather than an actual distribution because in practice no one draws consecutive samples from a population and plots their means. Statisticians have demonstrated that (1)

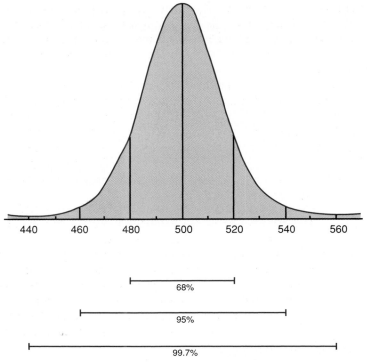

FIGURE 15.6 Sampling distribution of a mean.

sampling distributions of means follow a normal distribution and (2) the mean of a sampling distribution for an infinite number of sample means equals the population mean. In our example, the mean of the sampling distribution is 500, the same as the population mean.

Remember that when scores are normally distributed, 68% of the cases fall between +1 SD and –1 SD from the mean. Because a sampling distribution of means is normally distributed, the probability is 68 out of 100 that any randomly drawn sample mean lies between +1 SD and –1 SD of the population mean. The problem is to determine the standard deviation of the sampling distribution—which is called the **standard error of the mean** (or SEM). The word *error* signifies that the sample means contain some error as estimates of the population mean. The smaller the standard error (i.e., the less variable the sample means), the more accurate are the means as estimates of the population value.

Because no one actually constructs a sampling distribution, how can its standard deviation be computed? Fortunately, there is a formula for estimating the SEM from data from a single sample, using the sample's standard deviation and its size. In the present example, the SEM equals 20, as shown in Figure 15.6. This statistic is an estimate of how much sampling error there would be from one sample mean to another in an infinite number of samples of 25 nursing school applicants.

We can now estimate the probability of drawing a sample with a certain mean. With a sample size of 25 and a population mean of 500, the chances are about 95 out of

100 that a sample mean would fall between the values of 460 and 540—2 SDs above and below the mean. Only 5 times out of 100 would the mean of a randomly selected sample of 25 applicants be greater than 540 or less than 460. In other words, only 5 times out of 100 would we be likely to draw a sample whose mean deviates from the population mean by more than 40 points.

Because the SEM is partly a function of sample size, we need only increase sample size to increase the accuracy of our estimate. Suppose that instead of using a sample of 25 applicants to estimate the population mean, we used a sample of 100. With this many students, the standard error of the mean would be 10, not 20—and the probability would be about 95 in 100 that a sample mean would be between 480 and 520. The chances of drawing a sample with a mean very different from that of the population are reduced as sample size increases because large numbers promote the likelihood that extreme cases will cancel each other out.

You may be wondering why you need to learn about these abstract statistical notions. Consider, though, that what we are talking about concerns how likely it is that research results are accurate. As a consumer, you need to evaluate how believable research evidence is so that you can decide whether to incorporate it into your nursing practice. The concepts underlying the standard error are important in such an evaluation and are related to issues we stressed in Chapter 12 on sampling. First, the more homogeneous the population is on the critical attribute (i.e., the smaller the standard deviation), the more likely it is that results calculated from a sample will be accurate. Second, the larger the sample size, the greater is the likelihood of accuracy. The concepts discussed in this section are the basis for statistical hypothesis testing.

Hypothesis Testing

Statistical inference consists of two major techniques: estimation of parameters and hypothesis testing. **Estimation procedures** are used to estimate a single population characteristic, such as a mean value (e.g., patients' mean temperature). Researchers usually are more interested in relationships between variables than in estimating the accuracy of a single sample value, however. For this reason, we focus on hypothesis testing.

Statistical **hypothesis testing** provides objective criteria for deciding whether research hypotheses should be accepted as true or rejected as false. Suppose we hypothesized that maternity patients exposed to a film on breastfeeding would breastfeed longer than mothers who did not see the film. We find that the mean number of days of breastfeeding is 131.5 for 25 experimental subjects and 125.1 for 25 control subjects. Should we conclude that the hypothesis is supported? True, group differences are in the predicted direction, but perhaps in another sample the group means would be nearly identical. Two explanations for the observed outcome are possible: (1) the film is truly effective in encouraging breastfeeding, or (2) the difference in this sample was due to chance factors (e.g., differences in the two groups even before the film was shown, reflecting a selection bias).

The first explanation is the researcher's *research hypothesis*, and the second is the *null hypothesis*. The null hypothesis, it may be recalled, states that there is no relationship between the independent and dependent variables. Statistical hypothesis testing is basically a process of disproof or rejection. It cannot be demonstrated directly that the research hypothesis is correct. But it is possible to show, using theoretical sampling distributions, that the null hypothesis has a high probability of being incorrect, and such evidence lends support to the research hypothesis. Hypothesis testing helps researchers to make objective decisions about study results—that is, to decide which results likely reflect chance sample differences and which likely reflect true hypothesized effects in the population.

Researchers use **statistical tests** to test hypotheses. Although null hypotheses are accepted or rejected on the basis of sample data, the hypothesis is made about population values.

TYPE I AND TYPE II ERRORS

Researchers decide whether to accept or reject the null hypothesis by determining how probable it is that observed relationships are due to chance. Because information about the population is not available, it cannot be asserted flatly that the null hypothesis is or is not true. Researchers conclude that hypotheses are either *probably* true or *probably* false. Statistical inferences are based on incomplete information; there is always a risk of making an error.

Researchers can make two types of error, as summarized in Figure 15.7. Investigators make a **Type I error** by rejecting the null hypothesis when it is, in fact, true. For instance, if we concluded that the film was effective in promoting breastfeeding when, in fact, group differences were due to initial group differences, this would be a Type I error—a false positive conclusion. In the reverse situation, we might conclude that observed differences in breastfeeding were due to sampling fluctuations when the film actually *did* have an effect. Acceptance of a false null hypothesis is called a **Type II error**—a false negative conclusion.

LEVEL OF SIGNIFICANCE

Researchers do not know when an error in statistical decision making has been made. The validity of a null hypothesis could only be determined by collecting data from the population, in which case there would be no need for statistical inference.

	The actual situation is that the null hypothesis is:	
	True	False
True (Null accepted)	Correct decision	Type II error
False (Null rejected)	Type I error	Correct decision

The researcher calculates a test statistic and decides that the null hypothesis is:

FIGURE 15.7 Outcomes of statistical decision making.

Researchers control the degree of risk in making a Type I error by selecting a **level of significance**, which is the term used to signify the probability of making a Type I error. The two most frequently used levels of significance (referred to as **alpha or α**) are .05 and .01. With a .05 significance level, we accept the risk that out of 100 samples, a true null hypothesis would be wrongly rejected 5 times. In 95 out of 100 cases, however, a true null hypothesis would be correctly accepted. With a .01 significance level, the risk of making a Type I error is lower: In only one sample out of 100 would we wrongly reject the null hypothesis. By convention, the minimal acceptable alpha level is .05.

Naturally, researchers would like to reduce the risk of committing both types of error. Unfortunately, lowering the risk of a Type I error increases the risk of a Type II error. The stricter the criterion for rejecting a null hypothesis, the greater the probability of accepting a false null hypothesis. However, researchers can reduce the risk of a Type II error simply by increasing their sample size.

The probability of committing a Type II error, referred to as **beta (β)**, can be estimated through *power analysis,* the same procedure we mentioned in Chapter 12 in connection with sample size. *Power*, the ability of a statistical test to detect true relationships, is the complement of beta—that is, power equals $1 - β$. The standard criterion for an acceptable risk for a Type II error is .20, and thus researchers ideally use a sample size that gives them a minimum power of .80.

CONSUMER TIP

In many studies, the risk of a Type II error is high because of small sample size, suggesting a need for greater use of power analysis. If a research report indicates that a research hypothesis was not supported, consider whether a Type II error might have occurred as a result of inadequate sample size. ■

TESTS OF STATISTICAL SIGNIFICANCE

Researchers testing hypotheses use study data to compute a **test statistic**. For every test statistic, there is a theoretical sampling distribution, analogous to the sampling distribution of means. Hypothesis testing uses theoretical distributions to establish *probable* and *improbable* values for the test statistics, which are, in turn, used as a basis for accepting or rejecting the null hypothesis.

A simple (if contrived) example will illustrate the process. Suppose we wanted to test the hypothesis that the average entrance examination score (on a hypothetical standardized examination) for students applying to nursing schools in Ontario is higher than that for applicants in all provinces, whose mean score is 500. The null hypothesis is that there is no difference in the mean population scores of students applying to nursing schools in Ontario versus elsewhere. Let us say that the mean score for a sample of 100 nursing school applicants in Ontario is 525, with a standard deviation of 100. Using statistical procedures, we can test the hypothesis that the mean of 525 is not merely a chance fluctuation from the population mean of 500.

In hypothesis testing, researchers assume that the null hypothesis is true and then gather evidence to disprove it. Assuming a mean of 500 for the entire applicant population, a sampling distribution can be constructed with a mean of 500 and an SD of 10. In this example, 10 is the standard error of the mean, calculated from a formula that used the sample standard deviation of 100 for a sample of 100 students. This is shown in Figure 15.8. Based on normal distribution characteristics, we can determine probable and improbable values of sample means from the population. If, as is assumed according to the null hypothesis, the population mean for Ontario applicants is 500, 95% of all sample means would fall between 480 and 520 because 95% of the cases are within 2 SDs of the mean. The obtained sample mean of 525 lies in the region considered *improbable* if the null hypothesis were true, with an alpha level of .05 as the criterion of improbability. The improbable range beyond 2 SDs corresponds to only 5% (100% − 95%) of the sampling distribution. We would thus reject the null hypothesis that the mean of the Ontario applicant population equals 500. We would not be justified in saying that we have proved the research hypothesis because the possibility of a Type I error remains.

Researchers reporting the results of hypothesis tests state whether their findings are **statistically significant.** The word *significant* does not mean important or meaningful.

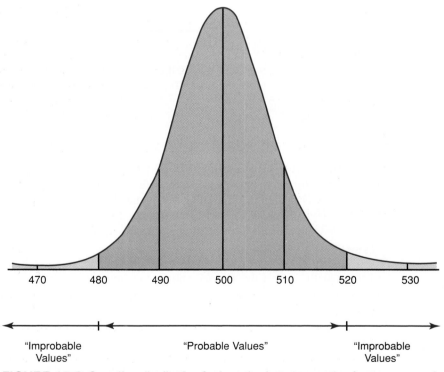

470	480	490	500	510	520	530

"Improbable Values" "Probable Values" "Improbable Values"

FIGURE 15.8 Sampling distribution for hypothesis test example of entrance examination scores.

In statistics, the term *significant* means that obtained results are not likely to have been due to chance, at a specified level of probability. A **nonsignificant result** means that an observed difference or relationship could have been the result of a chance fluctuation.

CONSUMER TIP

Inferential statistics are usually more difficult to understand than descriptive statistics. It may help to keep in mind that inferential statistics are just a tool to help us evaluate whether the results are likely to be real and replicable, or simply spurious. As recommended in Chapter 4, you can overcome much of the obscurity of the results section by translating the basic thrust of research findings into everyday language. ▬

PARAMETRIC AND NONPARAMETRIC TESTS

The bulk of the tests that we discuss in this chapter—and also most tests used by researchers—are **parametric tests**. Parametric tests have three attributes: (1) they focus on population parameters; (2) they require measurements on at least an interval scale; and (3) they involve other assumptions, such as the assumption that the variables in the analysis are normally distributed in the population.

Nonparametric tests, by contrast, do not estimate parameters and involve less restrictive assumptions about the shape of the distribution of the critical variables. Nonparametric tests are usually applied when the data have been measured on a nominal or ordinal scale. Parametric tests are more powerful than nonparametric tests and are generally preferred. Nonparametric tests are most useful when the research data cannot be construed as interval measures or when the data distribution is markedly skewed.

OVERVIEW OF HYPOTHESIS TESTING PROCEDURES

In the next section, a few statistical tests are discussed. The emphasis is on explaining their applications and on interpreting their meaning rather than on describing computations.

Each statistical test has a particular application and can be used only with certain kinds of data; however, the overall process of testing hypotheses is basically the same for all tests. The steps that researchers take are the following:

1. *Selecting an appropriate test statistic.* Researchers select a test based on such factors as the level of measurement of the variables and, if relevant, how many groups are being compared.
2. *Selecting the level of significance.* An α level of .05 is usually chosen, but sometimes the level is set more stringently at .01.
3. *Computing a test statistic.* Researchers then calculate a test statistic based on the collected data.
4. *Determining degrees of freedom.* The term **degrees of freedom** (*df*) refers to the number of observations free to vary about a parameter. The concept is too complex for elaboration here, but computing degrees of freedom is easy.

5. *Comparing the test statistic to a tabled value.* Theoretical distributions have been developed for all test statistics, and there are tables with distribution for specified degrees of freedom and levels of significance. The *tabled* value enables researchers to see whether the *computed* value of the statistic is beyond what is probable if the null hypothesis is true. If the absolute value of the computed statistic is larger than the tabled value, the results are statistically significant; if the computed value is smaller, the results are nonsignificant.

When a computer is used for the analysis, researchers follow only the first step and then give appropriate commands to the computer. The computer calculates the test statistic, degrees of freedom, and the *actual* probability that the relationship being tested is due to chance. For example, the computer may print that the probability *(p)* of an experimental group doing better on a measure of postoperative recovery than the control group on the basis of chance alone is .025. This means that fewer than 3 times out of 100 (or only 25 times out of 1000) would a group difference of the size observed occur by chance. This computed probability can then be compared with the desired level of significance. In the present example, if the significance level were .05, the results would be significant because .025 is more stringent than .05. If .01 was the significance level, the results would be nonsignificant (sometimes abbreviated *NS*). Any computed probability level greater than .05 (e.g., .20) indicates a nonsignificant relationship (i.e., one that could have occurred on the basis of chance in more than 5 out of 100 samples).

BIVARIATE STATISTICAL TESTS

Researchers use a variety of statistical tests to make inferences about the validity of their hypotheses. The most frequently used bivariate tests are briefly described and illustrated below.

t-Tests

A common research situation involves comparing scores on an outcome variable for two groups of people. The procedure used to test the statistical significance of a difference between the means of two groups is the parametric test called the *t*-test.

Suppose we wanted to test the effect of early discharge of maternity patients on their perceived maternal competence. We administer a scale of perceived maternal competence 1 week after delivery to 10 primiparas who were discharged early (i.e., within 24 hours of delivery) and to 10 others who remained in the hospital longer. Some hypothetical data for this example are presented in Table 15.8. The mean scores for the two groups are 19.0 and 25.0, respectively. Is this difference a true population difference—is it likely to be replicated in other samples of early-discharge and later-discharge mothers? Or is the group difference just the result of chance fluctuations in this sample? The 20 scores—10 for each group—vary from one person to another. Some variability reflects individual differences in perceived maternal competence. Some variability might be due to measurement error (e.g., the scale's low reliability), and so forth. The research question is: Is a portion of the variability attributable to the independent variable—time of discharge from the hospital? The *t*-test allows us to answer this question objectively.

TABLE 15.8	Fictitious Data for *t*-Test Example: Scores on a Perceived Maternal Competence Scale for Two Groups of Mothers	

REGULAR-DISCHARGE MOTHERS	EARLY-DISCHARGE MOTHERS
23	30
17	27
22	25
18	20
20	24
26	32
16	17
13	18
21	28
14	29
Mean = 19.0	Mean = 25.0

$t = 2.86$; $df = 18$; $p < .05$

The value for the *t* statistic is calculated based on group means, variability, and sample size. The computed value of *t* for the data in Table 15.8 is 2.86. Next, degrees of freedom are calculated. Here, *df* equals the total sample size minus 2 ($df = 20 - 2 = 18$). Then, the tabled value for *t* with 18 *df* is ascertained. For an α level of .05, the tabled value of *t* is 2.10. *This value establishes an upper limit to what is probable if the null hypothesis is true.* Thus, the calculated *t* of 2.86, which is larger than the tabled value of the statistic, is improbable (i.e., statistically significant). We can now say that the primiparas discharged early had significantly lower perceptions of maternal competence than those who were not discharged early. The group difference in perceived maternal competence is sufficiently large that it is unlikely to reflect merely chance fluctuations. In fewer than 5 out of 100 samples would a difference in means this great be found by chance alone.

The situation just described requires an *independent groups t-test*: mothers in the two groups were different people, independent of each other. There are situations in which this type of *t*-test is not appropriate. For example, if means for a single group of people measured before and after an intervention were being compared, researchers would compute a *paired t-test* (or a *dependent groups t-test*) with a different formula.

Example of a *t*-test

Dennis (2004) compared the use of maternal health services among women who either did or did not exhibit symptoms of postpartum depression. The results indicated that women with postpartum depression had significantly more visits with a public health nurse 2 months postpartum ($t = 3.11$, $df = 492$, $p = .002$) and significantly more visits to a walk-in clinic ($t = 2.66$, $df = 492$, $p = .008$) than nondepressed women.

Analysis of Variance

Analysis of variance (ANOVA) is a parametric procedure used to test mean group differences of three or more groups. ANOVA decomposes the variability of a dependent variable into two components: variability attributable to the independent variable (i.e., group status) and variability due to all other sources (e.g., individual differences, measurement error). Variation *between* groups is contrasted with variation *within* groups to yield the statistic called an *F* **ratio**.

Suppose we wanted to compare the effectiveness of different instructional techniques to teach high school students about AIDS. One group of students is exposed to an interactive Internet course on AIDS, a second group is given special lectures, and a control group receives no special instruction. The dependent variable is students' scores on an AIDS knowledge test after the intervention. The null hypothesis is that the group population means for AIDS knowledge test scores are the same, whereas the research hypothesis predicts that they are different.

Test scores for 60 students are shown in Table 15.9, according to treatment group. As this table shows, there is variation from one student to the next within a group, and there are also group differences. The mean test scores are 25.35, 24.75, and 20.35 for groups A, B, and C, respectively. These means are different, but are they significantly different—or do the differences reflect random fluctuations?

An ANOVA applied to these data yields an *F* ratio of 18.64. Two types of degree of freedom are calculated in ANOVA: between groups (number of groups minus 1) and within groups (total number of subjects minus the number of groups). In this example, $df = 2$ and 57. In a table of values for a theoretical *F* distribution, we would find that the value of *F* for 2 and 57 *df*, with an alpha of .05, is 3.16. Because our obtained *F* value of 18.64 exceeds 3.16, we reject the null hypothesis that the population means are equal. The mean group differences would be obtained by chance in fewer than 5 samples out of 100. (Actually, the probability of achieving an *F* of 18.64 by chance is less than 1 in 1000.)

TABLE 15.9 Fictitious Data for One-Way ANOVA: Effects of Instructional Mode on AIDS Knowledge Test Scores

INTERNET GROUP (A)		LECTURE GROUP (B)		CONTROL GROUP (C)	
26	25	22	24	15	22
20	29	24	25	26	19
16	30	27	21	24	20
25	27	23	27	18	22
25	29	23	25	20	18
23	28	26	21	20	24
26	26	22	24	19	18
25	25	24	29	21	23
24	27	24	28	17	20
23	28	30	26	17	24
Mean 25.35		24.75		20.35	

$F = 18.64$; $df = 2.57$; $p < .001$

The data in our example support the hypothesis that the instructional interventions affected students' knowledge about AIDS, but we cannot tell from these results whether treatment A was significantly more effective than treatment B. **Multiple comparison procedures** (also called *post hoc* **tests**) are needed to isolate the differences between group means that are responsible for rejecting the overall ANOVA null hypothesis. Note that it is *not* appropriate to use a series of *t*-tests (group A versus B, A versus C, and B versus C) in this situation because this would increase the risk of a Type I error.

ANOVA also can be used to test the effect of two (or more) independent variables on a dependent variable (e.g., when a factorial experimental design has been used). Suppose we wanted to test whether the two instructional techniques discussed previously (Internet versus lecture) were equally effective in helping male and female students acquire knowledge about AIDS. We could set up a design in which males and females would be randomly assigned, separately, to the two modes of instruction. Some hypothetical data, shown in Table 15.10, reveal the following about two *main effects*: On average, people in the Internet group scored higher than those in the lecture group (25.35 versus 24.75), and female students scored higher than male students (26.20 versus 23.90). In addition, there is an *interaction effect:* Females scored higher in the Internet group, whereas males scored higher in the lecture group. By performing a *two-way ANOVA* on these data, it would be possible to ascertain the statistical significance of these differences.

A type of ANOVA known as **repeated measures ANOVA** is used when the means being compared are means at different points in time (e.g., mean blood pressure at 2, 4, and 6 hours after surgery). This is analogous to a paired *t*-test, extended to three or more points of data collection, because it is the same people being measured multiple times.

Example of an ANOVA

Wilson (2002) studied dependency in dying persons in relation to their care setting. Three groups of patients who died were compared using ANOVA: (a) hospital inpatients, (b) home care clients who died at home, and (c) home care clients who died in the hospital. Wilson found that the mean number of days of dependency was highest among the transferred (group C) clients (mean = 81.3), and was especially high compared with hospital inpatients (mean = 13.8). The *F* test was significant at $p < .01$.

CONSUMER TIP

Experimental crossover designs (see Chapter 9) require either a dependent groups *t*-test or a repeated measures ANOVA because the same people are measured more than once after being randomly assigned to a different ordering of treatments. Repeated measures ANOVA can also be used in studies that do not involve an experimental crossover design (e.g., in one-group pre-experimental designs) if outcomes are measured more than once and the hypothesis concerns changes over time. ▪

TABLE 15.10	Fictitious Data for Two-Way (2 × 2) ANOVA Example: Instructional Mode and Gender in Relation to Test Scores					

	INSTRUCTIONAL MODE					
YEAR IN SCHOOL	Internet		Lecture			
Male	26 20 16 25 25 23 26 25 24 23	$\bar{X} = 23.3$	22 24 27 33 23 26 22 24 24 30	$\bar{X} = 24.5$	Male mean = 23.90	
Female	25 29 30 27 29 28 26 25 27 28	$\bar{X} = 27.4$	24 25 21 27 27 25 21 24 28 26	$\bar{X} = 25.0$	Female mean = 26.20	
Internet group mean	25.35	Lecture group mean	24.75		Grand mean = 25.05	

Chi-Squared Test

The **chi-squared** (χ^2) **test** is a nonparametric procedure used to test hypotheses about the proportion of cases that fall into various categories, as in a contingency table. Suppose we were interested in studying the effect of planned nursing instruction on patients' compliance with a medication regimen. The experimental group is instructed by nurses implementing a new instructional approach. Control group patients are cared for by nurses using the usual mode of instruction. The research hypothesis is that a higher proportion of people in the experimental than in the control group will comply with the regimen. Some hypothetical data for this example are presented in Table 15.11.

The chi-squared statistic is computed by summing differences between the *observed frequencies* in each cell and the *expected frequencies*—the frequencies that would be expected if there were no relationship between the two variables. In this example, the value of the χ^2 statistic is 18.18, which we can compare with the value from a theoretical

TABLE 15.11	Observed Frequencies for a Chi-Squared Example on Patient Compliance		
	EXPERIMENTAL	CONTROL	TOTAL
Compliant	60	30	90
Noncompliant	40	70	110
TOTAL	100	100	200
$\chi^2 = 18.18$; $df = 1$; $p < .001$.			

chi-squared distribution. For the chi-squared statistic, the *df* are equal to the number of rows minus 1 times the number of columns minus 1. In the present case, *df* = 1 × 1, or 1. With 1 *df*, the value that must be exceeded to establish significance at the .05 level is 3.84. The obtained value of 18.18 is substantially larger than would be expected by chance. Thus, we can conclude that a significantly larger percentage of patients in the experimental group (60%) than in the control group (30%) were compliant.

Example of a chi-squared test

Khanlou (2004) studied the self-esteem of adolescents in multicultural Canadian schools. She examined factors associated with high self-esteem and found, for example, that males were significantly more likely than females (33.1% versus 22.6%) to have high self-esteem (χ^2 = 14.85, *df* = 6, *p* = <.02).

Correlation Coefficients

Pearson's *r* is both descriptive and inferential. As a descriptive statistic, *r* summarizes the magnitude and direction of a relationship between two variables. As an inferential statistic, *r* tests hypotheses about population correlations; the null hypothesis is that there is no relationship between two variables, that is, that *r* = .00.

Suppose we were studying the relationship between patients' self-reported level of stress (higher scores mean more stress) and the pH level of their saliva. With a sample of 50 patients, we find that *r* = −.29. This value indicates a tendency for people with high stress scores to have low pH levels. But we need to ask whether this finding can be generalized to the population. Does the coefficient of −.29 reflect a random fluctuation, observed only in this particular sample, or is the relationship significant? Degrees of freedom for correlation coefficients are equal to the number of participants minus 2—48 in this example. The tabled value for *r* with *df* = 48 and α = .05 is .282. Because the absolute value of the calculated *r* is .29 and thus larger than .282, the null hypothesis can be rejected. There is a modest, significant relationship between patients' stress level and the acidity of their saliva.

Example of correlation coefficients

Gélinas and Fillion (2004) studied factors related to persistent fatigue following breast cancer treatment. They found, among other things, that fatigue was not significantly correlated with the women's age (*r* = −.09) nor their educational attainment (*r* = .06), but was significantly correlated with their level of pain (*r* = .30, *p* < .01).

Guide to Bivariate Statistical Tests

The selection of a statistical test depends on such factors as the number of groups and the levels of measurement of the variables. To aid you in evaluating the appropriateness of statistical tests used in studies, Table 15.12 summarizes major features of several tests. This table does not include every test you may encounter in research reports, but it does include the bivariate tests most often used by nurse researchers, including a few not discussed in this book.

CONSUMER TIP

Every time a report presents information about statistical tests such as those described in this section, it means that the researcher was testing hypotheses—whether those hypotheses were formally stated in the introduction or not. ■

MULTIVARIATE STATISTICAL ANALYSIS

Nurse researchers have become increasingly sophisticated, and many now use complex **multivariate statistics** to analyze their data. We use the term *multivariate* to refer to analyses dealing with at least three—but usually more—variables simultaneously. This evolution has resulted in better-quality evidence in nursing studies, but one unfortunate side effect is that it has become more challenging for novice consumers to understand research reports.

Given the introductory nature of this text, it is not possible to describe in detail the complex analytic procedures that now appear in nursing journals. However, we present some basic information that might assist you in reading reports in which two commonly used multivariate statistics are used: multiple regression and analysis of covariance (ANCOVA).

Multiple Regression

Correlations enable researchers to make predictions. For example, if the correlation between secondary school grades and nursing school grades were .60, nursing school admission committees could make predictions—albeit imperfect ones—about applicants' future performance. Because two variables are rarely perfectly correlated, researchers often strive to improve their ability to predict a dependent variable by including more than one independent variable in the analysis.

As an example, we might predict that infant birth weight is related to the amount of maternal prenatal care. We could collect data on birth weight and number of prenatal visits and then compute a correlation coefficient to determine whether a significant relationship between the two variables exists (i.e., whether prenatal care would help predict infant birth weight). Birth weight is affected by many other factors, however, such

TABLE 15.12   **Guide to Widely Used Bivariate Statistical Tests**

NAME	TEST STATISTIC	PURPOSE	MEASUREMENT LEVEL*	
			IV	DV
Parametric Tests				
t-test for independent groups	t	To test the difference between two independent group means	Nominal	Interval, ratio
t-test for dependent group	t	To test the difference between two dependent group means	Nominal	Interval, ratio
Analysis of variance (ANOVA)	F	To test the difference among the means of three or more independent groups, or of more than one independent variable	Nominal	Interval, ratio
Repeated measures ANOVA	F	To test the difference among means of three or more related groups or sets of scores	Nominal	Interval, ratio
Pearson's r	r	To test the existence of a relationship between two variables	Interval, ratio	Interval, ratio
Nonparametric Tests				
Chi-squared test	χ^2	To test the difference in proportions in two or more independent groups	Nominal	Nominal
Mann-Whitney U-test	U	To test the difference in ranks of scores of two independent groups	Nominal	Ordinal
Kruskal-Wallis test	H	To test the difference in ranks of scores of three or more independent groups	Nominal	Ordinal
Wilcoxon signed ranks test	T(Z)	To test the difference in ranks of scores of two related groups	Nominal	Ordinal
Friedman test	χ^2	To test the difference in ranks of scores of three or more related groups	Nominal	Ordinal
Phi coefficient	ϕ	To test the magnitude of a relationship between two dichotomous variables	Nominal	Nominal
Spearman's rank-order correlation	r_s	To test the existence of a relationship between two variables	Ordinal	Ordinal

*Measurement level of the independent variable (IV) and dependent variable (DV).

as gestational period and mothers' smoking behaviour. Many researchers, therefore, perform **multiple regression analysis** (or *multiple correlation analysis*), which allows them to use more than one independent variable to explain or predict a dependent variable. In multiple regression, the dependent variables are interval- or ratio-level variables. Independent variables (also called **predictor variables** in multiple regression) are either interval- or ratio-level variables or dichotomous nominal-level variables, such as male/female.

When several independent variables are used to predict a dependent variable, the resulting statistic is the **multiple correlation coefficient,** symbolized as *R*. Unlike the bivariate correlation coefficient *r*, *R* does not have negative values. *R* varies from .00 to 1.00, showing the *strength* of the relationship between several independent variables and a dependent variable, but not *direction*.

There are several ways to evaluate *R*. One is to determine whether *R* is statistically significant—that is, whether the overall relationship between the independent variables and the dependent variable is likely to be real or the result of chance fluctuations. This is done through the computation of an *F* statistic that can be compared with tabled *F* values.

A second way of evaluating *R* is to determine whether the addition of new independent variables adds further predictive power. For example, we might find that the *R* between infant birth weight on the one hand and maternal weight and prenatal care on the other is .30. By adding a third independent variable—let's say maternal smoking behaviour—*R* might increase to .36. Is the increase from .30 to .36 statistically significant? In other words, does knowing whether the mother smoked during her pregnancy improve our understanding of the birth-weight outcome, or does the larger *R* value simply reflect factors peculiar to this sample? Multiple regression provides a way of answering this question.

The magnitude of *R* is also informative. Researchers would like to predict a dependent variable perfectly. In our example, if it were possible to identify all the factors that affect infants' weight, we could collect the relevant data to obtain an *R* of 1.00. Usually, the value of *R* in nursing studies is much smaller—seldom higher than .70. An interesting feature of the *R* statistic is that, when squared, it can be interpreted as the proportion of the variability in the dependent variable accounted for or explained by the independent variables. In predicting infant birth weight, if we achieved an *R* of .60 ($R^2 = .36$), we could say that the independent variables accounted for about one third (36%) of the variability in infants' birth weights. Two thirds of the variability, however, was caused by factors not identified or measured. Researchers usually report multiple correlation results in terms of R^2 rather than *R*.

Example of multiple regression

Ing and Reutter (2003) studied sense of coherence (SOC) and other factors in the self-rated health of more than 6000 Canadian women. The SOC construct is a global orientation that enables a person to perceive world events as comprehensible and meaningful. Using multiple regression, the researchers found that SOC and several background characteristics were significant predictors of self-rated health. Overall, the R^2 between predictor variables and self-rated health was .15, $p < .001$.

We will use this study by Ing and Reutter to illustrate some additional features of multiple regression. First, multiple regressions yield information about whether each independent variable is related significantly to the dependent variable. In Table 15.13, the first column shows that the analysis used four independent variables to predict the health ratings: marital status, age, income, and SOC scores. (The first entry, "Constant," is a value we would need if we wanted to predict health ratings of women not in the sample, based on their scores on the predictor variables.) The next column shows the values for *b*, which are the *regression coefficients* associated with each predictor. These coefficients, which were computed from the raw study data, could be used to predict health ratings in other Canadian women; however, like the value for constant, they are not values you need to be concerned with in interpreting a regression table. The next column shows the standard error (SE) of the regression coefficients. When the regression coefficient (*b*) is divided by the standard error, the result is a value for the *t* statistic, which is used to determine the significance of individual predictors. In this table, the *t* values are not shown, but many regression tables in reports *do* present them. We can compute them, though, from information in the table; for example, the *t* value for the variable *age* is -2.67 ($-0.08 + .03 = -2.67$). This is highly significant, as shown in the last column: the probability (*p*) is less than 1 in 1000 (.000) that the relationship between age and health ratings is spurious. The results indicate that the older the woman, the lower the health ratings, as indicated by the negative regression coefficient. Income and SOC were also significantly related to self-rated health: women with higher income and higher SOC scores tended to have higher health ratings. Marital status was not significantly related to health rating (although this predictor narrowly missed being significant, $p = .062$).

Multiple regression analysis indicates whether an independent variable is significantly related to the dependent variable *even after* the other predictor variables are controlled—a concept we explain more fully in the next section. In this example, SOC was

TABLE 15.13	Example of Multiple Regression Analysis: Self-Rated Health in Canadian Women, Regressed on Marital Status, Age, Income, and Sense of Coherence				
PREDICTOR VARIABLE*	*b*	**SE**	**BETA (β)**		*p*
Constant	2.57	0.07			< .001
Marital status: Married or attached	−0.05	0.03	−0.02		.062
Age	−0.08	0.03	−0.20		< .001
Income	0.16	0.01	0.18		< .001
Sense of coherence	0.02	0.00	0.28		< .001
N = 6,222 women					
F = 266.51	*df* = 4, 6217	*p* < .001	*Adjusted R²* = .15		

*Self-rated health (1 = poor to 5 = excellent); marital status (1 = married or attached, 0 = unattached); age (5-year cohorts from 20–24 to 60–64); income (1 = lowest income category to 5 = highest income category); sense of coherence scale (possible range = 0 to 78).

Adapted from Ing, J. D., & Reutter, L. (2003). Socioeconomic status, sense of coherence, and health in Canadian women. *Canadian Journal of Public Health, 94,* 224–228, Table II.

a significant predictor of health ratings, even with the other three variables controlled. Thus, multiple regression, like analysis of covariance (discussed next), is a means of controlling extraneous variables statistically.

The fourth column of Table 15.13 shows the value of the *beta* (β) *coefficients* for each predictor. Although it is beyond the scope of this textbook to explain beta coefficients in detail, suffice it to say that, unlike the *b* regression coefficients, betas are all in the same measurement units, and their absolute values are sometimes used to compare the relative importance of predictors. In this particular sample, and with these particular predictors, the variable *SOC* was the best predictor of health ($\beta = .28$), and the variable *age* was the second best predictor ($\beta = -.20$).

At the bottom of the table, we see that the value of *F* for the overall regression equation, with 4 and 6217 *df*, was 266.51, which is highly significant, $p < .001$. The value of R^2, after adjustments are made for sample size and number of predictors, is .15. Thus, 15% of the variance in self-rated health status is explained by the combined effect of the four predictors. The remaining 85% of variation in health is explained by other factors—variables not in the analysis, such as genetic factors, lifestyle behaviours, and so on.

Analysis of Covariance

Analysis of covariance (ANCOVA), which is essentially a combination of ANOVA and multiple regression, is used to control extraneous variables statistically. This approach can be especially valuable in certain research situations, such as when a nonequivalent control group design is used. The initial lack of equivalence of the experimental and comparison groups in such studies is always a potential threat to internal validity. When control through randomization is lacking, ANCOVA offers the possibility of *post hoc* statistical control.

Because the concept of statistical control may mystify you, we will explain the underlying principle with a simple illustration. Suppose we were interested in testing the effectiveness of a special training program on physical fitness, using employees of two companies as subjects. Employees of one company receive the physical fitness intervention, and those of the second company do not. The employees' score on a physical fitness test is the dependent variable. The research question is: Can some of the group difference in performance on the physical fitness test be attributed to participation in the special program? Physical fitness is also related to other, extraneous characteristics of the study participants (e.g., their age)—characteristics that might differ between the two intact groups.

Figure 15.9 illustrates how ANCOVA works. The large circles represent total variability (i.e., the extent of individual differences) in physical fitness scores for both groups. A certain amount of variability can be explained by age differences: Younger people tend to perform better on the test than older ones. This relationship is represented by the overlapping small circle on the left in part A of Figure 15.9. Another part of the variability can be explained by participation in the physical fitness program, represented here by the overlapping small circle on the right. In part A, the fact that the two small circles (age and program participation) themselves overlap indicates that there is a relationship between these two variables. In other words, people in the experimental

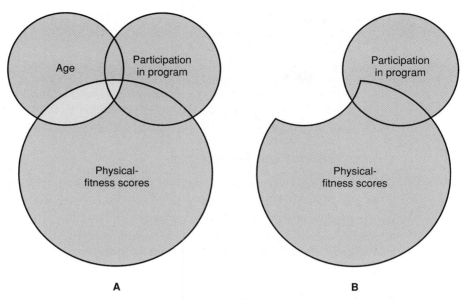

FIGURE 15.9 Schematic diagram illustrating the principle of analysis of covariance.

group are, on average, either older or younger than those in the comparison group. Because of this relationship, which could distort the results of the study, age should be controlled.

ANCOVA can do this by statistically removing the effect of the extraneous variable (age) on physical fitness, designated in part A of Figure 15.9 by the darkened area. Part B illustrates that the analysis would examine the effect of program participation on fitness scores *after* removing the effect of age (called a **covariate**). With the variability associated with age removed, we get a more precise estimate of the training program's effect on physical fitness. Note that even after removing variability resulting from age, there is still variability not associated with program participation (the bottom half of the large circle) that is not explained. This means that analytic precision could be further enhanced by controlling additional extraneous variables (e.g., nutritional habits, smoking status). ANCOVA can accommodate multiple extraneous variables.

Analysis of covariance tests the significance of differences between group means after adjusting scores on the dependent variable to eliminate the effect of covariates, using regression procedures. ANCOVA produces *F* statistics—one for evaluating the significance of the covariates and another for evaluating the significance of group differences—that can be compared with tabled values of *F* to determine whether to accept or reject the null hypothesis.

ANCOVA, like multiple regression analysis, is an extremely powerful and useful analytic technique for controlling extraneous influences on dependent measures. ANCOVA can be used with true experimental designs because randomization can never guarantee that groups are totally equivalent. Baseline measures of the dependent variables make particularly good covariates.

Example of ANCOVA

Johnston and Walker (2003) studied the short- and long-term effects of repeated pain during infancy on the later development of pain responses in rats. They used ANCOVA to test for differences in pain sensitivity among rat pups exposed to different pain conditions, controlling for duration of maternal grooming of the pups.

Other Multivariate Techniques

Other multivariate techniques are being used in nursing studies. We mention a few briefly to acquaint you with terms you might encounter in the research literature.

DISCRIMINANT FUNCTION ANALYSIS

In multiple regression, the dependent variable being predicted is a measure on either the interval or ratio scale. **Discriminant function analysis** is used to make predictions about membership in groups—that is, about a dependent variable measured on the nominal scale. For example, researchers might wish to use multiple independent variables to predict membership in such groups as compliant versus noncompliant cancer patients or patients with or without decubiti. In discriminant function analysis, as in multiple regression, the predictor variables and covariates are either interval- or ratio-level measures or dichotomous nominal variables (e.g., smoker versus nonsmoker).

LOGISTIC REGRESSION

Logistic regression (or *logit analysis*) analyzes the relationships between multiple independent variables and a nominal-level dependent variable. It is thus used in situations similar to discriminant function analysis, but it employs a different statistical estimation procedure that many prefer for nominal-level dependent variables. Logistic regression transforms the probability of an event occurring (e.g., that a woman will practice breast self-examination or not) into its *odds* (i.e., into the ratio of one event's probability relative to the probability of a second event). After further transformations, the analysis examines the relationship of the independent variables to the transformed dependent variable. For each predictor, the logistic regression yields an **odds ratio** (OR), which is the factor by which the odds change for a unit change in the predictors.

Example of logistic regression

Fisher, Wells, and Harrison (2004) conducted a study to identify predictors of pressure ulcers in adults in acute care hospitals. The researchers used data from nearly 2000 patients, about 12% of whom had a pressure ulcer. The logistic regression analysis revealed that age, male gender, nutrition, and several other variables were significant predictors. For example, the odds of having a pressure ulcer when nutrition was a deficit was twice as high for men as for women (OR = 2.29, *p* = .03).

FACTOR ANALYSIS

Factor analysis is widely used by researchers who develop, refine, or validate complex instruments. The purpose of factor analysis is to reduce a large set of variables into a smaller, more manageable set. Factor analysis disentangles complex interrelationships among variables and identifies which variables go together as unified concepts. For example, suppose we developed 50 Likert statements to measure men's attitudes toward a vasectomy. It would not be appropriate to combine all 50 items to form a scale score because there are various dimensions to men's attitudes toward vasectomy. One dimension may relate to the issue of masculine identity, another may concern the loss of ability to reproduce, and so on. These various dimensions should serve as the basis for scale construction, and factor analysis offers an objective, empirical method for doing so.

Example of factor analysis

Goulet, Polomeno, Laizner, Marcil, and Lang (2003) did a psychometric assessment of a French translation of Brown's Support Behaviors Inventory, a measure of satisfaction with social support in the perinatal period. The scale was administered to 271 Francophone respondents in Québec whose responses to scale items were factor analyzed. The analysis revealed two factors: satisfaction with partner support and satisfaction with the support of others.

MULTIVARIATE ANALYSIS OF VARIANCE

Multivariate analysis of variance (MANOVA) is the extension of ANOVA to more than one dependent variable. MANOVA is used to test the significance of differences between the means of two or more groups on two or more dependent variables, considered simultaneously. For instance, if we wanted to compare the effect of two alternative exercise treatments on both blood pressure and heart rate, then a MANOVA would be appropriate. Covariates can also be included, in which case the analysis would be a **multivariate analysis of covariance** (MANCOVA).

CAUSAL MODELING

Causal modeling involves the development and statistical testing of a hypothesized explanation of the causes of a phenomenon, usually with nonexperimental data. **Path analysis,** which is based on multiple regression, is a widely used approach to causal modeling. Alternative methods of testing causal models are also used by nurse researchers, the most important of which is **linear structural relations analysis,** more widely known as **LISREL.** Both LISREL and path analysis are highly complex statistical techniques whose utility relies on a sound underlying causal theory.

Guide to Multivariate Statistical Analyses

In selecting a multivariate analysis, researchers must attend to such issues as the number of independent variables, the number of dependent variables, the measurement level of all variables, and the desirability of controlling extraneous variables. Table 15.14 is an aid to help you evaluate the appropriateness of multivariate statistics used in research reports. This chart includes the major multivariate analyses used by nurse researchers.

READING AND UNDERSTANDING STATISTICAL INFORMATION

Statistical findings are communicated in the results section of research reports and are reported in the text as well as in tables (or, less frequently, figures). This section provides some assistance in reading and interpreting statistical information.

Tips on Reading Text With Statistical Information

The results section of a research report presents various types of statistical information. First, there are descriptive statistics (such as those shown in Table 15.4), which typically provide readers with a basic overview of participants' characteristics. Information about the subjects' background enables readers to draw conclusions about the groups to which findings might be generalized. Second, researchers may provide statistical information about biases. For example, researchers sometimes compare the characteristics of people who did and did not agree to participate in the study (e.g., using t-tests). Or, in a quasi-experimental design, statistics on the preintervention comparability of the experimental and comparison groups might be presented so that readers can evaluate internal validity. Inferential statistics relating to the research hypotheses are usually presented. Finally, supplementary analyses are sometimes included to help unravel the meaning of the results.

The text of research reports normally provides certain information about the statistical tests, including (1) which test was used, (2) the actual value of the calculated statistic, (3) the degrees of freedom, and (4) the level of statistical significance. Examples of how the results of various statistical tests would likely be reported in the text of a report are shown below.

t-test: $t = 1.68$; $df = 160$; $p = .09$
Chi-squared: $\chi^2 = 16.65$; $df = 2$; $p < .001$
Pearson's r: $r = .36$; $df = 100$; $p < .01$
ANOVA: $F = 0.18$; $df = 1, 69$, NS

Note that the significance level is sometimes reported as the *actual* computed probability that the null hypothesis is correct, as in example 1. In this case, the observed group differences could be found by chance in 9 out of 100 samples; thus, this result is not significant because the differences have an unacceptably high chance of being spurious. The probability level is sometimes reported simply as falling below or above a significance level, as in examples 2 and 3. In both cases, the results are statistically significant because the probability of obtaining such results by chance alone is less than 1 in 100. When results do not achieve statistical significance at the desired level, researchers simply may indicate that the results were not significant (NS), as in example 4.

Statistical information usually is noted parenthetically in a sentence describing the findings, as in the following example: Patients in the experimental group had a significantly lower rate of infection than those in the control group ($\chi^2 = 7.99$, $df = 1$, $p < .01$).

TABLE 15.14   Guide to Widely Used Multivariate Statistical Analyses

NAME	PURPOSE	MEASUREMENT LEVEL*			NUMBER OF:		
		IV	DV	COV	IVs	DVs	COVs
Multiple correlation, regression	To test the relationship between two or more IVs and one DV; to predict a DV from two or more IVs	N, I, R	I, R		2+	1	
Analysis of covariance (ANCOVA)	To test the difference between the means of two or more groups, while controlling for one or more covariate	N	I, R	N, I, R	1+	1	1+
Multivariate analysis of variance (MANOVA)	To test the difference between the means of two or more groups for two or more DVs simultaneously	N	I, R		1+	2+	
Multivariate analysis of covariance (MANCOVA)	To test the difference between the means of two or more groups for two or more DVs simultaneously, while controlling for one or more covariate	N	I, R	N, I, R	1+	2+	1+
Factor analysis	To determine the dimensionality or structure of a set of variables						
Discriminant analysis	To test the relationship between two or more IVs and one DV; to predict group membership; to classify cases into groups	N, I, R	N		2+	1	
Logistic regression	To test the relationship between two or more IVs and one DV; to predict the probability of an event, to estimate relative risk (odds ratios)	N, I, R	N		2+	1	

*Measurement level of the independent variable (IV), dependent variable (DV), and covariates (COV): N = nominal, I = interval, R = ratio.

In reading research reports, you do not need to absorb the numeric values for the actual test statistic. For example, the actual value of χ^2 has no inherent interest. What is important is to grasp whether the statistical tests indicate that the research hypotheses were accepted as probably true (as established by significant results) or rejected as probably false (as established by nonsignificant results).

Tips on Reading Statistical Tables

Tables allow researchers to condense a lot of statistical information in a compact space and also prevent redundancy. Consider, for example, putting information from a correlation matrix (see Table 15.7) into the text: "The correlation between caregivers' age and problematic behaviours was −.11; the correlation between caregivers' age and number of caregiving tasks was −.08. . . ."

Unfortunately, although tables are efficient, they may be daunting and difficult to decipher. Part of the problem is the lack of standardization of tables. There is no universally accepted method of presenting *t*-test information, for example, and so each table may present a new challenge. Another problem is that some researchers try to include an enormous amount of information in their tables; we deliberately used tables of relative simplicity as examples in this chapter.

We know of no magic solution for helping you to comprehend statistical tables, but we have some suggestions. First, read the text and the tables simultaneously—the text may help to unravel the tables. Second, before trying to understand the numbers in a table, try to glean as much information as possible from the words. Table titles and footnotes often communicate critical pieces of information. The table headings should be carefully reviewed because these indicate what the variables in the analyses are (often listed in the far left-hand column as row labels) and what statistical information is included (often specified in the top row as column headings). Third, you may find it helpful to consult the glossary of symbols in Box 15.1 to determine the meaning of a statistical symbol in a report table. Note that not all symbols in Box 15.1 were described in this chapter; therefore, it may be necessary to refer to a statistics textbook, such as that of Polit (1996), for further information. We recommend that you devote some extra time to making sure you have grasped what the tables are conveying and that you write out a sentence or two that summarizes some of the tabular information in "plain English."

CONSUMER TIP

In tables, probability levels associated with the significance tests are sometimes presented directly (e.g., $p < .05$), as in Table 15.13. Here, the significance of each test is indicated in the last column, headed "*p*". However, researchers often indicate significance levels in tables through asterisks placed next to the value of the test statistic. By convention, one asterisk usually signifies $p < .05$, two asterisks signify $p < .01$, and three asterisks signify $p < .001$ (there is usually a key at the bottom of the table that indicates what the asterisks mean). Thus, a table might show: $t = 3.00$, $p < .01$ *or* $t = 3.00$**. The absence of an asterisk would signify a nonsignificant result. ■

BOX 15.1   Glossary of Selected Statistical Symbols

This list contains some commonly used symbols in statistics. The list is in approximate alphabetical order, with English and Greek letters intermixed. Nonletter symbols have been placed at the end.

a	Regression constant, the intercept
α	Greek alpha; significance level in hypothesis testing, probability of Type I error
b	Regression coefficient, slope of the line
β	Greek beta, probability of a Type II error; also, a standardized regression coefficient (beta weights)
χ^2	Greek chi squared, a test statistic for several nonparametric tests
CI	Confidence interval around estimate of a population parameter
df	Degrees of freedom
η^2	Greek eta squared, index of variance accounted for in ANOVA context
f	Frequency (count) for a score value
F	Test statistic used in ANOVA, ANCOVA, and other tests
H_0	Null hypothesis
H_1	Alternative hypothesis; research hypothesis
λ	Greek lambda, a test statistic used in several multivariate analyses (Wilks' lambda)
μ	Greek mu, the population mean
M	Sample mean (alternative symbol for $\bar{X}$)
MS	Mean square, variance estimate in ANOVA
n	Number of cases in a subgroup of the sample
N	Total number of cases or sample members
p	Probability that observed data are consistent with null hypothesis
r	Pearson's product–moment correlation coefficient for a sample
r_s	Spearman's rank-order correlation coefficient
R	Multiple correlation coefficient
R^2	Coefficient of determination, proportion of variance in *dependent variable* attributable to *independent variables*
R_c	Canonical correlation coefficient
ρ	Greek rho, population correlation coefficient
SD	Sample standard deviation
SEM	Standard error of the mean
σ	Greek sigma (lowercase), population standard deviation
Σ	Greek sigma (uppercase), sum of
SS	Sum of squares
t	Test statistics used in t-tests (sometimes called Student's t)
U	Test statistic for the Mann-Whitney U-test
$\bar{X}$	Sample mean
x	Deviation score
Y'	Predicted value of Y, dependent variable in regression analysis
z	Standard score in a normal distribution
$\|$	Absolute value
$\leq$	Less than or equal to
$\geq$	Greater than or equal to
$\neq$	Not equal to

CRITIQUING QUANTITATIVE ANALYSES

It may be difficult for you to critique statistical analyses. We hope this chapter has helped to demystify statistics, but we also recognize the limited scope of this presentation. Although it would be unreasonable to expect you to now be adept at evaluating statistical analyses, there are certain things you should routinely look for in reviewing research reports. Some specific guidelines are presented in Box 15.2.

Researchers generally perform many more analyses than can be reported in a journal article. You should determine whether the statistical information adequately describes the sample and reports the results of statistical tests for all hypotheses. You might also consider whether the report included unnecessary statistical information. Another presentational issue concerns the researcher's judicious use of tables to summarize statistical information.

A thorough critique also addresses whether researchers used the appropriate statistics. Tables 15.12 and 15.14 provide summaries of the most frequently used statistical tests—although we do not expect that you will be able to determine the appropriateness of the tests used in a study without further statistical instruction. The major issues to consider are the number of independent and dependent variables, the levels of measurement of the research variables, the number of groups (if any) being compared, and the appropriateness of using a parametric test.

 BOX 15.2   Guidelines for Critiquing Quantitative Analyses

1. Does the report include any descriptive statistics? Do these statistics sufficiently describe the major characteristics of the researcher's data set?
2. Were the correct descriptive statistics used? (e.g., Were percentages reported when a mean would have been more informative?)
3. Does the report include any inferential statistical tests? If not, should it have (e.g., were groups compared without information on the statistical significance of group differences)?
4. Was a statistical test performed for each of the hypotheses or research questions?
5. Do the selected statistical tests appear to be appropriate (e.g., are the tests appropriate for the level of measurement of key variables)?
6. Were any multivariate procedures used? If not, should multivariate analyses have been conducted—would the use of a multivariate procedure strengthen the internal validity of the study?
7. Were the results of any statistical tests significant? Nonsignificant? What do the tests tell you about the plausibility of the research hypotheses? Can you draw any conclusions about the possibility that Type I or Type II errors were committed?
8. Was an appropriate amount of statistical information reported? Were important analyses omitted, or were unimportant analyses included?
9. Were tables used judiciously to summarize statistical information? Is information in the text and tables totally redundant? Are the tables clear, with a good title and carefully labeled headings?
10. Is the researcher sufficiently objective in reporting the results?

If researchers did not use a multivariate technique, you should consider whether the bivariate analysis adequately tests the relationship between the independent and dependent variables. For example, if a *t*-test or ANOVA was used, could the internal validity of the study have been enhanced through the statistical control of extraneous variables, using ANCOVA? The answer will almost always be "yes," even when an experimental design was used.

As we noted in Chapter 9, statistical analyses and design issues are sometimes intertwined, in the sense that both analytic and design decisions can affect statistical conclusion validity. When sample size is low, when an independent variable is weakly defined (or when participation in an intervention is low), and when a weak statistical procedure is used in lieu of a more powerful one, then the risk of drawing the wrong conclusion about the research hypotheses is heightened. You should pay particular attention to the possibility of statistical conclusion validity problems when research hypotheses are not supported.

The main task for beginning consumers in reading a results section of a research report is to understand the meaning of the statistical tests, but it is also important to consider the believability of the findings.

RESEARCH EXAMPLES — Critical Thinking Activities

 Example 1: Descriptive, Bivariate, and Multivariate Statistics

Aspects of a nursing study, featuring terms and concepts discussed in this chapter, are presented below, followed by some questions to guide critical thinking.

Study
"Efficacy of a psychoeducative group program for caregivers of demented persons living at home: A randomized controlled trial" (Hébert, Lévesque, Vézina, Lavoie, Ducharme, Gendron, Préville, Voyer, & Dubois, 2003)

Statement of Purpose
The goal of the study was to evaluate the effectiveness of a special psychoeducative program for the informal caregivers of persons with dementia. The 15-week program, which was designed to improve the caregivers' ability to cope with stress, was based on the theoretical framework of Lazarus and Folkman. The researchers hypothesized that the program would decrease the frequency of reactions to behaviour problems and decrease the caregiver's burden.

Research Design
The researchers undertook a multicentre clinical trial using a before–after experimental design. Study participants ($N = 158$) were randomly assigned to a 15-week intervention group or to a control group at six centres in the province of Québec. Control group members were referred to a regular support group program. The researchers used power analysis to estimate the sample size they needed to effectively test the study hypotheses. Participants were interviewed at baseline and

(Research Examples continue on page 382)

Critical Thinking Activities (continued)

16 weeks later by interviewers blinded to group assignment. Primary outcome variables included measures of caregivers' reaction to problem behaviours, perceived burden, and anxiety.

Descriptive Statistics
The researchers reported means and percentages to describe sample characteristics. For example, the caregivers in the experimental group were, on average, 59.8 years old (SD = 11.9), and the average age of the care-receiver was 73.6 (SD = 7.8). The majority of caregivers were women (80%), married (82%), and living in the same household as the relative (85%).

Bivariate Inferential Statistics
To evaluate the success of random assignment, the researchers used *t*-tests and chi-squared tests to compare participants in the experimental and control groups, in terms of both demographic characteristics and baseline measures of the dependent variables. These analyses indicated that, for the vast majority of variables, the two groups were equivalent. For example, the mean number of years of being a caregiver was 2.9 in the experimental group and 2.7 in the control group ($p = .69$). These analyses did reveal, however, that the two groups were significantly different in terms of baseline scores on a scale of personal efficacy and the desire to institutionalize the relative (52% of those in the treatment group compared to 31% in the control group expressed a significant desire to institutionalize at the outset of the study, $p = .02$).

Multivariate Analyses
To control for baseline differences (as well as to increase the precision of the analyses), the researchers used ANCOVA to test hypotheses about program effectiveness. Pretest measures were the covariates, and the two groups were compared in terms of posttest scores on the dependent variables. The results suggest that the program had several impacts. For example, the treatment group caregivers had a 14% decrease in their reactions to their relatives' behaviour problems, compared with a 5% decrease among control group caregivers ($p = .04$). There was also a significant, favourable effect on perceived burden, after controlling for initial levels of perceived burden ($p = .02$). Anxiety levels were not significantly different in the two groups ($p = .39$).

Conclusions
The researchers concluded that the findings were promising and that the program merits consideration by Alzheimer societies and health organizations.

*Critical Thinking Suggestions**
*See the Student Resource CD-ROM for a discussion of these questions.
1. Answer questions 1 through 7 from Box 15.2 regarding this study.
2. Also consider the following targeted questions, which may assist you in further assessing aspects of the study:

Critical Thinking Activities (continued)

    a. Do you think the statistical conclusion validity of this study is high? Why or why not?

    b. In what way (if at all) do the statistical analyses in this study affect its internal validity?

    c. One of the researchers' secondary outcomes was the caregivers' desire to institutionalize their relatives (operationalized as having/not having the desire). Which statistical test(s) would be appropriate for determining the program's effect on this outcome?

3. If the results of this study are valid and reliable, what are some of the uses to which the findings might be put in practice?

 EXAMPLE 2: Descriptive, Inferential, and Multivariate Statistics

1. Read the Results section from the study by Feeley and colleagues ("Mother–VLBW Infant Interaction") in Appendix A of this book, and then answer the relevant questions in Box 15.2.

2. Also consider the following targeted questions, which may further sharpen your critical thinking skills and assist you in assessing aspects of the study's merit:

    a. Does Table 1 present descriptive or inferential statistics? What is the level of measurement of the following variables in this table: infant's duration of hospitalization? oxygen in NICU? intraventricular hemorrhage?

    b. With regard to Table 2, did mothers receive more support at 3 months or at 9 months? At which of these two periods was there greater variability in scores? Does this table show whether changes in score over time were statistically significant? What statistical test was or would be used to test such changes?

    c. In Table 3, which two variables had the strongest correlation? What does this correlation mean? Which had the weakest correlation? How many correlations were statistically significant? Why do you think the researchers reported one of the correlations as $p = .055$? Comparing Table 3 and Table 4, the correlations between which pairs of variables were significant at 3 months that were not significant at 9 months?

    d. What were the independent variables in the multiple regression (Table 5)? Which of these variables were significant predictors of mother–infant interaction, given all other variables in the analysis? Once birth weight and severity of illness were in the regression, was the addition of education and state anxiety (step 2) significant? And then was the addition of the next two variables significant (step 3)? What was the overall R^2 (adjusted) for the multiple regression analysis? Was the overall predictive model statistically significant? Based on the standardized regression weights (the βs), which independent variable was most strongly correlated with mother–infant interaction?

CHAPTER REVIEW
Summary Points

▶ There are four major **levels of measurement:** (1) **nominal measurement**—the classification of attributes into mutually exclusive categories; (2) **ordinal measurement**—the ranking of objects based on their relative standing on an attribute; (3) **interval measurement**—indicating not only the ranking of objects but also the distance between them; and (4) **ratio measurement**—distinguished from interval measurement by having a rational zero point.

▶ **Descriptive statistics** enable researchers to synthesize and summarize quantitative data.

▶ In a **frequency distribution**, numeric values are ordered from lowest to highest, together with a count of the number (or percentage) of times each value was obtained.

▶ Data for a variable can be completely described in terms of the shape of its distribution, central tendency, and variability.

▶ The shape of a distribution can be **symmetric** or **skewed**, with one tail longer than the other; it can also be **unimodal** with one peak (i.e., one value of high frequency), or **multimodal** with more than one peak.

▶ A **normal distribution** (bell-shaped curve) is symmetric, unimodal, and not too peaked.

▶ Measures of **central tendency** indicate the average or typical value of a variable. The **mode** is the value that occurs most frequently in a distribution; the **median** is the point above which and below which 50% of the cases fall; and the **mean** is the arithmetic average of all scores. The mean is usually the preferred measure of central tendency because of its stability.

▶ Measures of **variability**—how spread out the data are—include the range and standard deviation. The **range** is the distance between the highest and lowest scores, and the **standard deviation** indicates how much, on average, scores deviate from the mean.

▶ A **contingency table** is a two-dimensional frequency distribution in which the frequencies of two nominal- or ordinal-level variables are **cross-tabulated**.

▶ **Correlation coefficients** describe the direction and magnitude of a relationship between two variables. The values range from −1.00 for a perfect negative correlation, to .00 for no relationship, to +1.00 for a perfect positive correlation. The most frequently used correlation coefficient is the **product–moment correlation coefficient (Pearson's r)**, used with interval- or ratio-level variables.

▶ **Inferential statistics**, which are based on *laws of probability*, allow researchers to make inferences about a population based on data from a sample; they offer a framework for deciding whether the sampling error that results from sampling fluctuation is too high to provide reliable population estimates.

▶ The **sampling distribution of the mean** is a theoretical distribution of the means of an infinite number of same-sized samples drawn from a population. Sampling distributions are the basis for inferential statistics.

▶ The **standard error of the mean**—the standard deviation of this theoretical distribution—indicates the degree of average error of a sample mean; the smaller the standard error, the more accurate are the estimates of the population value based on the sample mean.

▶ **Hypothesis testing** through statistical tests enables researchers to make objective decisions about relationships between variables.

▶ The *null hypothesis* states that no relationship exists between the variables and that any observed relationship is due to chance or sampling fluctuations; rejection of the null hypothesis lends support to the research hypothesis.

▶ A **Type I error** occurs if a null hypothesis is incorrectly rejected (false positives). A **Type II error** occurs when a null hypothesis is incorrectly accepted (false negatives).

▶ Researchers control the risk of making a Type I error by establishing a **level of significance** (or **alpha** level), which specifies the probability that such an error will occur. The .05 level means that in only 5 out of 100 samples would the null hypothesis be rejected when it should have been accepted.

▶ The probability of committing a Type II error, referred to as **beta** (β), can be estimated through *power analysis. Power,* the ability of a statistical test to detect true relationships, is the complement of beta (i.e., power equals $1 - \beta$). The standard criterion for an acceptable level of power is .80.

▶ Results from hypothesis tests are either significant or nonsignificant; **statistically significant** means that the obtained results are not likely to be due to chance fluctuations at a given probability level (***p* level**).

▶ **Parametric statistical tests** involve the estimation of at least one parameter, the use of interval- or ratio-level data, and an assumption of normally distributed variables; **nonparametric tests** are used when the data are nominal or ordinal and the normality of the distribution cannot be assumed.

▶ Two common statistical tests are the ***t*-test** and **analysis of variance** (ANOVA), both of which can be used to test the significance of the difference between group means; ANOVA is used when there are more than two groups.

▶ The most frequently used nonparametric test is the **chi-squared test**, which is used to test hypotheses about differences in proportions.

▶ Pearson's *r* can be used to test whether a correlation is significantly different from zero.

▶ **Multivariate statistics** are increasingly being used in nursing research to untangle complex relationships among three or more variables.

▶ **Multiple regression** is a method for understanding the effect of two or more **predictor** (independent) **variables** on a dependent variable. The **multiple correlation coefficient** (***R***), can be squared to estimate the proportion of variability in the dependent variable accounted for by the predictors.

▶ **Analysis of covariance** (ANCOVA) permits researchers to control extraneous variables (called **covariates**) before determining whether group differences are significant.

▶ Other multivariate procedures used by nurse researchers include discriminant function analysis, logistic regression, factor analysis, multivariate analysis of variance (MANOVA), multivariate analysis of covariance (MANCOVA), path analysis, and LISREL.

Additional Resources for Review

Chapter 15 of the *Study Guide to Accompany Essentials of Nursing Research,* 6th edition offers various exercises and study suggestions for reinforcing the concepts presented in this chapter. For additional review, see the Student Self-Study Review Questions section of the Student Resource CD-ROM provided with this book.

SUGGESTED READINGS

References for studies cited in the chapter appear at the end of the book.

Methodologic References

Jaccard, J., & Becker, M. A. (2001). *Statistics for the behavioral sciences* (4th ed.). Belmont, CA: Wadsworth.

McCall, R. B. (2000). *Fundamental statistics for behavioral sciences* (8th ed.). Belmont, CA: Wadsworth.

Polit, D. F. (1996). *Data analysis and statistics for nursing research.* Stamford, CT: Appleton & Lange.

Welkowitz, J., Ewen, R. B., & Cohen, J. (2000). *Introductory statistics for the behavioral sciences* (5th ed.). New York: Harcourt College.

Analyzing Qualitative Data

STUDENT OBJECTIVES

STUDENT OBJECTIVES

On completing this chapter, you will be able to:

▶ Distinguish prototypical qualitative analysis styles and describe the intellectual processes that play a role in qualitative analysis
▶ Describe activities that qualitative researchers perform to manage and organize their data
▶ Discuss the procedures used to analyze qualitative data, including both general procedures and those used in grounded theory, phenomenological, and ethnographic research
▶ Evaluate researchers' descriptions of their analytic procedures and assess the adequacy of those procedures
▶ Define new terms in the chapter

As we saw in Chapter 13, qualitative data are derived from narrative materials such as verbatim transcripts of in-depth interviews, field notes from participant observation, and personal diaries. This chapter describes methods for analyzing such qualitative data.

INTRODUCTION TO QUALITATIVE ANALYSIS

Qualitative analysis is a labour-intensive activity that requires creativity, conceptual sensitivity, and sheer hard work. Qualitative analysis is more complex and difficult to do well than quantitative analysis because it is less formulaic. In this section, we discuss some general issues relating to qualitative analysis.

Qualitative Analysis: General Considerations

The purpose of data analysis, regardless of the type of data or the underlying research tradition, is to organize, provide structure to, and elicit meaning from the data. Data analysis is particularly challenging for qualitative researchers, for three major reasons. First, there are no universal rules for analyzing and summarizing qualitative data. The absence of standard analytic procedures makes it difficult to present findings in such a way that their validity is apparent. Some of the procedures described in Chapter 14 (e.g., member checking and investigator triangulation) are important tools for enhancing the trustworthiness not only of the data themselves but also of the analyses and interpretation of those data.

The second challenge of qualitative analysis is the enormous amount of work required. The qualitative analyst must organize and make sense of pages and pages of narrative materials. In a recent multimethod study by one of us (Polit), the qualitative data consisted of transcribed, unstructured interviews with about 25 to 30 low-income women in four cities discussing life stressors and health problems over a 3-year period. The transcriptions ranged from 30 to 50 pages in length, resulting in thousands of pages that had to be read and reread and then organized, integrated, and interpreted.

The final challenge comes in reducing the data for reports. Quantitative results can often be summarized in two or three tables. Qualitative researchers, by contrast, must balance the need to be concise to adhere to journal requirements with the need to maintain the richness and evidentiary value of their data.

CONSUMER TIP

Qualitative analyses are often more difficult to do than quantitative ones, but qualitative findings are generally easier to understand than quantitative findings because the stories are often told in everyday language. However, qualitative analyses are harder to evaluate critically than quantitative analyses because readers cannot know first-hand if researchers adequately captured thematic patterns in the data. ■

Analysis Styles

Crabtree and Miller (1999) observed that there are nearly as many qualitative analysis strategies as there are qualitative researchers. However, they have identified three major styles that fall along a continuum. At one extreme is a style that is more systematic and standardized, and at the other is a style that is more intuitive, subjective, and interpretive. The three prototypical styles are as follows:

▶ **Template analysis style**. In this style, researchers develop a *template*—a category and analysis guide for sorting the narrative data. Researchers usually begin with a rudimentary template before collecting data, but the template undergoes constant revision as the data are gathered and analyzed. This style is most likely to be adopted by researchers whose research tradition is ethnography, ethology, discourse analysis, or ethnoscience.

▶ **Editing analysis style**. Researchers using an editing style act as interpreters who read through texts in search of meaningful segments. Once segments are identified and reviewed, researchers develop a category scheme and corresponding codes that can be used to sort and organize the data. The researchers then search for the patterns and structure that connect the thematic categories. Researchers whose research tradition is grounded theory, phenomenology, hermeneutics, or ethnomethodology use procedures within this analysis style.

▶ **Immersion/crystallization analysis style**. This style involves the analyst's total immersion in and reflection of the text materials, resulting in an intuitive crystallization of the data. This interpretive and subjective style is exemplified in personal case reports of a semianecdotal nature and is less frequently encountered in the nursing research literature than the other two styles.

Researchers seldom use terms like template analysis style or editing style in their reports—these terms are *post hoc* characterizations of styles that are adopted. However, King (1998) has described the process of undertaking a template analysis, and his approach has been adopted by some nurse researchers undertaking descriptive qualitative studies.

Example of a template analysis

Beardwood and French (2004) used a template to analyze their data in a study of the effectiveness of mediation in complaints against nurses, as carried out by the College of Nurses of Ontario. The study involved an analysis of 34 cases, semistructured interviews with 44 participants in the mediation process, and several focus group sessions.

The Qualitative Analysis Process

The analysis of qualitative data is an active and interactive process. Qualitative researchers typically scrutinize their data carefully and deliberatively. Insights cannot spring forth from the data unless the researchers are completely familiar with those data, and so they often read their narrative data over and over in search of meaning. Morse and Field (1995) note that qualitative analysis is "a process of fitting data together, of making the invisible obvious, of linking and attributing consequences to antecedents. It is a process of conjecture and verification, of correction and modification, of suggestion and defense" (p. 126). Morse and Field identified four cognitive processes that play a role in qualitative analysis:

▶ *Comprehending*. Early in the analytic process, qualitative researchers strive to make sense of the data and to learn "what is going on." When comprehension is achieved, researchers are able to prepare a thorough description of the phenomenon under study, and new data do not add much to that description. Thus, comprehension is completed when saturation has been attained.

▶ *Synthesizing.* Synthesizing involves a "sifting" of the data and inductively putting pieces together. At this stage, researchers get a sense of what is typical with regard to the phenomenon and of what variation is like. At the end of the synthesis process, researchers can make some general statements about the phenomenon and about study participants.

▶ *Theorizing.* Theorizing involves a systematic sorting of the data. During the theorizing process, researchers develop alternative explanations of the phenomenon under study and then hold these explanations up to determine their "fit" with the data. The theorizing process continues to evolve until the best and most parsimonious explanation is obtained.

▶ *Recontextualizing.* The process of *recontextualization* involves the further development of the theory such that its applicability to other settings or groups is explored.

Although the intellectual processes in qualitative analysis are not linear in the same sense that quantitative analysis is, these four processes follow a rough progression over the course of the study. Comprehension occurs primarily while in the field. Synthesis begins in the field but may continue well after the fieldwork has been completed. Theorizing and recontextualizing are processes that are difficult to undertake before synthesis has been completed.

QUALITATIVE DATA MANAGEMENT AND ORGANIZATION

The intellectual processes of qualitative analysis are supported and facilitated by early tasks that help to organize and manage the masses of narrative data.

Developing a Category Scheme

Qualitative researchers begin their analysis by organizing their data. The main organizational task is devising a method to classify and index the data. Researchers must design a means of gaining access to parts of the data, without having to repeatedly reread the data set in its entirety. This phase of data analysis is essentially reductionist—data must be converted to smaller, more manageable units that can be retrieved and reviewed.

The most widely used procedure is to develop a category scheme and to then code the data according to the categories. A category system (or template) is sometimes drafted before data collection, but more typically the qualitative analyst develops categories based on a scrutiny of the actual data.

There are, unfortunately, no straightforward or easy guidelines for this task. The development of a high-quality category scheme for qualitative data involves a careful reading of the data, with an eye to identifying underlying concepts and clusters of concepts.

Depending on the aims of the study, the nature of the categories may vary in level of detail or specificity as well as in level of abstraction.

Researchers whose aims are primarily descriptive tend to use concrete categories. The category scheme may focus on actions or events or on different phases in the unfolding of an experience. In developing a category scheme, related concepts are often grouped together to facilitate the coding process.

Example of a descriptive category scheme

The category scheme used by Polit, London, and Martinez (2000) to categorize data relating to food insecurity and hunger in low-income families is an example of a system that was concrete and descriptive. For example, one major coding category was "Strategies used to avoid hunger." The subcategories used to code the interview transcripts included eight strategies, such as "Stretching food, eating smaller portions" and "Eating old or unsafe food."

Studies aimed at theory development are more likely to develop abstract and conceptual categories. In designing conceptual categories, researchers must break the data into segments, closely examine them, and compare them to other segments for similarities and dissimilarities to determine what type of phenomena are reflected in them and what the meaning of those phenomena are. Researchers ask questions about discrete events, incidents, or thoughts, such as the following:

▶ What is this?
▶ What is going on?
▶ What does it stand for?
▶ What else is like this?
▶ What is this distinct from?

Important concepts that emerge from close examination of the data are then given a label that forms the basis for a category scheme. These category names are abstractions, but the labels are usually sufficiently graphic that the nature of the material to which the label refers is clear—and often provocative.

Example of a conceptual category scheme

Box 16.1 shows the category scheme developed by Beck (2004) to categorize data from her Internet interviews on birth trauma (See Appendix B). The coding scheme included four major thematic categories with subcodes. For example, an excerpt that described a mother's feelings of humiliation would be coded under category 1B (i.e., being stripped of her dignity).

BOX 16.1   **Beck's (2004) Coding Scheme for Birth Trauma**

Theme 1. To care for me: Was that too much to ask?
A. Feeling abandoned and alone
B. Stripped of dignity
C. Lack of interest in a woman as a unique person
D. Lack of support and reassurance

Theme 2. To communicate with me: Why was this neglected?
A. Labor and delivery staff failed to communicate with the patients.
B. Labor and delivery staff spoke as if the woman in labor was not present.
C. Clinicians failed to communicate among themselves.

Theme 3. To provide safe care: You betrayed my trust and I felt powerless.
A. Perceived unsafe care
B. Feared for their own safety and that of their unborn infants
C. Felt powerless

Theme 4. The end justifies the means: At whose expense? At what price?
A. Traumatic deliveries were glossed over.
B. Successful outcome of the baby took center stage.
C. The mother was made to feel guilty.
D. No one wanted to listen to the mother.

CONSUMER TIP

A good category scheme is crucial to the analysis of qualitative data. Without a high-quality category system, researchers cannot retrieve the narrative information that has been collected. Unfortunately, research reports rarely present the category scheme for readers to review, but they may provide other information that may help you evaluate its adequacy (e.g., researchers may say that the scheme was reviewed by peers or developed and independently verified by two or more researchers). ■

Coding Qualitative Data

After a category scheme has been developed, the data are then read in their entirety and coded for correspondence to the identified categories. The process of coding qualitative material is not an easy one. Researchers may have difficulty in deciding which code is most appropriate, or they may not fully comprehend the underlying meaning of some aspect of the data. It may take a second or third reading of the material to grasp its nuances.

Moreover, researchers often discover in going through the data that the initial category system was incomplete or inadequate. It is not unusual for some themes to emerge that were not initially conceptualized. When this happens, it is risky to assume that the topic failed to appear in previously coded materials. That is, a concept might not be identified as salient until it has emerged a third or fourth time in the data. In such a case, it would be necessary to reread all previously coded material to have a truly complete grasp of that category.

Another issue is that narrative materials are generally not linear. For example, paragraphs from transcribed interviews may contain elements relating to three or four different categories, embedded in a complex fashion.

Example of coding qualitative data

An example of a multitopic segment of an interview from Beck's (2004) phenomenological study of birth trauma is shown in Figure 16.1. The codes in the margin represent codes from the scheme presented in Box 16.1.

"At some point a fetal scalp monitor was introduced then what seemed to be very shortly after that, my own OB came in and said my baby was in fetal distress and that a c-section was probably needed given that I was only 6 cms. This floored me in every imaginable way-emotionally, physically, and mentally. I'd labored in what I thought was "well mannered" for 12 hours. NO ONE had told me they were monitoring my baby. NO ONE told me they suspected she was in distress. Then BOOM, my baby is in trouble and my almost picture-perfect labor is gone. After that point, things became blurry because I can only see them through what I describe as an emotional fog. I lost it in front of everybody which I rarely do. **[2 A]**

[2 A] As they wheeled me into the theatre, I asked again where was my husband. They said he was on his way. They wheeled me in and told me to curl my back for the epidural. There were a few nurses there and I remember them talking about me as if I wasn't **[2 B]**
[2 A] there. Didn't they realize that I could hear them? The needle must have gone in 4 or 5 times. I was crying. I was scared and the epidural hurt a bloody lot. Some one please help me. I felt all alone. And I was thinking that I don't want another baby and go through this again. I recall thinking how much more pain do I have to put up with? Was my baby going to be all right? I needed reassurance but none was given. **[1 D]**
Then another man took over the epidural and asked me to sit up and bend over while he put the needle in. I started to feel numb below my waist. I felt a pin prick and felt my tummy being pulled apart. It was awful as I couldn't see or feel anything.
[1 A] So my trauma was a result of that emergency caesarean. It happened so fast. Of feeling so scared and alone and having to go through it all alone with out my husband there. The nurses didn't tell me anything about what was going on. I felt powerless.
[3 C] I also felt the hospital staff could have given me some indication that I may have **[2 A]** had to have an emergency caesarean instead of letting me think that I was going to have a natural labor. I also wished that the doctor herself could have come to see
[1 C] how I was doing afterwards. I think it would have helped me a lot if she had come and talked about how I was doing and how I felt and why I had to have an emergency c-section. **[2 A]**
[4 B] All people kept telling me after my daughter was born was how lucky I was and that I could have lost her. I know I was lucky but telling that does not help how I felt. With them telling me that, I felt guilty for feeling the way I did. I wanted some attention too. I wanted to be looked after and listened to. I tried several times to bring up how **[4 C]**
[4 D] I felt but it was brushed away with the "I've been through that before and so what response." I really felt like I was in the wrong to feel the way I did because I had a healthy baby."

FIGURE 16.1 Coded excerpt from Beck's (2004) study.

Manual Methods of Organizing Qualitative Data

Various procedures have been used to organize qualitative data. Before the advent of computer programs for managing qualitative data, the most usual procedure was to develop **conceptual files**. This approach involves creating a physical file for each category, and then cutting out and inserting into the file all materials relating to that category. Researchers can then retrieve all of the content on a particular topic by reviewing the applicable file folder.

The creation of such conceptual files is a cumbersome and labour-intensive task, particularly when segments of the narrative materials have multiple codes (e.g., the excerpt shown in Figure 16.1). There would need to be, for example, three copies of the last paragraph—one for each file corresponding to the three codes used for this paragraph. Researchers must also be sensitive to the need to provide enough context that the cut-up material can be understood. Thus, it is often necessary to include material preceding or following the directly relevant materials.

Computer Programs for Managing Qualitative Data

Traditional manual methods of organizing qualitative data have a long and respected history, but sophisticated computer programs for managing qualitative data are now widely used. These programs permit the entire data file to be entered onto the computer, each portion of an interview or observational record coded, and then portions of the text corresponding to specified codes retrieved and printed (or shown on a screen) for analysis. The current generation of programs also has features that go beyond simple indexing and retrieval—they offer possibilities for actual analysis and integration of the data.

Computer programs remove the drudgery of cutting and pasting pages and pages of narrative material. However, some people prefer manual indexing because it allows them to get closer to the data. Others have raised concerns about using programs for the analysis of qualitative data, objecting to having a process that is basically cognitive turned into an activity that is mechanical. Despite these issues, some qualitative researchers have switched to computerized data management because it frees up their time and permits them to pay greater attention to important conceptual issues.

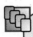

Example of using computers to manage qualitative data

Hyman, Guruge, Mason, Gould, Stuckless, Tang, Teffera, and Mekonnen (2004) studied postmigration changes in gender relations between Ethiopian husbands and wives living in Canada. Data came from in-depth interviews and focus group discussions with eight Ethiopian couples who had migrated to Toronto. Transcribed interviews were entered into a computer program called N6 (a version of the widely used NUD*IST program) for coding and organization.

CONSUMER TIP

A good category system is of little utility if the actual coding is not done with care. There is, of course, no way for you as a reader to know whether coding was diligently performed. However, you can have more confidence if the report mentions that two or more people were involved in coding the data, or at least portions of it, to ensure intercoder reliability. ■

ANALYTIC PROCEDURES

Data *management* in qualitative research is reductionist in nature because it converts large masses of data into smaller, more convenient units. By contrast, qualitative data *analysis* is constructionist: it involves putting segments together into a meaningful conceptual pattern. Although there are several approaches to qualitative data analysis, some elements are common to several of them. We provide some general guidelines, followed by a description of the procedures used by ethnographers, phenomenologists, and grounded theory researchers.

It should be noted that qualitative researchers who conduct studies that are not based on a specific research tradition sometimes say that a **content analysis** was performed. Qualitative content analysis is the analysis of narrative data to identify prominent themes and patterns among the themes.

Example of a content analysis

Letourneau, Neufeld, Drummond, and Barnfather (2003) explored parental decision making related to surgery for infants with isolated craniosyntosis. Using content analysis to analyze their focus group data, their analysis revealed four themes that encapsulated the process of parental decision making.

A General Analytic Overview

The analysis of qualitative materials generally begins with a search for recurring regularities or themes. DeSantis and Ugarriza (2000), in their thorough review of the way in which the term theme is used among qualitative researchers, offer this definition: "A **theme** is an abstract entity that brings meaning and identity to a current experience and its variant manifestations. As such, a theme captures and unifies the nature or basis of the experience into a meaningful whole" (p. 362).

Themes emerge from the data. They often develop within categories of data (i.e., within categories of the coding scheme used for indexing materials) but sometimes cut across them. For example, in Beck's (2004) study (see Figure 16.1), one theme that emerged was the clinicians' neglect of communication, including failure to communicate with their patients in labour and delivery (code 2A) and failure to communicate amongst themselves (code 2C).

The search for themes involves not only the discovery of commonalities but also a search for variation. Themes are never universal; researchers must attend not only to what themes arise but also to how they are patterned. Does the theme apply only to certain subsets of participants? In certain types of communities or in certain contexts? At certain periods? What are the conditions that precede an observed phenomenon, and what are the consequences of it? In other words, qualitative analysts must be sensitive to *relationships* within the data.

CONSUMER TIP

Major themes are often the subheadings used in the results section of qualitative reports. For example, in their phenomenological study of older Canadian women's experiences as they negotiated health care, Kinch and Jakubec (2004) identified four main themes that were used to organize their results section: "Femininity, relationships, and means of support," "Health information and the politics of access to care," "The supportive role of faith, religion, and tradition," and "Abuse and power." ■

Researchers' search for themes and regularities in the data can sometimes be facilitated by charting devices that enable them to summarize the evolution of behaviours and processes. For example, for qualitative studies that focus on dynamic experiences (e.g., decision making), it is often useful to develop flow charts or time-lines that highlight time sequences, major decision points, or events.

Example of a time-line

In Beck's (2002) grounded theory study of mothering twins during the first year of life, timelines that highlighted mothers' 24-hour schedule were helpful. Figure 16.2 presents an example for a 23-year-old mother of twins who had been born premature and were in the NICU for 2 months. At the time of the interview, the twins had recently been discharged from the hospital. Until they were 3 months old, the mother fed them on the same schedule they had been on in the hospital—every 3 hours. The time-line illustrates a typical 24-hour period for this mother.

A further step involves validation to determine whether the themes inferred are an accurate representation of the phenomenon. Several validation procedures can be used, as discussed in Chapter 14. If more than one researcher is working on the study, sessions in which the themes are reviewed and specific cases discussed can be highly productive. Investigator triangulation cannot ensure thematic validity, but it can minimize idiosyncratic biases. It is also useful to undertake member checks—that is, to present the preliminary thematic analysis to some informants, who can be encouraged to offer comments to support or contradict the analysis.

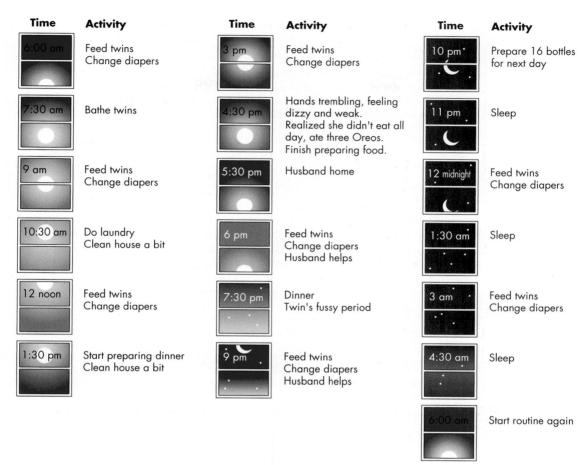

FIGURE 16.2 Example of a timeline for mothering multiples study.

At this point, some researchers introduce **quasi-statistics**—a tabulation of the frequency with which certain themes or patterns are supported by the data. The frequencies cannot be interpreted in the same way as frequencies generated in survey studies because of imprecision in the sampling of cases and enumeration of the themes. Nevertheless, as Becker (1970) pointed out:

> *Quasi-statistics may allow the investigator to dispose of certain troublesome null hypotheses. A simple frequency count of the number of times a given phenomenon appears may make untenable the null hypothesis that the phenomenon is infrequent. A comparison of the number of such instances with the number of negative cases—instances in which some alternative phenomenon that would not be predicted by his theory appears—may make possible a stronger conclusion, especially if the theory was developed early enough in the observational period to allow a systematic search for negative cases (p. 81).*

Example of tabulating qualitative data

Harrison, Kushner, Benzies, Rempel, and Kimak (2003) interviewed 47 women with a high-risk pregnancy to explore how satisfied they were with their personal involvement in health care decisions. The researchers tabulated some aspects of the women's experiences. For example, they noted that most women (n = 30 out of 47) wanted to be active partners in their care management decisions. Of these 30 women, 21 were satisfied with their active decisions, but 8 of the 21 had had to struggle with health professionals for increased involvement.

In the final analysis stage, researchers strive to weave the thematic pieces together into an integrated whole. The various themes need to be interrelated to provide an overall structure (such as a theory or integrated description) to the data. The integration task is a difficult one because it demands creativity and intellectual rigour to be successful.

CONSUMER TIP

Research reports vary in the amount of detail provided about qualitative analytic procedures. At one extreme, researchers say little more than "data were analyzed qualitatively." At the other extreme, researchers describe the steps they took to analyze their data and validate emerging themes. Most studies fall between the two extremes, but limited detail is more prevalent than abundant detail. ■

These general analytic procedures provide an overview of how qualitative researchers make sense of their data. However, variations in the goals and philosophies of qualitative researchers also lead to variations in analytic strategies. The next section describes data analysis in ethnographic studies.

Analysis of Ethnographic Data

Ethnographic analysis begins the moment the researcher sets foot in the field. Ethnographers are continually looking for *patterns* in the behaviour and thoughts of the participants, comparing one pattern against another, and analyzing many patterns simultaneously (Fetterman, 1989). As they analyze patterns of everyday life, ethnographers acquire a deeper understanding of the culture being studied. They analyze key events (e.g., social events) because these events provide a lens through which to view a culture. Maps, flow charts, and organizational charts are also useful analytic tools that help to crystallize and illustrate the data being collected.

Spradley's (1979) developmental research sequence is one method that is often used for data analysis in an ethnographic study. His method is based on the premise that language is the primary means that relates cultural meaning in a culture. The task of ethnographers is to describe cultural symbols and to identify their rules. His sequence of 12 steps, which includes both data collection and data analysis, is as follows:

1. Locating an informant
2. Interviewing an informant
3. Making an ethnographic record
4. Asking descriptive questions
5. Analyzing ethnographic interviews
6. Making a domain analysis
7. Asking structural questions
8. Making a taxonomic analysis
9. Asking contrast questions
10. Making a componential analysis
11. Discovering cultural themes
12. Writing the ethnography

Thus, in Spradley's method, there are four levels of data analysis: domain, taxonomic, componential, and theme. *Domain analysis* is the first level of analysis. **Domains**, which are units of cultural knowledge, are broad categories that encompass smaller categories. There is no preestablished number of domains to be uncovered in an ethnographic study. During this first level of data analysis, ethnographers identify relational patterns among terms in the domains that are used by members of the culture. Ethnographers focus on the cultural meaning of terms and symbols (objects and events) used in a culture and their interrelationships.

In *taxonomic analysis*, ethnographers decide how many domains the data analysis will encompass. Will only one or two domains be analyzed in depth, or will a number of domains be studied less intensively? After making this decision, a **taxonomy**—a system of classifying and organizing terms—is developed to illustrate the internal organization of a domain and the relationship among the subcategories of the domain.

In *componential analysis*, ethnographers analyze data for similarities and differences among cultural terms in a domain. Finally, in *theme analysis*, cultural themes are uncovered. Domains are connected in cultural themes, which help to provide a holistic view of the culture being studied. The discovery of cultural meaning is the outcome.

Example of a study with a taxonomic analysis

Hirst (2002) conducted a study designed to define resident abuse within the culture of long-term care institutions, as perceived by nurses working in those settings. Ten RNs working in five long-term institutions in Canada were interviewed on several occasions. Information from the first interview was used to create a set of cards on which key terms were printed. During the second interview, respondents sorted these cards into similar and dissimilar terms and then into subcategories. Participants were encouraged to verbalize their thinking as they sorted. Hirst then developed a taxonomy, which was refined from her understanding of the participants' structuring processes.

Other approaches to ethnographic analysis have also been developed. For example, in her ethnonursing research method, Leininger (2001) provided ethnographers with a data analysis guide to help systematically analyze large amounts of data from their fieldwork. There are four phases to Leininger's ethnonursing data analysis guide. In the first phase, ethnographers collect, describe, and record data. The second phase involves identifying and categorizing descriptors. In phase 3, data are analyzed to discover repetitive patterns in their context. The fourth and final phase involves abstracting major themes and presenting findings.

Example of a study using Leininger's ethnonursing method

DeOliveira and Hoga (2005) studied the process of seeking and undergoing surgical contraception by low-income Brazilian women. Using Leininger's ethnonursing research method, the researchers interviewed 7 key informants and 11 additional informants. The cultural theme was that "being *operada* was the realization of a great dream" (p. 5).

Phenomenological Analysis

Schools of phenomenology have developed different approaches to data analysis. Three frequently used methods of data analysis for descriptive phenomenology are the methods of Colaizzi (1978), Giorgi (1985), and Van Kaam (1966), all of whom are from the Duquesne school of phenomenology, based on Husserl's philosophy. Table 16.1 presents a comparison of the steps involved in these three methods of analysis. The basic outcome of all three methods is the description of the meaning of an experience, often through the identification of essential themes. The phenomenologist searches for common patterns shared by particular instances. However, there are some important differences among these three approaches. Colaizzi's method, for example, is the only one that calls for a validation of the results by returning to study participants (i.e., member checking). Giorgi's analysis relies solely on the researcher. His view is that it is inappropriate to either return to the participants to validate the findings or to use external judges to review the analysis. Van Kaam's method requires that intersubjective agreement be reached with other expert judges.

Example of a study using Colaizzi's method

Malinowski and Stamler (2003) explored the personal experiences of adolescent girls with an infant simulator; the nine 11th-grade girls had participated in a *Baby Think It Over* program. The adolescents were interviewed and invited to describe their experiences. The transcribed interviews were analyzed using Colaizzi's method, which involved "reading entire transcripts, extracting significant statements and formulating meanings for them, organizing clusters of themes and validating them by referring to original transcripts, documenting discrepancies, integrating results into an exhaustive description, and returning the findings to participants for validation" (p. 207).

TABLE 16.1   Comparison of Three Phenomenological Methods

COLAIZZI (1978)	GIORGI (1985)	VAN KAAM (1966)
1. Read all protocols to acquire a feeling for them.	1. Read the entire set of protocols to get a sense of the whole.	1. List and group preliminarily the descriptive expressions, which must be agreed upon by expert judges. Final listing presents percentages of these categories in that particular sample.
2. Review each protocol and extract significant statements.	2. Discriminate units from participants' description of phenomenon being studied.	2. Reduce the concrete, vague, and overlapping expressions of the participants to more descriptive terms. (Intersubjective agreement among judges needed.)
3. Spell out the meaning of each significant statement (i.e., formulate meanings).	3. Articulate the psychological insight in each of the meaning units.	3. Eliminate elements not inherent in the phenomenon being studied or that represent blending of two related phenomena.
4. Organize the formulated meanings into clusters of themes. a. Refer these clusters back to the original protocols to validate them. b. Note discrepancies among or between the various clusters, avoiding the temptation of ignoring data or themes that do not fit.	4. Synthesize all of the transformed meaning units into a consistent statement regarding participants' experiences (referred to as the "structure of the experience"); can be expressed on a specific or general level.	4. Write a hypothetical identification and description of the phenomenon being studied.
5. Integrate results into an exhaustive description of the phenomenon under study.		5. Apply hypothetical description to randomly selected cases from the sample. If necessary, revise the hypothesized description, which must then be tested again on a new random sample.
6. Formulate an exhaustive description of the phenomenon under study in as unequivocal a statement of identification as possible.		6. Consider the hypothesized identification as a valid identification and description once preceding operations have been carried out successfully.
7. Ask participants about the findings thus far as a final validating step.		

A second school of phenomenology is the Utrecht school. Phenomenologists using this Dutch approach combine characteristics of descriptive and interpretive phenomenology. Van Manen's (1990) method is an example of this combined approach in which researchers try to grasp the essential meaning of the experience being studied. According to Van Manen, themes can be uncovered from descriptions of an experience by three different means: (1) the holistic approach, (2) the selective or highlighting approach, and the (3) detailed or line-by-line approach. In the *holistic approach*, researchers view the text as a whole and try to capture its meanings. In the *selective approach*, researchers underline, highlight, or pull out statements or phrases that seem essential to the experience under study. In the *detailed approach*, researchers analyze every sentence. Once the themes have been identified, they become the objects of reflecting and interpreting through follow-up interviews with participants. Through this process, the essential themes are discovered. In addition to identifying themes from participants' descriptions, Van Manen's method also encourages gleaning thematic descriptions from artistic sources (e.g., from poetry, novels, and other art forms).

Example of a study using Van Manen's method

Evans and O'Brien (2005) conducted a phenomenological study of the experience and meaning of gestational diabetes. They described how Van Manen's thematic approach was used to analyze data from interviews with 12 women who were diagnosed with and being treated for diabetes in pregnancy. "We read each transcript in its entirety to analyze it for a sense of the whole before making any focus on particular components. Through inductive reasoning, we extracted words, statements and paragraphs to emulate all possible meanings of the pregnancy experience as described by the women. As we moved back and forth between parts and the whole of the written text, a dialectal process emerged" (p. 69).

Some qualitative researchers—especially phenomenologists—use *metaphors* as an analytic strategy. A metaphor, a figurative comparison, can be a powerfully creative and expressive tool for qualitative analysts. As a literary device, metaphors can permit greater

Example of a metaphor

"Data had been collected over the cold winter months and the researcher felt the intensity of the participants' descriptions translate into a powerful visual image. Their experience of feeling depressed as an adolescent mother following the birth of their babies was like being faced with a sudden storm. While some storm patterns are merely a nuisance—something you deal with—others have the potential to cripple entire regions of a country. Nor'easters in particular are strange weather systems that suddenly pop out of nowhere. It was this image that emerged from the participants' descriptions and is presented here as a metaphor to frame the thematic structure" (Clemmens, 2002, p. 556).

insight and understanding in qualitative data analysis in addition to helping link together parts to the whole. One researcher, who studied adolescent mothers' depression after giving birth, described the integration of a storm metaphor (which emerged from the adolescents' descriptions of their experiences) into her analysis.

A third school of phenomenology is the interpretive approach of Heideggerian hermeneutics. Central to analyzing data in a hermeneutic study is the notion of the **hermeneutic circle**. The circle (which is itself a metaphor) signifies a methodologic process in which, to reach understanding, there is continual movement between the parts and the whole of the text being analyzed. To interpret a text is to understand the possibilities that can be revealed by the text. Gadamer (1975) stressed that to interpret a text, researchers cannot separate themselves from the meanings of the text. Ricoeur (1981) broadened this notion of text to include not just the written text but also any human action or situation.

Example of Gadamerian hermeneutics

Tapp (2004) studied dilemmas of family support during cardiac recovery. Her data were derived from transcripts of videotaped clinical sessions with six families. Guided by Gadamer's writings, Tapp's interpretation of the text occurred at three levels: "First, the transcripts for each session were reviewed to identify salient events, meanings, and patterns related to experiences ... that ... illustrated attempts to offer or receive support. Second, all of the sessions for each family were then reviewed for thematic patterns across their unique situation.... Interpretive memoing traced emerging understandings of support within each family situation and within their relationships. Finally, the salient events, family concerns, and recurrent patterns were compared between and across the six family situations" (p. 566).

Diekelmann, Allen, and Tanner (1989) have proposed a seven-stage process of data analysis in hermeneutics that involves collaborative effort by a team of researchers. The goal of this process is to describe shared practices and common meanings. Diekelmann and colleagues' stages include the following:

1. Reading all interviews or texts for an overall understanding.
2. Preparing interpretive summaries of each interview.
3. Analyzing selected transcribed interviews or texts by a research team.
4. Resolving any disagreements on interpretation by going back to the text.
5. Identifying recurring themes that reflect common meanings and shared practices of everyday life by comparing and contrasting the texts.
6. Identifying emergent relationships among themes.
7. Presenting a draft of the themes, along with exemplars from texts, to the team; incorporating responses and suggestions into the final draft.

According to Diekelmann and colleagues, the discovery (step 6) of a **constitutive pattern**—a pattern that expresses the relationships among relational themes and is present in all the interviews or texts—forms the highest level of hermeneutical analysis. A situation is constitutive when it gives actual content or style to a person's self-understanding or to a person's way of being in the world.

Example of Diekelmann's hermeneutic analysis

Cheung and Hocking (2004) used Diekelmann's method to explore spousal caregivers' experience of caring for victims of multiple sclerosis in Australia. Data were obtained through interviews with 10 spousal caregivers. The researchers examined the data to identify a constitutive pattern that described the ways in which participants' experiences of caring for their partner had changed their way of living and their personal meanings. The constitutive pattern that emerged from the data was called "Weaving through a web of paradoxes."

Another data analytic approach for hermeneutic phenomenology is offered by Benner (1994). Her interpretive analysis consists of three interrelated processes: the search for paradigm cases, thematic analysis, and analysis of exemplars. **Paradigm cases** are "strong instances of concerns or ways of being in the world" (Benner, 1994, p. 113). Paradigm cases are used early in the analytic process as a strategy for gaining understanding. Thematic analysis is done to compare and contrast similarities across cases. Lastly, paradigm cases and thematic analysis can be enhanced by *exemplars* that illuminate aspects of a paradigm case or theme. The presentation of paradigm cases and exemplars in research reports allows readers to play a role in consensual validation of the results by deciding whether the cases support the researchers' conclusions.

Example of Benner's hermeneutic analysis

Raingruber and Kent (2003) conducted an interpretive phenomenological study of faculty and student experiences during traumatic clinical events. The researchers interviewed students and faculty in nursing and social work as well as psychiatrists. Using Benner's interpretive analysis, one paradigm case and 12 exemplars were described in support of their conclusion that faculty and students experienced strong physical sensations during traumatic situations in their practice. In the paradigm case, "Trina, a social work student, described suddenly feeling like her body was 'a ripe apple ready to drop from the tree when a little boy surprised her by calling her momma' " (p. 455).

Grounded Theory Analysis

As noted in Chapter 10, there are two major approaches to substantive grounded theory analysis. One grounded theory approach was developed by Glaser and Strauss (1967), and another by Strauss and Corbin (1998).

GLASER AND STRAUSS' GROUNDED THEORY METHOD

Grounded theory in both systems of analysis uses the **constant comparative** method of data analysis. This method involves a comparison of elements present in one data source (e.g., in one interview) with those identified in another. The process is continued until the content of each source has been compared to the content in all sources. In this fashion, commonalities are identified.

The concept of fit is an important element in Glaser and Strauss' grounded theory analysis. **Fit** is the process of identifying characteristics of one piece of data and comparing them with those of other data to determine whether they are similar. Fit is used to sort and reduce data; it enables researchers to determine whether data can be placed in the same category or if they can be related to one another (but data should not be forced or distorted to fit the developing category).

Coding in Glaser and Strauss' grounded theory approach is used to conceptualize data into patterns or concepts. The substance of the topic being studied is conceptualized though **substantive codes**, whereas **theoretical codes** provide insights into how the substantive codes relate to each other.

In the Glaser and Strauss approach, there are two types of substantive codes: open and selective. **Open coding**, used in the first stage of analysis, captures what is going on in the data. Open codes may be the actual words used by participants. Through open coding, data are broken down into incidents, and their similarities and differences are examined. During open coding, researchers ask, "What category or property of a category does this incident indicate?" (Glaser, 1978, p. 57).

There are three levels of open coding that vary in level of abstraction. **Level I codes** (or *in vivo codes*) are derived directly from the language of the substantive area. They have vivid imagery and "grab." Table 16.2 presents five level I codes from interviews in Beck's (2002) grounded theory study on mothering twins, and excerpts associated with those codes.

As researchers constantly compare new level I codes with previously identified ones, they condense them into broader categories—**level II codes**. For example, in Table 16.2, Beck's five level I codes were collapsed into the level II code, "Reaping the blessings." **Level III codes** (or theoretical constructs) are the most abstract codes. These constructs "add scope beyond local meanings" (Glaser, 1978, p. 70) to the generated theory. Collapsing level II codes aids in identifying constructs.

Example of open codes in grounded theory analysis

Dewar's (2003) grounded theory study explored strategies people use to live with catastrophic illnesses and injuries. Dewar identified one key strategy that she called "boosting"—the individuals' efforts to improve their self-esteem, which helped them to endure their circumstances. Dewar's report indicated that the participants' own words were used as a first level of coding. These *in vivo* codes later were combined into categories. For example, an early *in vivo* code was "it could be worse," but as the analysis proceeded it became "comparing self to others" and eventually became part of the large category called "boosting."

TABLE 16.2	Collapsing Level I Codes Into the Level II Code of "*REAPING THE BLESSINGS*" (Beck, 2002)

QUOTE	LEVEL I CODE
I enjoy just watching the twins interact so much. Especially now that they are mobile. They are not walking yet but they are crawling. I will tell you they are already playing. Like one will go around the corner and kind of peek around and they play hide and seek. They crawl after each other.	Enjoying Twins
With twins it's amazing. She was sick and she had a fever. He was the one acting sick. She didn't seem like she was sick at all. He was. We watched him for like 6–8 hours. We gave her the medicine and he started calming down. Like WOW! That is so weird. 'Cause you read about it but it's like, Oh come on! You know that doesn't really happen and it does. It's really neat to see.	Amazing
These days it's really neat 'cause you go to the store or you go out and people are like, "Oh, they are twins, how nice." And I say, "Yeah they are. Look, look at my kids."	Getting Attention
I just feel blessed to have two. I just feel like I am twice as lucky as a mom who has one baby. I mean that's the best part. It's just that instead of having one baby to watch grow and change and develop and become a toddler and school age child you have two.	Feeling Blessed
It's very exciting. It's interesting and it's fun to see them and how the twin bond really is. There really is a twin bond. You read about it and you hear about it but until you experience it, you just don't understand. One time they were both crying and they were fed. They were changed and burped. There was nothing wrong. I couldn't figure out what was wrong. So I said to myself, "I am just going to put them together and close the door." I put them in my bed together and they patty caked their hands and put their noses together and just looked at each other and went right to sleep.	Twin Bonding

Open coding ends when the core category is discovered, and then selective coding begins. The **core category** is a pattern of behaviour that is relevant or problematic for study participants. In **selective coding** (which can also have three levels of abstraction), researchers code only those data that are related to the core variable. One kind of core variable is a **basic social process** (BSP), which evolves over time in two or more phases. All BSPs are core variables, but not all core variables have to be BSPs.

Glaser (1978) provided nine criteria to help researchers decide on a core category:

1. It must be central, meaning that it is related to many categories.
2. It must reoccur frequently in the data.
3. It takes more time to saturate than other categories.
4. It relates meaningfully and easily to other categories.
5. It has clear and grabbing implications for formal theory.
6. It has considerable carry-through.
7. It is completely variable.
8. It is a dimension of the problem.
9. It can be any kind of theoretical code.

Theoretical codes help the grounded theorist to weave the broken pieces of coded data back together again. Glaser (1978) proposed 18 families of theoretical codes that researchers can use to conceptualize how substantive codes relate to each other. Five examples of the 18 families include the following:

▶ Process: stages, phases, passages, transitions
▶ Type: kinds, styles, forms
▶ Strategy: tactics, techniques, manoeuverings
▶ Cutting point: boundaries, critical junctures, turning points
▶ The six C's: causes, contexts, contingencies, consequences, covariances, and conditions

Example of theoretical codes

Weaver, Wuest, and Ciliska (2005) undertook a grounded theory study to understand women's recovery from anorexia nervosa. They noted that, in their theoretical coding, they used the following coding families to tease out properties and dimensions of the category of *sheltering:* types, strategies, consequences, and conditions. For example, sheltering strategies included isolating, conforming, and putting on a mask. Types of sheltering included families sheltering women as daughters and women sheltering themselves.

Throughout coding and analysis, grounded theory researchers document their ideas about the emerging conceptual scheme in *memos*. Memos preserve ideas that may initially not seem productive but may later prove valuable once further developed. Memos also encourage researchers to reflect on and describe patterns in the data, relationships between categories, and emergent conceptualizations.

Glaser and Strauss' grounded theory method is concerned with the *generation* of categories and hypotheses rather than testing them. The product of the typical grounded theory analysis is a theoretical model that explains a pattern of behaviour that is both relevant and/or problematic for the people in the study. Once the basic problem emerges, the grounded theorist goes on to discover the process these participants experience in coping with or resolving this problem.

Example of a Glaser & Strauss grounded theory analysis

Figure 16.3 presents the model developed by Beck (2002) in her grounded theory study that conceptualized "Releasing the pause button" as the core category and the process through which mothers of twins progressed as they attempted to resume their lives after giving birth. According to this model, the process involves four phases: "Draining power," "Pausing own life," "Striving to reset," and "Resuming own life." Beck used 10 coding families in her theoretical coding for the "Releasing the pause button" process. The family *cutting point* provides an illustration. Three months seemed to be the turning point for mothers, when life started to become more manageable. Here is an excerpt from an interview that Beck coded as a cutting point: "Three months came around and the twins sort of slept through the night and it made a huge, huge difference."

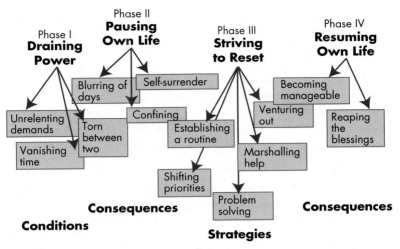

FIGURE 16.3 Beck's (2002) model of mothering twins.

STRAUSS AND CORBIN'S GROUNDED THEORY METHOD

The Strauss and Corbin (1998) approach to grounded theory analysis differs from the original Glaser and Strauss method with regard to method and outcomes. Table 16.3 summarizes major analytic differences between these two methods.

Glaser (1978) stressed that to generate a grounded theory, the basic problem must emerge from the data—it must be discovered. The theory is, from the very start, grounded in the data, rather than starting with a preconceived problem. Strauss and Corbin, however, argued that the research itself is only one of four possible sources of the research problem.

TABLE 16.3	**Comparison of Glaser's and Strauss/Corbin's Methods**	
	GLASER	**STRAUSS & CORBIN**
Initial data analysis	Breaking down and conceptualizing data involves comparison of incident to incident so patterns emerge	Breaking down and conceptualizing data includes taking apart a single sentence, observation, and incident
Types of coding	Open, selective, theoretical	Open, axial, selective
Connections between categories	18 coding families	Paradigm model (conditions, contexts, action/interactional strategies, and consequences)
Outcome	Emergent theory (discovery)	Conceptual description (verification)

Research problems can, for example, come from the literature or from researchers' personal and professional experience.

The Strauss and Corbin method involves three types of coding: open, axial, and selective coding. In **open coding**, data are broken down into parts and compared for similarities and differences. Similar actions and events are grouped together into categories. In open coding, the researcher focuses on generating categories and their properties. In **axial coding**, the analyst systematically develops categories and links them with subcategories. Strauss and Corbin (1998) term this process of relating categories and their subcategories as "axial because coding occurs around the axis of a category, linking categories at the level of properties and dimensions" (p. 123). **Selective coding** is a process in which the findings are integrated and refined. The first step in integrating the findings is to decide on the **central category** (or core category), which is the main theme of the research. Recommended techniques to facilitate identifying the central category are writing the storyline, using diagrams, and reviewing and organizing memos.

The outcome of the Strauss and Corbin approach is a full conceptual description. The original grounded theory method (Glaser & Strauss, 1967), by contrast, generates a theory that explains how a basic social problem that emerged from the data is processed in a social setting.

Example of a Strauss & Corbin grounded theory analysis

O'Brien, Evans, and White-McDonald (2002) used the Strauss and Corbin method in their study of women's coping with severe nausea and vomiting during pregnancy. Interviews with 24 women admitted to a large tertiary care hospital in western Canada were read and coded by at least two researchers. Lines, paragraphs and words were coded and emerging categories were discussed and finalized by consensus. "Data were then reconstructed by linking categories and subcategories within a set of relationships so that the context in which the experience occurred could be described (axial coding). A concept (i.e., core category) around which all emerging categories could be related was selected" (p. 304). The core category was the process (diagrammed in Figure 16.4) of increasingly complete isolation to cope with unrelenting and severe symptoms.

CRITIQUING QUALITATIVE ANALYSES

The task of evaluating a qualitative analysis is not an easy one, even for experienced researchers. The difficulty lies mainly in the fact that readers must accept largely on faith that researchers exercised good judgment and insight in coding the narrative materials, developing a thematic analysis, and integrating the materials into a meaningful whole. This is because researchers are seldom able to include more than a handful of examples of actual data in a research report and because the process of inductively abstracting meaning from data is difficult to describe.

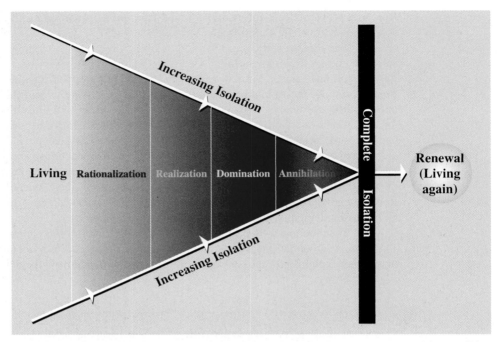

FIGURE 16.4 Isolated from living: process of coping with severe nausea, vomiting, and/or retching of pregnancy. (O'Brien, Evans, & White-McDonald, 2002).

In a critique of qualitative analysis, a primary task usually is determining whether researchers took sufficient steps to validate inferences and conclusions. A major focus of a critique of qualitative analyses, then, is whether the researchers have adequately documented the analytic process. The report should provide information about the approach used to analyze the data. For example, a report for a grounded theory study should indicate whether the researchers used the Glaser and Strauss or the Strauss and Corbin method.

Quantitative analyses can be evaluated in terms of the adequacy of specific analytic decisions (e.g., did the researcher use the appropriate statistical test?). Critiquing analytic decisions is substantially less clearcut in a qualitative study. For example, it typically would be inappropriate to critique a phenomenological analysis for following Giorgi's approach rather than Colaizzi's approach. Both are respected methods of conducting a phenomenological study and analyzing the resulting data (although phenomenologists themselves may have cogent reasons for preferring one approach over the other).

One aspect of a qualitative analysis that *can* be critiqued, however, is whether the researchers have documented that they have used one approach consistently and have been faithful to the integrity of its procedures. For example, if researchers say they are using the Glaser and Strauss approach to grounded theory analysis, they should not also include elements from the Strauss and Corbin method. An even more serious problem occurs when, as sometimes happens, the researchers "muddle" traditions. For example, researchers who describe their study as a grounded theory study should not have a presentation of *themes* because grounded theory analysis does not yield themes. Furthermore, researchers who

BOX 16.2 Guidelines for Critiquing Qualitative Analyses

1. Given the nature of the data, was the data analysis approach appropriate for the research design?
2. Is the category scheme described? If so, does the scheme appear logical and complete? Does there seem to be unnecessary overlap or redundancy in the categories?
3. Were manual methods used to index and organize the data, or was a computer program used?
4. Does the report adequately describe the process by which the actual analysis was performed? Does the report indicate whose approach to data analysis was used (e.g., Glaser & Strauss or Strauss & Corbin, in grounded theory studies)? Was this method consistently and appropriately applied?
5. What major themes or processes emerged? If excerpts from the data are provided, do the themes appear to capture the meaning of the narratives—that is, does it appear that the researcher adequately interpreted the data and conceptualized the themes? Is the analysis parsimonious—could two or more themes be collapsed into a broader and perhaps more useful conceptualization?
6. What evidence does the report provide that the analysis is accurate and replicable?
7. Were data displayed in a manner that allows you to verify the researcher's conclusions? Was a conceptual map, model, or diagram effectively displayed to communicate important processes?
8. Was the context of the phenomenon adequately described? Does the report give you a clear picture of the social or emotional world of study participants?
9. Did the analysis yield a meaningful and insightful picture of the phenomenon under study? Is the resulting theory or description trivial or obvious?

attempt to blend elements from two traditions may not have a clear grasp of the analytic precepts of either one. For example, a researcher who claims to have undertaken an ethnography using a grounded theory approach to analysis may not be well informed about the underlying goals and philosophies of these two traditions.

Some further guidelines that may be helpful in evaluating qualitative analyses are presented in Box 16.2.

RESEARCH EXAMPLES | Critical Thinking Activities

EXAMPLE 1: Analysis in a Grounded Theory Study

Aspects of a grounded theory study, featuring terms and concepts discussed in this chapter, are presented below, followed by some questions to guide critical thinking.

Study
"Reworking professional nursing identity" (MacIntosh, 2003)

Statement of Purpose
The purpose of this study was to explore experienced nurses' perceptions of how they became professional.

(Research Examples continue on page 412)

Critical Thinking Activities (continued)

Method
MacIntosh used Glaser and Strauss's grounded theory methods to explore how experienced nurses interpreted their professional development and how they addressed problems in that development. She conducted interviews with 21 nurses who had 3 to 34 years of nursing experience working in urban and rural communities in eastern Canada. Each interview was transcribed and analyzed before the next interview was conducted, providing MacIntosh with information for theoretical sampling and framing appropriate questions with subsequent participants. Data collection ended when saturation was achieved.

Analysis
Data analysis was ongoing as new interviews were conducted. Constant comparison among concepts and incidents was used to identify relevant processes, connections, and contextual conditions. In the substantive coding, MacIntosh chose words from the verbatim transcripts to represent each line of data, comparing these words with other codes and then clustering those with similar meanings into initial categories. At the theoretical level, MacIntosh sorted categories by similarities and differences, examined relationships among the categories, and asked questions of the data to "elevate them to a conceptual level" (p. 729). One of the families of theoretical codes that she used was the "strategy" family. For example, one of the strategies nurses used in the final stage of professionalization was mentoring other nurses. MacIntosh noted that she kept copious memos to record thoughts, insights, and questions. Her analysis was validated through several means, including member checks (second interviews with a sample of participants) and discussions of the analytic process with another researcher experienced in grounded theory analysis.

Key Findings
▶ The data revealed a three-stage process among nurses in addressing the problematic issue of dissonance between expectations and experiences as they became and sustained being professional. The process was called "Reworking professional identity."
▶ The three stages were "Assuming adequacy," "Realizing practice," and "Developing a reputation."
▶ The final stage, "Developing a reputation," involved the processes of establishing practice patterns, choosing standards, and helping to advance nursing. Mentoring other nurses was a strategy used in this stage, as exemplified by the following quote: "And once you have seen, or once it's opened for you to have advanced, you want to go around opening all the doors for everyone" (p. 736).

Critical Thinking Suggestions*
*See the Student Resource CD-ROM for a discussion of these questions.
1. Answer questions 1 through 9 from Box 16.2 regarding this study.
2. Also answer the following targeted questions, which may assist you in further assessing aspects of this study:

Critical Thinking Activities (continued)

    a. In the description of her analytic procedures, MacIntosh cited both Glaser and Strauss and Strauss and Corbin. Comment on this.

    b. MacIntosh analyzed data from interviews with experienced nurses in this study. What other data sources could have been used to augment and validate her understandings?

3. If the results of this study are trustworthy, what are some of the uses to which the findings might be put in clinical practice?

 EXAMPLE 2: Analysis in an Ethnographic Study

Aspects of an ethnographic nursing study, featuring terms and concepts discussed in this chapter, are presented below, followed by some questions to guide critical thinking.

Study
"Sources of practice knowledge among nurses" (Estabrooks, Rutakumwa, O'Leary, Profetto-McGrath, Milner, Levers, & Scott-Finlay, 2005)

Statement of Purpose
The purpose of this study was to explore and identify nurses' sources of practice knowledge.

Method
This report was based on two large studies that used an ethnographic case study design to examine factors that influence nurses' use of research in their practice. The cases for the first study were five paediatric units, and those for the second were two adult patient care units, drawn from four tertiary level hospitals in Alberta and Ontario. Data included transcribed individual and focus group interviews with nurses in the hospitals, as well as field notes from participant observation. Card-sorting interviews were also conducted to uncover the structure of the knowledge sources domain. In each setting, data were collected by a research assistant (a master's prepared nurse), who spent 6 months on the unit.

Analysis
Interview transcripts and field notes were entered into the computer program called NUD*IST for subsequent coding and analysis. Data were coded using a line-by-line process. Initial codes, which were based on a reading of the first interviews, were reviewed by the research team until consensus on the coding scheme was achieved. Spradley's procedures were used to develop a taxonomy. The process was a dynamic one, involving "repeated re-categorization of initial categories, and further sorting and analysis of each large (and saturated) category."

Key Findings
Nurses' sources of practice knowledge were categorized into four broad groupings, and these groupings formed the structure of the taxonomy.

(Research Examples continue on page 414)

Critical Thinking Activities (continued)

▶ The category of *social interactions* dominated the findings; these interactions are processes through which nurses communicate and exchange information between and among each other, other health care professionals, and patients.

▶ *Experiential knowledge*, the second category, is knowledge gained during the regular course of nursing practice.

▶ *Documentary sources* included written and printed materials, including unit-based sources (e.g., patients' charts) and off-unit sources (e.g., material in journals, on the Internet); use of these latter sources was limited.

▶ *A priori knowledge* is knowledge that a nurse brings to the unit, including knowledge gained in nursing school and from prior experiences.

Critical Thinking Suggestions
1. Answer questions 1 through 9 from Box 16.2 regarding this study.
2. Also answer the following targeted questions, which may assist you in further assessing aspects of this study:
    a. Comment on the amount of data that had to be analyzed in this study.
    b. What parts of Spradley's analytic method appear to have been followed in this study? What was the *domain* in this study?
3. If the results of this study are trustworthy, what are some of the uses to which the findings might be put in clinical practice?

 EXAMPLE 3: Analysis in a Phenomenological Study

1. Read the Method and Results section from the Beck study ("Birth Trauma") in Appendix B of this book, and then answer the relevant questions in Box 16.1.
2. Also consider the following targeted questions, which may further sharpen your critical thinking skills and assist you in assessing aspects of the study's merit:
    a. Comment on the amount of data that had to be analyzed in this study.
    b. If Beck had used Giorgi's method of phenomenological data analysis instead of Colaizzi's, would it have been appropriate for her to return to the mothers who participated in the study to validate the findings?

C H A P T E R   R E V I E W
S u m m a r y   P o i n t s

▶ Qualitative analysis is a challenging, labour-intensive activity, guided by few standardized rules.

▶ Although there are no universal strategies, three prototypical analytic styles have been identified: (1) a **template analysis style** that involves the development of an analysis guide (*template*) to sort the data; (2) an **editing analysis style** that involves an interpretation of the data on which a **category scheme** is based; and (3) an

immersion/crystallization style that is characterized by the analyst's total immersion in and reflection of text materials.

▶ Qualitative analysis typically involves four intellectual processes: comprehending, synthesizing, theorizing, and **recontextualizing** (exploration of the developed theory vis-à-vis its applicability to other settings or groups).

▶ The first major step in analyzing qualitative data is to organize and index the data for easy retrieval, typically by coding the content according to a category scheme.

▶ Traditionally, researchers have organized their coded data by developing **conceptual files**, which are physical files in which excerpts of data relevant to specific categories are placed. Now, however, computer programs are widely used to perform basic indexing functions and to facilitate data analysis.

▶ The actual analysis of data begins with a search for patterns, regularities, or **themes** in the data, which involves the discovery not only of commonalities across subjects but also of natural variation in the data.

▶ Another analytic step generally involves a validation of the thematic analysis. Some researchers use **quasi-statistics**, a tabulation of the frequency with which certain themes or relations are supported by the data.

▶ In a final analytic step, analysts try to weave thematic strands together into an integrated picture of the phenomenon under investigation.

▶ In ethnographies, analysis begins as the researcher enters the field. Ethnographers continually search for *patterns* in the behaviour and expressions of study participants.

▶ One approach to analyzing ethnographic data is Spradley's method, which involves four levels of data analysis: *domain analysis* (identifying **domains**, or units of cultural knowledge); *taxonomic analysis* (selecting key domains and constructing **taxonomies** or systems of classification); *componential analysis* (comparing and contrasting terms in a domain); and a *theme analysis* (to uncover cultural themes).

▶ Leininger's method for ethnonursing research involves four phases: collecting and recording data; categorizing descriptors; searching for repetitive patterns; and abstracting major themes.

▶ There are various approaches to phenomenological analysis, including the descriptive methods of Colaizzi, Giorgi, and Van Kaam, in which the goal is to find common patterns of experiences shared by particular instances.

▶ In Van Manen's approach, which involves efforts to grasp the essential meaning of the experience being studied, researchers search for themes using either a *holistic approach* (viewing text as a whole); *selective approach* (pulling out key statements and phrases); or a *detailed approach* (analyzing every sentence).

▶ Central to analyzing data in a hermeneutic study is the notion of the **hermeneutic circle**, which signifies a methodological process in which there is continual movement between the parts and the whole of the text under analysis.

▶ In hermeneutics, there are several choices for data analysis. Diekelmann's method calls for the discovery of a **constitutive pattern**, which expresses the relationships among themes. Benner's approach consists of three processes: searching for **paradigm cases**, thematic analysis, and analysis of *exemplars*.

▶ Grounded theory uses the **constant comparative** method of data analysis.

▶ One approach to grounded theory is the Glaser and Strauss method, in which there are two broad types of codes: **substantive codes** (in which the empirical substance of the topic is conceptualized) and **theoretical codes** (in which the relationships among the substantive codes are conceptualized).

▶ Substantive coding involves **open coding** to capture what is going on in the data, and then **selective coding**, (in which only variables relating to a core category is coded). The **core category**, a behaviour pattern that has relevance for participants, is sometimes a **basic social process** (BSP) that involves an evolutionary process of coping or adaptation.

▶ In the Glaser and Strauss method, open codes begin with **level I** (*in vivo*) **codes**, which are collapsed into a higher level of abstraction in **level II codes**. Level II codes are then used to formulate **level III codes**, which are theoretical constructs.

▶ The Strauss and Corbin method is an alternative grounded theory method whose outcome is a full conceptual description. This approach to grounded theory analysis involves three types of coding: open (in which categories are generated), **axial coding** (where categories are linked with subcategories), and selective (in which the findings are integrated and refined).

▶ Some researchers identify neither a specific approach nor a specific research tradition; rather, they might say that they used qualitative **content analysis** as their analytic method.

A d d i t i o n a l   R e s o u r c e s   f o r   R e v i e w

Chapter 16 of the *Study Guide to Accompany Essentials of Nursing Research,* 6th edition offers various exercises and study suggestions for reinforcing the concepts presented in this chapter. For additional review, see the Student Self-Study Review Questions section of the Student Resource CD-ROM provided with this book.

SUGGESTED READINGS

References for studies cited in the chapter appear at the end of the book.

Methodologic References
Becker, H. S. (1970). *Sociological work*. Chicago: Aldine.

Benner, P. (1994). The tradition and skill of interpretive phenomenology in studying health, illness, and caring practices (pp. 99–127). In P. Benner (Ed.), *Interpretive phenomenology*. Thousand Oaks, CA: Sage Publications.

Colaizzi, P. (1978). Psychological research as the phenomenologist views it. In R. Valle & M. King (Eds.), *Existential phenomenological alternatives for psychology*. New York: Oxford University Press.

Crabtree, B. F., & Miller, W. L., Eds. (1999). *Doing qualitative research* (2nd ed.). Newbury Park, CA: Sage Publications.

DeSantis, L., & Ugarriza, D. N. (2000). The concept of theme as used in qualitative nursing research. *Western Journal of Nursing Research, 22,* 351–372.

Diekelmann, N., Allen, D., & Tanner, C. (1989). *The NLN criteria for appraisal of baccalaureate programs: A critical hermeneutic analysis*. New York: NLN Press.

Fetterman, D. M. (1989). *Ethnography: Step by step*. Newbury Park, CA: Sage Publications.

Gadamer, H. G. (1975). *Truth and method*. (G. Borden & J. Cumming, Trans.). London: Sheed and Ward.

Giorgi, A. (1985). *Phenomenology and psychological research*. Pittsburgh: Duquesne University Press.

Glaser, B. G. (1978*). Theoretical sensitivity: Advances in the methodology of grounded theory*. Mill Valley, CA: Sociology Press.

Glaser, B. G., & Strauss, A. L. (1967). *The discovery of grounded theory: Strategies for qualitative research*. Chicago: Aldine.

King, N. (1998). Template analysis. In C. Cassell & G. Symon (Eds.), *Qualitative methods and analysis in organizational research* (pp. 118–134). London: Sage Publications.

Leininger, M. (2001). *Culture care diversity and universality: A theory of nursing*. Boston: Jones and Bartlett.

Morse, J. M., & Field, P. A. (1995). *Qualitative research methods for health professionals* (2nd ed.). Thousand Oaks, CA: Sage Publications.

Ricoeur, P. (1981). *Hermeneutics and the social sciences*. (J. Thompson, Trans. & Ed.). New York: Cambridge University Press.

Spradley, J. P. (1979). *The ethnographic interview.* New York: Holt, Rinehart, and Winston.

Strauss, A., & Corbin, J. (1998). *Basics of qualitative research: Techniques and procedures for developing grounded theory* (2nd ed.). Thousand Oaks, CA: Sage Publications.

Van Kaam, A. (1966). *Existential foundations of psychology*. Pittsburgh: Duquesne University Press.

Van Manen, M. (1990). *Researching lived experience*. New York: State University of New York.

Critical Appraisal and Utilization of Nursing Research

Critiquing Research Reports

STUDENT OBJECTIVES

On completion of this chapter, the student will be able to:

▶ Describe aspects of a study's findings important to consider in developing an interpretation of quantitative and qualitative findings
▶ Evaluate researchers' interpretation of their results
▶ Describe the purposes and dimensions of a research critique
▶ Conduct a comprehensive critique of a qualitative or quantitative research report
▶ Define new terms in the chapter

Throughout this book, we have provided questions and suggestions for critiquing various aspects of nursing research reports. This chapter describes the purposes of a research critique and offers further tips on how to evaluate research reports. One important aspect of a research critique involves the reviewer's interpretation of the study findings. Therefore, we begin this chapter by offering some suggestions on interpreting research results.

INTERPRETING STUDY RESULTS

The analysis of research data provides the study *results*, which need to be evaluated and interpreted—often a challenging task. *Interpretation* should take into account the study's aims, its theoretical underpinnings, the existing body of related research, and the limitations of the adopted research methods. The interpretive task involves a consideration of the following aspects of the study findings:

▶ The credibility and accuracy of the results
▶ The meaning of the results
▶ The importance of the results
▶ The extent to which the results can be generalized or have potential use in other contexts
▶ The implications for practice, theory, or research

In this section, we review issues relating to these interpretive aspects for quantitative and qualitative research reports.

Interpreting Quantitative Results

Quantitative research results often offer readers more interpretive opportunities than qualitative ones—in large part because a quantitative report summarizes most of the study data (e.g., in statistical tables), whereas qualitative reports contain only illustrative examples of the data. When reading quantitative reports, you will need to give careful thought to the possible meaning behind the numbers. Your interpretations can then be compared with those of the researchers, who discuss their views on the meaning and implications of the study results in the discussion section of their reports.

THE CREDIBILITY OF QUANTITATIVE RESULTS

One of the first tasks in interpreting quantitative results is assessing their accuracy. A thorough assessment of the credibility of the results relies on critical thinking skills and on your understanding of research methods. The evaluation should be based on an analysis of evidence, not on "gut feelings." Both external and internal evidence can be brought to bear. External evidence comes primarily from the body of prior research. If the results are consistent, the credibility of the findings is enhanced. If the results are inconsistent with prior research, possible reasons for the discrepancy should be sought. What was different about the way the data were collected, the sample was selected, key variables were operationalized, and so on? You should also consider whether the findings are consistent with common sense and with your own clinical experiences.

Internal evidence for the accuracy of the findings comes from an evaluation of the methods used. You will need to evaluate carefully all the major methodologic decisions made in executing the study to determine whether alternative decisions might have yielded different results. This issue is discussed later in this chapter.

A critical analysis of the research methods and conceptualization almost inevitably indicates some limitations. These limitations must be taken into account in interpreting the results and in contrasting your interpretation with that of the researchers themselves.

THE MEANING OF QUANTITATIVE RESULTS

Quantitative results are usually in the form of test statistic values and probability levels, which do not in and of themselves confer meaning. The statistical results must be translated conceptually and interpreted. In this section, we discuss the interpretation of research outcomes within a statistical hypothesis testing context.

CONSUMER TIP

Many research reports do not formally state hypotheses, but rather present research questions or purpose statements (see Chapter 6). However, every time researchers use an inferential statistic (e.g., a *t*-test), they are using statistics to test a hypothesis. The research hypothesis being tested almost invariable is that, in the population, the groups being compared are different or that variables are related. When hypotheses are not stated but statistical tests are performed, you have to infer the hypotheses. ■

Interpreting Hypothesized Significant Results

When statistical tests support the researcher's hypotheses, the task of interpreting the results may be straightforward because the rationale for the hypotheses typically offers an explanation of what the findings mean. However, hypotheses can be correct even when the researcher's explanation of what is going on is not. As a reviewer, you need to evaluate whether the researchers went beyond the data in interpreting the results. For example, suppose a nurse researcher hypothesized that a relationship exists between a pregnant woman's level of anxiety about the labour and delivery experience and the number of children she has already borne. The study data reveal that a negative relationship between anxiety levels and parity does exist ($r = -.40; p < .05$). The researcher concludes that childbirth experience reduces anxiety. Is this conclusion supported by the data? The conclusion seems logical, but, in fact, there is nothing within the data that leads to this interpretation. An important, indeed critical, research precept is: correlation does not prove causation. The finding that two variables are related offers no evidence about which of the two variables—if either—caused the other. Alternative explanations for the findings should always be considered. If competing interpretations can be excluded on the basis of the data or previous research findings, so much the better, but interpretations should always be given adequate competition.

Throughout the interpretation process, you should bear in mind that the support of research hypotheses through statistical testing never constitutes proof of their validity. Hypothesis testing is probabilistic, and it is always possible that obtained relationships were due to chance.

Example of corroboration of a hypothesis

Norris, Ghali, Galbraith, Graham, Jensen, and Knudtson, for the APPROACH Investigators (2004), hypothesized that women with coronary artery disease would report worse health-related quality-of-life outcomes compared with men 1 year after treatment. Their hypothesis was fully supported, even after they statistically controlled for demographic factors and disease severity.

This study is a good example of the challenges of interpreting quantitative findings in nonexperimental studies. There are several possible explanations for the pattern of findings. The researchers' interpretation was that men and women differ with respect to pretreatment levels of support and depression, a conclusion that they support with evidence from other studies. However, there is nothing in their data that would rule out other possible explanations.

Interpreting Nonsignificant Results

Nonsignificant results pose interpretive problems. Standard statistical procedures are geared toward disconfirmation of the null hypothesis. Failure to reject a null hypothesis (i.e., obtaining results indicating no relationship between the independent and dependent variables) could occur for either of two reasons: (1) because the null hypothesis is true (i.e., there really is no relationship among research variables), or (2) because the null hypothesis is false (i.e., a true relationship exists but the data failed to show it). Neither you nor the researchers know which is right. In the first situation (a true null hypothesis), the problem is likely to lie in the conceptualization that led the researcher to posit the hypotheses. The second situation (a false null hypothesis), by contrast, generally reflects methodologic limitations, such as internal validity problems, a small or atypical sample, or a weak statistical procedure. Thus, the interpretation must consider both substantive and methodologic reasons for nonsignificant results.

Whatever the underlying cause, there is never justification for interpreting a retained null hypothesis as proof of the absence of a relationship among variables. The safest interpretation is that nonsignificant findings represent a lack of evidence for either truth or falsity of the hypothesis.

Note, however, that there is a decided bias against publishing the results of studies in which the results are nonsignificant. This reflects the concern of those making publication decisions that nonsignificant results are likely to reflect methodologic limitations.

Example of nonsignificant results

Taylor, Oberle, Crutcher, and Norton (2005) conducted a pilot study of the effects of a nurse–physician collaborative approach on the care of patients with type 2 diabetes. Forty patients were randomly assigned to either the control group (standard care) or to an experimental group (standard care plus home visits from a nurse and consultation with an exercise specialist and/or nutritionist). Although there was a trend toward positive outcomes with regard to blood pressure, glycosylated hemoglobin, and quality of life, group differences were not statistically significant.

Because statistical procedures are designed to provide support for the *rejection* of null hypotheses, they are not well suited for testing actual research hypotheses about the *absence* of relationships between variables or about *equivalence* between groups. Yet sometimes this is exactly what researchers want to do—and this is especially true in clinical situations in which the goal is to determine whether one practice is just as effective as another. When the actual *research* hypothesis is null (i.e., a prediction of no group difference or no relationship), stringent additional strategies must be used to provide supporting evidence. For one thing, it is imperative to perform a power analysis to demonstrate that the risk of a Type II error is small. There may also be clinical standards that can be used to corroborate that nonsignificant—but predicted—results can be accepted as consistent with the research hypothesis.

Example of nonsignificant results supporting a hypothesis

Medves and O'Brien (2004) conducted a clinical trial to test the hypothesis that thermal stability would be comparable for infants bathed for the first time by a parent or by a nurse. As predicted, there was no difference in temperature change between newborns bathed by nurses or parents. The researchers provided additional support for concluding that heat loss is not associated with who bathes the newborn by noting that a power analysis had been used to determine sample size needs and that the parents in the two groups were comparable demographically at the outset. Also, although the prebath temperatures of the infants in the two groups were significantly different, the researchers used initial temperature as a covariate to control these differences. Finally, they made an *a priori* determination that a change in temperature of 1°C would be clinically significant; at four points in time after the bath, the group differences in temperature were never this large; thus, the differences were clinically insignificant.

Interpreting Unhypothesized Significant Results

Although this does not often happen, there are situations in which researchers obtain significant results that are the opposite of the research hypothesis—that is, *unhypothesized significant results.* For example, a researcher might predict a negative relationship between patient satisfaction with nursing care and the length of stay in the hospital, but a significant *positive* relationship might be found. In such cases, it is less likely that the methods are flawed than that the reasoning or theory is incorrect. In attempting to explain such findings, you should pay particular attention to the results of previous research and alternative theories. It is also useful to consider, however, whether there is anything unusual about the sample that might have led participants to behave or respond atypically.

Example of unhypothesized significant results

Provencher, Perreault, St.-Onge, and Rousseau (2003) studied predictors of psychological distress in Canadian family caregivers of relatives with psychiatric disabilities. Contrary to their hypothesis that social support would be beneficial, the researchers found that caregivers who perceived more support from friends experienced a higher level of distress than those who perceived less support. Also contrary to their predictions, relatives who had more contact with their relatives' primary mental health providers were more distressed than those with less contact.

Interpreting Mixed Results

The interpretive process is often complicated by *mixed results*: some hypotheses are supported by the data, whereas others are not. Or a hypothesis may be accepted when one measure of the dependent variable is used but rejected with a different measure. When only some results run counter to a conceptual scheme or prior findings, the research methods likely deserve critical scrutiny. Differences in the validity and reliability of the various measures may account for such discrepancies, for example. On the other hand, mixed results may suggest that a theory needs to be qualified, or that certain constructs within the theory need to be reconceptualized.

Example of mixed results

Davies, Hodnett, Hannah, O'Brien-Pallas, Pringle, and Wells (2002) studied the effectiveness of alternative means of reducing the use of electronic foetal monitoring (EFM) for healthy women in labour. There was a large decrease in the use of EFM in one intervention hospital, but not in the other. There were also site differences in improvements in other areas.

THE IMPORTANCE OF QUANTITATIVE RESULTS

In quantitative studies, results supporting the hypotheses are described as being significant. A careful analysis of study results involves an evaluation of whether, in addition to being statistically significant, they are important.

The fact that statistical significance was attained in testing the hypothesis does not necessarily mean the results were of value. Statistical significance indicates that the results were unlikely to be due to chance. This means that the observed group differences or relationships were probably real—but not necessarily important. With large samples, even modest relationships are statistically significant. For instance, with a sample of 500 subjects, a correlation coefficient of .10 is significant at the .05 level, but a relationship of this magnitude might have little practical value. As a reviewer, therefore, you should pay attention to the numeric values obtained in an analysis in addition to the significance level when assessing the implications of the findings.

Conversely, the absence of statistically significant results does not mean that the results are unimportant—although, because of problems in interpreting nonsignificant results, the case is more complex. Suppose we compared two methods of making a clinical assessment (e.g., pain) and retained the null hypothesis (i.e., found no statistically significant differences between the two methods). If the study involved a small sample, the nonsignificant results would be ambiguous. If a very large sample was used, however, the probability of a Type II error would be low. It might then reasonably be concluded that the two procedures yield equally accurate assessments. If one of these procedures were more efficient, less stressful, or less costly than the other, the nonsignificant findings could, indeed, be clinically important.

It should be noted that, especially in an evidence-based practice environment, research findings need not necessarily reveal new information to be consequential. To build a strong base of knowledge upon which practice decisions will be made, replicated findings are quite important.

THE GENERALIZABILITY OF QUANTITATIVE RESULTS

Another aspect of quantitative results that you should assess is their generalizability. The aim of most nursing research is to develop evidence for use in nursing practice. Therefore, an important interpretive question is whether the intervention will work or whether observed relationships will hold in other settings, with other people. Part of the interpretive process involves asking the question: To what groups, environments, and conditions can the results of the study be applied?

THE IMPLICATIONS OF QUANTITATIVE RESULTS

After you have formed conclusions about the accuracy, meaning, importance, and generalizability of the results, you are ready to draw inferences about their implications. You might consider the implications of the findings with respect to future research (What should other researchers working in this area do—what is the right "next step"?) or theory development (What are the implications for nursing theory?). However, you are most likely to consider the implications for nursing practice (How, if at all, should the results be used by other nurses in their practice—or by me in my own work as a nurse?). Of course, if you have reached the conclusion that the results have limited credibility or importance, they may be of little utility to your practice.

Interpreting Qualitative Results

It is usually difficult for readers of qualitative research reports to interpret qualitative findings thoroughly because the researchers have necessarily had to be selective in the amount and types of data included for perusal. Nevertheless, you should strive to consider the same five interpretive dimensions for a qualitative study as for a quantitative one.

THE CREDIBILITY OF QUALITATIVE RESULTS

As with the case of quantitative reports, you should question whether the results of a qualitative inquiry are believable. It is reasonable to expect authors of qualitative reports to provide evidence of the credibility of the findings, as described in Chapter 14—although this does not always happen. Because readers of qualitative reports are exposed to only a portion of the data, they must rely on researchers' efforts to corroborate findings through such mechanisms as peer debriefings, member checks, audits, and triangulation.

CONSUMER TIP

Even when peer debriefings or member checks have been undertaken, you should realize that they do not unequivocally establish proof that the results are believable. For example, member checks may not always be effective in illuminating flaws. Perhaps some participants are too polite to disagree with the researcher's interpretations. Or perhaps they become intrigued with a conceptualization they themselves would never have developed on their own—a conceptualization that is not necessarily accurate. ▬

In thinking about the believability of qualitative results—as with quantitative results—it is advisable to adopt the posture of a person who needs to be persuaded about the researcher's conceptualization and to expect the researcher to marshal solid evidence with which to persuade you. It is also appropriate to consider whether the researcher's conceptualization of the phenomenon is consistent with common experiences and with your own clinical insights.

THE MEANING OF QUALITATIVE RESULTS

In qualitative studies, interpretation and analysis of the data occur virtually simultaneously: researchers interpret the data as they categorize them, develop a thematic analysis, and integrate the themes into a unified whole. Efforts to validate the qualitative analysis are necessarily efforts to validate interpretations as well. Thus, unlike quantitative analyses, the meaning of the data flows from qualitative analysis.

Nevertheless, prudent qualitative researchers hold their interpretations up for closer scrutiny—self-scrutiny as well as review by peers and outside reviewers. Thus, for qualitative researchers as well as quantitative researchers, it is important to consider possible alternative explanations for the findings and to take into account methodologic or other limitations that could have affected study results.

Example of researcher self-scrutiny during analysis

Shoveller, Lovato, Young, and Moffat (2003) conducted a grounded theory study to understand how adolescents make decisions about becoming a sun tanner. They conducted in-depth interviews with 20 adolescents and their parents. The four researchers met regularly to discuss emergent categories and hypotheses. As noted in the report, "The researchers also documented their efforts to look for new data to test emerging ideas and discussed how their own values and assumptions related to sun tanning may have affected their interpretations of the data" (p. 303).

THE IMPORTANCE OF QUALITATIVE RESULTS

Qualitative research is especially productive when it is used to describe and explain poorly understood phenomena. But the amount of prior research on a topic is not a sufficient barometer for deciding whether the findings can make a contribution to nursing knowledge. The phenomenon must be one that merits rigourous scrutiny. For example, some people prefer the colour green and others like red. Colour preference may not, however, be a sufficiently important topic for an in-depth inquiry. Thus, you must judge whether the topic under study is important or trivial.

In a critical evaluation of a study's importance, you should also consider whether the findings themselves are trivial. Perhaps the topic is worthwhile, but you may feel after reading the report that nothing has been learned beyond what is common sense or everyday knowledge—which can result when the data are too "thin" or when the conceptualization is shallow. Qualitative researchers often attach catchy labels to their themes and processes, but you should ask yourself whether the labels have really captured an insightful construct.

THE TRANSFERABILITY OF QUALITATIVE RESULTS

Although qualitative researchers do not strive for generalizability, the application of the results to other settings and contexts must be considered. If the findings are only relevant to the people who participated in the study, they cannot be useful to nursing practice. Thus, in interpreting qualitative results, you should consider how transferable the findings are. In what other types of settings and contexts would you expect the phenomena under study to be manifested in a similar fashion? Of course, to make such an assessment, the author of the report must have described in sufficient detail the context in which the data were collected. Because qualitative studies are context bound, it is only through a careful analysis of the key parameters of the study context that the transferability of results can be assessed.

THE IMPLICATIONS OF QUALITATIVE RESULTS

If the findings are judged to be believable and important, and if you are satisfied with the interpretation of the results, you can consider what the implications of the findings might be. As with quantitative studies, the implications can be multidimensional. First, you can consider the implications for further research: Should a similar study be undertaken in a new setting? Can the study be expanded in productive ways? Do the results reveal an important construct that merits formal measurement? Does the emerging theory suggest hypotheses that could be tested through controlled research? Second, do the findings have implications for nursing practice? For example, could the health care needs of a subculture (e.g., the homeless) be identified and addressed more effectively as a result of the study? Finally, do the findings shed light on fundamental processes that are incorporated into nursing theory?

RESEARCH CRITIQUES

If nursing practice is to be based on research evidence, the worth of studies appearing in the nursing literature must be critically appraised. Consumers may mistakenly believe that if a research report was accepted for publication, the study must be completely sound. Unfortunately, this is not necessarily the case. Indeed, most studies have limitations, and thus no single study offers definitive answers to research questions. Nevertheless, the methods of disciplined inquiry continue to provide us with the best possible means of answering certain questions. Evidence is accumulated not by an individual researcher conducting a single study but rather through the conduct of several studies addressing the same or similar questions and through the subsequent critical appraisal of these studies by others. Thus, consumers who can thoughtfully critique research reports also play a role in the advancement of nursing knowledge.

Purposes of a Research Critique

A research **critique** is not just a summary of a study but rather a careful appraisal of its merits and flaws. Regardless of the scope or purpose of a critique, its function is not to hunt for and expose mistakes. A good critique objectively identifies areas of adequacy and inadequacy, virtues as well as faults. Sometimes, the need for this balance is obscured by the terms *critique* and *critical appraisal*, which connote unfavourable observations. The merits of a study are as important as its limitations in coming to conclusions about the worth of its findings. Therefore, a research critique should reflect a thoughtful, objective, and balanced consideration of the study's validity and significance.

Critiques can vary in scope, length, and form, depending on the underlying purpose. Three main types of critiques that are relevant to nursing research include critiques that are:

▶ undertaken by students to demonstrate their skills;
▶ conducted by other researchers (**peer reviewers**) to assist journal editors with publication decisions;
▶ conducted by researchers whose intent is to evaluate the strength of evidence of related studies as part of an integrative review (including meta-analyses and metasyntheses).

All three types attach great importance to whether the study focused on a problem of importance to the nursing profession, but other aspects of a study are of more concern to some types of critiques than to others. For example, a meta-analyst would not be as concerned about the ethical aspects of a study (e.g., was informed consent obtained?) as a student conducting a comprehensive critique. The emphases in a critique depend on the overall purpose of conducting it.

In this chapter we focus primarily on the type of critique that students undertake. We briefly describe the two other main types of critiques, however, because although you are developing skills now that are used primarily in student critiques, you may one day be part of an integrative review team or be called upon to be a peer reviewer.

STUDENT CRITIQUES

As a student, you are likely to be asked to prepare a critique of a research report as a course requirement. Such critiques are usually expected to be comprehensive, with attention paid to all five of the major dimensions of a report (substantive and theoretical; methodologic; ethical; interpretive; and presentational). The purpose of such a critique is to cultivate critical thinking, to induce you to use and demonstrate newly acquired skills in research methods, and to prepare you for a rewarding professional career in which research will almost surely play a role. Writing research critiques is an important step on the path to developing an evidence-based practice.

Although student critiques are comprehensive, involving the evaluation of all aspects of a report, there are a few critiquing questions that are typically less relevant for students than for others. For example, students are typically not required to be sufficiently knowledgeable about the substantive content of a report that they would be able to critically evaluate the thoroughness of its literature review. Students also may not be expected to evaluate the qualifications of a research team, an issue that might have greater salience in other types of critiques.

Much of the remainder of this chapter presents materials that are relevant to comprehensive reviews such as those you are likely to undertake. Appendices C and D—which contain a quantitative and qualitative research report, respectively—also include comprehensive critiques that you can use as models.

PEER REVIEWS

Most nursing journals that publish research reports have a policy of independent, anonymous (sometimes called **blind**) **reviews** by two or more peers who are experts in the field. By anonymous, we mean that the peer reviewers do not know the identity of the authors, and authors do not learn the identity of reviewers. Journals that have such a policy are

refereed journals, and are generally more prestigious than **nonrefereed journals**. The journals *Canadian Journal of Nursing Research (CJNR)*, *Nursing in Research & Health*, and many other journals cited in this book are refereed journals. Peer reviewers develop written critiques and make a recommendation about whether or not to publish the report.

Example of categories of recommendation for peer reviewers

The *Canadian Journal of Nursing Research (CJNR)* asks reviewers to make one of four recommendations to the editor pertaining to a manuscript under review: (1) acceptable as it is; (2) acceptable with minor revisions; (3) acceptable with major revisions; and (4) not at all acceptable. The reviewers also are asked to rate the manuscript, if acceptable, in terms of publication priority: low, medium, or high.

Peer reviewers' critiques can address a wide array of concerns, but they typically are brief and focus primarily on key substantive and methodologic issues. Reviewers may also comment on prominent presentational deficiencies (e.g., a confusing table) and noteworthy ethical issues. Peer reviewers' comments may be written in narrative, essay form or may take the form of a bulleted list of the study's strengths and weaknesses. Researchers typically revise their manuscripts based on the reviewers' critiques, addressing to the extent possible the reviewers' suggestions for improvement.

CRITIQUES FOR ASSESSING A BODY OF LITERATURE

Critiques of individual studies are sometimes undertaken as part of a formal, systematic evaluation of multiple studies on a topic. Such reviews are often undertaken with the aim of developing practice guidelines or drawing conclusions about the state of knowledge on which practice can be based. As described in Chapter 7, there are various ways of integrating findings on a topic from the research literature, including meta-analyses (for quantitative research) and metasyntheses (for qualitative ones). In both cases, reviewers must draw conclusions about what is known about a topic or phenomenon, and most consider the quality of the studies included in the review.

Chapter 18, which focuses on the utilization of nursing research for evidence-based practice, discusses the important role of systematic, integrative reviews. These reviews, rather than being comprehensive, focus on the methodologic dimension of studies and on the study findings. A person undertaking an integrative review as part of an EBP effort is not typically concerned with, for example, the thoroughness of the literature review in individual reports because it has no bearing on the quality of study's *evidence*.

Integrative reviews and critiques of a body of research typically do not involve written critiques of individual studies. More often, the people doing such reviews use a formal instrument for evaluating each study, often with quantitative ratings of different aspects of the study, so that appraisals across studies ("scores") can be compared. Many such instruments have been developed for use with quantitative research, as we discuss in Chapter 18.

Although less has been done to develop formal scoring systems for evaluating the quality of evidence in qualitative research, work in this area has begun. One example is the system developed by Cesario, Morin, and Santa-Donato (2002) as part of a project to develop clinical guidelines by the Association of Women's Health, Obstetric, and Neonatal Nurses (AWHONN). Another tool is the Primary Research Appraisal Tool, which was developed by Canadian nurse researchers for determining an individual study's eligibility for a meta-synthesis (Paterson, Thorne, Canam, & Jillings, 2001).

Dimensions of a Research Critique

This section offers guidance primarily to those preparing a detailed, comprehensive critique, such as the ones that students prepare in research courses. The goal of such critiques is to evaluate thoroughly the decisions the researcher made in conceptualizing, designing, and executing the study and in interpreting and communicating the results. Each researcher, in addressing the same or a similar research question, makes different decisions about how a study should be done, and researchers who have made different *methodologic decisions* may arrive at different answers to the same research question. It is precisely for this reason that you as a consumer must be knowledgeable about research methods. You must be able to evaluate research decisions so that you can determine how much faith should be put in the study findings. You must ask: What other approaches could have been used to study this research problem? and, If another approach had been used, would the results have been more credible or replicable? In other words, you need to evaluate the impact of the researcher's decisions on the study's ability to reveal the truth.

Much of this book has been designed to acquaint you with a range of methodologic options for the conduct of research—options on how to design a study, collect and analyze data, select a sample, and so on. We hope a familiarity with these options will provide you with the tools to challenge a researcher's decisions when it is appropriate to do so.

As previously noted, a comprehensive review involves an appraisal of five dimensions of a research report, each of which is discussed below. Specific critiquing guidelines for quantitative and qualitative studies are presented later in the chapter.

SUBSTANTIVE AND THEORETICAL DIMENSION

In preparing a critique, you need to assess whether the study was sound in terms of the significance of the problem, the appropriateness of the conceptual framework, and the insightfulness of the analysis and interpretation. The research problem should have clear relevance to some aspect of nursing.

Another issue that has both substantive and methodologic implications is the congruence between the study question and the methods used to address it. There must be a good fit between the research problem on the one hand and the research methods on the other. Questions that deal with poorly understood phenomena, with processes, with the dynamics of a situation, or with in-depth description, for example, are usually best addressed with flexible designs, unstructured methods of data collection, and qualitative analysis. Questions that involve the measurement of well-defined variables, cause-and-effect relationships, or the effectiveness of some specific intervention, however, are better suited to more structured, quantitative approaches using designs that maximize research control.

A final issue to consider is whether the researcher has appropriately placed the research problem into a larger theoretical context. As noted in Chapter 8, researchers do little to enhance the value of a study if the connection between the research problem and a conceptual framework is contrived. But a research problem that is genuinely framed as a part of a larger intellectual problem can often make an especially important contribution to nursing knowledge.

METHODOLOGIC DIMENSION

Researchers make a number of important decisions regarding how best to answer their research questions or test their research hypotheses. It is your job as consumer to evaluate critically the consequences of those decisions. In fact, the heart of a research critique lies in the appraisal of the researchers' methodologic decisions. The quality of evidence that a study yields is inextricably linked to the researchers' choice of methods and strategies for study design and for collecting and analyzing data.

One thing to keep in mind in assessing a study's methods is that, because of practical constraints, researchers almost always make compromises between what is ideal and what is feasible. For example, a quantitative researcher might ideally like to have a sample of 500 subjects, but resources may prohibit a sample larger than 200. A qualitative researcher might recognize that 3 years of fieldwork would yield an especially rich understanding of the phenomenon under study, but cannot afford to devote this much time to the effort. In doing a critique, you cannot realistically demand that researchers attain methodologic ideals, but you must evaluate how much damage has been done by failure to achieve them.

ETHICAL DIMENSION

In performing a comprehensive critique, you should consider whether there is evidence of ethical violations. If there are any potential ethical problems, you will need to consider the impact of those problems on the scientific merit of the study as well as on the subjects' well-being.

Sometimes ethical transgressions are inadvertent. For example, privacy and confidentiality can sometimes be compromised when interviews are conducted in participants' homes and other family members are nearby. In other cases, researchers are aware of potential ethical problems but consciously decide that the violation is minor in relation to the knowledge gained. For example, researchers may decide not to obtain informed consent from the parents of minor children attending a family planning clinic because such consent might discourage participation in the study and lead to a biased sample of clinic users; it could also violate the minors' right to confidential treatment at the clinic. When researchers knowingly elect not to follow the ethical principles outlined in Chapter 5, the decision itself, the researchers' rationale, and the likely effect of the decision of the study's rigour should be evaluated.

CONSUMER TIP

Sometimes ethical transgressions actually strengthen the methodologic rigour of a study, and so you may need to "pit" one dimension of the critique against another. ■

INTERPRETIVE DIMENSION

Research reports conclude with a discussion, conclusions, or implications section. In this final section, researchers offer an interpretation of the findings, consider whether the findings are congruent with a conceptual framework or earlier research, and discuss what the findings might imply for nursing.

As a reviewer, you should be somewhat wary if the discussion section fails to point out any limitations. Researchers are in the best position to detect and assess the impact of sampling deficiencies, practical constraints, data quality problems, and so on, and it is a professional responsibility to alert readers to these difficulties. Moreover, when researchers note methodologic or other shortcomings, readers know that these limitations were considered in interpreting the results.

Example of researcher-noted limitations

Estabrooks, Midodzi, Cummings, Ricker, and Giovannetti (2005) studied the impact of hospital nursing characteristics (e.g., nursing education and skill mix) on 30-day mortality for 18,000 patients discharged from 49 acute care hospitals in Alberta. The researchers were meticulous in noting several methodologic limitations. For example, they noted that "the study is vulnerable to the quality of the administrative data.... Second, one of the criticisms of aggregating data collected at one level to a higher level is that the relationships among the variables is typically different at each level.... Third, the selected sample only involves patients with a primary diagnosis of acute myocardial infarction, congestive heart failure, chronic obstructive pulmonary disease, stroke, or pneumonia. Patients in these diagnostic categories may differ from the general population of patients in Alberta hospitals" (p. 82).

Of course, researchers are unlikely to note all relevant shortcomings of their own work. Thus, the inclusion of comments about study limitations in the discussion section, although important, does not relieve you of the responsibility of appraising methodologic decisions. Your task as reviewer is to contrast your own interpretation and assessment of limitations with those of the researchers, to challenge conclusions that do not appear to be warranted by the results, and to indicate how the study's evidence could have been enhanced.

It may be especially difficult for you to determine the validity of qualitative researchers' interpretations. To help readers understand the lens from which they interpreted their data, qualitative researchers ideally should mention whether they kept field notes or a journal of their actions and emotions during the investigation, discuss their own behaviour and experiences in relation to the participants' experiences, and acknowledge any effects of their presence on data quality. You should look for such information in critiquing qualitative reports and drawing conclusions about the interpretations.

Your critique should also draw conclusions about the stated implications of the study. Some researchers offer unfounded recommendations on the basis of modest results. Some guidelines for evaluating researchers' interpretation and implications are offered in Box 17.1.

PRESENTATION AND STYLISTIC DIMENSION

Although the worth of the study is primarily reflected in the dimensions discussed thus far, the manner in which the information is communicated in the research report is also fair

BOX 17.1 Guidelines for Critiquing the Discussion Section of a Research Report

Interpretation of the Findings

1. Are all important results discussed? If not, what is the likely explanation for omissions?
2. Does the report discuss the limitations of the study and possible effects of the limitations on the results?
3. Are interpretations consistent with results? Do the interpretations take limitations into account? Do the interpretations suggest distinct biases?
4. What types of evidence are offered in support of the interpretation, and is that evidence persuasive? Are results interpreted in light of findings from other studies? Are results interpreted in terms of the study hypotheses and the conceptual framework?
5. In qualitative studies, are the findings interpreted within an appropriate social or cultural context?
6. Are alternative explanations for the findings mentioned, and is the rationale for their rejection presented?
7. In quantitative studies, does the interpretation distinguish between practical and statistical significance?
8. Are any unwarranted interpretations of causality made?
9. Are generalizations made that are not warranted?

Implications of the Findings and Recommendations

10. Do the researchers discuss the study's implications for clinical practice, nursing education, nursing administration, or nursing theory, or make specific recommendations?
11. If yes, are the stated implications appropriate, given the study's limitations and given the body of evidence from other studies? Are there important implications that the report neglected to include?

game in a comprehensive critical appraisal. Box 17.2 summarizes points that should be taken into account in evaluating the presentation of a research report.

An important consideration is whether the research report has provided sufficient information for a thoughtful critique of the other dimensions. For example, if the report does not describe how participants were selected, reviewers cannot comment on the adequacy of the sample, but they can criticize the report's failure to include information on sampling. When vital pieces of information are missing, researchers leave readers little choice but to assume the worst because this would lead to the most cautious interpretation of the worth of the evidence.

The writing in a research report, as in any published document, should be clear, grammatical, concise, and well organized. Unnecessary jargon should be minimized. Inadequate organization is another flaw in some reports: logical development of thoughts is critical to good communication of scientific information. Tables and figures should highlight key points and should be capable of "standing alone," without forcing readers to scrutinize the text to grasp what they mean.

Styles of writing do differ for qualitative and quantitative reports, and it is unreasonable to apply the standards considered appropriate for one paradigm to the other. Quantitative research reports are typically written in a more formal, impersonal fashion, using either the third person or passive voice to connote objectivity. Qualitative studies are likely to be written in a more literary style, using the first or second person and active voice

> ### BOX 17.2 Guidelines for Critiquing the Presentation of a Research Report
>
> 1. Does the report include a sufficient amount of detail to permit a thorough critique of the study's substantive, methodologic, ethical, and interpretive dimensions? Does the report neglect to include key aspects of the study's methods?
> 2. Is the report understandable to those with moderate research skills, or is it unnecessarily abstruse? Is research jargon or clinical jargon used when simpler language could have improved communication to a broad audience of nurses?
> 3. Does the report suggest any overt biases on the part of the researcher? Does the researcher convey the tentative nature of research findings (e.g., avoiding words like "demonstrated" or "proved")?
> 4. Is the report well organized, or is the presentation confusing? Is there a logical, orderly presentation of ideas? Are transitions smooth, and is the report characterized by continuity of thought and expression?
> 5. Is the report well written and grammatical?
> 6. Does the report avoid sexist language? Does the report suggest any insensitivity to racial, ethnic, or cultural groups?
> 7. Does the report title adequately capture key concepts and the target population? Does the abstract adequately summarize the research problem, study methods, and key findings?

to connote proximity and intimacy with the phenomenon under study. Regardless of style, however, you should, as a reviewer, be alert to indications of overt biases, exaggerations, emotionally laden comments, or melodramatic language.

In summary, a research report should be an account of how and why a problem was studied and what results were obtained. The report should be accurate, clearly written, cogent, and concise. It should reflect scholarship, but not pedantry, and it should be written in a manner that piques the reader's interest and curiosity.

GUIDELINES FOR CRITIQUING RESEARCH REPORTS

Most chapters in this book have presented guidelines for evaluating various research decisions and aspects of research reports. The guidelines presented detailed questions, whose primary function was to encourage you to read particular sections of research reports carefully and critically. Hopefully, these questions helped to reinforce the methodologic content of this book. However, you would seldom be expected to answer all of these questions in an overall critique of a research report. If you did this, the critique would be far longer than the report itself!

This section presents an abridged set of critiquing questions to assist you in evaluating quantitative and qualitative reports. We can begin by offering a few general suggestions. First, you will need to read the report you are critiquing at least twice, and you may need to read parts of it several times. It may be helpful to skim the section titled "Reading and Summarizing Research Reports" in Chapter 4, which offers suggestions on how to carefully and actively read research reports. Obviously, the first step in preparing a critique is to understand what the report is saying.

It is sometimes helpful to create a preliminary list of the aspects of the study that you thought were well done and those you viewed as problematic, without worrying too much initially about the organization of your thoughts. Once you have a preliminary list, you can organize it by arranging the items or bullets into a structure corresponding to the major sections of the report. You can then revise and augment your list by using the guidelines we provide later in this section.

When you are ready to write the critique, it may be useful to begin by preparing an abstract or introductory summary that will give you—and the person reading your critique—an overall "road map." The abstract should succinctly state what your final conclusions are about the merits of the study and the degree of confidence that can be placed in the study findings. Then in the body of the critique, you will need to document the specific features that led you to those conclusions.

An important thing to remember is that it is appropriate to assume the posture of a sceptic when you are critiquing a report. Just as a careful clinician seeks evidence from research findings that certain practices are or are not effective, you as a reviewer should demand evidence from the report that the researchers' substantive and methodologic decisions were sound.

Some additional broad tips for preparing a formal, written research critique are presented in Box 17.3.

Critiquing Quantitative Reports

Table 17.1 presents guidelines for critiquing quantitative research reports. The guidelines are organized using the IMRAD format, following the structure of most research reports (i.e., Introduction, Method, Results, and Discussion). The first column identifies the section of the report for which the questions are relevant. The next column provides cross-references to the more detailed guidelines in the earlier chapters of the book. And the final column lists some key critiquing questions that have broad applicability to quantitative studies.

BOX 17.3   General Guidelines for Conducting a Written Research Critique

1. The function of a critique is not to *describe* a study or to *summarize* the content of the report. A research critique should provide an appraisal of the worth of the study itself and the merits of the report.
2. Be sure to comment on the study's strengths *and* weaknesses. The critique should be a balanced analysis of the study's value, noting positive as well as negative aspects.
3. Avoid vague generalizations—give specific examples of the study's strengths and limitations, providing direct references or quotes with page numbers.
4. Justify your criticisms. Offer a rationale for how a limitation affected the quality of the study, and suggest an alternative approach that could have eliminated the prob̶ but be sure that your suggestions are practical.
5. Be as objective as possible. Try not to be overly critical of a study simply beca̶ example, your world view is inconsistent with the underlying paradigm or be̶ field of specialization is different from that of the researchers.
6. If you are writing a critique that the report authors themselves will receive, b̶ to your tone and the sharpness of your criticisms, and avoid sarcasm.

TABLE 17.1		**Guide to an Overall Critique of a Quantitative Research Report**

ASPECT OF THE REPORT	DETAILED CRITIQUING GUIDELINES	BASIC QUESTIONS FOR A CRITIQUE
Title		▶ Was the title a good one, suggesting the research problem and the study population?
Abstract		▶ Does the abstract clearly and concisely summarize the main features of the report?
Introduction Statement of the problem	Box 6.1, page 112	▶ Is the problem stated unambiguously, and is it easy to identify? ▶ Does the problem statement make clear the concepts and the population under study? ▶ Does the problem have significance for nursing? ▶ Is there a good match between the research problem and the paradigm and methods used? Is a quantitative approach appropriate?
Literature review	Box 7.1, page 147	▶ Is the literature review thorough, up-to-date, and based mainly on primary sources? ▶ Does the review summarize knowledge on the dependent and independent variables and the relationship between them? ▶ Does the literature review lay a solid basis for the new study?
Conceptual/ theoretical framework	Box 8.1, page 165	▶ Are key concepts adequately defined conceptually? ▶ Is there a conceptual/theoretical framework, and is it appropriate? If not, is the absence of one justified?
Hypotheses or research questions	Box 6.1, page 112	▶ Are research questions and/or hypotheses explicitly stated? If not, is their absence justified? ▶ Are questions and hypotheses appropriately worded? ▶ Are the questions/hypotheses consistent with the literature review and the conceptual framework?
Method Research design	Box 9.1, page 200	▶ Was the most rigorous possible design used, given the study purpose? ▶ Were appropriate comparisons made to enhance interpretability of the findings? ▶ Was the number of data collection points appropriate? ▶ Did the design minimize threats to the internal and external validity of the study?
Population and sample	Box 12.1, page 271	▶ Was the population identified and described? Was the sample described in sufficient detail? ▶ Was the best possible sampling design used to enhance the sample's representativeness? ▶ Was the sample size adequate? Was a power analysis used to estimate sample size needs?
Data collection and measurement	Box 13.2, page 296; Box 13.4, page 305	▶ Are the operational and conceptual definitions congruent? ▶ Were key variables operationalized using the best possible method (e.g., interviews, observations, and so on)?

TABLE 17.1   Guide to an Overall Critique of a Quantitative Research Report (Continued)

ASPECT OF THE REPORT	DETAILED CRITIQUING GUIDELINES	BASIC QUESTIONS FOR A CRITIQUE
	Box 13.5, page 308; Box 14.1, page 331	▶ Were the specific instruments adequately described, and were they good choices? ▶ Did the report provide evidence that the data collection methods yielded data that were high on reliability and validity?
Procedures	Box 13.6, page 309; Box 5.2, page 103	▶ If there was an intervention, was it adequately described, and was it properly implemented? ▶ Were data collected in a manner that minimized bias? Were data collection staff appropriately trained? ▶ Were appropriate procedures used to safeguard the rights of study participants?
Results Data analysis	Box 15.2, page 380	▶ Were analyses undertaken to address each research question or test each hypothesis? ▶ Were appropriate statistical methods used, given the level of measurement of the variables, number of groups being compared, and so on? ▶ Was the most powerful analytic method used? (e.g., Did the analysis help to control for extraneous variables)?
Findings	Box 15.2, page 380	▶ Were the findings adequately summarized, with good use of tables and figures? ▶ Do the findings provide strong evidence regarding the research questions? Were Type I and Type II errors minimized?
Discussion Interpretation of the findings	Box 17.1, page 435	▶ Are all major findings interpreted and discussed within the context of prior research and/or the study's conceptual framework? ▶ Are the interpretations consistent with the results and with the study's limitations? ▶ Does the report address the issue of the generalizability of the findings?
Implications/ recommendations	Box 17.1, page 435	▶ Do the researchers discuss the implications of the study for clinical practice or further research—and are those implications reasonable and complete?
Global Issues Presentation	Box 17.2, page 436	▶ Was the report well written, well organized, and sufficiently detailed for critical analysis? ▶ Were you able to understand the study? Was the report written in a manner that makes the findings accessible to practicing nurses?
Summary assessment		▶ Despite any identified limitations, do the study findings appear to be valid—do you have confidence in the *truth* value of the results? ▶ Does the study contribute any meaningful evidence that can be used in nursing practice or that is useful to the nursing discipline?

A few comments about these guidelines are in order. First, the wording of the questions calls for a yes or no answer (although for some, it may well be that your answer will be "Yes, *but* ..."). In all cases, the desirable answer is "yes"—that is, a "no" suggests a possible limitation, and a "yes" suggests a strength. Therefore, the more "yeses" a study gets, the stronger it is likely to be. Thus, these guidelines can cumulatively suggest a global assessment: a report that has 25 "yeses" is likely to be superior to one that has only 10.

However, it is also important to realize that not all "yeses" are equal. Some elements are far more important in drawing conclusions about the rigour of a study than others. For example, the inadequacy of a literature review is far less damaging to the validity of the study findings than the use of a design with internal validity problems. In general, the questions addressing the researchers' methodologic decisions (i.e., the questions under "Method," as well as questions relating to the statistical analysis) are especially important in evaluating the integrity of a study's evidence.

Although the questions in Table 17.1 elicit yes or no responses, your critique will obviously need to do more than point out what the study did and did not do. Each relevant issue needs to be discussed—and you will need to supply supporting evidence for your conclusions. For example, if you answered "no" to the question about whether the design minimized threats to the study's internal validity, your critique should elaborate on why you said this—for example, by pointing out that the design was vulnerable to self-selection bias because the groups being compared might not have been comparable at the outset. Each time you answered one of the questions negatively, it might be profitable to review the more detailed questions presented in earlier chapters of the book.

CONSUMER TIP

There are many questions in these guidelines for which there are no totally objective answers. Even experts sometimes disagree about what the best methodologic strategies for a study are. Thus, you should not be afraid to "stick out your neck" to express an evaluative opinion—but do be sure that your comments have some basis in methodologic principles discussed in this book. ■

We must acknowledge that our simplified guidelines have a number of shortcomings. In particular, the guidelines are generic despite the fact that critiquing cannot really use a one-size-fits-all list of questions. Critiquing questions that are relevant to certain types of studies (e.g., experiments) do not fit into a set of general questions for all quantitative studies. For example, we have not included a question about whether subjects or research staff were blinded to experimental treatments because this question would not be relevant to most studies, which are nonexperimental. Furthermore, many supplementary questions would be needed to thoroughly assess certain types of research—for example, mixed method studies. Thus, you will need to use some judgment about whether the guidelines are sufficiently comprehensive for the type of study you are critiquing.

Another word of caution is that we developed these guidelines based on our years of experience as researchers and research methodologists. They do not represent a formal, rigourously developed set of questions that can be used for a formal EBP-type critique. They should, however, facilitate your beginning efforts to critically appraise nursing studies.

Critiquing Qualitative Reports

Table 17.2 presents guidelines for you to use in critiquing qualitative research reports. These guidelines, like the ones in Table 17.1, are organized using the IMRAD format. Although qualitative reports are somewhat less likely than quantitative ones to follow this format, many of them do. In any event, it would still be possible to organize your critique using this structure, regardless of how the report is organized. Table 17.2 also presents, for each section, a series of questions and cross-references to more in-depth critiquing questions.

The comments about the guidelines for quantitative studies presented in the previous section are also relevant for critiquing qualitative ones. In particular, the difficulty with a "one-size-fits-all" approach is also salient for critiques of qualitative studies. Supplementary questions may be needed to fully critique studies within specific qualitative research traditions. Additional questions would be relevant for comprehensive critiques of, say, grounded theory studies (e.g., Did the categories describe the full range or continuum of the process?).

In undertaking a critique of a qualitative study, you should keep in mind that richness and thoroughness of description are especially important. Rich detail is required in the description of the methods in part because of the lack of standardization in qualitative studies—readers need to have sufficient information with which to judge the researchers' approach. For example, in a quantitative study, it might be sufficient to say that the data analysis involved a series of t-tests, whereas in a qualitative report, it is important to know, for example, how the data were coded, how coding categories were combined, who did the coding, whether there was intercoder agreement, and so on. Vivid description is also needed in presenting results in qualitative studies because without descriptive clarity and eloquence, readers cannot grasp the nuances and complexities of the phenomenon under study. Qualitative studies can be a "gold mine for clinical insights" (Kearney, 2001, p. 146) only when the presentation is richly detailed and powerfully narrated.

As noted earlier, formal systems have been proposed to evaluate the quality of evidence in qualitative studies, and these approaches are typically not organized according to sections of a report but rather according to a number of cross-cutting themes. For example, Cesario and her colleagues (2002), who were involved with the AWHONN practice guideline development project, used five broad categories that were suggested by Burns (1989) for rating the quality of qualitative studies: descriptive vividness, methodologic congruence, analytic precision, theoretical connectedness, and heuristic relevance. Our guidelines cover most of the same issues and questions as were included in this rating system, but we think students may have an easier time using our less abstract structure.

TABLE 17.2   Guide to an Overall Critique of a Qualitative Research Report

ASPECT OF THE REPORT	DETAILED CRITIQUING GUIDELINES	BASIC QUESTIONS FOR A CRITIQUE
Title		▶ Was the title a good one, suggesting the key phenomenon and the group or community under study?
Abstract		▶ Does the abstract clearly and concisely summarize the main features of the report?
Introduction Statement of the problem	Box 6.1, page 112	▶ Is the phenomenon of interest clearly identified? ▶ Is the problem stated unambiguously, and is it easy to identify? ▶ Does the problem have significance for nursing? ▶ Is there a good match between the research problem and the paradigm and methods used? Is a qualitative approach appropriate?
Literature review	Box 7.1, page 147	▶ Does the report summarize the existing body of knowledge related to the problem or phenomenon of interest? ▶ Is the literature review adequate? ▶ Does the literature review lay a solid basis for the new study?
Conceptual underpinnings	Box 8.1, page 165	▶ Are key concepts adequately defined conceptually? ▶ Is the philosophical basis, underlying tradition, conceptual framework, or ideological orientation made explicit, and is it appropriate for the problem?
Research questions	Box 6.1, page 112	▶ Are research questions explicitly stated? If not, is their absence justified? ▶ Are the questions consistent with the study's philosophical basis, underlying tradition, conceptual framework, or ideological orientation?
Method Research design and research tradition	Box 10.1, page 225	▶ Is the identified research tradition (if any) congruent with the methods used to collect and analyze data? ▶ Was an adequate amount of time spent in the field or with study participants? ▶ Did the design unfold in the field, allowing researchers to capitalize on early understandings? ▶ Was there evidence of reflexivity in the design? ▶ Was there an adequate number of contacts with study participants?
Sample and setting	Box 12.2, page 271	▶ Was the group or population of interest adequately described? Were the setting and sample described in sufficient detail? ▶ Was the approach used to gain access to the site or to recruit participants appropriate? ▶ Was the best possible method of sampling used to enhance information richness and address the needs of the study? ▶ Was the sample size adequate? Was saturation achieved?

TABLE 17.2	Guide to an Overall Critique of a Qualitative Research Report (Continued)	
ASPECT OF THE REPORT	**DETAILED CRITIQUING GUIDELINES**	**BASIC QUESTIONS FOR A CRITIQUE**
Data collection	Box 13.2, page 296; Box 13.4, page 305	▶ Were the methods of gathering data appropriate? Were data gathered through two or more methods to achieve triangulation? ▶ Did the researcher ask the right questions or make the right observations, and were they recorded in an appropriate fashion? ▶ Was a sufficient amount of data gathered? Was the data of sufficient depth and richness?
Procedures	Box 13.6, page 309; Box 5.2, page 103	▶ Were data collection and recording procedures adequately described, and do they appear appropriate? ▶ Were data collected in a manner that minimized bias or behavioral distortions? Were data collection staff appropriately trained? ▶ Were appropriate procedures used to safeguard the rights of study participants?
Enhancement of rigour	Box 14.2, page 331	▶ Were methods used to enhance the trustworthiness of the data (and analysis), and was the description of those methods adequate? ▶ Were the methods used to enhance credibility appropriate and sufficient? ▶ Did the researcher document research procedures and decision processes sufficiently that findings are auditable and confirmable?
Results Data analysis	Box 16.1, page 392	▶ Were the data management (e.g., coding) and data analysis methods sufficiently described? ▶ Was the data analysis strategy compatible with the research tradition and with the nature and type of the data gathered? ▶ Did the analysis yield an appropriate "product" (e.g., a theory, taxonomy, thematic pattern, etc.)? ▶ Did the analytic procedures suggest the possibility of biases?
Findings	Box 16.1, page 392	▶ Were the findings effectively summarized, with good use of excerpts? ▶ Do the themes adequately capture the meaning of the data? Does it appear that the researcher satisfactorily conceptualized the themes or patterns in the data? ▶ Did the analysis yield an insightful, provocative, and meaningful picture of the phenomenon under investigation?
Theoretical integration	Box 16.1, page 392	▶ Are the themes or patterns logically connected to each other to form a convincing and integrated whole? ▶ Were figures, maps, or models used effectively to summarize conceptualizations? ▶ If a conceptual framework or ideological orientation guided the study, are the themes or patterns linked to it in a cogent manner?
Discussion Interpretation of the findings	Box 17.1, page 435	▶ Are the findings interpreted within an appropriate social or cultural context?

table continues on pa

TABLE 17.2 Guide to an Overall Critique of a Qualitative Research Report (Continued)

ASPECT OF THE REPORT	DETAILED CRITIQUING GUIDELINES	BASIC QUESTIONS FOR A CRITIQUE
		▶ Are major findings interpreted and discussed within the context of prior studies? ▶ Are the interpretations consistent with the study's limitations? ▶ Does the report address the issue of the transferability of the findings?
Implications/ recommendations	Box 17.1, page 435	▶ Do the researchers discuss the implications of the study for clinical practice or further inquiry—and are those implications reasonable?
Global Issues Presentation	Box 17.2, page 436	▶ Was the report well written, well organized, and sufficiently detailed for critical analysis? ▶ Was the description of the methods, findings, and interpretations sufficiently rich and vivid?
Summary assessment		▶ Do the study findings appear to be trustworthy—do you have confidence in the *truth* value of the results? ▶ Does the study contribute any meaningful evidence that can be used in nursing practice or that is useful to the nursing discipline?

RESEARCH EXAMPLES   **Critical Thinking Activities**

 EXAMPLE 1: Interpretation of Quantitative Findings

1. Read the Discussion section from the study by Feeley and colleagues ("Mother–VLBW Infant Interaction") in Appendix A of this book and then answer the relevant questions in Box 17.1.
2. Also consider the following targeted questions, which may further sharpen your critical thinking skills and assist you in assessing aspects of the report's merit:
   a. Comment on the information in the paragraph that begins "One subgroup of mothers..." (third paragraph of the discussion).
   b. If you were making a recommendation for how a future study on this topic should be designed, what would you suggest in terms of research design, sampling, data collection, and analysis?

 EXAMPLE 2: Interpretation of Qualitative Findings

1. Read the Discussion section from Beck's study ("Birth Trauma") in Appendix B of this book, and then answer the relevant questions in Box 17.1.
2. Also consider the following targeted questions, which may further sharpen your critical thinking skills and assist you in assessing aspects of the study's merit:

Critical Thinking Activities (continued)

   a. Suggest two future studies that researchers could conduct based on the findings of Beck's birth trauma study. One study should be quantitative and one study should be qualitative.

   b. Suggest a qualitative study that would increase the transferability of Beck's findings.

EXAMPLE 3: Critique of a Quantitative Study

Read the full study "Postoperative arm massage: A support for women with lymph node dissection" by Forchuk and colleagues in Appendix C, and then address the following activities and questions.

1. Before reading our critique, which accompanies the full report, either write your own critique or prepare a list of what you think are the major strengths and weaknesses of the study. Then contrast your critique or list with ours. Remember that you (or your instructor) do not necessarily have to agree with all of the points made in our critique and that you may identify strengths and weaknesses that we overlooked.

2. Using the guidelines in Table 17.1, how many "yes" ratings would you give the study? Compare your "score" with that of other classmates.

3. In selecting studies to include in this textbook, we avoided choosing a poor-quality study—which would have been much easier to critique. We did not, however, wish to create a publicly embarrassing situation for any member of the nursing research community. In the questions below, we offer some "pretend" scenarios in which the researchers for this study made different methodologic decisions than the ones they in fact did make. Write a paragraph or two critiquing these "pretend" decisions, pointing out how these alternatives would have affected the quality of the study.

   a. Pretend that the researchers had been unable to randomize subjects to treatments and had also been unable to measure pain, family stress and strengths, and shoulder function preoperatively. The design, in other words, would be a posttest-only preexperiment, with the intervention administered to patients who were not in special treatment on a random basis.

   b. Pretend that the sample size was only 30 patients (15 per group).

   c. Pretend that the researchers had only collected pain data on the first postoperative day.

EXAMPLE 4: Critique of a Qualitative Study

Read the full study "Redefining parental identity: Caregiving and schizophrenia" by Milliken and Northcutt in Appendix D, and then address the following activities and questions.

(Research Examples continue on page 446)

Critical Thinking Activities (continued)

1. Before reading our critique, which accompanies the full report, either write your own critique or prepare a list of what you think are the major strengths and weaknesses of the study. Then contrast your critique or list with ours. Remember that you (or your instructor) do not necessarily have to agree with all of the points made in our critique and that you may identify strengths and weaknesses that we overlooked.

2. Using the guidelines in Table 17.2, how many "yes" ratings would you give the study? Compare your "score" with that of other classmates.

3. As noted in Example 3, we purposely selected good-quality studies to feature in this textbook. In the questions below, we offer some "pretend" scenarios in which the researchers for this study made different methodologic decisions than the ones they in fact did make. Write a paragraph or two critiquing these "pretend" decisions, pointing out how these alternatives would have affected the quality of the study.

a. Pretend that Milliken and Northcott had used structured questionnaires rather than unstructured interviews to gather their data.

b. Pretend that Milliken and Northcott had not used theoretical sampling.

c. Pretend that Milliken and Northcott had used a sample of 10 parent caregivers.

d. Pretend that the researchers had done a descriptive qualitative study, not in the grounded theory tradition.

C H A P T E R   R E V I E W

S u m m a r y   P o i n t s

▶ The *interpretation* of research findings is a search for the broader meaning and implications of the results of an investigation.

▶ Interpretation of both qualitative and quantitative results typically involves: (1) analyzing the credibility of the results; (2) determining their meaning; (3) considering their importance; (4) determining the generalizability or transferability of the findings; and (5) assessing the implications in regard to nursing practice, theory, and future research.

▶ A research **critique** is a careful, critical appraisal of the strengths and limitations of a study to draw conclusions about the worth of the evidence and its significance to nursing.

▶ Critiques are done for a variety of purposes, including critiques by students to demonstrate their research skills; assessments by **peer reviewers** to assist journal editors with publication decisions; and critiques done as part of an integrated review.

▶ Peer reviewers who critique studies for a **refereed journal** often do **blind reviews** in which the reviewers do not learn the identity of the researchers, and *vice versa*.

▶ Critiques of individual studies done in an effort to come to conclusions about a body of literature (e.g., those done by a meta-analyst) often involve the use of a structured instrument or scale to rate aspects of study quality.

▶ A reviewer preparing a comprehensive review should consider five major dimensions of the study: the substantive and theoretical, methodologic, ethical, interpretive, and presentation and stylistic dimensions.

▶ Researchers designing a study must make a number of important *methodologic decisions* that affect the quality and rigour of the research. Consumers preparing a critique must evaluate these decisions to determine how much faith can be placed in the results.

▶ When undertaking a critique, it is appropriate to assume the posture of a sceptic who demands evidence from the report that the conclusions are credible and significant.

Additional   Resources   for   Review

Chapter 17 of the *Study Guide to Accompany Essentials of Nursing Research,* 6th edition offers various exercises and study suggestions for reinforcing the concepts presented in this chapter. For additional review, see the Student Self-Study Review Questions section of the Student Resource CD-ROM provided with this book.

SUGGESTED READINGS

* References for studies cited in the chapter appear at the end of the book.

Methodologic References

Beck, C. T. (1990). The research critique: General criteria for evaluating a research report. *Journal of Obstetric, Gynecologic, and Neonatal Nursing, 19,* 18–22.

Beck, C. T. (1993). Qualitative research: The evaluation of its credibility, fittingness, and auditability. *Western Journal of Nursing Research, 15,* 263–266.

Burns, N. (1989). Standards for qualitative research. *Nursing Science Quarterly, 2,* 254–260.

Cesario, S., Morin, K., & Santa-Donato, A. (2002). Evaluating the level of evidence of qualitative research. *Journal of Obstetrics, Gynecologic, & Neonatal Nursing, 31,* 708–714.

Kearney, M. H. (2001). Levels and applications of qualitative research evidence. *Research in Nursing & Health, 24,* 145–153.

Paterson, B. L., Thorne, S. E., Canam, C., & Jillings, C. (2001). *Meta-study of qualitative health research.* Thousand Oaks, CA: Sage Publications.

Using Research in Evidence-Based Nursing Practice

STUDENT OBJECTIVES

On completion of this chapter, you will be able to:

▶ Distinguish research utilization (RU) and evidence-based practice (EBP) and discuss their current status within nursing
▶ Identify barriers to EBP and strategies for improving it
▶ Identify several models that have relevance for EBP and describe the general steps in an EBP project
▶ Discuss the role that integrative reviews play in EBP and describe basic steps in undertaking such a review
▶ Critique an integrative review
▶ Define new terms in the chapter

Most nurse researchers would like to have their findings incorporated into nursing protocols and curricula, and most nurses in clinical settings are aware of the benefits of research-based practice. There is a growing interest in basing nursing actions on solid evidence confirming that the actions are clinically appropriate, cost-effective, and beneficial for clients. In this chapter, we discuss various issues related to the use of nursing research to support an evidence-based practice.

RESEARCH UTILIZATION AND EVIDENCE-BASED PRACTICE

The term **research utilization** is sometimes used synonymously with **evidence-based practice**. There is an overlap between the two concepts, but they are, in fact, distinct. Evidence based practice (EBP), the broader of the two terms, involves making clinical decisions based on the best possible evidence. The best evidence usually comes from rigorous research, but EBP also uses other sources of information. A basic feature of EBP is that it de-emphasizes decision making based on custom or authority opinion. Rather, the emphasis is on identifying the best available research evidence and *integrating* it with clinical expertise, patient input, and existing resources.

Broadly speaking, research utilization (RU) refers to the use of the findings from a disciplined study or set of studies in a practical application that is unrelated to the original research. In research utilization projects, the goal is to translate empirically based knowledge into real-world applications. Figure 18.1 provides a basic schema of how RU and EBP are interrelated. This section further explores and distinguishes the two concepts.

The Utilization of Nursing Research

During the 1980s and early 1990s, RU became an important buzz word. Several changes in nursing education and nursing research were prompted by the desire to develop a knowledge base for nursing practice. Nursing schools increasingly began to include courses on research methods so that students would become skilful research consumers, and researchers shifted their focus to clinical problems. These changes, coupled with the completion of several large research utilization projects, played a role in sensitizing the nursing community to the desirability of using research as a basis for practice; the changes were not enough, however, to lead to widespread integration of research findings into the delivery of nursing care. Research utilization, as the nursing community has come to recognize, is a complex and nonlinear phenomenon that poses professional challenges.

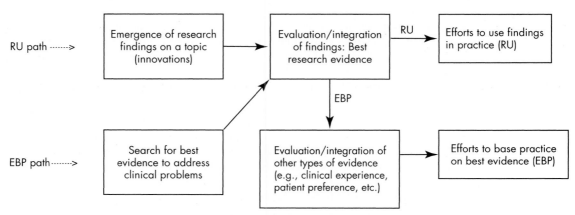

FIGURE 18.1 Research utilization (RU) and evidence-based practice (EBP).

THE RESEARCH UTILIZATION CONTINUUM

As Figure 18.1 indicates, the start-point of research utilization is new knowledge and new ideas that emerge from research. When studies are completed, knowledge on a topic accumulates and works its way into use—to varying degrees and at differing rates.

Theorists who have studied knowledge development and the diffusion of ideas recognize a continuum in terms of the specificity of the use to which research findings are put. At one end is **instrumental utilization** (Caplan & Rich, 1975), which refers to discrete, identifiable attempts to base specific actions on research findings. For example, a series of studies in the 1960s and 1970s demonstrated that the optimal placement time of a glass thermometer for accurate oral temperature determination is 9 minutes. When nurses specifically altered their behaviour from shorter placement times to the empirically based recommendation of 9 minutes, this constituted instrumental utilization.

Research findings can, however, be used in a more diffuse manner—in a way that promotes cumulative awareness or understanding. Caplan and Rich (1975) refer to this end of the utilization continuum as **conceptual utilization**. As an example, a nurse may read a qualitative research report describing *courage* among individuals with chronic illness as a dynamic process that includes efforts to accept reality and to develop problem-solving skills. The nurse may be reluctant to alter his or her own behaviour based on the results, but the study may make the nurse more observant in working with patients with chronic illnesses; it may also lead to informal efforts to promote problem-solving skills. Conceptual utilization, then, refers to situations in which users are influenced in their thinking about an issue based on research findings but do not put the findings to any specific use.

The middle ground of this continuum involves the partial use of research findings on nursing actions, reflecting what Weiss (1980) has termed knowledge creep and decision accretion. *Knowledge creep* refers to an evolving "percolation" of research ideas and findings. *Decision accretion* refers to the manner in which momentum for a decision builds over a period of time based on accumulated information gained through readings, discussions, and so on. Increasingly, however, nurses *are* making conscious decisions to use research in their clinical practice, and the EBP movement has contributed to this change.

Estabrooks (1999) studied research utilization by collecting survey data from 600 Canadian nurses. She found evidence to support three distinct types of research utilization: (1) *indirect research utilization*, involving changes in nurses' thinking—analogous to conceptual utilization; (2) *direct research utilization*, involving the direct use of findings in giving patient care—analogous to instrumental utilization; and (3) *persuasive utilization*, involving the use of findings to persuade others to make changes in policies or practices relevant to nursing care.

These varying ways of thinking about research utilization suggest that both qualitative and quantitative research can play key roles in improving nursing practice. Estabrooks (2001) has argued that the process of using research findings in practice is essentially the same for both quantitative and qualitative research, but she claims that qualitative research may have a privileged position: clinicians do not need a background in statistics to understand qualitative research, and thus using qualitative results is more readily accomplished.

RESEARCH UTILIZATION IN NURSING PRACTICE

During the 1980s and 1990s, there was considerable concern that nurses had failed to use research findings as a basis for making clinical decisions. This concern was based on early studies suggesting that nurses were not always aware of research results or did not use results in their practice. For example, Helen Shore (1972), a Canadian nurse, was one of the first to study this problem; she studied the adoption of six nursing practices presented in a nursing institute and learned that whereas there were some "adopters," there were also "laggards" who resisted new ideas. Ketefian (1975) reported on nurses' oral temperature determination practices. As noted, there was solid evidence that the optimal placement time with glass thermometers is 9 minutes. In Ketefian's study, only 1 out of 87 nurses reported the correct placement time, suggesting that these practicing nurses were unaware of or ignored the research findings. Other studies in the 1980s (e.g., Kirchhoff, 1982), were similarly discouraging.

Coyle and Sokop (1990) investigated practicing nurses' adoption of 14 strong, empirically based innovations that had been reported in the literature. A sample of 113 nurses from 10 hospitals completed questionnaires that measured the nurses' awareness and use of the findings. There was wide variation across the 14 innovations, with awareness of them ranging from 34% to 94%. Coyle and Sokop categorized each innovation according to stage of adoption: awareness (indicating knowledge of the innovation); persuasion (indicating the nurses' belief that nurses *should* use the innovation in practice); occasional use in practice; and regular use in practice. Only 1 of the 14 innovations was at the regular use stage of adoption, but six were in the persuasion stage.

A study by Varcoe and Hilton (1995) with 183 Canadian nurses found that 9 of the 10 research-based practices investigated were used by 50% or more of the acute care nurses at least sometimes. Similar results have been reported in a survey of nearly 1000 nurses from 25 hospitals in Scotland (Rodgers, 2000).

Example from Rodgers' study

One of the innovations included in Rodgers' (2000) study was the following: "Maintaining a closed drainage system for urinary catheters is one of the most important steps in the prevention of urinary tract infections in patients with indwelling catheters," a finding reported in several studies during the 1980s. This innovation was at the "regular use" stage of adoption, with 85% of respondents saying they always used these findings. By contrast, the following was in the "occasional use" stage of adoption, with 51% saying they used the findings sometimes: "The use of deliberative touch for therapeutic means (e.g., holding of hands or hugging) has been shown to promote psychological well-being in some patients."

The results of the recent studies are more encouraging than the earlier ones because they suggest that, on average, practicing nurses are aware of many research findings, are persuaded that the innovations should be used, and are beginning to use them, at least on occasion.

EFFORTS TO IMPROVE UTILIZATION OF NURSING RESEARCH

The desire to reduce the gap between nursing research and nursing practice has led to formal attempts to bridge the gap. The best-known of several early nursing RU projects is the

Conduct and Utilization of Research in Nursing (CURN) **Project**, a 5-year project awarded to the Michigan Nurses' Association in the 1970s. CURN's major objective was to increase the use of research findings in nursing practice by disseminating research findings, facilitating organizational changes, and encouraging collaborative clinical research. CURN project staff saw RU as primarily an organizational process, with the commitment of organizations that employ nurses as essential to the research utilization process (Horsley, Crane, & Bingle, 1978). The CURN project team concluded that RU by practicing nurses is feasible, but only if the research is relevant to practice and if the results are broadly disseminated. The CURN project generated considerable international interest. For example, the Cross Cancer Institute in Edmonton, Alberta used the CURN model as a framework to integrate research findings into nursing practice (Alberta Association of Registered Nurses, 1997).

During the 1980s and 1990s, utilization projects were undertaken by a growing number of hospitals and organizations, and project descriptions began to appear in the nursing research literature worldwide. These projects were usually institutional attempts to implement changes in nursing practice on the basis of research findings and to evaluate the effects of the innovation. For example, Logan, Harrison, Graham, Dunn, & Bissonnette (1999) described a project implemented at three Ottawa health care settings during a time of multiple restructuring changes. The **Ottawa Model of Research Use**, which we describe in a later section, was applied in an effort to increase evidence-based decision making in the three project sites. Multiple approaches aimed at research transfer were used, with a major emphasis on educational activities such as workshops.

These early utilization projects often did not have the hoped-for impact on the use of research in nursing practice, but during the 1990s, the call for research utilization began to be superseded by the push for EBP.

Evidence-Based Nursing Practice

The RU process begins with an empirically based innovation or new idea that gets scrutinized for possible adoption in practice settings. Evidence-based practice, by contrast, begins with a search for information about how best to solve specific problems (see Figure 18.1). Findings from rigorous research are considered the best source of information, but EBP also draws on other sources of evidence.

The evidence-based practice movement has given rise to considerable debate. Supporters of EBP argue that a rational approach is needed to provide the best possible care to the most people, with the most cost-effective use of resources. Critics worry that the advantages of EBP are exaggerated and that clinical judgments and patient inputs are being devalued. Although there is a need for close scrutiny of how the EBP journey unfolds, it seems likely that the EBP path is one that health care professions are likely to follow in the 21st century.

OVERVIEW OF THE EBP MOVEMENT

In the 1970s, British epidemiologist Archie Cochrane published an influential book that drew attention to the dearth of solid evidence about the effects of health care. He called for efforts to make research summaries available to health care decision makers. This eventually led to the development of the Cochrane Centre in Oxford in 1992 and the **Cochrane**

Collaboration, with centres established in 15 locations throughout the world. The aim of the collaboration is to help people make good decisions about health care by preparing, maintaining, and disseminating systematic reviews of the effects of health care interventions.

At about the same time as the Cochrane Collaboration got underway, a group from McMaster Medical School developed a clinical learning strategy they called evidence-based medicine (EBM). Dr. David Sackett, a pioneer of EBM at McMaster, defined evidence-based medicine as "the conscientious, explicit, and judicious use of current best evidence in making decisions about the care of individual patients. The practice of evidence-based medicine means integrating individual clinical expertise with the best available external evidence from systematic research" (Sackett, Rosenberg, Gray, Haynes, & Richardson, 1996, p. 71). The EBM movement has shifted over time to a broader conception of using best evidence by all health care practitioners (not just doctors) in a multidisciplinary team.

TYPES OF EVIDENCE AND EVIDENCE HIERARCHIES

There is no consensus about what constitutes good evidence for EBP, but there is general agreement that findings from rigourous studies are paramount. In the early years of the EBP movement, there was a strong bias toward reliance on evidence from randomized clinical trials (RCTs)—a bias that led to some resistance to EBP by nurses who felt that evidence from qualitative and non-RCT studies would be ignored.

Positions about what constitutes useful evidence have loosened, but there have nevertheless been efforts to develop **evidence hierarchies** that rank studies according to the strength of evidence they provide. Several such hierarchies have been developed, many based on the one proposed by Archie Cochrane. Most hierarchies put meta-analyses of RCT studies at the pinnacle and other types of nonresearch evidence (e.g., clinical expertise) at the base. As one example, Stetler, Morsi, Rucki, Broughton, Corrigan, Fitzgerald, Giuliano, Havener, and Sheridan (1998) developed a six-level evidence hierarchy. The levels (from strongest to weakest) are as follows: (I) meta-analyses of RCTs; (II) individual experimental studies; (III) quasi-experimental studies or matched case-control studies; (IV) nonexperimental studies (e.g., correlational studies, qualitative studies); (V) research utilization studies, quality improvement projects, case reports; and (VI) opinions of respected authorities and of expert committees.

To date, there have been relatively few published RCT studies in nursing, and even fewer published meta-analyses of RCT nursing studies. Therefore, evidence from other types of research will play an important role in evidence-based nursing practice. Many clinical questions of importance to nurses can best be answered with rich descriptive and qualitative data from level IV and V studies.

Thus, nurses and other health care professionals must be able to locate evidence, evaluate it, and integrate it with clinical judgment and patient preferences to determine the most clinically effective solutions to health problems. Note that an important feature of EBP is that it does not necessarily imply practice changes: the best evidence may confirm that existing practices are effective and cost-efficient.

Barriers to Research Utilization and EBP in Nursing

Studies done in Canada and in many other countries have explored nurses' perceptions of barriers to research utilization and have yielded remarkably similar results about constraints clinical nurses face (e.g., Gerrish & Clayton, 2004; Graham, Logan, Davies, & Nimrod, 2004; Hutchinson & Johnston, 2004; McCleary & Brown, 2003a).

RESEARCH-RELATED BARRIERS

For some nursing problems, research knowledge is at a rudimentary level. Research findings may not warrant use in practice if studies are flawed or small in number. Thus, one impediment to research utilization is that, for some problems, a solid base of trustworthy study results has not been developed.

As we have stressed, most studies have flaws of one type or another, and so if nurses were to wait for perfect studies before basing clinical decisions on research evidence, they would have a long wait. Replication is essential: when repeated efforts to address a research question in different settings yield similar results, there can be greater confidence in the evidence. Single studies rarely provide an adequate basis for making practice changes. Therefore, another utilization constraint is the dearth of published replications.

As a consumer, you should evaluate the extent to which researchers have adopted strategies to enhance RU/EBP. These include working collaboratively with clinicians, communicating clearly so that practicing nurses can evaluate studies, and describing clinical implications in the discussion section of their reports.

NURSE-RELATED BARRIERS

Nurses are increasingly sophisticated and able to appreciate research findings. Indeed, a recent survey in Scotland suggests that nurses may have better skills to carry out literature reviews and evaluate research evidence than other health care professionals in primary care (O'Donnell, 2004). However, studies have also found that nurses prefer to use knowledge gained through personal experiences and interactions with co-workers rather than through textbooks and journal articles (e.g., Estabrooks, Chong, Brigidear, & Profetto-McGrath, 2005; Gerrish & Clayton, 2004).

Nurses' education and research skills have consistently been found to constrain the use of research evidence in practice (e.g., McCleary & Brown, 2003b). Many clinical nurses have not had formal instruction in research and may lack the skills to evaluate a study. Courses on research methods are now offered in most baccalaureate nursing programs, but the ability to critique a study is not necessarily sufficient for effectively incorporating research evidence into daily decision making.

Nurses' attitudes toward research and their motivation to engage in EBP have also been identified as potential barriers. Studies have found that the more positive the attitude, the more likely is the nurse to use research in practice. Fortunately, there is growing evidence from international surveys that many nurses value nursing research and want to be involved in research-related activities.

ORGANIZATIONAL BARRIERS

Many of the impediments to using research in practice stem from the organizations that train and employ nurses. Organizations, perhaps to an even greater degree than individuals, resist change unless there is a strong organizational perception that there is something fundamentally wrong with the status quo. To challenge tradition and accepted practices, a spirit of intellectual curiosity and openness must prevail.

CONSUMER TIP

Every nurse can play a role in using research evidence. Here are some strategies:

▶ *Read widely.* Professionally accountable nurses keep abreast of new developments. You should read journals relating to your specialty, including research reports in them.
▶ *Attend professional conferences.* Many nursing conferences include presentations of studies that have clinical relevance. At a conference, you can meet researchers and explore practice implications.
▶ *Learn to expect evidence that a procedure is effective.* Every time you are told about a standard nursing procedure, you have a right to ask, why? Nurses should develop expectations that their clinical decisions are based on sound rationales.
▶ *Become involved in a journal club.* Many organizations that employ nurses sponsor journal clubs that meet to review studies that have potential relevance to practice.
▶ *Pursue and participate in RU/EBP projects.* Sometimes ideas for RU or EBP projects come from staff nurses (e.g., ideas may emerge in a journal club). Studies have found that nurses who are involved in research-related activities (e.g., data collection efforts) develop more positive attitudes toward research and EBP.

In many practice settings, administrators have systems to reward competence in nursing practice, but few have instituted a system to reward nurses for critiquing studies, using research in practice, or discussing research findings with clients. Thus, organizations have failed to motivate nurses for RU/EBP. Organizations may also be reluctant to expend resources for RU/EBP projects. Resources may be required for outside consultants, staff release time, library materials, and so on. With the push toward cost containment in health care settings, resource constraints may pose a barrier to change—unless cost containment is an explicit project goal.

EBP will become part of organizational norms only if there is a commitment on the part of managers and administrators. Strong leadership in health care organizations is essential to making evidence-based practice happen.

THE PROCESS OF USING RESEARCH IN NURSING PRACTICE

In the years ahead, many of you are likely to be engaged in individual and institutional efforts to use research as a basis for clinical decisions. This section describes how that might be accomplished. We begin with a description of some RU and EBP models developed by nurses.

Models for Evidence-Based Nursing Practice

A number of different models of research utilization have been developed by nurse researchers in Canada, the United States, the United Kingdom, and other countries during the past few decades. These models, which offer guidelines for designing and implementing RU and EBP projects in practice settings, include the following:

▶ Stetler Model of Research Utilization (Stetler 1994, 2001)
▶ Iowa Model of Research in Practice (Titler, Kleiber, Steelman, Goode, Rakel, Barry-Walker, Small, & Buckwalter 1994; Titler, Kleiber, Steelman, Rakel, Budreau, Everett, Buckwalter, Tripp-Reimer, & Goode, 2001)
▶ Ottawa Model of Research Use (Logan & Graham, 1998)
▶ Evidence-Based Multidisciplinary Practice Model (Goode & Piedalue, 1999)
▶ Model for Change to Evidence-Based Practice (Rosswurm & Larrabee, 1999)

The most prominent of these models have been the Stetler, Iowa, and Ottawa Models. The first two models were originally developed in an environment that emphasized RU and have been updated to incorporate EBP processes.

THE STETLER MODEL

According to a recent study by Canadian researchers Estabrooks and colleagues (2004), Cheryl Stetler continues to be one of the most often-cited authors in the research utilization field. The **Stetler Model** (originally developed with Marram in 1976 and then refined in 1994) has an underlying assumption that RU can be undertaken not only by organizations but also by individual clinicians and managers. The model was designed to facilitate critical thinking about the application of research findings in practice. The updated model is based on many of the same assumptions and strategies as the original but provides "an enhanced approach to the overall application of research in the service setting" (Stetler, 2001, p. 273). Stetler's model, presented graphically in Figure 18.2, involves five sequential phases of an EBP effort:

1. *Preparation.* In this phase, nurses define the underlying purpose of the project; search for and select sources of research evidence; consider external factors that can influence potential application and internal factors that can diminish objectivity; and affirm the clinical significance of solving the perceived problem.
2. *Validation.* The second phase involves a utilization-focused critique of each evidence source, focusing on whether it is sufficiently sound for potential use in practice. The process stops at this point if the evidence sources are rejected.
3. *Comparative evaluation and decision making.* This phase involves a synthesis of findings and the application of four criteria that are used to determine the desirability and feasibility of applying findings from validated sources to nursing practice. These criteria (fit of setting, feasibility, current practice, and substantiating evidence) are summarized in Box 18.1. The end result of this phase is to make a decision about using the evidence.
4. *Translation/application.* This phase involves confirming how the findings will be used (e.g., formally or informally), spelling out the operational details of the application, and then implementing the plan. The latter might involve the development of a guideline or plan of action, possibly including a proposal for formal organizational change.
5. *Evaluation.* In the final phase, the application would be evaluated. Informal versus formal use of the innovation would lead to different evaluative strategies.

Although the Stetler Model was designed as a tool for individual practitioners, it has also been the basis of formal RU and EBP projects by groups of nurses.

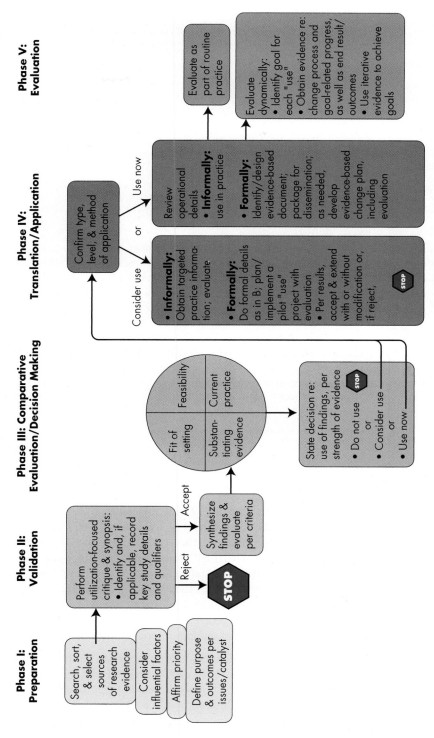

FIGURE 18.2 Stetler Model of Research Utilization to facilitate evidence-based practice. (Adapted from Stetler, C.B. [1994]. Refinement of the Stetler/Marram model for application of research findings into practice. *Nursing Outlook, 42,* 15–25.)

BOX 18.1   **Criteria for Comparative Evaluation Phase of Stetler's Model**

1. **Fit of Setting**

   Similarity of characteristics of sample to your client population
   Similarity of study's environment to the one in which you work

2. **Feasibility**

   Potential risks of implementation to patients, staff, and the organization
   Readiness for change among those who would be involved in a change in practice
   Resource requirements and availability

3. **Current Practice**

   Congruency of the study with your theoretical basis for current practice behaviour

4. **Substantiating Evidence**

   Availability of confirming evidence from other studies
   Availability of confirming evidence from a meta-analysis or integrative review

Adapted from Stetler, C. B. (1994). Refinement of the Stetler/Marram model for application of research findings into practice. *Nursing Outlook, 42,* 15–25.

Example of an application of the Stetler Model

Bauer, Bushey, and Amaros (2002) applied the five phases of the Stetler Model to pressure ulcer prevention and care by nurses in home health care environments.

THE IOWA MODEL

Efforts to use research evidence to improve nursing practice are often addressed by groups of nurses interested in a critical practice issue, using a model such as the Iowa Model of Research in Practice (Titler et al., 1994). This model, like the Stetler Model, was revised recently and renamed the **Iowa Model of Evidence-Based Practice to Promote Quality Care** (Titler et al., 2001). The current version of the Iowa Model, shown in Figure 18.3, acknowledges that a formal RU/EBP project begins with a *trigger*—an impetus to explore possible changes to practice. The start-point can be either (a) a *knowledge-focused trigger* that emerges from awareness of an innovation (and thus follows a more traditional RU path, as in the top panel of Figure 18.3); or (b) a *problem-focused trigger* that has its roots in a clinical or organizational problem (and thus follows a path that more closely resembles an EBP intent). The model outlines a series of activities with three decision points:

1. Deciding whether the problem is a sufficient priority for the organization exploring possible changes; if yes, a team is formed to proceed with the project;
2. Deciding whether there is a sufficient research base; if yes, the innovation is piloted in the practice setting (if no, the team would either search for other sources of evidence or conduct its own research); and

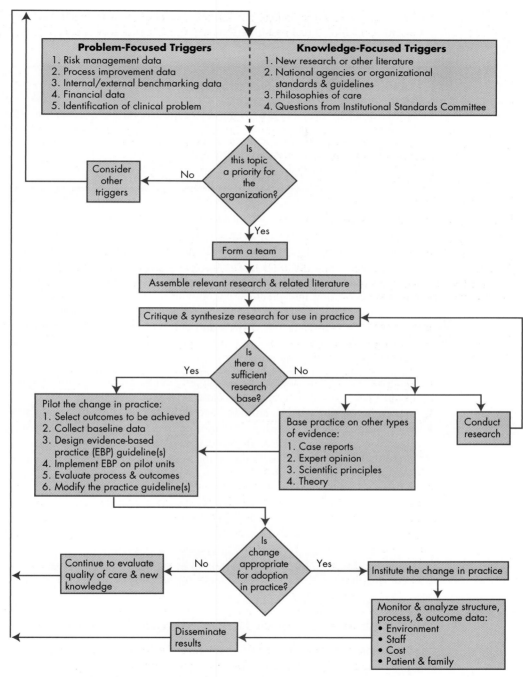

FIGURE 18.3 Iowa Model of Evidence-Based Practice to Promote Quality Care (Adapted from Titler. et al. [2001]. The Iowa Model of Evidence-Based Practice to Promote Quality Care. *Critical Care Nursing Clinics of North America, 13*, 497–509.)

3. Deciding whether the change is appropriate for adoption in practice; if yes, a change would be instituted and monitored.

Examples of application of the Iowa Model

Numerous EBP projects are underway at the University of Iowa, including an initiative focused on pain management in acute care and outpatient settings, and another focused on facilitation of pet visitation in acute care settings (*http://www.uihealthcare.com/depts/nursing/rqom/evidencebasedpractice/currentprojects.html*).

THE OTTAWA MODEL OF RESEARCH USE (OMRU)

The OMRU, developed by Logan & Graham (1998), consists of six key components interrelated through the process of evaluation. The six components deal with "the practice environment, the potential research adopter (administrators and clinical staff), the evidence-based innovation (the research intended for use in practice), strategies for transferring the innovation into practice, adoption/use of the evidence, and health and other outcomes" (Logan, et al., 1999, p. 39). Systematic assessment, monitoring, and evaluation (AME) are central to the OMRU and are applied to each of the six components before, during, and after any effort to transfer research findings. The data gathered through AME serves several purposes:

▶ to determine potential barriers to and supports for research use associated with the practice environment (structural, social, patients, and others);
▶ to consider the knowledge, attitudes, and skills possessed by potential adopters;
▶ to offer direction for choosing and tailoring transfer strategies to surmount the recognized barriers and enhance strategies that were deemed supportive; and
▶ to evaluate the evidence-based innovation used and the influence it had on the outcomes of interest.

Example of an application of the Ottawa Model

Graham and Logan (2004) used the OMRU to guide the implementation of clinical practice guidelines for skin care in a surgical program of a tertiary care hospital.

Activities in a Research Utilization or EBP Project

As the various models of RU/EMP imply, formal efforts to use research to improve nursing practice involves a series of activities, decisions, and assessments. In this section, we discuss some of the major activities that are typical in an RU/EBP project. The three models described in the previous section are used as a basis for discussing key activities to support RU and EBP.

SELECTING A TOPIC OR PROBLEM

As noted in the Iowa Model, there are two types of stimulus for an EBP or RU endeavour—identification of a clinical practice problem needing solution, and discovery of an innovation in the literature. Problem-focused triggers may arise in the normal course of clinical practice or in the context of quality improvement efforts. This approach is likely to have staff support if the problem is one that numerous nurses have encountered, and it is likely to have considerable clinical relevance because a specific clinical situation generated interest in the problem in the first place.

Gennaro, Hodnett, and Kearney (2001) advise nurses following this approach to begin by clarifying the practice problem that needs to be solved and framing it as a question. The goal can be to find the most effective way to anticipate a problem (how to diagnose it) or the best way to solve a problem (how to intervene). Clinical practice questions may well take the form of, "What is the best way to . . ."—for example, "What is the best way to manage hospitalized children's pain?"

A second catalyst for an RU/EBP project is the research literature, that is, knowledge-focused triggers. For example, a utilization project could emerge as a result of discussions within a journal club. In this approach, a preliminary assessment needs to be made of the clinical relevance of the research. The central issue is whether a significant nursing problem will be solved by making some change. Five questions relating to clinical relevance (shown in Box 18.2) can be applied to a research report or set of related reports. If the answer is yes to any of these questions, the next step can be pursued.

With both types of triggers, it is important to ensure that there is a consensus about the importance of the problem and the need for change. Titler and colleagues (2001) include as the first decision point in their model the resolution of whether the topic is a priority for the organization considering practice changes. They advise that the following issues be taken into account when initiating an EBP project: the topic's fit with the organization's strategic plan, magnitude of the problem, number of people invested in the problem, support of nurse leaders and of those in other disciplines, costs, and possible barriers to change.

CONSUMER TIP

The method of selecting a topic does not appear to have any bearing on the success of an RU/EBP project. What is important, however, is that the nurses who will implement an innovation are involved in the topic selection and that key stakeholders are "on board." ■

ASSEMBLING AND EVALUATING EVIDENCE

Once a clinical practice question has been selected and a team has been formed to work on the project, the next step is to search for and assemble evidence on the topic. Chapter 7 provided information about locating research information, and Chapter 17 discussed research critiques, but some additional issues are relevant.

In doing a literature review for a new study, the central goal is to discover how best to advance knowledge. For EBP or RU projects, which typically have as end products

BOX 18.2   **Criteria for Evaluating the Clinical Relevance of a Body of Research**

1. Does the research have the potential to help solve a problem that is currently being faced by practitioners?
2. Does the research have the potential to help with clinical decision making with respect to (a) making appropriate observations, (b) identifying client risks or complications, or (c) selecting an appropriate intervention?
3. Are clinically relevant theoretical propositions tested by the research?
4. If the research involves an intervention, does the intervention have potential for implementation in clinical practice? Do nurses have control over the implementation of such interventions?
5. Can the measures used in the study be used in clinical practice?

Adapted from Tanner, C. A. (1987). Evaluating research for use in practice: Guidelines for the clinician. *Heart & Lung, 16,* 424–430.

prescriptive practice protocols or clinical guidelines, literature reviews are typically much more rigourous and formalized. The emphasis is on gathering comprehensive information on the topic, weighing pieces of evidence, and integrating information to draw conclusions about the evidence base. *Integrative reviews* thus play a crucial role in developing an evidence-based practice. If nurses are to glean best practices from research findings, they must take into account as much of the evidence as possible, organized and synthesized in a rigorous manner.

High-quality integrative reviews are a critical tool for RU/EBP, and if the project team has the skills to complete one, this is valuable. It is, however, unlikely that every clinical organization will be able to assemble the skills needed to do a high-quality critical review of research literature on a chosen topic. Fortunately, many researchers and organizations have taken on the responsibility of preparing integrative reviews and making them available for EBP.

Cochrane reviews are an especially important resource. These reports, which are based mainly on meta-analyses, describe the background and objectives of the review; the methods used to search for, select, and evaluate studies; the main results; and, importantly, the reviewers' conclusions. Cochrane reviews are checked and updated regularly.

Example of a Cochrane review

Hodnett, Gates, Hofmeyr, and Sakala (2003) did a Cochrane review to critically appraise the evidence relating to the effects of continuous, one-to-one support for women during childbirth. Data from 15 clinical trials involving nearly 13,000 women were included in the review. The review found that women who had continuous intrapartum support were less likely than women who did not to have analgesia or operative birth to report dissatisfaction with their childbirth experience.

Another important resource for integrative reviews is the Agency for Healthcare Research and Quality (AHRQ) in the United States. This agency awarded 12 5-year contracts in 1997 to establish Evidence-Based Practice Centres at institutions in the United States and Canada (e.g., at McMaster University), and new 5-year contracts were awarded in 2002. Each centre issues *evidence reports* that are based on rigourous integrative reviews of relevant scientific literature; dozens of these reports are now available to help "improve the quality, effectiveness, and appropriateness of clinical care" (AHRQ website, *http://www.ahrq.gov*). In Canada, the Ontario Ministry of Health and Long-Term Care has sponsored the Effective Public Health Practice Project (EPHPP), a project that also undertakes and disseminates integrative reviews on a broad array of health topics (*http://www.hamilton.ca/phcs/ephpp*).

If an integrative review has been prepared, it is possible that a formal evidence-based clinical guideline has been developed and can be used directly in an RU/EBP project. AHRQ, for example, has developed such guidelines on pain management, continence, and other problems of relevance to nurses (*http://www.guidelines.gov*). Nursing organizations have also developed clinical practice guidelines on several topics. For example, the Registered Nurses Association of Ontario (RNAO) launched its Nursing Best Practice Guidelines (NBPG) Project in 1999. Funded as a multiyear project by the Ontario Ministry of Health and Long Term Care, the project team has developed 21 guidelines to date and are available at *http://www.rnao.org/bestpractices* (Grinspun, Virani, & Bajnok, 2001–2002). Five guidelines were undergoing stakeholder review as of March 2005, and an additional four guidelines were in progress.

In some cases, it may be possible to develop a new practice guideline based on a published integrative review. However, it is always wise to make sure that the review is up-to-date and that new findings published after the review are taken into consideration. Moreover, even a published integrative review needs to be critiqued and the validity of its conclusions assessed. Of course, there are many clinical questions for which integrative reviews are not available, and so the RU/EBP team might need to prepare its own integrative review. Some information about conducting and critiquing integrative reviews is presented later in this chapter.

An integrative review or synthesis of research evidence is used by the RU/EBP team to draw conclusions about the sufficiency of the research base for guiding clinical practice. Adequacy of research evidence depends on such factors as the consistency of findings across studies, the quality and rigour of the studies, the strength of observed effects, the transferability of the findings to clinical settings, and cost-effectiveness.

Conclusions about a body of evidence can lead to different decisions for further action. First, if the research base is small—or if there is a large base with ambiguous conclusions—the team might decide to pursue a different problem. A second option (preferable in the EBP environment) is to assemble other types of evidence (e.g., through consultation with experts, surveys of clients, and so on) and assess whether that evidence suggests a practice change. Finally, another possibility is to pursue an original clinical study to directly address the practice question, thereby gathering new evidence and contributing to the base of practice knowledge. This last course may well be impractical for many and would clearly result in years of delay before any further conclusions could be drawn.

A solid research base also could point in different directions. The evidence might, for example, support existing practices—which might lead to an analysis of why the practice question emerged and what might make existing practices work better. Another possibility is that there would be compelling evidence that a clinical change is warranted, which would lead to the activities described next.

ASSESSING IMPLEMENTATION POTENTIAL

Some models of RU/EBP move directly from the conclusion that evidence supports a change in practice to the pilot testing of the innovation. Others include steps to first evaluate the appropriateness of the innovation within the specific organizational context; in some cases, such an assessment (or aspects of it) may be warranted even before embarking on efforts to assemble best evidence. We think a preliminary assessment of the **implementation potential** of an innovation is often sensible.

In determining the implementation potential of an innovation in a particular setting, several issues should be considered, particularly the transferability of the innovation, the feasibility of implementing it, and the cost/benefit ratio. Box 18.3 presents some assessment questions for these categories.

▶ *Transferability.* The main question relating to transferability is whether it makes good sense to implement the innovation in the new practice setting. If there is some aspect of the practice setting that is fundamentally incongruent with the innovation in terms of its philosophy, types of client served, personnel, or administrative structure, it may not be prudent to try to adopt the innovation, even if it has been shown to be effective in other contexts.

▶ *Feasibility.* The feasibility questions in Box 18.3 address various practical concerns about the availability of staff and resources, the organizational climate, the availability of external assistance, and the potential for clinical evaluation. An important issue here is whether nurses will have (or share) control over the innovation. When nurses do not have full control over the new procedure, it is important to recognize the interdependent nature of the project and to proceed as early as possible to establish necessary cooperative arrangements.

▶ *Cost/Benefit Ratio.* A critical part of any decision to proceed with an RU/EBP project is a careful assessment of the costs and benefits of the innovation. The *cost–benefit assessment* should encompass likely costs and benefits to various groups, including clients, staff, and the overall organization. Clearly, the most important factor is the client. If the degree of risk in introducing a new procedure is high, then the potential benefits must be great, and the knowledge base must be very sound. A cost–benefit assessment should consider the opposite side of the coin as well: the costs and benefits of *not* implementing the innovation. It is sometimes easy to forget that the status quo bears its own risks and that failure to change, especially when such change is based on rigorous evidence, is also costly.

If the assessment suggests that there might be problems in testing the innovation within that particular practice setting, the team might consider devising a plan to improve the implementation potential (e.g., seeking external resources if costs are the inhibiting factor).

BOX 18.3 Criteria for Evaluating the Implementation Potential of an Innovation Under Scrutiny

Transferability of the Findings

1. Will the innovation "fit" in the proposed setting?
2. How similar are the target populations in the research and in your setting?
3. Is the philosophy of care underlying the innovation fundamentally different from the philosophy prevailing in your setting? How entrenched is the prevailing philosophy?
4. Is there a sufficiently large number of clients in your setting who could benefit from the innovation?
5. Will the innovation take too long to implement and evaluate?

Feasibility

1. Will nurses have the freedom to carry out the innovation? Will they have the freedom to terminate the innovation if it is considered undesirable?
2. Will the implementation of the innovation interfere inordinately with current staff functions?
3. Does the administration support the innovation? Is the organizational climate conducive to research utilization?
4. Is there a fair degree of consensus among the staff and among the administrators that the innovation could be beneficial and should be tested? Are there major pockets of resistance or uncooperativeness that could undermine efforts to implement and evaluate the innovation?
5. To what extent will the implementation of the innovation cause friction within your organization? Does the utilization project have the support and cooperation of departments outside the nursing department?
6. Are the skills needed to carry out the utilization project (both the implementation and the clinical evaluation) available in the nursing staff? If not, how difficult will it be to collaborate with or to secure the assistance of others with the necessary skills?
7. Does your organization have the equipment and facilities necessary for the innovation? If not, is there a way to obtain the needed resources?
8. If nursing staff need to be released from other practice activities to learn about and implement the innovation, what is the likelihood that this will happen?
9. Are appropriate measuring tools available for a clinical evaluation of the innovation?

Cost/Benefit Ratio of the Innovation

1. What are the risks to which clients would be exposed during the implementation of the innovation and what are the potential benefits to clients?
2. What are the risks of maintaining current practices (i.e., the risks of *not* trying the innovation)?
3. What are the material costs of implementing the innovation? What are the costs in the short term during utilization, and what are the costs in the long run, if the change is to be institutionalized?
4. What are the material costs of *not* implementing the innovation (i.e., could the new procedure result in some efficiencies that could lower the cost of providing service)?
5. What are the potential nonmaterial costs and benefits of implementing the innovation to the organization (e.g., in terms of lower staff morale, staff turnover, absenteeism)?

DEVELOPING, IMPLEMENTING AND EVALUATING THE INNOVATION

If the implementation criteria are met, the next phase of the project would involve the following activities:

▶ Developing a written EBP guideline or protocol based on the synthesis of the evidence, preferably a guideline that is clear and user-friendly and that uses such devices as flow charts and decision trees;

▶ Training relevant staff in the use of the new guideline and, if necessary "marketing" the innovation to users so that it is given a fair test;

▶ Developing an evaluation plan (e.g., identifying outcomes to be achieved, determining how many clients to involve, deciding when and how often to take measurements);

▶ Collecting baseline data relating to those outcomes, to develop a counterfactual against which the outcomes of the innovation would be assessed;

▶ Trying out the guideline in some units or with a sample of clients; and

▶ Evaluating the pilot project, in terms of both process (e.g., how was the innovation received, to what extent were the guidelines actually followed, what implementation problems were encountered?) and outcomes (in terms of clinical outcomes and cost effectiveness).

Evaluation data should be gathered over a sufficiently long period (typically, 6 to 12 months) to allow for a true test of a "mature" innovation. The end result of this process is a decision about whether to adopt the innovation, to modify it for ongoing use, or to revert to prior practices.

Examples of Evidence-Based Nursing Projects

Many EBP and RU projects are underway in practice settings, and some that have been described in the nursing literature offer information about planning and implementing such an endeavour. For example, Thurston and King (2004) described their use of Russworm and Larrabee's EBP model with 10 nursing teams in a region-wide mentorship program aimed at enabling clinical nurses to understand and implement an evidence-based approach to practice. As another example, Clarke, Barbour, White, and MacIntyre (2005) collaborated in a 2-year project to evaluate the use of computer-assisted strategies for implementing clinical practice guidelines for prevention and optimal treatment of pressure ulcers.

The Association of Women's Health, Obstetric, and Neonatal Nurses (AWHONN) has conducted several major RU/EBP projects as part of its Research-Based Practice program. Each project has resulted in the development and testing of evidence-based nursing protocols. For example, one project is focusing on a smoking cessation counselling strategy for pregnant women in clinical settings (Maloni, Albrecht, Thomas, Halleran, & Jones, 2003), and another is focusing on the management of cyclic perimenstrual pain and discomfort (Collins-Sharp, Taylor, Thomas, Killeen, & Dawood, in press). And yet another group, under the leadership of neonatal clinical nurse specialist Carolyn H. Lund, undertook a 4-year project designed to develop and evaluate an evidence-based clinical practice guideline for assessment and routine care of neonatal skin (Lund, Kuller, Lane, Lott, Raines, & Thomas, 2001a; Lund, Osborne, Kuller, Lane, Lott, & Raines, 2001b). The project also sought to educate nurses about the scientific basis for the recommended skin care practices and designed procedures to facilitate using the guideline in practice.

INTEGRATIVE REVIEWS

Evidence-based practice relies on meticulous integration and critical evaluation of research evidence on a topic. This section is not specifically designed to teach you how to do an integrative review because the conduct of such reviews requires methodologic sophistication. However, it is important for you to have some skills in critiquing and appraising integrative reviews so that you can decide how much confidence to place in the reviewers' conclusions. To critique integrative reviews, you will need to learn a bit about how they are done.

Steps in Doing an Integrative Review

An **integrative review** is in itself a systematic inquiry that follows many of the same rules as those for primary studies. In other words, those doing an integrative review develop research questions or hypotheses, devise a sampling plan and data collection strategy, collect relevant data, and analyze and interpret those data.

It should be noted that integrative reviews are sometimes done by individuals, but it is far preferable to have at least two reviewers. Multiple reviewers not only share the workload but also help to minimize subjectivity. Reviewers should have substantive and clinical knowledge of the problem and sufficiently strong methodologic skills to evaluate study quality.

RESEARCH QUESTIONS AND HYPOTHESES IN INTEGRATIVE REVIEWS

An integrative review begins with a problem statement and a research question or hypothesis. In critiquing an integrative review, you should determine whether the problem statement and questions are clearly worded and sufficiently specific, whether the variables or phenomena under study are adequately defined, and whether the population has been stated. Whether the review is a traditional narrative review, a meta-analysis, or a metasynthesis, the reviewers should clearly communicate their purpose and their rationale for undertaking it.

Example of a statement of purpose from a metasynthesis

An extensive metasynthesis was undertaken by Barbara Paterson and her colleagues for the following purpose: "... to develop an understanding of fatigue in chronic illness as it has been depicted in the existing body of qualitative health research" and "to create a comprehensive picture of how fatigue is described and experienced" (Paterson, Canam, Joachim, & Thorne, 2003, p. 120).

Questions for an integrative review can be narrow, focusing, for example, on a particular type of intervention, or more inclusive, examining a range of alternative interventions or practices. Forbes (2003) described an integrative review guided by the question, "What strategies, within the scope of nursing, are effective in managing the behavioral symptoms associated with Alzheimer's disease?" (p. 182). She noted that "in retrospect, selecting specific interventions would have made the review more manageable" (p. 182). The broader the question, the more complex and costly the integrative review becomes. In some cases, the broader the question, the less appropriate it is to integrate studies—just as in primary research, there must be an identifiable independent and dependent variable (for quantitative studies) or phenomenon (in qualitative studies).

SAMPLING IN INTEGRATIVE REVIEWS

In an integrative review, the "sample" involves primary studies that have addressed the same or a similar research question. In most cases, the reviewers try first to identify the full population of relevant studies, only some of which (a sample) may actually be used in the review.

Reviewers must make a number of upfront decisions regarding the sample, which they should share in their review so that readers can evaluate the rigour and generalizability of their conclusions. Sampling decisions include the following:

▶ What are the exclusion and/or inclusion criteria for the search?
▶ Will both published and unpublished reports be assembled?
▶ What databases and other retrieval mechanisms will be used to locate the sample?
▶ What key words or search terms will be used to identify relevant studies?

Example of sampling decisions for an integrative review

Chiu, Emblen, Van Hofwegen, Sawatzky, and Meyerhoff (2004) used both qualitative and quantitative approaches in their integration of the research on spirituality in the health literature. They decided to sample reports only from English-language journals published between January 1990 and September 2000. Studies had to provide an operational or conceptual definition of spirituality and had to relate spirituality to health. They made a conscious decision to search for various terms relating to *spirituality* (e.g., spiritual well-being, spiritual health), but not to search for terms relating to *religiosity*.

Eligibility criteria cover substantive, methodologic, and practical factors. Substantively, the criteria must stipulate what specific variables (or phenomena) are going to be studied. For example, if the review is integrating material about the effectiveness of a nursing intervention, what outcomes (dependent variables) must the researchers have studied? Another substantive issue concerns the study population. For example, will certain age groups of study participants (e.g., children, the elderly) be excluded? Methodologically, the

Example of eligibility criteria for an integrative review

Forbes (2003), in her meta-analysis of interventions for Alzheimer's disease patients, stipulated five criteria. The study must have (1) been published or conducted between January 1985 and May 1997, (2) evaluated a nonpharmacologic intervention for individuals aged 65 or older with Alzheimer's disease, (3) involved an intervention within the scope of nursing practice, (4) measured at least one outcome of a stipulated type (e.g., wandering, agitation), and (5) incorporated a control group or changes over time.

criteria might specify that (for example) only studies that used an experimental design would be included. From a practical standpoint, the criteria might exclude, for example, reports written in a language other than English, or reports published before a certain date.

There is some disagreement about whether reviewers should limit their sample to published studies or cast as wide a net as possible and include *grey literature*—that is, studies with a more limited distribution, such as dissertations, unpublished reports, and so on. Some people use only published reports in peer-reviewed journals, as a proxy for study rigour. Conn, Valentine, Cooper, and Rantz (2003) conducted a study on this matter, however, and concluded that the exclusion of grey literature can lead to certain types of biases, such as overestimating effects.

In searching for a comprehensive sample of research reports, reviewers usually need to use techniques more exhaustive than simply doing a computerized literature search of key databases, and this is especially true if the sample is to include grey literature. Five search methods described in path-breaking work by Cooper (1984) include the *ancestry approach* ("footnote chasing" of cited studies); the *descendancy approach* (searching forward in citation indexes for subsequent references to key studies), online searches (including Internet searches), informal contacts at research conferences, and the more traditional searches of bibliographic databases.

Example of a search strategy for an integrative review

Dennis and Stewart (2004) did a meta-analysis of studies on biologic interventions for postpartum depression. They noted that, "Databases searched for this review included MEDLINE, PubMed, CINAHL, PsychINFO, EMBASE, ProQuest, the Cochrane Library, and the WHO Reproductive Health Library from 1996 to 2003.... Tables of contents for key journals were hand-searched for the previous two years (2001–2003), reference lists of included studies and relevant reviews were examined, and key postpartum depression researchers were contacted via e-mail" (p. 1242).

When a potential pool of studies has been identified, reviewers then screen them for appropriateness. Typically, many located studies are discarded because they turn out not to be relevant or do not meet the eligibility criteria. Yet another reason for excluding studies from the initial pool (particularly for meta-analyses) is that some provide insufficient information to perform the necessary analyses. All decisions relating to exclusions (preferably made by at least two reviewers to ensure objectivity) should be well documented and justified.

EVALUATING PRIMARY STUDIES FOR INTEGRATIVE REVIEWS

In any integrative review, each study must be evaluated to determine how much confidence to place in the findings. Strong studies need to be given more weight than weaker ones in coming to conclusions about the state of knowledge. There are different strategies for doing this, however. Some reviewers use methodologic quality as an exclusion criterion—for example, excluding non-RCT studies or studies with a low quality rating. Others, however, include studies regardless of quality but incorporate information about quality into the analysis.

> ### Example of excluding low-quality studies in an integrative review
>
> Peacock and Forbes (2003) did a systematic review of interventions for care-givers of persons with dementia. A total of 36 relevant studies were rated according to various methodologic criteria; the scores then were used to categorize the studies as strong, moderate, weak, or poor. Only the 11 "strong" studies were included in the review.

For metasyntheses, Paterson, Thorne, Canam, and Jillings (2001) have developed the Primary Research Appraisal Tool as a systematic means of reviewing and evaluating qualitative studies. This protocol covers such aspects of a qualitative study as the sampling procedure, data gathering strategy, data analysis, researcher credentials, and researcher reflexivity. At the end of the process, the reviewer makes a decision to include the qualitative study in the metasynthesis or to reject it.

In meta-analyses, the evaluation usually involves a quantitative rating of the scientific merit of each study. AHRQ (2002) has published a guide that describes and evaluates various systems and instruments to rate the strength of evidence in quantitative medical and health studies. Based on a comprehensive review of the literature, the authors identified 121 instruments or systems, only 19 of which fully address quality domains AHRQ deemed to be essential. One of these 19 was developed by a British team working at the Royal College of Nursing Institute at the University of Oxford (Sindhu, Carpenter, & Seers, 1997). Deeks, Dinnes, D'Amico, Sowden, Sakarovitch, Song, Petticrew, and Altman (2003) reviewed 194 instruments for assessing the rigour of nonexperimental intervention studies and recommended only 6 for future use; one of these was developed by a team from Ontario that included nurse researchers (Thomas, Ciliska, Dobbins, & Micucci, 2004).

> ### Example of quality assessment tool
>
> The goal of the previously mentioned Effective Public Health Practice Project (EPHPP) is to assess research evidence to support the development of practice guidelines. The project team undertakes integrative reviews and has developed a quality assessment tool appropriate for evaluating various research designs. The EPHPP instrument provides explicit rules for ratings of *strong, moderate,* or *weak* for six components of the study under review: sample selection, study design, treatment of confounders, blinding, reliability and validity of measures, and withdrawals and dropouts. Studies with no *weak* ratings and at least four *strong* ratings are considered strong studies (Thomas, Ciliska, Dobbins, & Micucci, 2004).

Quality assessments in integrative reviews should involve ratings by two or more qualified individuals. If there are disagreements between the two raters, there should be a discussion until a consensus has been reached, or, if necessary, a third rater should be asked to help resolve the difference. Indexes of interrater reliability are often calculated to demonstrate to readers that rater agreement was adequate.

EXTRACTING AND RECORDING DATA FOR INTEGRATIVE REVIEWS

The next step in an integrative review is to extract and record relevant information about study characteristics, methods, and findings. Reviewers often use a written protocol to record such information. The goal of this task is to produce a *data set*, and procedures similar to those used in creating a data set with raw data from individual participants also apply. Examples of the type of methodologic information that reviewers record for each study include type of research design and sample size. Characteristics of the study participants (e.g., age, gender) are usually recorded, as well as information about the data source (e.g., year of publication, country where the study took place). For a meta-analysis, all information would be numerically coded for statistical analysis.

Finally, and most importantly, information about the results must be extracted and recorded. In a narrative review, results are usually noted with a verbal summary or simple classification (e.g., nonsignificant versus significant group difference). In a metasynthesis, the information to be recorded includes the key metaphors, themes, or categories from each study. In a meta-analysis, as we subsequently discuss, the information to be recorded might include group means and standard deviations, and, most importantly, the **effect size**, that is, the index summarizing the magnitude of the relationship between the independent and dependent variables.

As with ratings of quality, extraction and coding of information ideally should be completed by two or more people, at least for a portion of the studies in the sample. This allows for an assessment of interrater agreement, which should be sufficiently high to persuade readers of the review that the recorded information is accurate.

Example of interrater agreement

DiCenso, Guyatt, Willan, and Griffith (2002) did a meta-analysis of interventions to reduce unintended pregnancies among adolescents. Two independent reviewers extracted data from 22 reports and assessed methodologic quality using a formal rating tool. Discrepancies were resolved by joint review and consensus. The assessments were also shared with authors of the primary studies, who provided additional information when necessary.

ANALYZING DATA IN INTEGRATIVE REVIEWS

In narrative integrative reviews, reviewers interpret the pattern of findings, draw conclusions about the evidence, and derive implications for practice and further research. There are various methods of qualitatively analyzing the data for narrative reviews, although many reviewers appear to rely primarily on judgments and do not make clear the rules of inference they used. Stetler and her colleagues (1998) have argued that analysis and synthesis in narrative integrative reviews should be a group process and that a whole review team should meet to discuss their conclusions after reviewing synopsised studies.

In a metasynthesis, data analysis involves transforming individual findings into a new conceptualization. Noblit and Hare (1988) provide one approach to metasynthesis. Their method consists of making a list of key metaphors from each study and determining their relation to each other. Are the metaphors, for example, directly comparable (reciprocal)? Are they in opposition to each other (refutational)? Next, the studies' metaphors are translated into each other. Noblit and Hare noted that "translations are especially unique syntheses because they protect the particular, respect holism, and enable comparison. An adequate translation maintains the central metaphors and/or concepts of each account in their relation to other key metaphors or concepts in that account" (1988, p. 28). This synthesis of qualitative studies creates a whole that is more than the sum of the parts of the individual studies.

Example of data analysis in a metasynthesis

Beck (2002) used Noblit and Hare's approach in her metasynthesis of 18 qualitative studies on postpartum depression. As part of the analysis, key metaphors were listed for each study and organized under four overarching themes, one being "spiraling downward." For instance, in one study included in the metasynthesis, the key metaphors listed under this theme included "total isolation; façade of normalcy; obsessive thoughts; pervasive guilt; panic/overanxious/feels trapped; completely overwhelmed by infant demands; anger" (p. 459).

Meta-analysts analyze their data quantitatively using objective, standardized procedures. The essence of a meta-analysis is the calculation of a common metric—an *effect size*—for every study. The effect size represents the magnitude of the impact of an intervention on an outcome, or the degree of association between variables. Formulas for effect size differ depending on the nature of the statistical test used in the original analysis. The simplest formula to understand is the effect size for the difference between two means (e.g., an experimental group versus a control group). In this situation, the effect size for an outcome variable equals the mean for one group, minus the mean for the second group, divided by the overall standard deviation. Effect sizes for individual studies are then pooled across studies and averaged to yield estimates of population effects. These average effect sizes yield information about not only the *existence* of a relationship between variables but also the *magnitude*. Meta-analysts can, for example, draw conclusions about how big an effect an intervention has (with a specified probability of accuracy), which can yield estimates of the intervention's cost-effectiveness.

Meta-analysts can also examine whether there are **moderator effects** (or **subgroup effects**), that is, whether the relationship between an independent variable and a dependent variable is *moderated* by a third variable. For example, effect sizes can be computed separately for key subgroups (e.g., men versus women, children versus adolescents) to determine whether effects or relationships differ for segments of a population or variants of an intervention.

Some meta-analysts exclude studies that fail to meet a specified level of quality. Others prefer to retain methodologically weak studies in the dataset, and then to "downweight"

CONSUMER TIP

It is difficult to provide explicit guidance on whether an effect size is "large" because it depends on the circumstances. However, it might help to know that effect sizes for comparing two group means are in standard deviation units. Thus, an effect size of 1.0 in an experimental–control group comparison would mean that the experimental group's average score was a full standard deviation higher (or lower) than that for the control group. This would be considered a very large effect size. An effect size of .50 typically would be considered a moderate effect. ■

Example of subgroup analysis in a meta-analysis

Dennis and Creedy (2004) did a Cochrane review on the effectiveness of interventions for preventing postpartum depression (PPD). The meta-analysis of 15 clinical trials indicated that, overall, such interventions were no more effective than standard care in reducing the risk of PPD. However, subgroup analyses suggested that certain *types* of interventions were more effective than standard care (e.g., intensive postpartum support by nurses).

them in the analysis. For example, weights proportional to the quality rating can be assigned so that more rigorous studies "count" more in developing estimates of effects. Another approach is to conduct **sensitivity analyses**. This involves doing the statistical analyses twice, first including low-quality studies and then excluding them to see if including them changes the conclusions, or comparing the effect sizes for low-quality versus higher-quality studies.

Example of a sensitivity analysis

Devine (2003) conducted a meta-analyses of 25 studies that examined the effect of psychoeducational interventions on pain in adults with cancer. When analyzed across all studies, there was a significant, beneficial effect on pain. Study quality was quite varied, however. When Devine limited her analysis to studies with the best methodologic quality, the effect on pain continued to be significant.

EVALUATING THE BODY OF EVIDENCE

The emphasis on evidence-based practice has led to the development of systems not only for appraising and rating individual studies but also for evaluating the strength of a body of evidence. The report by AHRQ (2002) identified seven such systems as being especially useful, four of which were specifically created for use in developing practice guidelines. As an example, one system was developed by the Institute for Clinical Systems Improvement (ICSI), a collaboration of 17 medical groups in Minnesota (Greer, Mosser, Logan, & Halaas, 2000). ICSI has used its system to develop numerous practice guidelines and technology assessment reports. An example of an ICSI guideline developed in 2004 is "The Assessment and Management of Acute Pain" (*http://www.icsi.org*).

The AHRQ report identified three domains that are important in systems to grade the strength of a body of evidence on a topic: (1) *quality*—the aggregate of quality ratings for individual studies; (2) *quantity*—the magnitude of effect, number of studies, and aggregate sample size; and (3) *consistency*—the extent to which similar findings are reported using similar and different study designs. The ICSI system addresses all three domains.

Meta-analysts do not typically apply a formal system such as the one developed by ICSI to the body of evidence under review. However, their conclusions should include comments about the three domains of quality, quantity, and consistency.

THE WRITTEN INTEGRATIVE REVIEW

Reports for integrative reviews typically follow the same format as a research report for a primary study. That is, there is typically an introduction, method section, results section, and discussion. An abstract summarizing the major features of the review project is important. The method section should be thorough: readers of the review need to be able to assess the validity of the findings by understanding and critiquing the procedures the reviewers used.

A well-written and thorough conclusion or discussion section is especially crucial in integrative reviews. The discussion should include an overall summary of the findings, the reviewers' assessment of the strength and limitations of the body of evidence, what further research should be undertaken to extend the evidence base, and what the implications of the review are for clinicians and patients.

The review should also discuss the consistency of findings across studies and provide an interpretation of why there might be inconsistency. Did the samples, research designs, or data collection strategies in the studies differ in important ways? Or do differences reflect substantive differences, such as variation in the interventions or outcomes themselves?

Dissemination efforts for integrative reviews are even more important than for primary studies. Ideally, the review should be made available in a variety of formats and to a wide audience.

Critiquing Integrative Reviews

Like primary studies, integrative reviews should be thoroughly critiqued before the findings are deemed trustworthy and relevant to clinicians. Box 18.4 offers guidelines for evaluating integrative reviews.

Although these guidelines are fairly broad, not all questions apply equally well to all integrative reviews. For example, the question on subgroups under the "Data Analysis" questions is relevant primarily for integrative reviews of quantitative studies. Moreover, questions in Box 18.4 are not necessarily comprehensive. Supplementary questions might be needed for certain types of review.

In drawing conclusions about an integrative review, one issue is to evaluate whether the reviewer did a good job in pulling together and summarizing the evidence, as suggested by the questions in Box 18.4. Another aspect, however, is drawing inferences about how you might use the evidence in your own practice. It is not the reviewer's job, for example, to consider such issues as barriers to making use of the evidence, acceptability of an innovation, costs and benefits of change in various settings, and so on. These are issues for practicing nurses seeking to maximize the effectiveness of their actions and decisions.

BOX 18.4   Guidelines for Critiquing Integrative Reviews

The Problem

Does the review clearly state the research problem and/or research questions? Is the topic of the review important for the nursing profession? Is the scope of the review appropriate? Are concepts, variables, or phenomena adequately defined?

Search Strategy

Does the review clearly describe the criteria for selecting primary studies, and are those criteria reasonable? Are the databases the reviewers used identified, and are they appropriate? Are key words identified, and are they appropriate? Did the reviewers use adequate supplementary efforts to identify relevant studies, including nonpublished studies?

The Sample

Did the search strategy yield an adequate sample of studies? Did the studies include an adequate sample of participants? If an original report was lacking key information, did the reviewers attempt to contact the original researchers for additional information—or did the study have to be excluded? If studies were excluded for reasons other than insufficient information, did the reviewers provide a rationale for the decision? Did the reviewers retrieve primary source materials (i.e., the actual study reports), or did they draw their data from secondary sources?

Quality Appraisal

Did the reviewers determine the methodologic comparability of the studies in the review? Did the reviewers use appropriate procedures for appraising the quality of individual studies? Were formal criteria used in the appraisal, and were those criteria explicit? Were the criteria appropriate for the type of studies in the sample? Did two or more raters do the appraisals, and was interrater reliability reported?

The Data Set

Were two or more coders used to extract and record information for analysis? Was adequate information extracted about substantive, methodologic, and administrative aspects of the study? Was sufficient information extracted to permit subgroup analysis (if appropriate)? In a meta-analysis, was it possible to compute effect sizes for a sufficient number of studies in the sample?

Data Analysis

Do the reviewers explain their method of pooling and integrating their data? In a meta-synthesis, do the reviewers describe the techniques they used to compare the findings of each study, and do they explain their method of interpreting their data? Was the analysis of data objective and thorough? Were appropriate procedures used to address differences in methodologic quality among studies in the sample? Were appropriate subgroup analyses undertaken—or was the absence of subgroup analyses justified?

Conclusions

Did the reviewers draw reasonable conclusions about the quality, quantity, and consistency of evidence? In a metasynthesis, did the synthesis achieve a fuller understanding of the phenomenon to advance knowledge? Are limitations of the review noted? Are implications for nursing practice and further research clearly stated?

RESEARCH EXAMPLES | **Critical Thinking Activities**

EXAMPLE 1: A Meta-Analytic Integrative Review

Aspects of a meta-analysis, featuring terms and concepts discussed in this chapter, are presented below, followed by some questions to guide critical thinking.

Study
"Reducing venipuncture and intravenous insertion pain with eutectic mixture of local anesthetic" (Fetzer, 2002)

Purpose
The purpose of the study was to identify and synthesize research on the effectiveness of a eutectic mixture of local anaesthetics (EMLA) on venipuncture (VE) and intravenous (IV) insertion pain. The study also explored whether the effect is moderated by various other factors (e.g., patients' age, duration of application, research design, date of the research).

Eligibility Criteria
A primary study was included in the sample if (1) the design was a true experiment or repeated measures, (2) EMLA was administered as the intervention, (3) the control group received a placebo cream without active compounds (i.e., not with a different anaesthetic treatment), (4) the procedure involved needle puncture of the skin and underlying vein, (5) pain was measured by self-report, (6) adequate information was available to compute an effect size, (7) the report was in English, and (8) the report was published between 1980 and 2000.

Search Strategy
Fetzer used a variety of search procedures, including online databases (CINAHL, Medline), online journals, citations in bibliographies (the ancestry method), dissertation abstracts, and networking at conferences. The key words used in searches were EMLA, eutectic mixture local anaesthesia, lidocaine and prilocaine cream, dermal anaesthesia, VE pain, and IV insertion pain.

Sample
Twenty-two reports met the inclusion criteria, but three had to be eliminated (e.g., one was a duplicate of another study), yielding 19 reports for the meta-analysis. There were 7 studies on VE pain, with data based on 542 subjects in Canada, the United States, and Europe. There were 13 studies on IV pain, with more than 600 subjects from Canada, the United States, Europe, and Asia.

Quality Assessments
A quality index for each study was calculated using a scoring system adapted from Beck. Scores could range, theoretically, from 6 to 26. The actual range of scores for the 19 studies was 13 to 20.

Critical Thinking Activities (continued)

Data Extraction and Coding

A formal protocol was used to extract information about each study. The variables included substantive ones (e.g., health status of subjects, age and gender of subjects, puncture site); methodologic ones (sample size, research design, pain measurement method); and miscellaneous factors (e.g., country and date of study). Each study was independently coded by two nurse researchers. Rate of agreement on variables ranged from 97% to 100%, and discrepancies were resolved.

Data Analysis

Computer software was used to calculate effect sizes, which were computed three ways: unweighted, weighted by sample size, and weighted by quality rating. The effect size was found to be smallest when weighted by sample size, and these were the results reported.

Key Findings

▶ The beneficial effect of EMLA on pain was substantial across studies for both VE and IV. The mean effect sizes were 1.05 for VE pain and 1.04 for IV pain.

▶ The effect sizes for VE and IV pain were not moderated by any substantive variable; that is, effects were similarly beneficial for patients of different ages, with different health statuses, and so on.

Discussion

Fetzer concluded that EMLA cream has a large effect on both VE and IV insertion pain and that the effectives of EMLA did not appear to be diminished in relation to patient characteristics or insertion technique. Fetzer did note, however, that caution is appropriate in interpreting the moderator findings because the number of studies in the various subgroups was limited. Fetzer recommended the use of EMLA cream to reduce pain, especially for patients at highest risk of insertion pain and associated side effects.

Critical Thinking Suggestions*

*See the Student Resource CD-ROM for a discussion of these questions.

1. Answer appropriate questions from Box 18.4 regarding this study.
2. Also consider the following targeted questions, which may assist you in further assessing aspects of the study:
   a. Comment on Fetzer's decision to include studies from countries outside North America.
   b. As it turns out, all of the studies in the meta-analysis were in published journals. Comment on what this might mean.
3. If the results of this study are valid and reliable, what are some of the uses to which the findings might be put in clinical practice?

(Research Examples continue on page 478)

Critical Thinking Activities (continued)

 ### EXAMPLE 2: A Metasynthesis

Aspects of a metasynthesis, featuring terms and concepts discussed in this chapter, are presented below, followed by some questions to guide critical thinking.

Study
"Adolescent motherhood: A meta-synthesis of qualitative studies" (Clemmens, 2003)

Purpose
The purpose of the study was to synthesize qualitative studies on the phenomenon of adolescent motherhood.

Eligibility Criteria
A study was included if the phenomenon under investigation was the experience of adolescent motherhood and if a qualitative approach was used, regardless of research tradition. Studies were excluded if the focus was on depression in adolescent mothers or if the study findings were not organized into themes or metaphors on the experience of adolescent motherhood.

Search Strategy
Clemmens searched the following databases for studies published between 1990 and 2001 with the keywords "adolescent motherhood" and "qualitative studies": CINAHL, Medline, PsychINFO, ERIC, Sociological Abstracts, and Dissertation Abstracts.

Sample
Of the 50 studies initially identified, 18 met the sample inclusion and exclusion criteria. The 18 studies included 7 descriptive studies, 5 interpretive/phenomenological studies, 3 grounded theory studies, and 3 ethnographies. Thirteen were from published journal articles, and 5 were from dissertations. The combined sample of participants included 257 adolescent mothers from Canada, the United States, Australia, England, and China.

Data Extraction and Analysis
Noblit and Hare's (1988) comparative approach was used to compare study findings. The original metaphors, themes, concepts, and phrases from each of the 18 studies were organized into a grid and then reciprocally translated, one into the other, resulting in the construction of an initial list of metaphors. The complexity of experiences required a second level of analysis that revealed five overarching metaphors.

Key Findings
The five overarching metaphors were:
❱ The reality of motherhood brings hardships;
❱ Living in the two worlds of adolescence and motherhood;

Critical Thinking Activities (continued)

▶ Motherhood as positively transforming;
▶ Baby as a stabilizing influence; and
▶ Supportive context as turning point for future.

Discussion

Clemmens concluded that the metasynthesis provides nurses with a comprehensive picture of adolescent motherhood. She argued that nurses working in hospital, home care, and school settings can use the results to help develop appropriate interventions, and she offered some examples. She noted that the regularity of the themes and metaphors was important considering the diversity of racial backgrounds and cultures in the original studies.

Critical Thinking Suggestions

1. Answer appropriate questions from Box 18.4 regarding this study.
2. Also consider the following targeted questions, which may assist you in further assessing aspects of the study:
   a. Comment on Clemmens' decision to include studies from countries outside of North America.
   b. Comment on Clemmens' decision to include studies from various qualitative research traditions.
3. If the results of this study are trustworthy, what are some of the uses to which the findings might be put in clinical practice?

CHAPTER REVIEW
Summary Points

▶ **Research utilization** (RU) and **evidence-based practice** (EBP) are overlapping concepts that concern efforts to use research as a basis for clinical decisions. RU starts with research findings that get evaluated for possible use in practice. EBP starts with a search for the best possible evidence for a clinical problem, with emphasis on research-based evidence.

▶ Research utilization exists on a continuum, with direct utilization of some specific innovation at one end (**instrumental utilization**) and more diffuse situations in which users are influenced in their thinking about an issue based on some research (**conceptual utilization**) at the other end.

▶ Several major utilization projects have been implemented (e.g., the **Conduct and Utilization of Research in Nursing**—or CURN—**project**), which have demonstrated that research utilization can be increased but which have also shed light on barriers to utilization.

▶ EBP, which de-emphasizes clinical decision making based on custom or ritual, integrates the best available research evidence with other sources of data, including clinical expertise and patient preferences.

▶ In nursing, EBP and RU efforts often face various barriers, including methodologically weak or unreplicated studies, nurses' limited training in research and EBP, lack of organizational support, resource constraints, and limited communication and collaboration between practitioners and researchers.

▶ Many models of RU and EBP have been developed, including models for individual clinicians (e.g., the **Stetler Model**) and models for organizations or groups of clinicians (e.g., the **Iowa Model of Evidence-Based Practice to Promote Quality Care**, the **Ottawa Model of Research Use**).

▶ Most models of utilization involve the following steps: selecting a topic or problem; assembling and evaluating evidence; assessing the **implementation potential** of an evidence-based innovation; implementing the innovation and evaluating outcomes; and deciding whether to adopt or modify the innovation or revert to prior practices.

▶ Assessing implementation potential includes the dimensions of transferability of findings, the feasibility of using the findings in the new setting, and the cost/benefit ratio of a new practice.

▶ EBP relies on integration of research evidence on a topic through **integrative reviews**, which are rigorous, systematic inquiries with many similarities to original primary studies.

▶ Integrative reviews can involve either qualitative, narrative approaches to integration (including metasynthesis of qualitative studies), or quantitative (meta-analytic) methods.

▶ Integrative reviews typically involve the following activities: developing a question or hypothesis; assembling a review team; searching for and selecting a sample of studies to be included in the review; doing quality assessments of the studies; extracting and recording data from the sampled studies; analyzing the data; and writing up the review.

▶ Quality assessments (which may involve formal quantitative ratings) are sometimes used to exclude weak studies from integrative reviews but can also be used in **sensitivity analyses** to determine whether including or excluding weaker studies changes conclusions.

▶ Meta-analysis involves the computation of an **effect size** (which quantifies the magnitude of relationship between the independent and dependent variables) for every study in the sample, and averaging across studies. Meta-analysts can also test for **moderator** (or **subgroup**) **effects**, that is, whether effects are moderated by a third variable.

Additional Resources for Review

Chapter 18 of the *study Guide to Accompany Essentials of Nursing Research,* 6th edition offers various exercises and study suggestions for reinforcing the concepts presented in this chapter. Also, the *Study Guide* includes two full integrative reviews (a meta-analysis and a metasynthesis) reproduced in their entirety. For additional review, see the Student Self-Study Review Questions section of the Student Resource CD-ROM provided with this book.

SUGGESTED READINGS

References for studies cited in this chapter appear at the end of the book.

Methodologic and Nonempirical References

Agency for Healthcare Research and Quality. (2002). *Systems to rate the strength of scientific evidence.* Washington, DC: Author.

Alberta Association of Registered Nurses. (1997). Nursing research dissemination and utilization. Retrieved October, 2003, from Alberta Association of Registered Nurses Website, *http://www.nurses.ab.ca/publications/papers/html.*

Beck, C. T. (1997). Use of meta-analysis as a teaching strategy in nursing research courses. *Journal of Nursing Education, 36,* 87–90.

Caplan, N., & Rich, R. F. (1975). *The use of social science knowledge in policy decisions at the national level.* Ann Arbor, MI: Institute for Social Research, University of Michigan.

Cooper, H. (1984). The integrative research review: A social science approach. Beverly Hills, CA: Sage Publications.

Deeks, J. J., Dinnes, J., D'Amico, R., Sowden, A. J., Sakarovitch, C., Song, F., Pettigrew, M., & Altman, D. G. (2003). Evaluating non-randomized intervention studies. *Health Technology Assessment, 7,* 1–173.

Estabrooks, C. E. (2001). Research utilization and qualitative research. In J. M. Morse, J. M. Swanson, & A. J. Kuzel (Eds), *The nature of qualitative evidence* (pp. 275–298). Thousand Oaks, CA: Sage Publications.

Gennaro, S., Hodnett, E., & Kearney, M. (2001). Making evidence-based practice a reality in your institution. *Maternal Child Nursing, 26,* 236–244.

Goode, C., & Piedalue, F. (1999). Evidence based clinical practice. *Journal of Nursing Administration, 29*(6), 15–21.

Greer, N., Mosser, G., Logan, G., & Halaas, G. W. (2000). A practical approach to evidence grading. *Joint Commission Journal on Quality Improvement, 26,* 700–712.

Grinspun, D., Virani, T., & Bajnok, I. (2001–2002). Nursing best practice guidelines: The RNAO (Registered Nurses Association of Ontario) project. *Hospital Quarterly, 5*(2), 56–60.

Logan, J., & Graham, I. (1998). Toward a comprehensive interdisciplinary model of health care research use. *Science Communication, 20,* 227–246.

Logan, J., Harrison, M. B., Graham, I. D., Dunn, K., & Bissonnette, J. (1999). Evidence-based pressure-ulcer practice: The Ottawa Model of Research Use. *Canadian Journal of Nursing Research, 31,* 37–52.

Noblit, G. & Hare, R. D. (1988). *Meta-ethnography: Synthesizing qualitative studies.* Newbury Park, CA: Sage Publications.

Paterson, B. L., Thorne, S. E., Canam, C., & Jillings, C. (2001). *Meta-study of qualitative health research.* Thousand Oaks, CA: Sage Publications.

Rosenfeld, P., Duthie, E., Bier, J., Bower-Ferres, S., Fulmer, T., Iervolino, L., McClure, M., McGivern, D., & Roncoli, M. (2000). Engaging staff nurses in evidence-based research to identify nursing practice problems and solutions. *Applied Nursing Research, 13,* 197–203.

Rosswurm, M. A., & Larrabee, J. H. (1999). A model for change to evidence-based practice. *Image: Journal of Nursing Scholarship, 31,* 317–322.

Sackett, D. L., Rosenberg, W., Gray, J. A., Haynes, R., & Richardson, W. (1996). Evidence based medicine: What it is and what it isn't. *British Medical Journal, 312,* 71–72.

Sandelowski, M. (2004). Using qualitative research. *Qualitative Health Research, 14,* 1366–1386.

Sindhu, F., Carpenter, L., & Seers, K. (1997). Development of a tool to rate the quality assessment of randomized controlled trials using a Delphi technique. *Journal of Advanced Nursing, 25,* 1262–1268.

Stetler, C. B. (1994). Refinement of the Stetler/Marram model for application of research findings into practice. *Nursing Outlook, 42,* 15–25.

Stetler, C. B. (2001). Updating the Stetler Model of Research Utilization to facilitate evidence-based practice. *Nursing Outlook, 49,* 272–279.

Stetler, C. B., Morsi, D., Rucki, S., Broughton, S., Corrigan, B., Fitzgerald, J., Giuliano, K., Havener, P., & Sheridan, E. A. (1998). Utilization-focused integrative reviews in a nursing service. *Applied Nursing Research, 11,* 195–206.

Thomas, B. H., Ciliska, D., Dobbins, M., & Micucci, B. A. (2004). A process for systematically reviewing the literature: Providing the research evidence for public health nursing interventions. *Worldviews on Evidence Based Nursing, 1,* 176–184.

Thorne, S., Jensen, L., Kearney, M. H., Noblit, G., & Sandelowski, M. (2004). Qualitative metasynthesis: Reflections on methodological orientation and ideological agenda. *Qualitative Health Research, 14,* 1342–1354.

Titler, M. G., Kleiber, C., Steelman, V., Goode, C., Rakel, B., Barry-Walker, J., Small, S., & Buckwalter, J. (1994). Infusing research into practice to promote quality care. *Nursing Research, 43,* 307–313.

Titler, M. G., Kleiber, C., Steelman, V., Rakel, B., Budreau, G., Everett, L., Buckwalter, K., Tripp-Reimer, T., & Goode, C. (2001). The Iowa Model of Evidence-Based Practice to Promote Quality Care. *Critical Care Nursing Clinics of North America, 13,* 497–509.

Weiss, C. (1980). Knowledge creep and decision accretion. *Knowledge: Creation, Diffusion, Utilization, 1,* 381–404.

World Wide Web Sites

▶ AHCPR/AHRQ Clinical Practice Guidelines
   http://www.ahrq.gov and *http://www.guidelines.gov*
▶ The Cochrane Collaboration
   http://www.cochrane.org/
▶ Evidence Based Clinical Practice (McMaster University, Hamilton, Ontario)
   http://www-hsl.mcmaster.ca/ebcp
▶ Health Care Guidelines
   http://evidence.ahc.umn.edu/health_care_guidelines.htm
▶ Registered Nurses Association of Ontario Best Practice Guidelines
   http://www.rnao.org/bestpractices
▶ University of Alberta University of Alberta's "Evidence-Based Medicine Tool Kit"
   http://www.med.ualberta.ca/ebm/ebm.htm
▶ University of Iowa's Evidence Based Practice Center
   http://www.uihealthcare.com/depts/nursing/rqom/evidencebasedpractice/toolkit.html
▶ University of Sheffield (United Kingdom), "Netting the Evidence"
▶ *http://www.shef.ac.uk/scharr/ir/netting/*

Studies Cited in Chapters

Adlaf, E. M., Gliksman, L., Demers, A., & Newton-Taylor, B. (2003). Illicit drug use among Canadian university undergraduates. *Canadian Journal of Nursing Research, 35,* 24–43. (Chapter 13)

Aïta, M., & Goulet, C. (2003). Assessment of neonatal nurses' behaviors that prevent overstimulation in preterm infants. *Intensive and Critical Care Nursing, 19,* 109–118. (Chapter 8)

Angus, J., Evans, S., Lapum, J., Rukholm, E., St. Onge, R., Nolan, R., & Michel, I. (2005). "Sneaky disease": The body and health knowledge for people at risk for coronary heart disease in Ontario, Canada. *Social Science & Medicine, 60,* 2117–2128. (Chapter 1)

Angus, J., Kontos, P., Dyck, I., McKeever, P., & Poland, B. (2005). The personal significance of home: Habitus and the experience of receiving long-term home care. *Sociology of Health & Illness, 27,* 161–187. (Chapter 10)

Babenko-Mould, Y., Andrusyszen, M., & Goldenberg, D. (2004). Effects of computer-based clinical conferencing on nursing students' self-efficacy. *Journal of Nursing Education, 43,* 149–155. (Chapter ?)

Bailey, P. H. (2004). The dyspnea-anxiety-dyspnea cycle—COPD patients' stories of breathlessness: "It's scary/when you can't breathe." *Qualitative Health Research, 14,* 760–778. (Chapter 1)

Banister, E. M., Jakubec, S. L., & Stein, J. A. (2003). 'Like what am I supposed to do?': Adolescent girls' health concerns in their dating relationships. *Canadian Journal of Nursing Research, 35,* 16–33. (Chapter 5, 14)

Bartfay, W. J., & Bartfay, E. (2002). Decreasing effects of iron toxicosis on selenium and glutathione peroxidase activity. *Western Journal of Nursing Research, 24,* 119–131. (Chapter 5)

Bauer, N., Bushey, F., & Amaros, D. (2002). Diffusion of responsibility and pressure ulcers. *World Council of Enterostomal Therapist Journal, 22*(3), 9–18. (Chapter 18)

Beardwood, B. A., & French, S. E. (2004). Mediating complaints against nurses: A consumer-oriented educational approach. *Canadian Journal of Nursing Research, 36*(1), 122–141. (Chapter 16)

Beck, C. T. (1992). The lived experience of postpartum depression. *Nursing Research, 41,* 166–170. (Chapter 14)

Beck, C. T. (1993). Teetering on the edge: A substantive theory of postpartum depression. *Nursing Research, 42,* 42–48. (Chapter 6, 14)

Beck, C. T. (1996). Postpartum depressed mothers' experiences interacting with their children. *Nursing Research, 45,* 98–104. (Chapter 6, 14)

Beck, C. T. (2001). Predictors of postpartum depression: An update. *Nursing Research, 50,* 275–285. (Chapter 6)

Beck, C. T. (2002). Postpartum depression: A metasynthesis. *Qualitative Health Research, 12,* 453–472. (Chapter 18)

Beck, C. T. (2002). Releasing the pause button: Mothering twins during the first year of life. *Qualitative Health Research, 12,* 593–608. (Chapter 3, 12, 13, 16)

Beck, C. T. (2004). Birth trauma: In the eye of the beholder. *Nursing Research, 53,* 28–35. (Chapter 16)

Beck, C. T. (2005). Benefits of participating in Internet interviews: Women helping women. *Qualitative Health Research, 15,* 411–422. (Chapter 5)

Beck, C. T., & Gable, R. K. (2000). Postpartum Depression Screening Scale: Development and psychometric testing, *Nursing Research, 49,* 272–282. (Chapter 3, 14)

Beck, C. T., & Gable, R. K. (2001). Ensuring content validity: An illustration of the process. *Journal of Nursing Measurement, 9,* 201–215. (Chapter 2)

Beck, C. T., & Gable, R. K. (2001). Further validation of the Postpartum Depression Screening Scale. *Nursing Research, 50,* 155–164. (Chapter 3, 14)

Beck, C. T., & Gable, R. K. (2002). Postpartum Depression Screening Scale manual. Los Angeles: Western Psychological Services. (Chapter 6)

Beck, C. T., & Gable, R. K. (2003). Postpartum Depression Screening Scale—Spanish Version. *Nursing Research, 52,* 296–306. (Chapter 6, 14)

Benzies, K. M., Harrison, M. J., & Magill-Evans, J. (2004a). Parenting and childhood behavior problems: Mothers' and fathers' voices. *Issues in Mental Health Nursing, 25,* 9–24. (Chapter 11)

Benzies, K. M., Harrison, M. J., & Magill-Evans, J. (2004b). Parenting stress, marital quality, and child behavior problems at age 7 years. *Public Health Nursing, 21,* 111–121. (Chapter 9, 11)

Bérubé, M., & Loiselle, C. G. (2003). L'incertitude, le coping et l'espoir chez les blessés médullaires. [Uncertainty, coping and hope among individuals with a spinal cord injury.] *L'Infirmière du Québec, 10,* 16–23. (Chapter 8)

Billinghurst, F., Morgan, B., & Arthur, H. M. (2003). Patient and nurse-related implications of remote cardiac telemetry. *Clinical Nursing Research, 12,* 356–370. (Chapter 13)

Black, C., & Ford-Gilboe, M. (2004). Adolescent mothers: Resilience, family health work and health-promoting practices. *Journal of Advanced Nursing, 48,* 351–360. (Chapter 6, 8)

Bluvol, A., & Ford-Gilboe, M. (2004). Hope, health work and quality of life in families of stroke survivors. *Journal of Advanced Nursing, 48,* 322–332. (Chapter 6, 8)

Boechler, V., Harrison, M. J., & Magill-Evans, J. (2003). Father-child teaching interactions: The relationship to father involvement in caregiving. *Journal of Pediatric Nursing, 18,* 46–51. (Chapter 9)

Bottorff, J. L., Ratner, P. A., Richardson, C., Balneaves, L. G., McCullum, M., Hack, T., Chalmers, K., & Buxton, J. (2003). The influence of question wording on assessments of interest in genetic testing for breast cancer risk. *Psychooncology, 12,* 720–728. (Chapter 11)

Bournes, D. A. (2002). Having courage: A lived experience of human becoming. *Nursing Science Quarterly, 15,* 220–229. (Chapter 8)

Brathwaite, A. C., & Cooper, C. C. (2004). Childbirth experiences of professional Chinese Canadian women. *Journal of Obstetric, Gynecologic, & Neonatal Nursing, 33,* 748–75. (Chapter 14)

Brooks, D., Sidani, S., Graydon, J., McBride, S., Hall, L., & Weinacht, K. (2003). Evaluating the effects of music on dyspnea during exercise in individuals with chronic obstructive pulmonary disease. *Rehabilitation Nursing, 28,* 192–196. (Chapter 9)

Browne, A. J., & Fiske, J. (2001). First Nations women's encounters with mainstream health services. *Western Journal of Nursing Research, 23,* 126–147. (Chapter 10)

Bruce, B. S., Lake, J. P., Eden, V. A., & Denney, J. C. (2004). Children at risk of injury. *Journal of Pediatric Nursing, 19,* 121–127. (Chapter 6)

Bryanton, J., Walsh, D., Barrett, M., & Gaudet, D. (2004). Tub bathing versus traditional sponge bathing for the newborn. *Journal of Obstetric, Gynecologic, & Neonatal Nursing, 33,* 704–712. (Chapter 13)

Care, W. D., & Udod, S. A. (2003). Perceptions of first-line nurse managers: What competencies are needed to fulfill this role? *Nursing Leadership Forum, 7,* 109–115. (Chapter 13)

Cesario, S.' K. (2004). Reevaluation of Friedman's labor curve: A pilot study. *Journal of Obstetric, Gynecologic, & Neonatal Nursing, 33,* 713–722. (Chapter 15)

Chalmers, K., Gupton, A., Katz, A., Hack, T., Hildes-Ripstein, E., Brown, J., McMillan, D., Labossiere, D., Mackay, M., Pickerl, C., Savard-Preston, Y., Vincent, J. A., Morris, H. M., & Cann, B. (2004). The description and evaluation of a longitudinal pilot study of a smoking relapse/reduction intervention for perinatal women. *Journal of Advanced Nursing, 45,* 162–171. (Chapter 11)

Cheung, J., & Hocking, P. (2004). The experience of spousal carers of people with multiple sclerosis. *Qualitative Health Research, 14,* 153–166. (Chapter 16)

Chin-Peuckert, L., Rennick, J. E., Jednak, R., Capolicchio, J., & Salle, J. L. (2004). Should warm infusion solution be used for urodynamic studies in children? A prospective randomized study. *Journal of Urology, 172,* 1657–1661. (Chapter 13)

Chiu, L., Emblem, J. D., Van Hofwegen, L., Sawatzky, R., & Meyerhoff, H. (2004). An integrative review of the concept of spirituality in the health sciences. *Western Journal of Nursing Research, 26,* 405–428. (Chapter 2, 18)

Chouinard, M., Ntetu, A. L., Lapierre, R., Gagnon, D., & Hudon, M. (2004). [Evaluation by patients receiving nursing services in a cardiovascular disease prevention clinics network.] *Canadian Journal of Cardiovascular Nursing, 14*(2), 33–41. (Chapter 12)

Clark, A. M., Barbour, R. S., White, M., & MacIntyre, P. D. (2004). Promoting participation in cardiac rehabilitation: Patient choices and experiences. *Journal of Advanced Nursing, 47,* 5–14. (Chapter 13, 18)

Clemmens, D. A. (2002). Adolescent mothers' depression after the birth of their babies: Weathering the storm. *Adolescence, 37,* 551–565. (Chapter 16)

Clemmens, D. (2003). Adolescent motherhood: A metasynthesis of qualitative studies. *MCN The American Journal of Maternal/Child Nursing, 28,* 93–99. (Chapter 18)

Collins-Sharp, B. A., Taylor, D. L., Thomas, K. K., Killeen, M. B., & Dawood, M. Y. (In press). Cyclic perimenstrual pain and discomfort: The scientific basis for practice. *Journal of Obstetric, Gynecologic, & Neonatal Nursing, 33,* 637–649. (Chapter 18)

Conn, V. S., Valentine, J. C., Cooper, H. M., & Rantz, M. J. (2003). Grey literature in meta-analyses. *Nursing Research, 52,* 256–261. (Chapter 18)

Cossette, S., Frasure-Smith, N., & Lespérance, F. (2002). Nursing approaches to reducing psychological distress in men and women recovering from myocardial infarction. *International Journal of Nursing Studies, 39,* 479–494. (Chapter 8)

Côté, J. K., & Pepler, C. (2002). A randomized trial of a cognitive coping intervention for acutely ill HIV-positive men. *Nursing Research, 51,* 237–244. (Chapter 1, 8)

Côté, J. K., & Pepler, C. (2005). Cognitive coping intervention for acutely ill HIV-positive men. *Journal of Clinical Nursing, 14,* 321–326. (Chapter 1, 8)

Coulson, L., & Doran, D. M. (2003). Nurses' integration of outcomes assessment data into practice. *Outcomes Management, 8,* 13–18. (Chapter 13)

Coulson, I., Strang, V., Mariño, R., & Minichiello, V. (2004). Knowledge and lifestyle behaviors of healthy older adults related to modifying the onset of vascular dementia. *Archives of Gerontology and Geriatrics, 39,* 43–58. (Chapter 15)

Coyle, L. A., & Sokop, A. G. (1990). Innovation adoption behavior among nurses. *Nursing Research, 39,* 176–180. (Chapter 18)

Cummings, G., Hayduk, L., & Estabrooks, C. (2005). Mitigating the impact of hospital restructuring on nurses:

The responsibility of emotionally intelligent leadership. *Nursing Research, 54,* 2–12. (Chapter 1)

Davies, B. L., & Hodnett, E. (2002). Labor support Nurses' self-efficacy and views about factors influencing implementation. *Journal of Obstetric, Gynecologic, & Neonatal Nursing, 31,* 48–56. (Chapter 14)

Davies, B., Hodnett, E., Hannah, M., O'Brien-Pallas, L., Pringle, D., & Wells, G. (2002). Fetal health surveillance: A community-wide approach versus a tailored intervention for the implementation of clinical practice guidelines. *Canadian Medical Association Journal, 167,* 469–474. (Chapter 17)

Davison, B. J., & Degner, L. F. (2002). Feasibility of using a computer-assisted intervention to enhance the way women with breast cancer communicate with their physicians. *Cancer Nursing, 25,* 417–424. (Chapter 9)

Davison, B. J., Goldenberg, L., Gleave, M. E., & Degner, L. F. (2003). Provision of individualized information to men and their partners to facilitate treatment decision making in prostate cancer. *Oncology Nursing Forum, 30,* 107–114. (Chapter 5)

Degner, L. F., Hack, T., O'Neil, J., & Kristjanson, L. J. (2003). A new approach to eliciting meaning in the context of breast cancer. *Cancer Nursing, 26,* 169–178. (Chapter 1, 11)

DeJong-Watt, W. J., & Arthur, H. M. (2004). Anxiety and health-related quality of life in patients awaiting elective coronary angiography. *Heart & Lung, 33,* 237–248. (Chapter 1)

Dennis, C. L. (2002). Breastfeeding peer support: Maternal and volunteer perceptions from a randomized controlled trial. *Birth, 19,* 169–176. (Chapter 9)

Dennis, C. L. (2003). The Breastfeeding Self-Efficacy Scale: Psychometric assessment of the short form. *Journal of Obstetric, Gynecologic, & Neonatal Nursing, 32,* 734–744. (Chapter 14)

Dennis, C. L. (2004). Influence of depressive symptomatology on maternal health service utilization and general health. *Archives of Women's Mental Health, 7,* 183–191. (Chapter 15)

Dennis, C. L., & Creedy, D. (2004). Psychosocial and psychological interventions for preventing postpartum depression. *Cochrane Database of Systematic Reviews,* No. CD001134. (Chapter 18)

Dennis, C. L., & Stewart, D. E. (2004). Treatment of postpartum depression, Part 1: A critical review of biological interventions. *Journal of Clinical Psychiatry, 65,* 1242–1251. (Chapter 7, 18)

DeOliveira, E. A., & Hoga, L. A. (2005). The process of seeking and undergoing surgical contraception: An ethnographic study in a Bazilian community. *Journal of Transcultural Nursing, 16,* 5–14. (Chapter 16)

Devine, E. C. (2003). Meta-analysis of the effect of psycho-educational interventions on pain in adults with cancer. *Oncology Nursing Forum, 30,* 75–89. (Chapter 18)

Dewar, A. (2003). Boosting strategies: Enhancing the self-esteem of individuals with catastrophic illnesses and injuries. *Journal of Psychosocial Nursing & Mental Health Services, 41,* 24–32. (Chapter 1, 16)

Dewar. A. L., & Lee, F. A. (2000). Bearing illness and injury. *Western Journal of Nursing Research, 22,* 912–926. (Chapter 10)

DiCenso, A., Guyatt, G., Willan, A., & Griffith, L. (2002). Interventions to reduce unintended pregnancies among adolescents: Systematic review of randomised trials. *British Medical Journal, 324,* 1426–1436. (Chapter 18)

Dodd, V. L. (2005). Implications of kangaroo care for growth and devepment in preterm infants. *Journal of Obstetric, Gynecologic, & Neonatal Nursing, 34,* 218–232. (Chapter 1)

Doiron-Maillet, N., & Meagher-Stewart, D. (2003). The uncertain journey: Women's experiences following a myocardial infarction. *Canadian Journal of Cardiovascular Nursing, 13*(2), 14–23. (Chapter 12)

Drummond, J., Fleming, D., McDonald, L., & Kysela, G. M. (2005). Randomized controlled trial of a family problem-solving intervention. *Clinical Nursing Research, 14,* 57–80. (Chapter 13)

Duchscher, J. E., & Cowin, L. S. (2004). The experience of marginalization in new nursing graduates. *Nursing Outlook, 52,* 289–296. (Chapter 2)

Duggleby, W., & Wright, K. (2004). Elderly palliative care cancer patients' descriptions of hope-fostering strategies. *International Journal of Palliative Nursing, 10,* 352–359. (Chapter 6)

DuMont, J., & Parnis, D. (2003). Forensic nursing in the context of sexual assault: Comparing the opinions and practices of nurse examiners and nurses. *Applied Nursing Research, 16,* 173–183. (Chapter 5)

Durbin, J., Goering, P., Streiner, D. L., & Pink, G. (2004). Continuity of care: Validation of a new self-report measure for individuals using mental health services. *Journal of Behavioral Health Services and Research, 31,* 279–296. (Chapter 14)

Durbin, J., Goering, P., Streiner, D. L., & Pink, G. (2004). Program structure and continuity of mental health care. *Canadian Journal of Nursing Research, 36*(2), 12–37. (Chapter 12)

Egan, E., Clavarino, A., Burridge, L., Teuwen, M., & White, E. (2002). A randomized control trial of nursing-based case management for patients with chronic obstructive pulmonary disease. *Lippincott's Case Management, 7,* 170–179. (Chapter 11)

Epstein, I., Stinson, J., & Stevens, B. (2005). The effects of camp on health-related quality of life in children with chronic illnesses: A review of the literature. *Journal of Pediatric Oncology Nursing, 22,* 89–103. (Chapter 7)

Espin, S. L., & Lingard, L. A. (2001). Time as a catalyst for tension in nurse-surgeon communication. *AORN Journal, 74,* 672–682. (Chapter 10)

Estabrooks, C. A. (1999). The conceptual structure of research utilization. *Research in Nursing & Health, 22,* 203–216. (Chapter 18)

Estabrooks, C. A., Chong, H., Brigidear, K., Profetto-McGrath, J. (2005). Profiling Canadian nurses' preferred knowledge sources for clinical practice. *Canadian Journal of Nursing Research.* (Chapter 18)

Estabrooks, C. A., Midodzi, W. K., Cummings, G. G., Ricker, K. L., & Giovannetti, P. (2005). The impact of hospital nursing characteristics on 30-day mortality. *Nursing Research, 54,* 74–84. (Chapter 17)

Estabrooks, C. A., Rutakumwa, W., O'Leary, K. A., Profetto-McGrath, J., Milner, M., Levers, M. J., & Scott-Finlay, S. (2005). Sources of practice knowledge among nurses.

Qualitative Health Research, 15, 460–476. (Chapter 13, 16)

Estabrooks, C. A., Winther, C., & Derksen, L. (2004). Mapping the field: A bibliometric analysis of the research utilization literature in nursing. *Nursing Research, 53,* 293–313. (Chapter 18)

Evans, M. K., & O'Brien, B. (2005). Gestational diabetes: The meaning of an at-risk pregnancy. *Qualitative Health Research, 15,* 66–81. (Chapter 16)

Fergus, K. D., Gray, R. E., Fitch, M. I., Labreque, M., & Phillips, C. (2002). Active consideration: Conceptualizing patient-provided support for spouse caregivers in the context of prostate cancer. *Qualitative Health Research, 12,* 492–514. (Chapter 8)

Fetzer, S. J. (2002). Reducing venipuncture and intravenous insertion pain with eutectic mixture of local anesthetic. *Nursing Research, 51,* 119–124. (Chapter 18)

Fillion, L., Gélinas, C., Simard, S., Savard, J., & Gagnon, P. (2003). Validation evidence for the French Canadian adaptation of the Multidimensional Fatigue Inventory as a measure of cancer-related fatigue. *Cancer Nursing, 26,* 143–153. (Chapter 14)

Fisher, A. R., Wells, G., & Harrison, M. B. (2004). Factors associated with pressure ulcers in adults in acute care hospitals. *Advances in Skin & Wound Care, 17,* 80–90. (Chapter 15)

Fitch, M. I., Deane, K., & Howell, D. (2003). Living with ovarian cancer: Women's perspectives on treatment and treatment decision-making. *Canadian Oncology Nursing Journal, 13,* 8–20. (Chapter 11)

Fitch, M. I., Gray, R. E., DePetrillo, D., Franssen, E., & Howell, D. (1999). Canadian women's perspectives on ovarian cancer. *Cancer Prevention & Control, 3,* 52–60. (Chapter 11)

Fitch, M. I., Gray, R. E., & Franssen, E. (2000). Women's perspectives regarding the impact of ovarian cancer. *Cancer Nursing, 23,* 359–366. (Chapter 11)

Forbes, D. A. (2003). An example of the use of systematic reviews to answer an effectiveness question. *Western Journal of Nursing Research, 25,* 179–192. (Chapter 18)

Forbes, D. A., Stewart, N., Morgan, D., Anderson, M., Parent, K., & Janzen, B. L. (2003). Individual determinants of home-care nursing and housework assistance. *Canadian Journal of Nursing Research, 35,* 14–36. (Chapter 11)

Forchuk, C., Baruth, P., Prendergast, M., Holliday, R., Bareham, R., Brimmer, S., Schulz, V., Chan, Y. C., & Yammine, N. (2004). Postoperative arm massage: A support for women with lymph node dissection. *Cancer Nursing, 27,* 25–33. (Chapter 4)

Forchuk, C., Baruth, P., Prendergast, M., Holliday, R., Brimner, S., Bareham, R., Schulz, V., & Chan, L. (2001). Oral paper presentation. Post-Operative arm massage: A support for women with lymph node dissection and their families at the ICN 22nd Quadrennial Congress, June 10, 2001, Copenhagen, Denmark. (Chapter 4)

Forchuk, C., Baruth, P., Prendergast, M., Holliday, R. L., Brimner, S., Bareham, R., Schultz, V., & Chan, L. (2001). Poster presentation. Post-operative arm massage: A support for women with lymph node dissection and their families. University of Toronto Faculty of Nursing, International Research Conference, May 4, 2001, Toronto, Ontario, Canada. (Chapter 4)

Fortin, M., Lapointe, L., Hudon, C., Vanasse, A., Ntetu, A. L., & Maltais, D. (2004). Multimorbidity and quality of life in primary care. *Health & Quality of Life Outcomes, 2,* 51–61. (Chapter 7)

Fulford, A., & Ford-Gilboe, M. (2004). An exploration of the relationships between health promotion practices, health work, and flet stigma in families headed by adolescent mothers. *Canadian Journal of Nursing Research, 36*(4), 46–72. (Chapter 6, 8)

Gage-Rancoeur, D. M., & Purden, M. A. (2003). Daughters of cardiac patients: The process of caregiving. *Canadian Journal of Nursing Research, 35*(2), 90–105. (Chapter 13)

Gagnon, J., & Grenier, R. (2004). Élaboration et validation d'indicateurs de la qualité des soins relatifs à l'empowerment dans un context de maladie complexe à caractère chronique. [Evaluation and validation of quality care indicators relative to empowerment in complex chronic disease.] *Recherche en Soins Infirmiers, 76,* 50–67. (Chapter 8, 12)

Gagnon, J., Legendre-Parent, A., Vigneault, B., Marquis, F., Paquet, J., Michaud, D., & Gauyin, M. C. (2004). The impact of a case management approach for total hip and knee arthroplasty patients. *Perspectives Infirmières, 1,* 12–21. (Chapter 2)

Gaudine, A. P., & Saks, A. M. (2004). A longitudinal quasi-experiment on the effects of posttraining transfer interventions. *Human Resource Development Quarterly, 15,* 57–76. (Chapter 9)

Gaudine, A. P., & Beaton, M. R. (2002). Employed to go against one's values: Nurse managers' accounts of ethical conflict with their organization. *Canadian Journal of Nursing Research, 34*(2), 17–34. (Chapter 14)

Gaudine, A., Sturge-Jacobs, M., & Kennedy, M. (2003). The experience of waiting and life during breast cancer follow-up. *Research and Theory for Nursing Practice, 17,* 153–168. (Chapter 2)

Gélinas, C., & Fillion, L. (2004). Factors related to persistent fatigue following completion of breast cancer treatment. *Oncology Nursing Forum, 31,* 269–278. (Chapter 15)

Gélinas, C., Fortier, M., Viens, C., Fillion, L., & Puntillo, K. (2004). Pain assessment and management in critically ill intubated patients: A retrospective study. *American Journal of Critical Care, 13,* 126–135. (Chapter 13)

Gerrish, K., & Clayton, J. (2004). Promoting evidence-based practice: An organizational approach. *Journal of Nursing Management, 12,* 114–123. (Chapter 18)

Gibbins, S., Stevens, B., Hodnett, E., Pinelli, J., Ohlsson, A., & Darlington, G. (2002). Efficacy and safety of sucrose for procedural pain relief in preterm and term neonates. *Nursing Research, 51,* 375–382. (Chapter 13)

Goulet, C., Lampron, A., Marcil, I., & Ross, L. (2003). Attitudes and subjective norms of male and female adolescents toward breastfeeding. *Journal of Human Lactation, 19,* 402–410. (Chapter 8)

Goulet, C., Polomeno, V., Laizner, A. M., Marcil, I., & Lang, A. (2003). Translation and validation of a French version of Brown's Support Behaviors Inventory in perinatal health. *Western Journal of Nursing Research, 25,* 561–582. (Chapter 15)

Graham, I., & Logan, J. (2004). Using the Ottawa Model of Research Use to implement a skin care program. *Journal of Nursing Care Quality, 19,* 18–24. (Chapter 18)

Graham, I. D., Logan, J., Davies, B., & Nimrod, C. (2004). Changing the use of electronic fetal monitoring and labor support: A case study of barriers and facilitators. *Birth, 31*, 293–301. (Chapter 11, 18)

Grypma, S. (2004). Neither angels of mercy nor foreign devils: Revisioning Canadian missionary nurses in China, 1935–1947. *Nursing History Review, 12*, 97–119. (Chapter 10)

Hack, T. F., & Degner, L. F. (2004). Coping responses following breast cancer diagnosis predict psychological adjustment three years later. *Psychooncology, 13*, 235–247. (Chapter 6)

Hack, T. F., Degner, L. F., Watson, P., & Sinha, L. (2005). Do patients benefit from participating in medical decision making? Longitudinal follow-up of women with breast cancer. *Psychooncology, 24*. (Chapter 1)

Hall, L. M., & Doran, D. (2004). Nurse staffing, care delivery model, and patient care quality. *Journal of Nursing Care Quality, 19*, 27–33. (Chapter 11)

Hall, L. M., Doran, D., Baker, G. R., Pink, G. H., Sidani, S., O'Brien-Pallas, L., & Donner, G. J. (2003). Nurse staffing models as predictors of patient outcomes. *Medical Care, 41*, 1096–1109. (Chapter 11)

Hall, L. M., Doran, D., & Pink, G. H. (2004). Nurse staffing models, nursing hours, and patient safety outcomes. *Journal of Nursing Administration, 34*, 41–45. (Chapter 9)

Hall, W. A., & Callery, P. (2003). Balancing personal and family trajectories: An international study of dual-earner couples with pre-school children. *Internatioanal Journal of Nursing Studies, 40*, 401–412. (Chapter 12)

Hamilton, D. M., & Haennel, R. G. (2004). The relationship of self-efficacy to selected outcomes. *Canadian Journal of Cardiovascular Nursing, 14*(2), 23–32. (Chapter 8)

Harkness, K., Morrow, L., Smith, K., Kiczula, M., & Arthur, H. M. (2003). The effect of early education on patient anxiety while waiting for elective cardiac catheterization. *European Journal of Cardiovascular Nursing, 2*, 113–121. (Chapter 11)

Harrison, M. J., Kushner, K. E., Benzies, K., Rempel, G., & Kimak, C. (2003). Women's satisfaction with their involvement in health care decisions during a high-risk pregnancy. *Birth, 30*, 109–115. (Chapter 16)

Harrison, M. J., Magill-Evans, J., & Sadoway, D. (2001). Scores on the Nursing Child Assessment Teaching Scale for father-toddler dyads. *Public Health Nursing, 18*, 94–100. (Chapter 13)

Hayne, Y. M. (2003). Experiencing psychiatric diagnosis: Client perspectives on being named mentally ill. *Journal of Psychiatric & Mental Health Nursing, 10*, 722–729. (Chapter 3)

Hébert, R. Lévesque, L., Vézina, J., Lavoie, J., Ducharme, F., Gendron, C., Préville, M., Voyer, L., & Dubois, M. (2003). Efficacy of a psychoeducative group program for caregivers of demented persons living at home: A randomized controlled trial. *Journal of Gerontology: Social Sciences, 58B*, S58–S67. (Chapter 15)

Hentz, P. (2002). The body remembers: Grieving and a circle of time. *Qualitative Health Research, 12*, 161–172. (Chapter 5)

Hirst, S. P. (2002). Defining resident abuse within the culture of long-term care institutions. *Clinical Nursing Research, 11*, 267–284. (Chapter 10, 16)

Hodnett, E. D., Gates, S., Hofmeyr, G. J., & Sakala, C. (2003). Continuous support for women during childbirth. *Cochrane Database of Systematic Reviews, 3*, No. CD003766. (Chapter 18)

Hodnett, E. D., Lowe, N. K., Hannah, M. E., Willan, A. R., Stevens, B., Weston, J. A., Ohlsson, A., Gafni, A., Muir, H. A., Myhr, T. L., Stremler, R., & Nursing Supportive Care in Labor Trial Group. (2002). Effectiveness of nurses as providers of birth labor support in North American hospitals: A randomized controlled trial. *Journal of the American Medical Association, 288*, 1373–1381. (Chapter 11)

Holmes, D., Kennedy, S. L., & Perron, A. (2004). The mentally ill and social exclusion: A critical examination of the use of seclusion from the patient's perspective. *Issues in Mental Health Nursing, 25*, 559–578. (Chapter 6)

Horsley, J. A., Crane, J., & Bingle, J. D. (1978). Research utilization as an organizational process. *Journal of Nursing Administration, 8*, 4–6. (Chapter 18)

Howell, D., Fitch, M. I., & Deane, K. A. (2003a). Women's experience with recurrent ovarian cancer. *Cancer Nursing, 26*, 10–17. (Chapter 11)

Howell, D., Fitch, M. I., & Deane, K. A. (2003b). Impact of ovarian cancer perceived by women. *Cancer Nursing, 26*, 1–9. (Chapter 11)

Hutchinson, A. M., & Johnston, L. (2004). Bridging the divide: A survey of nurses' opinions regarding barriers to, and facilitators of, research utilization in the practice setting. *Journal of Clinical Nursing, 13*, 304–315. (Chapter 18)

Hyman, I., Guruge, S., Mason, R., Gould, J., Stuckless, N., Tang, T., Teffera, H., & Mekonnen, G. (2004). Post-migration changes in gender relations among Ethiopian couples living in Canada. *Canadian Journal of Nursing Research, 36*(4), 74–89. (Chapter 16)

Ing, J. D., & Reutter, L. (2003). Socioeconomic status, sense of coherence, and health in Canadian women. *Canadian Journal of Public Health, 94*, 224–228. (Chapter 13, 15)

Ingram, C., & Brown, J. K. (2004). Patterns of weight and body composition change in premenopausal women with early stage breast cancer: Has weight gain been overestimated? *Cancer Nursing, 27*, 483–490. (Chapter 7)

Iwasiw, C., Goldenberg, D., Bol, N., & MacMaster, E. (2003). Resident and family perspectives. The first year in a long-term care facility. *Journal of Gerontologic Nursing, 29*, 45–54. (Chapter 10)

Jack, S. M., DiCenso, A., & Lohfeld, L. (2005). A theory of maternal engagement with public health nurses and family visitors. *Journal of Advanced Nursing 49*, 182–190. (Chapter 10)

Janssen, P. A., Iker, C. E., & Carty, E. A. (2003). Early labour assessment and support at home: A randomized controlled trial. *Journal of Obstetrics and Gynaecology Canada, 25*, 734–741. (Chapter 15)

Jensen, L., Rebeyka, D., Urquhart, G., & Roschkov, S. (2004). Pain in adults post surgical repair of congenital heart defects. *Canadian Journal of Cardiovascular Nursing, 14*, 8–17. (Chapter 9)

Johnson, J. L., Bottorff, J. L., Browne, A. J., Grewal, S., Hilton, B. A., & Clarke, H. (2004). Othering and being othered in the context of health care services. *Health Communication, 16*, 253–271. (Chapter 3)

Johnson, J. L., Bottorff, J. L., Moffat, B., Ratner, P. A., Shoveller, J., & Lovato, C. Y. (2003). Tobacco dependence: Adolescents' perspectives on the need to smoke. *Social Science & Medicine, 56,* 1481–1492. (Chapter 11)

Johnson, J. L., Ratner, P. A, Bottorff, J. L., & Hayduk, L. A. (1993). An exploration of Pender's Health Promotion Model using LISREL. *Nursing Research, 42,* 132–138. (Chapter 1)

Johnson, J. L., Ratner, P. A, Bottorff, J. L., Hall, W., & Dahinten, S. (2000). Preventing smoking relapse in postpartum women. *Nursing Research, 49,* 44–52. (Chapter 1)

Johnson, J. L., Ratner, P. A., Tucker, R. S., Bottorff, J. L., Zumbo, B., Prkachin, K. M., & Shoveller, J. (2005). Development of a multidimensional measure of tobacco dependence in adolescence. *Addictive Behaviors, 30,* 510–515. (Chapter 1, 11)

Johnson, J. L., Tucker, R. S., Ratner, P. A., Bottorff, J. L., Prkachin, K. M., Shoveller, J., & Zumbo, B. (2004). Sociodemographic correlates of cigarette smoking among high school students: Results from the British Columbia Youth Survey on Smoking and Health. *Canadian Journal of Public Health, 95,* 268–271. (Chapter 1)

Johnston, C. C., Filion, F., Snider, L., Majnemer, A., Limperopoulos, C., Walker, C., Veilleux, A., Pelausa, E., Cake, H., Stone, S., Sherrard, A., & Boyer, K. (2003). Routine sucrose during the first week of life in neonates younger than 31 weeks' postconceptual age. *Pediatrics, 110,* 523–528. (Chapter 9)

Johnston, C. C., Stevens, B., Pinelli, J., Gibbins, S., Filion, F., Jack, A., Steele, S., Boyer, K., & Veilleux, A. (2003). Kangaroo care is effective in diminishing pain response in preterm neonates. *Archives of Pediatrics & Adolescent Medicine, 157,* 1084–8. (Chapter 1)

Johnston, C. C., & Walker, C. (2003). The effects of exposure to repeated minor pain during the neonatal period on formalin pain behavior and thermal withdrawal latencies. *Pain Research & Management, 8,* 213–217. (Chapter 15)

Jonas-Simpson, C. M. (2003). The experience of being listened to: A human becoming study with music. *Nursing Science Quarterly, 16,* 232–238. (Chapter 8)

Kaasalainen, S., & Crook, J. (2004). An exploration of seniors' ability to report pain. *Clinical Nursing Research, 13,* 199–215. (Chapter 12)

Kearney, M. H., & O'Sullivan, J. (2003). Identity shifts as turning points in health behavior change. *Western Journal of Nursing Research, 25,* 134–152. (Chapter 10)

Keller, S., Hunter, D., & Shortt, S. E. (2004). The impact of hospital restructuring on home care nursing. *Canadian Journal of Nursing Leadership, 17,* 82–89. (Chapter 9)

Ketefian, S. (1975). Application of selected nursing research findings into nursing practice. *Nursing Research, 24,* 89–92. (Chapter 18)

Khanlou, N. (2004). Influences on adolescent self-esteem in multicultural Canadian secondary schools. *Public Health Nursing, 21,* 404–411. (Chapter 15)

Kinch, J. L., & Jakubec, S. (2004). Out of the multiple margins: Older women managing their health care. *Canadian Journal of Nursing Research, 36*(4), 90–108. (Chapter 16)

King, K. M., Ghali, W. A., Faris, P. D., Curtis, M. J., Galbraith, P. D., Graham, M. M., & Knudtson, M. L. (2004). Sex differences in outcomes after cardiac catheterization. *Journal of the American Medical Association, 291,* 1220–1225. (Chapter 15)

Kirchhoff, K. T. (1982). A diffusion survey of coronary precautions. *Nursing Research, 31,* 196–201. (Chapter 18)

Kirk-Gardner, R., & Steven, D. (2003). Hearts for Life: A community program on heart health promotion. *Canadian Journal of Cardiovascular Nursing, 13,* 5–10. (Chapter 9)

Kirkham, S. R. (2003). The politics of belonging and intercultural health care. *Western Journal of Nursing Research, 25,* 762–780. (Chapter 12)

Kolanowski, A. M., Litaker, M. S., & Catalano, P. A. (2002). Emotional well-being in a person with dementia. *Western Journal of Nursing Research, 24,* 28–48. (Chapter 11)

Koop, P. M., & Strang, V. R. (2003). The bereavement experience following home-based family caregiving for persons with advanced cancer. *Clinical Nursing Research, 12,* 127–144. (Chapter 6)

Kreulen, G. J., & Braden, C. J. (2004). Model test of the relationship between self-help promoting nursing interventions and self-care and health status outcomes. *Research in Nursing & Health, 27,* 97–109. (Chapter 8)

Kushner, K. (2005). Embodied context: Social institutional influences on employed mothers' health decision making. *Health Care for Women International, 26,* 69–86. (Chapter 10)

Lam, P., & Beaulieu, M. (2004). Experiences of families in the neurological ICU: A "bedside" phenomenon. *Journal of Neuroscience Nursing, 36,* 142–146, 151–155. (Chapter 1)

Lang, A., Goulet, C., & Amsel, R. (2004). Explanatory model of health in bereaved parents post-fetal/infant death. *International Journal of Nursing Studies, 41,* 869–880. (Chapter 1)

Larden, C. N., Palmer, M. L., & Janssen, P. (2004). Efficacy of therapeutic touch in treating pregnant inpatients who have a chemical dependency. *Journal of Holistic Nursing, 22,* 320–332. (Chapter 7)

Laudenbach, L., & Ford-Gilboe, M. (2004). Psychometric testing of the Health Options Scale with adolescents. *Journal of Family Nursing, 10,* 121–138. (Chapter 8)

Lauterbach, S. S. (2001). Longitudinal phenomenology: An example of "doing" phenomenology over time. Phenomenology of maternal mourning: Being-a-mother in another world (1992) and five years later (1997) (pp. 185–208). In P. L. Munhall (Ed.), *Nursing research: A qualitative perspective.* Sudbury, MA: Jones & Bartlett. (Chapter 10)

Lavorato, L., Grypma, S., Spenceley, S., Hagen, B., & Nowatzky, N. (2003). Positive outcomes in cardiac rehabilitation: The little program that could. *Canadian Journal of Cardiovascular Nursing, 13,* 13–19. (Chapter 11)

Lebel, S., Jakubovits, G., Rosberger, Z., Loiselle, C., Seguin, C., Cornaz, C., Ingram, J., August, L., & Lisbona, A. (2003). Waiting for a breast biopsy: Psychosocial consequences and coping strategies. *Journal of Psychosomatic Research, 55,* 437–443. (Chapter 15)

Leipert, B. D., & Reutter, L. (2005). Developing resilience: How women maintain their health in northern geographically isolated settings. *Qualitative Health Research, 15,* 49–65. (Chapter 2)

Leslie, W. D., Derksen, S., Metge, C., Lix, L., Salamon, E., Steinman, P., & Roose, L. (2005). Demographic risk factors for fractures in First Nations people. *Canadian Journal of Public Health, 96,* S45–50. (Chapter 9)

Letourneau, N., Neufeld, S., Drummong, J., & Barnfather, A. (2003). Deciding on surgery: Supporting parents of infants with craniosynostosis. *Axone, 24*(3), 24–29. (Chapter 16)

Lipson, J. G. (2001). We are the canaries: Multiple chemical sensitivity sufferers. *Qualitative Health Research, 11,* 103–116. (Chapter 10)

Lipson, J. G., Weinstein, H. M., Gladstone, E. A., & Sarnoff, R. H. (2003). Bosnian and Soviet refugees' experiences with health care. *Western Journal of Nursing Research, 25,* 854–871. (Chapter 11)

Lobchuk, M. M., & Vorauer, J. D. (2003). Family caregiver perspective-taking and accuracy in estimating cancer patient symptom experiences. *Social Science & Medicine, 57,* 2379–2384. (Chapter 13)

Loiselle, C. G., Semenic, S., & Côté, B. (2005). Sharing empirical knowledge to improve breastfeeding promotion and support: A research findings dissemination project. *Worldviews on Evidence-Based Nursing, 2,* 25–32. (Chapter 6)

Loiselle, C. G., Semenic, S. E., Côté, B., Lapointe, M., & Gendron, R. (2001). Impressions of breastfeeding information and support among first-time mothers within a multiethnic community. *Canadian Journal of Nursing Research, 33*(3), 31–46. (Chapter 6)

Loo, R., & Thorpe, K. (2005). Relationships between critical thinking and attitudes toward women's roles in society. *Journal of Psychology, 139,* 47–55. (Chapter 6)

Low, G., & Gutman, G. (2003). Couples' ratings of chronic obstructive pulmonary disease patients' quality of life. *Clinical Nursing Research, 12,* 28–48. (Chapter 8)

Lund, C. H., Kuller, J., Lane, A. T., Lott, J. W., Raines, D. A., & Thomas, K. K. (2001a). Neonatal skin care: Evaluation of the AWHONN/NANN research-based practice project on knowledge and skin care practices. *Journal of Obstetric, Gynecologic, & Neonatal Nursing, 30,* 30–40. (Chapter 18)

Lund, C. H., Osborne, J. W., Kuller, J., Lane, A. T., Lott, J. W., & Raines, D. A. (2001b). Neonatal skin care: Clinical outcomes of the AWHONN/NANN evidence-based clinical practice guideline. *Journal of Obstetric, Gynecologic, & Neonatal Nursing, 30,* 41–51. (Chapter 18)

MacIntosh, J. (2003). Reworking professional nursing identity. *Western Journal of Nursing Research, 25,* 725–741. (Chapter 16)

MacKinnon, K., McIntyre, M., & Quance, M. (2005). The meaning of the nurse's presence during childbirth. *Journal of Obstetric, Gynecologic, & Neonatal Nursing, 34,* 28–36. (Chapter 1)

Majumdar, B., Browne, G., Roberts, J., & Carpio, B. (2004). Effects of cultural sensitivity training on health care provider attitudes and patient outcomes. *Journal of Nursing Scholarship, 36,* 161–166. (Chapter 11)

Malinowski, A., & Stamler, L. L. (2003). Adolescent girls' personal experience with *Baby Think It Over* infant simulator. *MCN: The American Journal of Maternal/Child Nursing, 28,* 205–211. (Chapter 16)

Maloni, J. A., Albrecht, S. A., Thomas, K. K., & Halleran, J., & Jones, R. (2003). Implementing evidence-based practice: Reducing risk for low birth weight through pregnancy

smoking cessation. *Journal of Obstetric, Gynecologic, & Neonatal Nursing, 32,* 676–682. (Chapter 18)

Martens, P. J. (2001). The effect of breastfeeding education on adolescent beliefs and attitudes: A randomized school intervention in the Canadian Ojibwa community of Sagkeeng. *Journal of Human Lactation, 17,* 245–255. (Chapter 9)

McBride, K. L., White, C. L., Sourial, R., & Mayo, N. (2004). Postdischarge nursing interventions for stroke survivors and their families. *Journal of Advanced Nursing, 47,* 192–200. (Chapter 11)

McCleary, L., & Brown, G. T. (2003a). Barriers to paediatric nurses' research utilization. *Journal of Advanced Nursing, 42,* 364–372. (Chapter 18)

McCleary, L., & Brown, G. T. (2003b). Association between nurses' education about research and their research use. *Nurse Education Today, 23,* 556–565. (Chapter 18)

McCleary, L., & Sanford, M. (2002). Parental expressed emotion in depressed adolescents: Prediction of clinical course and relationship to comorbid disorders and social functioning. *Journal of Child Psychology and Psychiatry, 43,* 587–595. (Chapter 9)

McClement, S. E., Chochinov, H. M., Hack, T., Kristjanson, L. J., & Harlos, M. (2004). Dignity conserving care: Application of research findings to practice. *International Journal of Palliative Nursing, 10,* 173–179. (Chapter 11)

McCloskey, R. (2004). Functional and self-efficacy changes of patients admitted to a Geriatric Rehabilitation Unit. *Journal of Advanced Nursing, 46,* 186–193. (Chapter 4)

McDonald, D. D., Wiczorek, M., & Walker, C. (2004). Factors affecting learning during health education sessions. *Clinical Nursing Research, 13,* 156–167. (Chapter 9)

McGilton, K. S. (2003). Development and psychometric evaluation of Supportive Leadership Scales. *Canadian Journal of Nursing Research, 35,* 72–86. (Chapter 14)

McGilton, K. S., O'Brien-Pallas, L. L., Darlington, G., Evans, M., Wynn, F., & Pringle, D. M. (2003). Effects of a relationship-enhancing program of care on outcomes. *Journal of Nursing Scholarship, 35,* 151–156. (Chapter 9)

McGilton, K. S., Rivera, T. M., & Dawson, P. (2003). Can we help persons with dementia find their way in a new environment? *Aging & Mental Health, 7,* 363–371. (Chapter 2)

Medves, J. M., & Davies, B. L. (2005). Sustaining rural maternity care: Don't forget the RNs. *Canadian Journal of Rural Medicine, 10,* 29–35. (Chapter 10)

Medves, J. M., & O'Brien, B. (2004). The effect of bather and location of first bath on maintaining thermal stability in newborns. *Journal of Obstetric, Gynecologic, & Neonatal Nursing, 33,* 175–182. (Chapter 17)

Metcalfe, K. A. (2004). Prophylactic bilateral mastectomy for breast cancer prevention. *Journal of Women's Health, 13,* 822–829. (Chapter 7)

Mill, J. E. (2003). Shrouded in secrecy: Breaking the news of HIV infection to Ghanaian women. *Journal of Transcultural Nursing, 14,* 6–16. (Chapter 10)

Miller, C. E., Ratner, P. A., & Johnson, J. L. (2003). Reducing cardiovascular risk: Identifying predictors of smoking relapse. *Canadian Journal of Cardiovascular Nursing, 13,* 7–12. (Chapter 9)

Miller, J. L. (2004). Level of RN educational preparation: Its impact on collaboration and the relationship between collaboration and professional identity. *Canadian Journal of Nursing Research, 36,* 132–147. (Chapter 6, 12)

Milliken, P. J., & Northcott, H. C. (2003). Redefining parental identity: Caregiving and schizophrenia. *Qualitative Health Research, 13,* 100–113. (Chapter 1)

Minore, B., Boone, M., & Hill, M. E. (2004). Finding temporary relief: Strategy for nursing recruitment in northern Aboriginal communities. *Canadian Journal of Nursing Research, 36*(2), 148–163. (Chapter 12)

Miranda, J. (2004). An exploration of participants' treatment preferences in a partial RCT. *Canadian Journal of Nursing Research, 36*(3), 100–114. (Chapter 11)

Mitchell, L. M. (2004). Women's experience of unexpected ultrasound findings. *Journal of Midwifery & Women's Health, 49,* 228–234. (Chapter 10)

Molzahn, A. E., Starzomski, R., McDonald, M., & O'Loughlin, C. (2005). Chinese Canadian beliefs toward organ donation. *Qualitative Health Research, 15,* 82–98. (Chapter 14)

Momtahan, K., Berkman, J., Sellick, J., Kearns, S. A., & Lauzon, N. (2004). Patients' understanding of cardiac risk factors: A point-prevalence study. *Journal of Cardiovascular Nursing, 19,* 13–20. (Chapter 12)

Montbriand, M. J. (2004). Seniors' life histories and perceptions of illness. *Western Journal of Nursing Research, 26,* 242–260. (Chapter 2)

Montbriand, M. J. (2004). Seniors' survival trajectories and the illness connection. *Qualitative Health Research, 14,* 449–461. (Chapter 10)

Monteith, B., & Ford-Gilboe, M. (2002). The relationships among mother's resilience, family health work, and mother's health-promoting lifestyle practices in families with preschool children. *Journal of Family Nursing, 8,* 383–407. (Chapter 6, 8)

Morgan, D. G., & Stewart, N. J. (2002). Theory building through mixed-method evaluation of a dementia special care unit. *Research in Nursing & Health, 25,* 479–488. (Chapter 11)

Morse, J. M., Beres, M. A., Spiers, J. A., Mayan, M., & Olson, K. (2003). Identifying signals of suffering by linking verbal and facial cues. *Qualitative Health Research, 13,* 1063–1077. (Chapter 1, 13)

Morse, J. M., Bottorff, J. L., & Hutchinson, S. (1994). The phenomenology of comfort. *Journal of Advanced Nursing, 20,* 189–195. (Chapter 1)

Morse, J. M., & Mitcham, C. (1997). Compathy: The contagion of physical distress. *Journal of Advanced Nursing, 26,* 649–657. (Chapter 1)

Morse, J. M., & Mitcham, C. (1998). The experience of agonizing pain and signals of disembodiment. *Journal of Psychosomatic Research, 44,* 667–680. (Chapter 1)

Morse, J. M., & Pooler, C. (2002). Patient-family-nurse interactions in the trauma-resuscitation room. *American Journal of Critical Care, 11,* 240–249. (Chapter 1)

Moules, N. J., Simonson, K., Prins, M., Angus, P., & Bell, J. M. (2004). Making room for grief: Walking backwards and living forward. *Nursing Inquiry, 11,* 99–107. (Chapter 13)

Myrick, F., & Yonge, O. (2004). Enhancing critical thinking in the preceptorship experience in nursing education. *Journal of Advanced Nursing, 45,* 371–380. (Chapter 2)

Nemeth, K. A., Harrison, M. B., Graham, I. D., & Burke, S. (2004). Understanding venous leg ulcer pain: Results of a longitudinal study. *Ostomy & Wound Management, 50,* 34–46. (Chapter 3)

Nemeth, K. A., Harrison, M. B., Graham, L. D., & Burke, S. (2003). Pain in pure and mixed aetiology venous leg ulcers: A three-phase point prevalence study. *Journal of Wound Care, 12,* 334–340. (Chapter 13)

Neufeld, A., & Harrison, M. J. (2003). Unfulfilled expectations and negative interactions: Nonsupport in the relationships of women caregivers. *Journal of Advanced Nursing, 41,* 323–331. (Chapter 5)

Neufeld, A., Harrison, M., Rempel, G. R. Larocque, S., Dublin, S., Stewart, M., & Hughes, K. (2004). Practical issues in using a card sort in a study of nonsupport and family caregiving. *Qualitative Health Research, 13,* 1418–1428. (Chapter 13)

Norris, C. M., Ghali, W. A., Galbraith, P. D., Graham, M. M., Jensen, L. A., Knudtson, M. L., & the APPROACH Investigators. (2004). Women with coronary artery disease report worse health-related quality of life outcomes compared to men. *Health and Quality of Life Outcomes, 2,* 21–32. (Chapter 17)

O'Brien, B., Evans, M., & White-McDonald, E. (2002). Isolation from "being alive": Coping with severe nausea and vomiting of pregnancy. *Nursing Research, 51,* 302–308. (Chapter 16)

O'Brien, J., & Fothergill-Bourbonnais, F. (2004). The experience of trauma resuscitation in the emergency room: Themes from seven patients. *Journal of Emergency Nursing, 30,* 216–224. (Chapter 10)

O'Donnell, C. A. (2004). Attitudes and knowledge of primary care professionals toward evidence-based practice. *Journal of Evaluation in Clinical Practice, 10,* 197–205. (Chapter 18)

Olson, K., Hanson, J., Hamilton, J., Stacey, D., Eades, M., Gue, D., Plummer, H., Janes, K., Fitch, M., Bakker, D., Baker, P., & Oliver, C. (2004). Assessing the reliability and validity of the revised WCCNR stomatitis staging system for cancer therapy-induced stomatitis. *Canadian Oncology Nursing Journal, 14,* 168–182. (Chapter 14)

Olson, K., Hanson, J., Michaud, M. (2003). A phase II trial of Reiki for the management of pain in advanced cancer patients. *Journal of Pain & Symptom Management, 26,* 990–997. (Chapter 11)

Olson, K., Rennie, R. P., Hanson, J., Ryan, M., Gilpin, J., Falsetti, M., Heffner, T., & Gaudet, S. (2004). Evaluation of a no-dressing intervention for tunneled central venous catheter exit sites. *Journal of Infusion Nursing, 27,* 37–44. (Chapter 9, 13)

Olson, K., Tom, B., Hewitt, J., Whittingham, J., Buchanan, L., & Ganton, G. (2002). Evolving routines: Preventing fatigue associated with lung and colorectal cancer. *Qualitative Health Research, 12,* 655–670. (Chapter 10)

Ostry, A. S., Tomlin, K. M., Cvitkovich, Y., Ratner, P. A., Park, I. H., Tate, R. B., & Yassi, A. (2004). Choosing a model of care for patients in alternative level care: Caregiver perspectives with respect to staff injury. *Canadian Journal of Nursing Research, 36*(1), 142–157. (Chapter 6)

Pasco, A. C. Y., Morse, J. M., & Olson, J. K. (2004). Cross-cultural relationships between nurses and Filipino

Canadian patients. *Journal of Nursing Scholarship, 36,* 239–246. (Chapter 6)

Paterson, B. L. (2001). The shifting perspectives model of chronic illness. *Journal of Nursing Scholarship, 33,* 21–26. (Chapter 8)

Paterson, B. L. (2003). The koala has claws: Applications of the Shifting Perspectives Model in research of chronic illness. *Qualitative Health Research, 13,* 987–994. (Chapter 8)

Paterson, B., Canam, C., Joachim, G., & Thorne, S. (2003). Embedded assumptions in qualitative studies of fatigue. *Western Journal of Nursing Research, 25,* 119–133. (Chapter 7, 18)

Patterson, C., Kaczorowski, J., Arthur, H., Smith, K., Mills, D. A. (2003). Complementary therapy practice: Defining the role of advanced nurse practitioners. *Journal of Clinical Nursing, 12,* 816–823. (Chapter 12)

Peacock, S. C., & Forbes, D. A. (2003). Interventions for caregivers of persons with dementia: A systematic review. *Canadian Journal of Nursing Research, 35,* 88–107. (Chapter 18)

Perreault, A., Fothergill-Bourbonnais, F., & Fiset, V. (2004). The experience of family members caring for a dying loved one. *International Journal of Palliative Nursing, 10,* 133–143. (Chapter 10)

Perry, J. (2002). Wives giving care to husbands with Alzheimer's disease: A process of interpretive caring. *Research in Nursing & Health, 25,* 307–316. (Chapter 12)

Perry, J. J. (2004). Daughters giving care to mothers who have dementia: Mastering the 3 R's of (re)calling, (re)learning, and (re)adjusting. *Journal of Family Nursing, 10,* 50–69. (Chapter 4)

Peter, E. H., Macfarlane, A. V., O'Brien-Pallas, L. L. (2004). Analysis of the moral habitability of the nursing work environment. *Journal of Advanced Nursing, 47,* 356–367. (Chapter 7)

Pilkington, F. B., & Mitchell, G. J. (2004). Quality of life for women living with a gynecologic cancer. *Nursing Science Quarterly, 17,* 147–155. (Chapter 8)

Polit, D. F., London, A. S., & Martinez, J. M. (2000). *Food security and hunger in poor, mother-headed families in four U. S. cities.* New York: MDRC. Available at *http//www.mdrc.org.* (Chapter 11, 16)

Polit, D. F., London, A. S., & Martinez, J. M. (2001). *The health of poor urban women.* New York: MDRC. Available at *http://www.mdrc.org.* (Chapter 11)

Profetto-McGrath, J. (2003). The relationship of critical thinking skills and critical thinking dispositions of baccalaureate nursing students. *Journal of Advanced Nursing, 43,* 569–577. (Chapter 9)

Provencher, H. L., Perreault, M., St. Onge, M., & Rousseau, M. (2003). Predictors of psychological distress in family caregivers of persons with psychiatric disabilities. *Journal of Psychiatric and Mental Health Nursing, 10,* 592–607. (Chapter 15, 17)

Raingruber, B., & Kent, M. (2003). Attending to embodied responses: A way to identify practice based and human meanings associated with secondary trauma. *Qualitative Health Research, 13,* 449–468. (Chapter 16)

Rashid, S. F. (2001). Indigenous notions of the workings of the inner body: Conflicts and dilemmas with Norplant use

in rural Bengladesh. *Qualitative Health Research, 11,* 85–102. (Chapter 10)

Ratner, P. A., Johnson, J. L., Richardson, C. G., Bottorff, J. L., Moffat, B., Mackay, M., Fofonoff, D., Kingsbury, K., Miller, C., & Budz, B. (2004). Efficacy of a smoking-cessation intervention for elective-surgical patients. *Research in Nursing & Health, 27,* 148–161. (Chapter 1, 9)

Ratner, P. S., Bottorff, J. L., Johnson, J. L., & Hayduk, L. A. (1994). The interaction effects of gender within the health promotion model. *Research in Nursing and Health, 17,* 341–350. (Chapter 1)

Regehr, M., Kjerulf, M., Popova, S. R., & Baker, A. J. (2004). Trauma and tribulation: The experiences and attitudes of operating room nurses working with organ donors. *Journal of Clinical Nursing, 13,* 430–437. (Chapter 3)

Rempel, G. R., Cender, L. M., Lynam, M. J., Sandor, G. G., & Farquharson, D. (2004). Parents' perspectives on decision-making after antenatal diagnosis of congenital heart disease. *Journal of Obstetric, Gynecologic, & Neonatal Nursing, 33,* 64–70. (Chapter 14)

Rempel, L. A. (2004). Factors influencing the breastfeeding decisions of long-term breastfeeders. *Journal of Human Lactation, 20,* 306–318. (Chapter 8)

Rennick, J. E., Morin, I., Kim, D., Johnston, C., Dougherty, G., & Platt, R. (2004). Identifying children at high risk for psychological sequelae after pediatric intensive care unit hospitalization. *Pediatric Critical Care Medicine, 5,* 358–363. (Chapter 5)

Reutter, L. I., Sword, W., Meagher-Stewart, D., & Rideout, E. (2004). Nursing students' beliefs about poverty and health. *Journal of Advanced Nursing, 48,* 299–309. (Chapter 2)

Robinson, J. R., Clements, K., & Land, C. (2003). Workplace stress among psychiatric nurses. Prevalence, distribution, correlates, & predictors. *Journal of Psychosocial Nursing and Mental Health Services, 41,* 32–41. (Chapter 11)

Rodgers, S. E. (2000). The extent of nursing research utilization in general medical and surgical wards. *Journal of Advanced Nursing, 32,* 182–193. (Chapter 18)

Roshkov, S., & Jensen, L. (2004). Coronary artery bypass graft patients' pain perception during epicardial pacing wire removal. *Canadian Journal of Cardiovascular Nursing, 14*(3) 32–38. (Chapter 12)

Ross-Kerr, J. C.. Warren, S., Schalm, C., Smith, D., & Godkin, M. D. (2003). Adult day programs: Are they needed? *Journal of Gerontological Nursing, 29*(12), 1–7. (Chapter 15)

Ryan, C. J., & Zerwic, J. J. (2004). Knowledge of symptom clusters among adults at risk for acute myocardial infarction. *Nursing Research, 53,* 363–369. (Chapter 13)

Schafer, P., & Peternelj-Taylor (2003). Therapeutic relationships and boundary maintenance: The perspective of forensic patients enrolled in a treatment program for violent offenders. *Issues in Mental Health Nursing, 24,* 605–625. (Chapter 14)

Secco, M. L., & Moffat, M. E. (2003). The home environment of Metis, First Nations, and Caucasian adolescent mothers: An examination of quality and influences. *Canadian Journal of Nursing Research, 35,* 106–126. (Chapter 1)

Semenic, S. E., Callister, L. C., & Feldman, P. (2004). Giving birth: The voice of Orthodox Jewish women living in

Canada. *Journal of Obstetric, Gynecologic, & Nenonatal Nursing, 33,* 80–87. (Chapter 10)

Sgarbossa, D., & Ford-Gilboe, M. (2004). Mother's friendship quality, parental support, quality of life, and family health work in families led by adolescent mothers with preschool children. *Journal of Family Nursing, 10,* 232–261. (Chapter 6, 8)

Shamian, J., Kerr, M. S., Laschinger, H. K., & Thomson, D. (2002). A hospital-level analysis of the work environment and workforce health indicators for registered nurses in Ontario's acute-care hospital. *Canadian Journal of Nursing Research, 33,* 35–50. (Chapter 10)

Shields, S. A., Wong, T., Mann, J., Jolly, A. M., Haase, D., Mahaffey, S., Moses, S., Morin, M., Patrick, D. M., Predy, G., Rossi, M., & Sutherland, D. (2004). Prevalence and correlates of Chlamydia infection in Canadian street youth. *Journal of Adolescent Health, 34,* 384–390. (Chapter 5)

Shore, H. L., (1972). Adopters and laggards. *Canadian Nurse, 68,* 36–39. (Chapter 18)

Shoveller, J. A., Lovato, C. Y., Young, R. A., & Moffat, B. (2003). Exploring the development of sun-tanning behavior: A grounded theory study of adolescents' decision-making experiences with becoming a sun tanner. *International Journal of Behavioral Medicine, 10,* 299–314. (Chapter 17)

Shyu, Y., Liang, J., Lu, J., & Wu, C. (2004). Environmental barriers and mobility in Taiwan: Is the Roy adaptation model applicable? *Nursing Science Quarterly, 17,* 165–170. (Chapter 8)

Sinding, C., Barnoff, L., & Grassau, P. (2004). Homophobia and heterosexism in cancer care: The experiences of lesbians. *Canadian Journal of Nursing Research, 36*(4), 170–188. (Chapter 14)

Sinding, C., Gray, R., Fitch, M., & Greenberg, M. (2002). Staging breast cancer, rehearsing metastatic disease. *Qualitative Health Research, 12,* 61–73. (Chapter 10)

Skillen, D. L., Anderson. M. C., & Knight, C. L. (2001). The created environment for physical assessment by case managers. *Western Journal of Nursing Research, 23,* 72–89. (Chapter 8)

Sloan, J. A., Scott-Finlay, S., Nemecek, A., Blood, P., Trylinski, C., Whittaker, H., El Sayed, S., Clinch, J., & Khoo, K. (2004). Mapping the journey of cancer patients through health care system. *Canadian Journal of Oncology Nursing, 14,* 183–186. (Chapter 6)

Small, S. P., Brennan-Hunter, A. L., Best, D. G., & Solberg, S. M. (2002). Struggling to understand: The experience of nonsmoking parents with adolescents who smoke. *Qualitative Health Research, 12,* 1202–1219. (Chapter 10)

Spiers, J. A. (2002). The interpersonal contexts of negotiating care in home care nurse-patient interactions. *Qualitative Health Research, 12,* 1033–1057. (Chapter 5)

Steel-O'Connor, K. O., Mowat, D. L., Scott, H. M., Carr, P. A., Dorland, J. L., Young-Tai, K. F. (2003). A randomized trial of two public health nurse follow-up programs after early obstetrical discharge. *Canadian Journal of Public Health, 94,* 98–103. (Chapter 11)

Steven, D., Fitch, M., Dhaliwal, H., Kirk-Gardner, R., Sevean, P., Jamieson, J., & Woodbeck, H. (2004). Knowledge, attitudes, beliefs, and practices regarding breast and cervical cancer screening in selected ethnocultural groups in northwestern Ontario. *Oncology Nursing Forum, 31,* 305–311. (Chapter 2)

Stewart, N. J., D'Arcy, C., Pitblado, J. R., Morgan, D. G., Forbes, D., Remus, G., Smith, B., Andrews, M. E., Kosteniuk, J., Kulig, J. C., & MacLeod, M. (2005). A profile of registered nurses in rural and remote Canada. *Canadian Journal of Nursing Research, 37*(1), 122–145. (Chapter 1)

Struthers, R. (2003). The artistry and ability of traditional women healers. *Health Care for Women International, 24,* 340–354. (Chapter 12)

Sword, W. (2003). Prenatal care use among women of low income: A matter of "taking care of self." *Qualitative Health Research, 13,* 319–332. (Chapter 4)

Tapp, D. M. (2004). Dilemmas of family support during cardiac recovery: Nagging as a gesture of support. *Western Journal of Nursing Research, 26,* 561–580. (Chapter 16)

Tarrant, M., & Gregory, D. (2003). Exploring childhood immunization uptake with First Nations mothers in northwestern Ontario, Canada. *Journal of Advanced Nursing, 41,* 63–72. (Chapter 10)

Taylor, K. I., Oberle, K. M., Crutcher, R. A., & Norton, P. G. (2005). Promoting health in type 2 diabetes: Nurse-physician collaboration in primary care. *Biological Research for Nursing, 6,* 207–215. (Chapter 3, 17)

Taylor-Piliae, R. E., & Froelicher, E. S. (2004). Effectiveness of Tai Chi exercise in improving aerobic capacity: A meta-analysis. *Journal of Cardiovascular Nursing, 19,* 48–57. (Chapter 7)

Then, K. L., Rankin, J. A., & Fofonoff, D. A. (2001). Atypical presentation of acute myocardial infarction in 3 age groups. *Heart & Lung, 30,* 285–293. (Chapter 12)

Thomas, B.H., Ciliska, D., Dobbins, M., & Micucci, B.A (2004). A process for systematically reviewing the literature: providing the research evidence for public health nursing interventions. *Worldviews on Evidence Based Nursing, 1,* 176–184. (Chapter 18)

Thorne, S., Con, A., McGuinness, L., McPerson, G., & Harris, S. R. (2004). Health care communication issues in multiple sclerosis: An interpretive description. *Qualitative Health Research, 14,* 5–22. (Chapter 11)

Thorne, S., Paterson, B., & Russell, C. (2003). The structure of everyday self-care decision making in chronic illness. *Qualitative Health Research, 13,* 1337–1352. (Chapter 14)

Thurston, N. E., & King, K. M. (2004). Implementing evidence-based practice: Walking the talk. *Applied Nursing Research, 17,* 239–47. (Chapter 18)

Tourangeau, A. E., & McGilton, K. (2004). Measuring leadership practices of nurses using the Leadership Practices Inventory. *Nursing Research, 53,* 182–189. (Chapter 14)

Tranmer, J. E., Minard, J., Fox, L. A., & Rebelo, L. (2003). The sleep experience of medical and surgical patients. *Clinical Nursing Research, 12,* 159–173. (Chapter 1)

Tranmer, J. E., & Parry, M. J. E., (2004). Enhancing postoperative recovery of cardiac surgery patients: A randomized clinical trial of an advanced practice nursing intervention. *Western Journal of Nursing Research, 26,* 515–532. (Chapter 9)

Tweedell, D., Forchuk, C., Jewell, J., & Steinnagel, L. (2004). Families' experience during recovery or nonrecovery from psychosis. *Archives of Psychiatric Nursing, 18,* 17–25. (Chapter 12)

Valente, S., & Saunders, J. M. (2004). Barriers to suicide risk management in clinical practice: A national survey of oncology nurses. *Issues in Mental Health Nursing, 25,* 629–648. (Chapter 13)

Van den Brink, Y. (2003). Diversity in care values and expression among Turkish family caregivers and Dutch community nurses in The Netherlands. *Journal of Transcultural Nursing, 14,* 146–154. (Chapter 8)

Varcoe, C., & Hilton, A. (1995). Factors affecting acute-care nurses' use of research findings. *Canadian Journal of Nursing Research, 27*(4), 51–71. (Chapter 18)

Vissandjee, B., Desmeules, M., Cao, Z., Abdool, S., & Kazanjian, A. (2004). Integrating ethnicity and migration as determinants of Canadian women's health. *BMC Women's Health, 25,* S32. (Chapter 9)

Voyer, P., Landreville, P., Moisan, J., Tousignant, M., & Préville, M. (2005). Insomnia, depression and anxiety disorders and their association with benzodiazepine drug use among the community-dwelling elderly: Implications for mental health nursing. *International Journal of Psychiatric Nursing Research, 10,* 1093–1116. (Chapter 4)

Voyer, P., McCubbin, M., Preville, M., & Boyer, R. (2003). Factors in duration of anxiolytic, sedative, and hypnotic drug use in the elderly. *Canadian Journal of Nursing Research, 35*(4), 126–149. (Chapter 15)

Voyer, P., Verreault, R., Mengue, N. P., Laurin, D., Rochette, L., Martin, L. S., & Baillargeon, L. (2005). Determinants of neuroleptic drugs use in long-term care facilities for elderly persons. *Journal of Applied Gerontology.* (Chapter 3)

Walker, C. D., Kudreikis, K., Sherrard, A., & Johnston, C. C. (2003). Repeated neonatal pain influences maternal behavior, but not stress responsiveness in rat offspring. *Developmental Brain Research, 140,* 253–261. (Chapter 13)

Ward-Griffin, C., Bol, N., Hay, K., & Dashney, I. (2003). Relationships between families and registered nurses in long-term care facilities: A critical analysis. *Canadian Journal of Nursing Research, 35,* 150–174. (Chapter 6)

Warren, S., Kerr, J. R., Smith, D., & Godkin, D., & Schalm, C. (2003). The impact of adult day programs on family caregivers of elderly relatives. *Journal of Community Health Nursing, 20,* 209–221. (Chapter 9)

Watson, C. P., Moulin, D., Watt-Watson, J., Gordon, A., & Eisenhoffer, J. (2003). Controlled-release oxycondone relieves neuropathic pain: A randomized controlled trial in painful diabetic neuropathy. *Pain, 105,* 71–78. (Chapter 9)

Watt-Watson, J., Chung, F., Chan, V. W. S., & McGillion, M. (2004). Pain management following discharge after ambulatory same-day surgery. *Journal of Nursing Management, 12,* 153–161. (Chapter 5)

Watt-Watson, J., Stevens, B., Katz, J., Costello, J., Reid, G. J., & David, T. (2004). Impact of preoperative education on pain outcomes after coronary artery bypass graft surgery. *Pain, 109,* 73–85. (Chapter 2)

Weaver, K., Wuest, J., & Ciliska, D. (2005). Understanding women's journey of recovering from anorexia nervosa. *Qualitative Health Research, 15,* 188–206. (Chapter 16)

Weinstein, H. M., Sarnoff, R., Gladstone, E., & Lipson, J. (2000). Physical and psychological health issues of resettled refugees in the United States. *Journal of Refugee Studies, 13,* 303–327. (Chapter 11)

Westerman, E., Aubrey, B., Gauthier, D., Aung, M., Beanlands, R. S., Ruddy, T. D., Davies, R. A., De Kemp, R. A., & Woodend, K. (2004). Positron emission tomography: A study of PET test-related anxiety. *Canadian Journal of Cardiovascular Nursing, 14*(2), 42–48. (Chapter 6)

Wilson, D. M. (2002). The duration and degree of end-of-life dependency of home care clients and hospital inpatients. *Applied Nursing Research, 15,* 81–86. (Chapter 15)

Winterburn, S., & Fraser, R. (2000). Does the duration of postnatal stay influence breastfeeding rates at one month in women giving birth for the first time? A randomized control trial. *Journal of Advanced Nursing, 32,* 1152–57. (Chapter 9)

Woodgate, R. L. (2005). A different way of being: Adolescents' experiences with cancer. *Cancer Nursing, 28*(1), 8–15. (Chapter 7)

Woodgate, R. L., & Degner, L. F. (2004). Cancer symptom transition periods of children and families. *Journal of Advanced Nursing, 46,* 356–368. (Chapter 3)

Woodgate, R. L., & Degner, L. F. (2004). "Nothing is carved in stone!": Uncertainty in children with cancer and their families. *European Journal of Oncology Nursing, 6,* 191–202. (Chapter 1)

Woodgate, R.H. Degner, L., & Yanofsky R. (2003). A different perspective to approaching cancer symptoms in children. *The Journal of Pain and Symptom Management, 26*(3), 800–817. (Chapter 10)

Wright, B. W. (2004). Trust and power in adults: An investigation using Rogers' Science of Unitary Human Beings. *Nursing Science Quarterly, 17,* 139–146. (Chapter 8)

Wuest, J. (2001). Precarious ordering: Toward a formal theory of women's caring. *Health Care for Women International, 22,* 167–193. (Chapter 12)

Wuest, J., Ford-Gilboe, M., Merritt-Gray, M., & Berman, H. (2003). Intrusion: The central problem for family health promotion among children and single mothers after leaving an abusive partner. *Qualitative Health Research, 13,* 597–622. (Chapter 5)

Wuest, J., Merritt-Gray, M., & Ford-Gilboe, M. (2004). Regenerating family: Strengthening the emotional health of mothers and children in the context of intimate partner violence. *Advances in Nursing Science, 27,* 257–274. (Chapter 10)

Wyatt, P. A., & Ratner, P. A. (2004). Evaluating treatment-seeking for acute myocardial infarction in women. *Canadian Journal of Cardiovascular Nursing, 14*(1), 39–45. (Chapter 8)

Yassi, A., Cohen, M., Cvitkovich, Y., Park, I., Ratner, P. A., Ostry, A. S., Village, J., & Pollak, N. (2004). Factors associated with staff injuries in intermediate care facilities in British Columbia, Canada. *Nursing Research, 53,* 87–97. (Chapter 6)

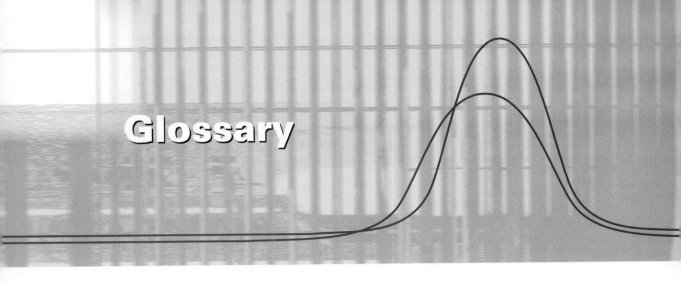

Glossary

Note: Entries preceded by an asterisk (*) are terms that were not explained in this book, but they are included here because you might come across them in the research literature. For further explanation of these terms, please refer to Polit and Beck (2004), *Nursing Research: Principles and Methods* (7th ed.), Philadelphia, PA: Lippincott Williams & Wilkins.

abstract A brief description of a completed or proposed study, usually located at the beginning of the report or proposal.

accessible population The population of people available for a particular study; often a nonrandom subset of the target population.

accidental sampling Selection of the most readily available persons as study participants; also called *convenience sampling.*

acquiescence response set A bias in self-report instruments, especially in psychosocial scales, created when study participants characteristically agree with statements ("yea-say") independent of their content.

*adjusted mean The mean group value for the dependent variable, after statistically removing the effect of covariates.

after-only design An experimental design in which data are collected from subjects only after an experimental intervention has been introduced.

alpha (α) (1) In tests of statistical significance, the level designating the probability of committing a Type I error; (2) in estimates of internal consistency, a reliability coefficient, as in Cronbach's alpha.

*alternative hypothesis In hypothesis testing, a hypothesis different from the one being tested—usually, different from the null hypothesis.

analysis The process of organizing and synthesizing data so as to answer research questions and test hypotheses.

analysis of covariance (ANCOVA) A statistical procedure used to test mean differences among groups on a dependent variable, while controlling for one or more extraneous variables (covariates).

analysis of variance (ANOVA) A statistical procedure for testing mean differences among three or more groups by comparing variability between groups to variability within groups.

*analysis triangulation The use of two or more analytic techniques to analyze the same set of data.

anonymity Protection of participants in a study such that even the researcher cannot link individuals with the information provided.

applied research Research designed to find a solution to an immediate practical problem.

assent The affirmative agreement of a vulnerable subject (e.g., a child) to participate in a study.

associative relationship An association between two variables that cannot be described as causal (i.e., one variable *causing* the other).

assumption A basic principle that is accepted as being true based on logic or reason, but without proof or verification.

asymmetric distribution A distribution of data values that is skewed, i.e., has two halves that are not mirror images of the each other.

*attribute variables Preexisting characteristics of study participants, which the researcher simply observes or measures.

attrition The loss of participants over the course of a study, which can create bias and undermine internal validity by changing the composition of the sample—particularly if more participants are lost from one group (e.g., experimentals) than another (e.g., controls).

*audio-CASI (computer-assisted self-interview) An approach to collecting self-report data in which respondents listen to questions being read over headphones and respond by entering information directly onto a computer.

auditability The extent to which an external reviewer or reader can follow a qualitative researcher's steps and decisions and draw conclusions about the analysis and interpretation of the data.

audit trail The systematic documentation of material that allows an independent auditor of a qualitative study to draw conclusions about the trustworthiness of the data.

auto-ethnography Ethnographic studies in which researchers study their own culture or group.

axial coding The second level of coding in a grounded theory study using the Strauss and Corbin approach, involving the process of categorizing, recategorizing, and condensing all first-level codes by connecting a category and its subcategories.

*back-translation The translation of a translated text back into the original language, so that a comparison of the original and back-translated version can be made.

baseline data Data collected before an intervention, including pretreatment data from a measure of the dependent variable.

basic research Research designed to extend the base of knowledge in a discipline for the sake of knowledge production or theory construction, rather than for solving an immediate problem.

basic social process (BSP) The central social process emerging through an analysis of grounded theory data.

before–after design An experimental design in which data are collected from research subjects both before and after the introduction of an experimental intervention.

beneficence A fundamental ethical principle that seeks to prevent harm and exploitation of, and maximize benefits for, study participants.

beta (β) (1) In multiple regression, the standardized coefficients indicating the relative weights of the independent variables in the regression equation; (2) in statistical testing, the probability of a Type II error.

between-subjects design A research design in which there are separate groups of people being compared (e.g., smokers and nonsmokers).

bias Any influence that produces a distortion in the results of a study.

bimodal distribution A distribution of data values with two peaks (high frequencies).

bivariate statistics Statistics derived from analyzing two variables simultaneously to assess the empirical relationship between them.

"blind" review The review of a manuscript or proposal such that neither the author nor the reviewer is identified to the other party.

blinding The masking or withholding of information (e.g., from research subjects, research personnel, or reviewers) to reduce the possibility of certain biases.

borrowed theory A theory borrowed from another discipline to guide nursing practice or research.

bracketing In phenomenological inquiries, the process of identifying and holding in abeyance any preconceived beliefs and opinions about the phenomena under study.

bricolage The tendency in qualitative research to assemble a complex array of data from a variety of sources, using a variety of methods.

*calendar question A question used to obtain retrospective information about the chronology of events and activities in people's lives.

*canonical analysis A statistical procedure for examining the relationship between two or more independent variables *and* two or more dependent variables.

carry-over effect The influence that one treatment can have on subsequent treatments.

case-control design A nonexperimental research design involving the comparison of a "case" (i.e., a person with the condition under scrutiny, such as lung cancer) and a matched control (a similar person without the condition).

case study A research method involving a thorough, in-depth analysis of an individual, group, institution, or other social unit.

categorical variable A variable with discrete values (e.g., gender) rather than values along a continuum (e.g., weight).

category system In observational studies, the prespecified plan for organizing and recording the behaviours and events under observation; in qualitative studies, the system used to sort and organize narrative data.

causal modeling The development and statistical testing of an explanatory model of hypothesized causal relationships among phenomena.

causal (cause-and-effect) relationship A relationship between two variables such that the presence or absence of one variable (the "cause") determines the presence or absence, or value, of the other (the "effect").

cell (1) The intersection of a row and column in a table with two or more dimensions; (2) in an experimental design, the representation of an experimental condition in a schematic diagram.

census A survey covering an entire population.

central (core) category The main theme of the research in a Strauss and Corbin grounded theory analysis.

central tendency A statistical index of the "typicalness" of a set of scores, derived from the centre of the score distribution; indexes of central tendency include the mode, median, and mean.

chi-squared test A nonparametric test of statistical significance used to assess whether a relationship exists between two nominal-level variables. Symbolized as χ^2.

clinical relevance The degree to which a study addresses a problem of significance to the practice of nursing.

clinical research Research designed to generate knowledge to guide clinical practice in nursing and other health care fields.

clinical trial A study designed to assess the safety and effectiveness of a new clinical treatment, sometimes involving several phases, one of which (Phase III) is a randomized clinical trial using an experimental design and, often, a large and heterogeneous sample of subjects.

closed-ended question A question that offers respondents a set of mutually exclusive and jointly exhaustive alternative response options, from which the one most closely approximating the "right" answer must be chosen.

*cluster analysis A multivariate statistical procedure used to cluster people or things based on patterns of association.

*cluster randomization The random assignment of intact groups of subjects—rather than individual subjects—to treatment conditions.

cluster sampling A form of sampling in which large groupings ("clusters") are selected first (e.g., nursing schools), with successive subsampling of smaller units (e.g., nursing students).

code of ethics The fundamental ethical principles established by a discipline or institution to guide researchers' conduct in research with human (or animal) subjects.

*codebook A record documenting categorization and coding decisions.

coding The process of transforming raw data into standardized form for data processing and analysis; in quantitative research, the process of attaching numbers to categories; in qualitative research, the process of identifying recurring words, themes, or concepts within the data.

coefficient alpha (Cronbach's alpha) A reliability index that estimates the internal consistency or homogeneity of a measure composed of several items or subparts.

coercion In a research context, the explicit or implicit use of threats (or excessive rewards) to gain people's cooperation in a study.

cohort study A kind of trend study that focuses on a specific subpopulation (which is often an age-related subgroup) from which different samples are selected at different points in time (e.g., the cohort of nursing students who graduated between 1970 and 1974).

comparison group A group of subjects whose scores on a dependent variable are used to evaluate the outcomes of the group of primary interest (e.g., nonsmokers as a comparison group for smokers); term often used in lieu of control group when the study design is not a true experiment.

*computer-assisted personal interviewing (CAPI) In-person interviewing in which the interviewers read questions from, and enter responses onto, a laptop computer.

*computer-assisted telephone interviewing (CATI) Interviewing done over the telephone in which the interviewers read questions from, and enter responses onto, a computer.

concealment A tactic involving the unobtrusive collection of research data without participants' knowledge or consent, used to obtain an accurate view of naturalistic behaviour when the known presence of an observer would distort the behaviour of interest.

concept An abstraction based on observations of—or inferences from—behaviours or characteristics (e.g., stress, pain).

conceptual definition The abstract or theoretical meaning of the concepts being studied.

conceptual file A manual method of organizing qualitative data, by creating file folders for each category in the coding scheme and inserting relevant excerpts from the data.

conceptual model Interrelated concepts or abstractions assembled together in a rational scheme by virtue of their relevance to a common theme; sometimes called *conceptual framework*.

conceptual utilization The use of research findings in a general, conceptual way to broaden one's thinking about an issue, without putting the knowledge to any specific, documentable use.

concurrent validity The degree to which scores on an instrument are correlated with some external criterion, measured at the same time.

***confidence interval** The range of values within which a population parameter is estimated to lie.

***confidence level** The estimated probability that a population parameter lies within a given confidence interval.

confidentiality Protection of participants in a study such that individual identities are not linked to information provided and are never publicly divulged.

confirmability A criterion for evaluating the quality of qualitative research, referring to the objectivity or neutrality of the data or the analysis and interpretation.

***confirmatory factor analysis** A factor analysis, based on maximum likelihood estimation, designed to confirm a hypothesized measurement model.

consent form A written agreement signed by a study participant and a researcher concerning the terms and conditions of voluntary participation in a study.

constant comparison A procedure often used in a grounded theory analysis wherein newly collected data are compared in an ongoing fashion with data obtained earlier, to refine theoretically relevant categories.

constitutive pattern In hermeneutic analysis, a pattern that expresses the relationships among relational themes and is present in all the interviews or texts.

construct An abstraction or concept that is deliberately invented (constructed) by researchers for a scientific purpose (e.g., health locus of control).

construct validity The degree to which an instrument measures the construct under investigation.

consumer An individual who reads, reviews, and critiques research findings and who attempts to use and apply the findings in his or her practice.

***contact information** Information obtained from study participants in longitudinal studies that facilitates their relocation at a future date.

***contamination** The inadvertent, undesirable influence of one experimental treatment condition on another treatment condition.

content analysis The process of organizing and integrating narrative, qualitative information according to emerging themes and concepts.

content validity The degree to which the items in an instrument adequately represent the universe of content for the concept being measured.

content validity index (CVI) An indicator of the degree to which an instrument is content valid, based on average ratings of a panel of experts.

contingency table A two-dimensional table that permits a crosstabulation of the frequencies of two categorical variables.

continuous variable A variable that can take on an infinite range of values along a specified continuum (e.g., height).

control The process of holding constant possible influences on the dependent variable under investigation.

control group Subjects in an experiment who do not receive the experimental treatment and whose performance provides a baseline against which the effects of the treatment can be measured (see also *comparison group*).

convenience sampling Selection of the most readily available persons as participants in a study; also called *accidental sampling*.

***convergent validity** An approach to construct validation that involves assessing the degree to which two methods of measuring a construct are similar (i.e., converge).

core variable (category) In a grounded theory study, the central phenomenon that is used to integrate all categories of the data.

correlation An association or connection between variables, such that variation in one variable is related to variation in another.

correlation coefficient An index summarizing the degree of relationship between variables, typically ranging from $+1.00$ (for a perfect positive relationship) through 0.0 (for no relationship) to -1.00 (for a perfect negative relationship).

correlation matrix A two-dimensional display showing the correlation coefficients between all pairs of a set of study variables.

correlational research Research that explores the interrelationships among variables of interest without any active intervention by the researcher.

cost–benefit analysis An evaluation of the monetary costs of a program or intervention relative to the monetary gains attributable to it.

***counterbalancing** The process of systematically varying the order of presentation of stimuli or treatments to control for ordering effects, especially in a crossover design.

counterfactual The condition or group used as a basis of comparison in a study.

covariate A variable that is statistically controlled (held constant) in analysis of covariance. The covariate is typically an extraneous, confounding influence on the dependent variable or a preintervention measure of the dependent variable.

covert data collection The collection of information in a study without participants' knowledge.

*Cramér's *V* An index describing the magnitude of the relationship between nominal-level data, used when the contingency table to which it is applied is larger than 2×2.

credibility A criterion for evaluating data quality in qualitative studies, referring to confidence in the truth of the data.

criterion sampling A sampling approach in qualitative research that involves selecting cases that meet a predetermined criterion of importance.

criterion variable The criterion against which the effect of an independent variable is tested; sometimes used instead of *dependent variable*.

criterion-related validity The degree to which scores on an instrument are correlated with some external criterion.

*critical case sampling A sampling approach used by qualitative researchers involving the purposeful selection of cases that are especially important or illustrative.

critical ethnography An ethnography that focuses on raising consciousness in the group or culture under study in the hope of effecting social change.

critical incident technique A method of obtaining data from study participants by in-depth exploration of specific incidents and behaviours related to the topic under study.

*critical region The area in the sampling distribution representing values that are "improbable" if the null hypothesis is true.

critical theory An approach to viewing the world that involves a critique of society, with the goal of envisioning new possibilities and effecting social change.

critique An objective, critical, and balanced appraisal of a research report's various dimensions (e.g., conceptual, methodologic, ethical).

Cronbach's alpha A widely used reliability index that estimates the internal consistency or homogeneity of a measure composed of several subparts; also called *coefficient alpha*.

crossover design An experimental design in which one group of subjects is exposed to more than one condition or treatment in random order; sometimes called a *repeated measures design*.

cross-sectional design A study design in which data are collected at one point in time; sometimes used to infer change over time when data are collected from different age or developmental groups.

crosstabulation A determination of the number of cases occurring when two variables are considered simultaneously (e.g., gender—male/ female—crosstabulated with smoking status—smoker/nonsmoker). The results are typically presented in a table with rows and columns divided according to the values of the variables.

data The pieces of information obtained in the course of a study (singular is *datum*).

data analysis The systematic organization and synthesis of research data and, in most quantitative studies, the testing of research hypotheses using those data.

data collection The gathering of information to address a research problem.

data collection protocols The formal procedures researchers develop to guide the collection of data in a standardized fashion in most quantitative studies.

data saturation See *saturation*.

data set The total collection of data on all variables for all study participants.

data source triangulation The use of multiple data sources for the purpose of validating conclusions.

debriefing Communication with study participants after participation is complete regarding various aspects of the study.

deception The deliberate withholding of information, or the provision of false information, to study participants, usually to reduce potential biases.

deductive reasoning The process of developing specific predictions from general principles (see also *inductive reasoning*).

degrees of freedom (*df*) A concept used in statistical testing, referring to the number of sample values free to vary (e.g., with a given sample mean, all but one value would be free to vary); degrees of freedom is often $N - 1$, but different formulas are relevant for different tests.

*Delphi technique A method of obtaining written judgments from a panel of experts about an issue of concern; experts are questioned individually in several rounds, with a summary of the panel's views circulated between rounds, to achieve some consensus.

*demonstration A test of an innovative intervention, often on a large scale, to determine its effectiveness and the desirability of making practice or policy changes.

dependability A criterion for evaluating data quality in qualitative data, referring to the stability of data over time and over conditions.

dependent variable The variable hypothesized to depend on or be caused by another variable (the *independent variable*); the outcome variable of interest.

descriptive phenomenology A type of phenomenology, developed by Husserl, that emphasizes the careful description of ordinary conscious experience of everyday life.

descriptive research Research studies that have as their main objective the accurate portrayal of the characteristics of persons, situations, or groups, and/or the frequency with which certain phenomena occur.

descriptive statistics Statistics used to describe and summarize data (e.g., means, standard deviations).

descriptive theory A broad characterization that thoroughly accounts for a single phenomenon.

determinism The belief that phenomena are not haphazard or random, but rather have antecedent causes; an assumption in the positivist paradigm.

*deviation score A score computed by subtracting the mean of a set of scores from an individual score.

dichotomous variable A variable having only two values or categories (e.g., gender).

directional hypothesis A hypothesis that makes a specific prediction about the direction and nature of the relationship between two variables.

discourse analysis A qualitative tradition, from the discipline of sociolinguistics, that seeks to understand the rules, mechanisms, and structure of conversations.

*discrete variable A variable with a finite number of values between two points.

discriminant function analysis A statistical procedure used to predict group membership or status on a categorical (nominal level) variable on the basis of two or more independent variables.

*discriminant validity An approach to construct validation that involves assessing the degree to which a single method of measuring two constructs yields different results (i.e., discriminates the two).

disproportionate sample A sample in which the researcher samples differing proportions of study participants from different population strata to ensure adequate representation from smaller strata.

domain In ethnographic analysis, a unit or broad category of cultural knowledge.

double-blind experiment An experiment in which neither the subjects nor those who administer the treatment know who is in the experimental or control group.

*dummy variable Dichotomous variables created for use in many multivariate statistical analyses, typically using codes of 0 and 1 (e.g., female = 1, male = 0).

ecological psychology A qualitative tradition that focuses on the environment's influence on human behaviour and attempts to identify principles that explain the interdependence of humans and their environmental context.

editing analysis style An approach to the analysis of qualitative data, in which researchers read through texts in search of meaningful segments and develop a categorization scheme that is used to sort and organize the data.

effect size A statistical expression of the magnitude of the relationship between two variables, or the magnitude of the difference between two groups, with regard to some attribute of interest.

*eigenvalue In factor analysis, the value equal to the sum of the squared weights for each factor.

electronic database Bibliographic files that can be accessed by computer for the purpose of conducting a literature review.

element The most basic unit of a population from which a sample is drawn—typically humans in nursing research.

eligibility criteria The criteria used to designate the specific attributes of the target population, and by which people are selected for participation in a study.

emergent design A design that unfolds in the course of a qualitative study as the researcher makes ongoing design decisions reflecting what has already been learned.

*emergent fit A concept in grounded theory that involves comparing new data and new categories with previously existing conceptualizations (e.g., from the literature).

emic perspective A term used by ethnographers to refer to the way members of a culture themselves view their world; the "insider's view."

empirical evidence Evidence rooted in objective reality and gathered using one's senses as the basis for generating knowledge.

*endogenous variable In path analysis, a variable whose variation is determined by other variables within the model.

error of measurement The deviation between true scores and obtained scores of a measured characteristic.

*error term The mathematic expression (typically in a regression analysis) that represents all unknown or immeasurable attributes that can affect the dependent variable.

estimation procedures Statistical procedures that have as their goal the estimation of population parameters based on sample statistics.

*eta squared In ANOVA, a statistic calculated to indicate the proportion of variance in the dependent variable explained by the independent variables, analogous to R in multiple regression.

ethics A system of moral values that is concerned with the degree to which research procedures adhere to professional, legal, and social obligations to the study participants.

ethnography A branch of human inquiry, associated with the field of anthropology, that focuses on the culture of a group of people, with an effort to understand the world view of those under study.

ethnomethodology A branch of human inquiry, associated with sociology, that focuses on the way in which people make sense of their everyday activities and come to behave in socially acceptable ways.

ethnonursing research The study of human cultures, with a focus on a group's beliefs and practices relating to nursing care and related health behaviours.

etic perspective A term used by ethnographers to refer to the "outsider's" view of the experiences of a cultural group.

evaluation research Research that investigates how well a program, practice, or policy is working.

event sampling In observational studies, a sampling plan that involves the selection of integral behaviours or events.

evidence hierarchy A ranked arrangement of the validity and dependability of evidence based on the rigour of the design that produced it.

evidence-based practice A practice that involves making clinical decisions on the best available evidence, with an emphasis on evidence from disciplined research.

ex post facto research Nonexperimental research conducted after variations in the independent variable have occurred in the natural course of events and, therefore, any causal explanations are inferred "after the fact."

exclusion criteria The criteria that specify characteristics that a population does *not* have.

*exogenous variable In path analysis, a variable whose determinants lie outside the model.

experiment A study in which the researcher controls (manipulates) the independent variable and—in a true experiment—randomly assigns subjects to different conditions.

experimental group Subjects in a study who receive the experimental treatment or intervention.

experimental intervention (experimental treatment) See *intervention*; *treatment*.

*exploratory factor analysis A factor analysis undertaken to determine the underlying dimensionality of a set of variables.

exploratory research A study that explores the dimensions of a phenomenon or that develops or refines hypotheses about relationships between phenomena.

*external criticism In historical research, the systematic evaluation of the authenticity and genuineness of data.

external validity The degree to which study results can be generalized to settings or samples other than the one studied.

extraneous variable A variable that confounds the relationship between the independent and dependent variables and that needs to be controlled either in the research design or through statistical procedures to clarify relationships.

extreme case sampling A sampling approach used by qualitative researchers that involves the purposeful selection of the most extreme or unusual cases.

extreme response set A bias in self-report instruments, especially in psychosocial scales, created when participants select extreme response alternatives (e.g., "strongly agree"), independent of the item's content.

F-ratio The statistic obtained in several statistical tests (e.g., ANOVA) in which variation attributable to different sources (e.g., between groups and within groups) is compared.

face validity The extent to which a measuring instrument looks as though it is measuring what it purports to measure.

factor analysis A statistical procedure for reducing a large set of variables into a smaller set of variables with common characteristics or underlying dimensions.

*factor extraction The first phase of a factor analysis, which involves the extraction of as much variance as possible through the successive creation of linear combinations of the variables in the analysis.

*factor loading In factor analysis, the weight associated with a variable on a given factor.

*factor rotation The second phase of factor analysis, during which the reference axes for the factors are moved such that variables more clearly align with a single factor.

*factor score A person's score on a latent variable (factor).

factorial design An experimental design in which two or more independent variables are simultaneously manipulated, permitting a separate analysis of the main effects of the independent variables, plus the interaction effects of those variables.

feasibility study A small-scale test to determine the feasibility of a larger study (see also *pilot study*).

feminist research Research that seeks to understand, typically through qualitative approaches, how gender and a gendered social order shapes women's lives and their consciousness.

field diary A daily record of events and conversations in the field; also called a *log*.

field notes The notes taken by researchers describing the unstructured observations they have made in the field and their interpretation of those observations.

field research Research in which the data are collected "in the field" from individuals in their normal roles, with the aim of understanding the practices, behaviours, and beliefs of individuals or groups as they normally function in real life.

fieldwork The activities undertaken by researchers (usually qualitative researchers) to collect data out in the field (i.e., in natural settings outside the research environment).

findings The results of the analysis of research data.

*Fisher's exact test A statistical procedure used to test the significance of the difference in proportions, used when the sample size is small or cells in the contingency table have no observations.

fit In grounded theory analysis, the process of identifying characteristics of one piece of data and comparing them with the characteristics of another datum to determine similarity.

fittingness In an assessment of the transferability of findings from a qualitative study, the degree of congruence between the research sample and another group or setting of interest.

fixed alternative question A question that offers respondents a set of prespecified responses, from which the respondent must choose the alternative that most closely approximates the correct response.

focus group interview An interview with a group of individuals assembled to answer questions on a given topic.

focused interview A loosely structured interview in which an interviewer guides the respondent through a set of questions using a topic guide; also called a *semi-structured interview*.

follow-up study A study undertaken to determine the outcomes of individuals with a specified condition or who have received a specified treatment.

forced-choice question A question that requires respondents to choose between two statements that represent polar positions or characteristics.

formal grounded theory A theory developed at a highly abstract level of theory by compiling several substantive grounded theories.

framework The conceptual underpinnings of a study; often called a *theoretical framework* in studies based on a theory, or a *conceptual framework* in studies rooted in a specific conceptual model.

frequency distribution A systematic array of numeric values from the lowest to the highest, together with a count of the number of times each value was obtained.

frequency polygon Graphic display of a frequency distribution in which dots connected by a straight line indicate the number of times score values occur in a data set.

*Friedman test A nonparametric analog of ANOVA, used with paired-groups or repeated-measures situations.

full disclosure The communication of complete information to potential study participants about the nature of the study, the right to refuse participation, and the likely risks and benefits that would be incurred.

functional relationship A relationship between two variables in which it cannot be assumed that one variable caused the other, but it can be said that one variable changes values in relation to changes in the other variable.

gaining entrée The process of gaining access to study participants in qualitative field studies through the cooperation of key actors in the selected community or site.

generalizability The degree to which the research methods justify the inference that the findings are true for a broader group than study participants; in particular, the inference that the findings can be generalized from the sample to the population.

*"going native" A pitfall in qualitative research wherein a researcher becomes too emotionally involved with participants and therefore loses the ability to observe rationally and objectively.

grand theory A broad theory aimed at describing large segments of the physical, social, or behavioural world; also called a *macrotheory*.

grand tour question A broad question asked in an unstructured interview to gain a general overview of a phenomenon on the basis of which more focused questions are subsequently asked.

*graphic rating scale A scale in which respondents are asked to rate something (e.g., a concept or an issue) along an ordered bipolar continuum (e.g., "excellent" to "very poor").

grounded theory An approach to collecting and analyzing qualitative data that aims to develop theories and theoretical propositions grounded in real-world observations.

Hawthorne effect The effect on the dependent variable resulting from subjects' awareness that they are participants under study.

hermeneutic circle In hermeneutics, the qualitative circle signifies a methodologic process in which, to reach understanding, there is continual movement between the parts and the whole of the text that are being analyzed.

hermeneutics A qualitative research tradition, drawing on interpretive phenomenology, that focuses on the lived experiences of humans and on how they interpret those experiences.

heterogeneity The degree to which objects are dissimilar (i.e., characterized by high variability) with respect to some attribute.

*hierarchical multiple regression A multiple regression analysis in which predictor variables are entered into the equation in steps that are prespecified by the analyst.

*histogram A graphic presentation of frequency distribution data.

historical research Systematic studies designed to discover facts and relationships about past events.

history threat The occurrence of events external to an intervention (or other independent variable) but occurring concurrent with it, which can affect the dependent variable and threaten the study's internal validity.

homogeneity (1) In terms of the reliability of an instrument, the degree to which its subparts are internally consistent (i.e., are measuring the same critical attribute); (2) more generally, the degree to which objects are similar (i.e., characterized by low variability).

homogenous sampling A sampling approach used by qualitative researchers involving the deliberate selection of cases with limited variation.

hypothesis A prediction, usually a statement of predicted relationships between variables.

hypothesis testing A statistical procedure that involves the comparison of empirically observed sample findings with theoretically expected findings that would be expected if the null hypothesis were true.

impact analysis An evaluation of the effects of a program or intervention on outcomes of interest, net of other factors influencing those outcomes.

implementation analysis In an evaluation, a description of the process by which a program or intervention was implemented in practice.

implementation potential The extent to which an innovation is amenable to implementation in a new setting, an assessment of which is usually made in an evidence-based practice (or research utilization) project.

implied consent Consent to participate in a study that a researcher assumes has been given based on certain actions of the participant (such as returning a completed questionnaire).

IMRAD format The organization of a research report into four sections: the Introduction, Methods, Research, and Discussion sections.

*incidence rate The rate of new "cases" with a specified condition, determined by dividing the number of new cases over a given period of time by the number at risk of becoming a new case (i.e., free of the condition at the outset of the time period).

independent variable The variable that is believed to cause or influence the dependent variable; in experimental research, the manipulated (treatment) variable.

inductive reasoning The process of reasoning from specific observations to more general rules (see also *deductive reasoning*).

inferential statistics Statistics that permit inferences on whether relationships observed in a sample are likely to occur in the larger population.

informant A term used to refer to those individuals who provide information to researchers about a phenomenon under study (usually in qualitative studies).

informed consent An ethical principle that requires researchers to obtain the voluntary participation of subjects, after informing them of possible risks and benefits.

inquiry audit An independent scrutiny of qualitative data and relevant supporting documents by an external reviewer to determine the dependability and confirmability of qualitative data.

insider research Research on a group or culture—usually in an ethnography—by a member of the group or culture.

Institutional Review Board (IRB) In the United States, the name for the group of individuals from an institution who convene to review proposed and ongoing studies with respect to ethical considerations.

instrument The device used to collect data (e.g., questionnaire, test, observation schedule).

instrumental utilization Clearly identifiable attempts to base some specific action or intervention on the results of research findings.

*instrumentation threat The threat to the internal validity of the study that can arise if the researcher changes the measuring instrument between two points of data collection.

integrative review A review of research that amasses comprehensive information on a topic, weighs pieces of evidence, and integrates information to draw conclusions about the state of knowledge.

*intensity sampling A sampling approach used by qualitative researchers involving the purposeful selection of intense (but not extreme) cases.

*intention to treat A principle for analyzing data that involves the assumption that each person received the treatment to which he or she was assigned; contrary to *on-protocol analysis.*

interaction effect The effect of two or more independent variables acting in combination (interactively) on a dependent variable rather than as unconnected factors.

intercoder reliability The degree to which two coders, operating independently, agree in their coding decisions.

internal consistency The degree to which the subparts of an instrument are all measuring the same attribute or dimension, as a measure of the instrument's reliability.

*internal criticism In historical research, an evaluation of the worth of the historical evidence.

internal validity The degree to which it can be inferred that the experimental treatment (or independent variable), rather than extraneous factors, is responsible for observed effects.

interpretation The process of making sense of the results of a study and examining their implications.

interpretive phenomenology An approach to phenomenology in which interpreting and understanding—and not just describing—human experience is stressed; also called *hermeneutics.*

interrater (interobserver) reliability The degree to which two raters or observers, operating independently, assign the same ratings or values for an attribute being measured or observed.

*interrupted time series design. See *time series design.*

*interval estimation A statistical estimation approach in which the researcher establishes a range of values that are likely, within a given level of confidence, to contain the true population parameter.

interval measurement A level of measurement in which an attribute of a variable is rank-ordered on a scale that has equal distances between points on that scale (e.g., Fahrenheit degrees).

intervention An experimental treatment or manipulation.

intervention protocol In experimental research, the specification of exactly what the treatment and the alternative condition (the counterfactual) will be, and how treatments are to be administered.

*intervention research A systematic research approach distinguished not so much by a particular research methodology as by a distinctive *process* of planning, developing, implementing, testing, and disseminating interventions.

interview A method of data collection in which one person (an interviewer) asks questions of another person (a respondent); interviews are conducted either face-to-face or by telephone.

interview schedule The formal instrument, used in structured self-report studies, that specifies the wording of all questions to be asked of respondents.

intuiting The second step in descriptive phenomenology, which occurs when researchers remain open to the meaning attributed to the phenomenon by those who experienced it.

inverse relationship A relationship characterized by the tendency of high values on one variable to be associated with low values on the second variable; also called a *negative relationship.*

investigator triangulation The use of two or more researchers to analyze and interpret a data set to enhance the validity of the findings.

item A single question on a test or questionnaire, or a single statement on an attitude or other scale (e.g., a final examination might consist of 100 items).

*item analysis A type of analysis used to assess whether items are tapping the same construct and are sufficiently discriminating.

joint interview An interview in which two or more people are interviewed simultaneously, typically using either a semistructured or unstructured interview.

*jottings Short notes jotted down quickly in the field so as to not distract researchers from their observations or their role as participating members of a group.

journal article A report appearing in professional journals such as *Nursing Research.*

journal club A group that meets (often in clinical settings) to discuss and critique research reports appearing in journals, sometimes to assess the potential use of the findings in practice.

judgmental sampling A type of nonprobability sampling method in which the researcher selects study participants based on personal judgment about who will be most representative or informative; also called *purposive sampling.*

*Kendall's tau A correlation coefficient used to indicate the magnitude of a relationship between ordinal-level variables.

key informant A person well-versed in the phenomenon of research interest and who is willing to share the information and insight with the researcher.

keyword An important concept or term used to search for references on a topic (e.g., in an electronic bibliographic database).

known-groups technique A technique for estimating the construct validity of an instrument through an analysis of the degree to which the instrument separates groups predicted to differ based on known characteristics or theory.

*****Kruskal-Wallis test** A nonparametric test used to test the difference between three or more independent groups, based on ranked scores.

*****Kuder-Richardson (KR-20) formula** A method of calculating an internal consistency reliability coefficient for a scaled set of items when the items are dichotomous.

*****latent variable** An unmeasured variable that represents an underlying, abstract construct (usually in the context of a LISREL analysis).

*****law** A theory that has accrued such persuasive empirical support that it is accepted as true (e.g., Boyle's law of gases).

*****least-squares estimation** A commonly used method of statistical estimation in which the solution minimizes the sums of squares of error terms; also called OLS (*ordinary least-squares*).

level of measurement A system of classifying measurements according to the nature of the quantitative information and the type of mathematical operations to which they are amenable; the four levels are nominal, ordinal, interval, and ratio.

level of significance The risk of making a Type I error in a statistical analysis, established by the researcher beforehand (e.g., the .05 level).

life history A narrative self-report about a person's life experiences vis-à-vis a theme of interest.

*****life table analysis** A statistical procedure used when the dependent variable represents a time interval between an initial event (e.g., onset of a disease) and an end event (e.g., death); also called *survival analysis*.

Likert scale A composite measure of attitudes involving the summation of scores on a set of items that are rated by respondents for their degree of agreement or disagreement.

*****linear regression** An analysis for predicting the value of a dependent variable by determining a straight-line fit to the data that minimizes the sum of squared deviations from the line.

LISREL The widely used acronym for linear structural relation analysis, typically used for testing causal models.

literature review A critical summary of research on a topic of interest, often prepared to put a research problem in context.

log In participant observation studies, the observer's daily record of events and conversations that took place.

logical positivism The philosophy underlying the traditional scientific approach; see also *positivist paradigm*.

logistic regression A multivariate regression procedure that analyzes relationships between multiple independent variables and categorical dependent variables; also called *logit analysis*.

*****logit** The natural log of the odds, used as the dependent variable in logistic regression; short for logistic probability unit.

longitudinal study A study designed to collect data at more than one point in time, in contrast to a cross-sectional study.

macrotheory A broad theory aimed at describing large segments of the physical, social, or behavioural world; also called a *grand theory*.

main effects In a study with multiple independent variables, the effects of a single independent variable on the dependent variable.

*****manifest variable** An observed, measured variable that serves as an indicator of an underlying construct (i.e., a latent variable), usually in the context of a LISREL analysis.

manipulation An intervention or treatment introduced by the researcher in an experimental or quasi-experimental study to assess its impact on the dependent variable.

*****manipulation check** In experimental studies, a test to determine whether the manipulation was implemented as intended.

*****Mann-Whitney U test** A nonparametric statistic used to test the difference between two independent groups, based on ranked scores.

MANOVA See *multivariate analysis of variance*.

matching The pairing of subjects in one group with those in another group, based on their similarity on one or more dimension, to enhance the overall similarity of comparison groups.

maturation threat A threat to the internal validity of a study that results when changes to the outcome measure (dependent variable) result from the passage of time.

*****maximum likelihood estimation** An estimation approach (sometimes used in lieu of the least-squares approach) in which the estimators are ones that estimate the parameters most likely to have generated the observed measurements.

maximum variation sampling A sampling approach used by qualitative researchers involving the purposeful selection of cases with a wide range of variation.

*McNemar test A statistical test for comparing differences in proportions when values are derived from paired (nonindependent) groups.

mean A descriptive statistic that is a measure of central tendency, computed by summing all scores and dividing by the number of subjects.

measurement The assignment of numbers to objects according to specified rules to characterize quantities of an attribute.

*measurement model In LISREL, the model that stipulates the hypothesized relationships among the manifest and latent variables.

median A descriptive statistic that is a measure of central tendency, representing the exact middle value in a score distribution; the value above and below which 50% of the scores lie.

*median test A nonparametric statistical test involving the comparison of median values of two independent groups to determine whether the groups are from populations with different medians.

mediating variable A variable that mediates or acts like a "go-between" in a chain linking two other variables (e.g., coping skills mediate the relationship between stressful events and anxiety).

member check A method of validating the credibility of qualitative data through debriefings and discussions with informants.

meta-analysis A technique for quantitatively integrating the findings from multiple studies on a given topic.

meta-matrix A device sometimes used in mixed-method studies that permits researchers to recognize important patterns and themes across data sources and to develop hypotheses.

metasynthesis The theories, grand narratives, generalizations, or interpretive translations produced from the integration or comparison of findings from multiple qualitative studies.

method triangulation The use of multiple methods of data collection about the same phenomenon to enhance the validity of the findings.

methodologic notes In observational field studies, the researcher's notes about the methods used in collecting data.

methodologic research Research designed to develop or refine methods of obtaining, organizing, or analyzing data.

methods (research) The steps, procedures, and strategies for gathering and analyzing data in a research investigation.

middle-range theory A theory that focuses on only a piece of reality or human experience involving a selected number of concepts (e.g., theories of stress).

minimal risk Anticipated risks that are no greater than those ordinarily encountered in daily life or during the performance of routine tests or procedures.

*missing values Values missing from a data set for some study participants, due, for example, to refusals, researcher error, or skip patterns in an instrument.

*mixed-mode strategy An approach to collecting survey data in which efforts are first made to conduct the interview by telephone, but then in-person interviewing is used if a telephone interview cannot be completed.

modality A characteristic of a frequency distribution describing the number of peaks (i.e., values with high frequencies).

mode A descriptive statistic that is a measure of central tendency; the score or value that occurs most frequently in a distribution of scores.

model A symbolic representation of concepts or variables and interrelationships among them.

moderator effect The effect that a third variable (a *moderator variable*) has on the relationship between the independent and dependent variables.

mortality threat A threat to the internal validity of a study, referring to the differential loss of participants (attrition) from different groups.

multimethod (mixed-method) research Generally, research in which multiple approaches are used to address a problem; often used to designate studies in which both qualitative and quantitative data are collected and analyzed.

multimodal distribution A distribution of values with more than one peak (high frequency).

*multiple classification analysis A variant of multiple regression and ANCOVA that yields group means on the dependent variable adjusted for the effects of covariates.

multiple comparison procedures Statistical tests, normally applied after an ANOVA indicates statistically significant group differences, that compare different pairs of groups; also called *post hoc tests*.

multiple correlation coefficient An index (symbolized as R) that summarizes the degree of relationship between two or more independent variables and a dependent variable.

multiple regression analysis A statistical procedure for understanding the simultaneous effects of two or more independent (predictor) variables on a dependent variable.

multistage sampling A sampling strategy that proceeds through a set of stages from larger to smaller sampling units (e.g., from states, to nursing schools, to faculty members).

***multitrait–multimethod matrix method** A method of establishing the construct validity of an instrument that involves the use of multiple measures for a set of subjects; the target instrument is valid to the extent that there is a strong relationship between it and other measures purporting to measure the same attribute (convergence) and a weak relationship between it and other measures purporting to measure a different attribute (discriminability).

multivariate analysis of variance (MANOVA) A statistical procedure used to test the significance of differences between the means of two or more groups on two or more dependent variables, considered simultaneously.

multivariate statistics Statistical procedures designed to analyze the relationships among three or more variables; commonly used multivariate statistics include multiple regression, analysis of covariance, and factor analysis.

N The symbol designating the total number of subjects (e.g., "the total *N* was 500").

n The symbol designating the number of subjects in a subgroup or cell of a study (e.g., "each of the four groups had an *n* of 125, for a total *N* of 500").

***narrative analysis** A type of qualitative approach that focuses on the story as the object of the inquiry.

***natural experiment** A nonexperimental study that takes advantage of some naturally occurring event or phenomenon (e.g., an earthquake) that is presumed to have implications for people's behaviour or condition, typically by comparing people exposed to the event with those not exposed.

naturalistic paradigm An alternative paradigm to the traditional positivist paradigm that holds that there are multiple interpretations of reality, and that the goal of research is to understand how individuals construct reality within their context; often associated with qualitative research.

naturalistic setting A setting for the collection of research data that is natural to those being studied (e.g., homes, places of work, and so on).

***needs assessment** A study designed to describe the needs of a group, a community, or an organization, usually as a guide to policy planning and resource allocation.

negative case analysis A method of refining a hypothesis or theory in a qualitative study that involves the inclusion of cases that appear to disconfirm earlier hypotheses.

negative relationship A relationship between two variables in which there is a tendency for higher values on one variable to be associated with lower values on the other (e.g., as temperature increases, people's productivity may decrease); also called an *inverse relationship.*

negative results Research results that fail to support the researcher's hypotheses.

negatively skewed distribution An asymmetric distribution of data values with a disproportionately high number of cases having high values—that is, falling at the upper end of the distribution; when displayed graphically, the tail points to the left.

***net effect** The effect of an independent variable on a dependent variable after controlling for the effect of one or more covariates through multiple regression or ANCOVA.

network sampling The sampling of participants based on referrals from others already in the sample; also called *snowball sampling* and *nominated sampling.*

***nocebo effect** Adverse side effect experienced by those receiving a placebo treatment.

nominal measurement The lowest level of measurement involving the assignment of characteristics into categories (e.g., males, category 1; females, category 2).

nominated sampling A sampling method in which researchers ask early informants to make referrals to other study participants; called *snowball sampling* and *network sampling.*

nondirectional hypothesis A research hypothesis that does not stipulate in advance the expected direction of the relationship between variables.

nonequivalent control group design A quasi-experimental design involving a comparison group that was not developed on the basis of random assignment, but from whom preintervention data usually are obtained to assess the initial equivalence of the groups.

nonexperimental research Studies in which the researcher collects data without introducing an intervention.

nonparametric statistical tests A class of inferential statistical tests that do not involve rigorous assumptions about the distribution of critical variables; most often used with nominal or ordinal data.

nonprobability sampling The selection of sampling units (e.g., participants) from a population using nonrandom procedures, as in convenience, judgmental, and quota sampling.

***nonrecursive model** A causal model that predicts reciprocal effects (i.e., a variable can be both the cause of and an effect of another variable).

nonresponse bias A bias that can result when a non-random subset of people invited to participate in a study fail to participate.

nonsignificant result The result of a statistical test indicating that group differences or a relationship between variables could have occurred as a result of chance at a given level of significance; sometimes abbreviated as *NS*.

normal distribution A theoretical distribution that is bell shaped, symmetric, and not too peaked or flat; also called a *normal curve*.

norms Test performance standards, based on test score information from a large, representative sample.

null hypothesis A hypothesis stating no relationship between the variables under study; used primarily in statistical testing as the hypothesis to be rejected.

nursing research Systematic inquiry designed to develop knowledge about issues of importance to the nursing profession.

objectivity The extent to which two independent researchers would arrive at similar judgments or conclusions (i.e., judgments not biased by personal values or beliefs).

*oblique rotation In factor analysis, a rotation of factors such that the reference axes are allowed to move to acute or oblique angles, and hence the factors are allowed to be correlated.

observational notes An observer's in-depth descriptions about events and conversations observed in naturalistic settings.

observational research Studies in which data are collected by observing and recording behaviours or activities of interest; medical researchers sometimes use this term to refer to nonexperimental research.

observed (obtained) score The actual score or numeric value assigned to a person on a measure.

odds The ratio of two probabilities, namely, the probability of an event occurring to the probability that it will not occur.

odds ratio (OR) The ratio of one odds to another odds; used in logistic regression as a measure of association and as an estimate of relative risk.

*on-protocol analysis A principle for analyzing data that includes data only from those members of a treatment group who actually received the treatment; contrary to an *intention-to-treat* analysis.

*one-tailed test A test of statistical significance in which only values at one extreme (tail) of a distribution are considered in determining significance; used when the researcher can predict the direction of a relationship (see *directional hypothesis*).

open coding The first level of coding in a grounded theory study, referring to the basic descriptive coding of the content of the narrative data.

open-ended question A question in an interview or questionnaire that does not restrict respondents' answers to preestablished alternatives.

operational definition The definition of a concept or variable in terms of the procedures by which it is to be measured.

operationalization The process of translating research concepts into measurable phenomena.

*oral history An unstructured self-report technique used to gather personal recollections of events and their perceived causes and consequences.

ordinal measurement A level of measurement that rank-orders phenomena along some dimension.

ordinary least-squares (OLS) regression Regression analysis that uses the least-squares criterion for estimating the parameters in the regression equation.

*orthogonal rotation In factor analysis, a rotation of factors such that the reference axes are kept at a right angle, and hence the factors remain uncorrelated.

outcome analysis An evaluation of what happens with regard to outcomes of interest after implementing a program or intervention, without using an experimental design to assess net effects; see also *impact analysis*.

outcome measure A term sometimes used to refer to the dependent variable, i.e., the measure that captures the outcome of an intervention.

outcomes research Research designed to document the effectiveness of health care services and the end results of patient care.

p value In statistical testing, the probability that the obtained results are due to chance alone; the probability of committing a Type I error.

pair matching See *matching*.

panel study A type of longitudinal study in which data are collected from the same people (a *panel*) at two or more points in time, often in the context of a survey.

paradigm A way of looking at natural phenomena that encompasses a set of philosophical assumptions and that guides one's approach to inquiry.

paradigm case In a hermeneutic analysis following the precepts of Benner, a strong exemplar of the phenomenon under study, often used early in the analysis to gain understanding of the phenomenon.

parameter A characteristic of a population (e.g., the mean age of all Japanese citizens).

parametric statistical tests A class of inferential statistical tests that involve (a) assumptions about the distribution of the variables, (b) the estimation of a parameter, and (c) the use of interval or ratio measures.

participant See *study participant*.

participant observation A special approach to collecting observational data in which researchers immerse themselves in the world of study participants and participate in that world insofar as possible.

participatory action research A research approach with an ideological perspective based on the premise that the use and production of knowledge can be political and used to exert power.

path analysis A regression-based procedure for testing causal models, typically using nonexperimental data.

*path coefficient The weight representing the impact of one variable on another in a path analytic causal model.

*path diagram A graphic representation of the hypothesized linkages and causal flow among variables in a causal relationship.

Pearson's *r* A widely used correlation coefficient designating the magnitude of the relationship between two variables measured on at least an interval scale; also called the *product–moment correlation*.

peer debriefing Sessions with peers to review and explore various aspects of a study—typically in a qualitative study.

peer reviewer A person who reviews and critiques a research report or proposal, who himself or herself is a researcher (usually working on similar types of research problems as those under review), and who makes a recommendation about publishing or funding the research.

perfect relationship A correlation between two variables such that the values of one variable permit perfect prediction of the values of the other; designated as 1.00 or −1.00.

persistent observation In qualitative research, the researcher's intense focus on the aspects of a situation that are relevant to the phenomena being studied.

*person triangulation The collection of data from different levels of persons, with the aim of validating data through multiple perspectives on the phenomenon.

personal interview A face-to-face interview between an interviewer and a respondent.

personal notes In field studies, written comments about the observer's own feelings during the research process.

phenomenology A qualitative research tradition, with roots in philosophy and psychology, that focuses on the lived experience of humans.

phenomenon The abstract concept under study, most often used by qualitative researchers in lieu of the term "variable."

*phi coefficient A statistical index describing the magnitude of the relationship between two dichotomous variables.

*photo elicitation An interview stimulated and guided by photographic images.

pilot study A small-scale version, or trial run, done in preparation for a major study.

placebo A sham or pseudo-intervention, often used as a control condition.

placebo effect Changes in the dependent variable attributable to the placebo condition.

*point estimation A statistical estimation procedure in which the researcher uses information from a sample to estimate the single value (statistic) that best represents the value of the population parameter.

*point prevalence rate The number of people with a condition or disease divided by the total number at risk, multiplied by the number of people for whom the rate is being established (e.g., per 1000 population).

population The entire set of individuals or objects having some common characteristics (e.g., all RNs in South Africa); sometimes called a *universe*.

positive relationship A relationship between two variables in which there is a tendency for high values on one variable to be associated with high values on the other (e.g., as physical activity increases, pulse rate also increases).

positive results Research results that are consistent with the researcher's hypotheses.

positively skewed distribution An asymmetric distribution of values with a disproportionately high number of cases having low values—that is, falling at the lower end of the distribution; when displayed graphically, the tail points to the right.

positivist paradigm The traditional paradigm underlying the scientific approach, which assumes that there is a fixed, orderly reality that can be objectively studied; often associated with quantitative research.

poster session A session at a professional conference in which several researchers simultaneously present visual displays summarizing their studies, while conference attendees circulate around the room perusing the displays.

post hoc test A test for comparing all possible pairs of groups following a significant test of overall group differences (e.g., in an ANOVA).

postpositivist paradigm A modification of the traditional positivist paradigm that acknowledges the impossibility of total objectivity; postpositivists appreciate the impediments to knowing reality with certainty and therefore seek *probabilistic* evidence.

posttest The collection of data after introducing an experimental intervention.

posttest-only design An experimental design in which data are collected from subjects only after the experimental intervention has been introduced; also called an *after-only design*.

power A research design's ability to detect relationships that exist among variables.

power analysis A procedure for estimating either the likelihood of committing a Type II error or sample size requirements.

prediction The use of empirical evidence to make forecasts about how variables will behave in a new setting and with different individuals.

predictive validity The degree to which an instrument can predict some criterion observed at a future time.

predictor variables In a regression analysis (and other multivariate analyses), the independent variables entered into the analysis to predict the dependent variable.

preexperimental design A research design that does not include mechanisms to compensate for the absence of either randomization or a control group.

pretest (1) The collection of data before the experimental intervention; sometimes called *baseline data*; (2) the trial administration of a newly developed instrument to identify flaws or assess time requirements.

pretest–posttest design An experimental design in which data are collected from research subjects both before and after introducing the experimental intervention; also called a *before–after design*.

*prevalence study A study undertaken to determine the prevalence rate of some condition (e.g., a disease or behaviour, such as smoking) at a particular point in time.

primary source First-hand reports of facts, findings, or events; in research, the primary source is the original research report prepared by the investigator who conducted the study.

*principal investigator (PI) The person who is the lead researcher and who will have primary responsibility for overseeing the project.

probability sampling The selection of sampling units (e.g., participants) from a population using random procedures, as in simple random sampling, cluster sampling, and systematic sampling.

*probing Eliciting more useful or detailed information from a respondent in an interview than was volunteered in the first reply.

problem statement The statement of the research problem, often phrased in the form of a research question.

process analysis An evaluation focusing on the process by which a program or intervention gets implemented and used in practice.

process consent In a qualitative study, an ongoing, transactional process of negotiating consent with study participants, allowing them to play a collaborative role in the decision making regarding their continued participation.

product–moment correlation coefficient (*r*) A widely-used correlation coefficient, designating the magnitude of the relationship between two variables measured on at least an interval scale; also called *Pearson's r*.

*projective technique A method of measuring psychological attributes (values, attitudes, personality) by providing respondents with unstructured stimuli to which to respond.

prolonged engagement In qualitative research, the investment of sufficient time during data collection to have an in-depth understanding of the group under study, thereby enhancing data credibility.

*proportional hazards model A model applied in multivariate analyses in which independent variables are used to predict the risk (hazard) of experiencing an event at a given point in time.

proportionate sample A sample that results when the researcher samples from different strata of the population in proportion to their representation in the population.

proposal A document specifying what the researcher proposes to study; it communicates the research problem, its significance, planned procedures for solving the problem, and, when funding is sought, how much the study will cost.

prospective design A study design that begins with an examination of presumed causes (e.g., cigarette smoking) and then goes forward in time to observe presumed effects (e.g., lung cancer).

psychometric assessment An evaluation of the quality of an instrument, based primarily on evidence of its reliability and validity.

psychometrics The theory underlying principles of measurement and the application of the theory in the development of measuring tools.

purposive (purposeful) sampling A nonprobability sampling method in which the researcher selects participants based on personal judgment about which ones will be most representative or informative; also called *judgmental sampling*.

Q sort A data collection method in which participants sort statements into a number of piles (usually 9 or 11) along a bipolar dimension (e.g., most like me/least like me; most useful/ least useful).

qualitative analysis The organization and interpretation of nonnumeric data for the purpose of discovering important underlying dimensions and patterns of relationships.

qualitative data Information collected in narrative (nonnumeric) form, such as the transcript of an unstructured interview.

***qualitative outcome analysis (QOA)** An approach to address the gap between qualitative research and clinical practice, involving the identification and evaluation of clinical interventions based on qualitative findings.

qualitative research The investigation of phenomena, typically in an in-depth and holistic fashion, through the collection of rich narrative materials using a flexible research design.

quantitative analysis The manipulation of numeric data through statistical procedures for the purpose of describing phenomena or assessing the magnitude and reliability of relationships among them.

quantitative data Information collected in a quantified (numeric) form.

quantitative research The investigation of phenomena that lend themselves to precise measurement and quantification, often involving a rigorous and controlled design.

quasi-experiment A study involving an intervention in which subjects are not randomly assigned to treatment conditions, but the researcher exercises certain controls to enhance the study's internal validity.

quasi-statistics An "accounting" system used to assess the validity of conclusions derived from qualitative analysis.

questionnaire A method of gathering self-report information from respondents through self-administration of questions in a paper-and-pencil format.

quota sampling The nonrandom selection of participants in which the researcher prespecifies characteristics of the sample to increase its representativeness.

r The symbol for a bivariate correlation coefficient, summarizing the magnitude and direction of a relationship between two variables.

R The symbol for a multiple correlation coefficient, indicating the magnitude (but not direction) of the relationship between the dependent variable and multiple independent variables, taken together.

R^2 The squared multiple correlation coefficient, indicating the proportion of variance in the dependent variable accounted for or explained by a group of independent variables.

random assignment The assignment of subjects to treatment conditions in a random manner (i.e., in a manner determined by chance alone); also called *randomization*.

random number table A table displaying hundreds of digits (from 0 to 9) set up in such a way that each number is equally likely to follow any other.

random sampling The selection of a sample such that each member of a population has an equal probability of being included.

randomization The assignment of subjects to treatment conditions in a random manner (i.e., in a manner determined by chance alone); also called *random assignment*.

***randomized block design** An experimental design involving two or more factors (independent variables), only one of which in experimentally manipulated.

randomized clinical trial (RCT) A full experimental test of a new treatment, involving random assignment to treatment groups and, typically, a large and diverse sample (also known as a Phase III clinical trial).

randomness An important concept in quantitative research, involving having certain features of the study established by chance rather than by design or personal preference.

range A measure of variability, computed by subtracting the lowest value from the highest value in a distribution of scores.

rating scale A scale that requires ratings of an object or concept along a continuum.

ratio measurement A level of measurement with equal distances between scores and a true meaningful zero point (e.g., weight).

raw data Data in the form in which they were collected, without being coded or analyzed.

reactivity A measurement distortion arising from the study participant's awareness of being observed, or, more generally, from the effect of the measurement procedure itself.

***readability** The ease with which research materials (e.g., a questionnaire) can be read by people with varying reading skills, often empirically determined through readability formulas.

***receiver operating characteristic curve (ROC curve)** A method used in developing and refining screening instruments to determine the best cut-off point for "caseness."

***recursive model** A path model in which the causal flow is unidirectional, without any feedback loops; opposite of a nonrecursive model.

refereed journal A journal in which decisions about the acceptance of manuscripts are made based on recommendations from peer reviewers.

reflective notes Notes that document a qualitative researcher's personal experiences, reflections, and progress in the field.

reflexive journal A journal maintained by qualitative researchers during data collection and data analysis to document their self-analysis of both how they affected the research and how the research affected them.

reflexivity In qualitative studies, critical self-reflection about one's own biases, preferences, and preconceptions.

regression analysis A statistical procedure for predicting values of a dependent variable based on the values of one or more independent variables.

relationship A bond or a connection between two or more variables.

***relative risk** An estimate of risk of "caseness" in one group compared to another, computed by dividing the rate for one group by the rate for another.

reliability The degree of consistency or dependability with which an instrument measures the attribute it is designed to measure.

reliability coefficient A quantitative index, usually ranging in value from .00 to 1.00, that provides an estimate of how reliable an instrument is; it is computed through such procedures as Cronbach's alpha technique, the split-half technique, the test–retest approach, and interrater approaches.

repeated measures design An experimental design in which one group of subjects is exposed to more than one condition or treatment in random order; also called a *crossover design.*

replication The deliberate repetition of research procedures in a second investigation for the purpose of determining if earlier results can be repeated.

representative sample A sample whose characteristics are comparable to those of the population from which it is drawn.

research Systematic inquiry that uses orderly, disciplined methods to answer questions or solve problems.

research control See *control.*

research design The overall plan for addressing a research question, including specifications for enhancing the study's integrity.

Research Ethics Board (REB) A group established within Canadian universities, hospitals, and other institutions where research is conducted to ensure that ethical principles are applied to research involving human subjects.

research hypothesis The actual hypothesis a researcher wants to test (as opposed to the *null hypothesis*), stating the anticipated relationship between two or more variables.

research methods The techniques used to structure a study and to gather and analyze information in a systematic fashion.

research misconduct Fabrication, falsification, plagiarism, or other practices that seriously deviate from those that are commonly accepted within the scientific community for proposing, conducting, or reporting research.

research problem A situation involving an enigmatic, perplexing, or conflictful condition that can be investigated through disciplined inquiry.

research proposal See *proposal.*

research question A statement of the specific query the researcher wants to answer to address a research problem.

research report A document summarizing the main features of a study, including the research question, the methods used to address it, the findings, and the interpretation of the findings.

research utilization The use of some aspect of a study in an application unrelated to the original research.

researcher credibility The faith that can be put in a researcher, based on his or her training, qualifications, and experience.

***residuals** In multiple regression, the error term or unexplained variance.

respondent In a self-report study, the study participant responding to questions posed by the researcher.

response rate The rate of participation in a study, calculated by dividing the number of persons participating by the number of persons sampled.

response set bias The measurement error introduced by the tendency of some individuals to respond to items in characteristic ways (e.g., always agreeing), independently of the items' content.

results The answers to research questions, obtained through an analysis of the collected data; in a quantitative study, the information obtained through statistical tests.

retrospective design A study design that begins with the manifestation of the dependent variable in the present (e.g., lung cancer) and then searches for the presumed cause occurring in the past (e.g., cigarette smoking).

risk/benefit ratio The relative costs and benefits, to an individual subject and to society at large, of participation in a study; also, the relative costs and benefits of implementing an innovation.

rival hypothesis An alternative explanation, competing with the researcher's hypothesis, to account for the results of a study.

sample A subset of a population, selected to participate in a study.

sample size The total number of study participants participating in a study.

sampling The process of selecting a portion of the population to represent the entire population.

sampling bias Distortions that arise when a sample is not representative of the population from which it was drawn.

sampling distribution A theoretical distribution of a statistic (e.g., a mean), using the values of the statistic computed from an infinite number of samples as the data points in the distribution.

sampling error The fluctuation of the value of a statistic from one sample to another drawn from the same population.

sampling frame A list of all the elements in the population from which the sample is drawn.

sampling plan The formal plan specifying a sampling method, a sample size, and procedures for recruiting subjects.

saturation The collection of data in a qualitative study to the point at which a sense of closure is attained because new data yield redundant information.

scale A composite measure of an attribute, involving the combination of several items that have a logical and empirical relationship to each other, resulting in the assignment of a score to place people on a continuum with respect to the attribute.

*scatter plot A graphic representation of the relationship between two variables.

scientific merit The degree to which a study is methodologically and conceptually sound.

scientific method A set of orderly, systematic, controlled procedures for acquiring dependable, empirical—and typically quantitative—information; the methodologic approach associated with the positivist paradigm.

screening instrument An instrument used to determine whether potential subjects for a study meet eligibility criteria (or for determining whether a person has a specified condition).

secondary analysis A form of research in which the data collected by one researcher are reanalyzed, usually by another investigator, to answer new research questions.

secondary source Second-hand accounts of events or facts; in a research context, a description of a study or studies prepared by someone other than the original researcher.

selective coding A level of coding in a grounded theory study that begins after the core category is discovered and involves systematically integrating relationships between the core category and other categories and validating those relationships.

selection threat (self-selection) A threat to the internal validity of the study resulting from preexisting differences between groups under study; the differences affect the dependent variable in ways extraneous to the effect of the independent variable.

self-determination A person's ability to voluntarily decide whether or not to participate in a study.

self-report A method of collecting data that involves a direct report of information by the person who is being studied (e.g., by interview or questionnaire).

semantic differential A technique used to measure attitudes that asks respondents to rate a concept of interest on a series of bipolar rating scales.

semistructured interview An interview in which the researcher has listed topics to cover rather than specific questions to ask.

sensitivity The ability of screening instruments to correctly identify a "case" (i.e., to correctly diagnose a condition).

sensitivity analysis In a meta-analysis, a method to determine whether conclusions are sensitive to the quality of the studies included.

*sequential clinical trial A clinical trial in which data are continuously analyzed and "stop rules" are used to decide when the evidence about the intervention's efficacy is sufficiently strong that the experiment can be stopped.

setting The physical location and conditions in which data collection takes place in a study.

significance level The probability that an observed relationship could be caused by chance (i.e., as a result of sampling error); significance at the .05 level indicates the probability that a relationship of the observed magnitude would be found by chance only 5 times out of 100.

*sign test A nonparametric test for comparing two paired groups based on the relative ranking of values between the pairs.

simple random sampling The most basic type of probability sampling, wherein a sampling frame is created by enumerating all members of a population and then selecting a sample from the sampling frame through completely random procedures.

*simultaneous multiple regression A multiple regression analysis in which all predictor variables are entered into the equation simultaneously; sometimes called *direct* or *standard* multiple regression.

*single-subject experiment A study that tests the effectiveness of an intervention with a single subject, typically using a time series design.

site The overall location where a study is undertaken.

skewed distribution The asymmetric distribution of a set of data values around a central point.

snowball sampling The selection of participants through referrals from earlier participants; also called *network sampling* or *nominated sampling.*

social desirability response set A bias in self-report instruments created when participants have a tendency to misrepresent their opinions in the direction of answers consistent with prevailing social norms.

*Solomon four-group design An experimental design that uses a before–after design for one pair of experimental and control groups, and an after-only design for a second pair.

*space triangulation The collection of data on the same phenomenon in multiple sites to enhance the validity of the findings.

*Spearman-Brown prophecy formula An equation for making corrections to a reliability estimate calculated by the split-half technique.

Spearman's rank-order correlation (Spearman's rho) A correlation coefficient indicating the magnitude of a relationship between variables measured on the ordinal scale.

specificity The ability of a screening instrument to correctly identify noncases.

split-half technique A method for estimating internal consistency reliability by correlating scores on half of the instrument with scores on the other half.

standard deviation The most frequently used statistic for measuring the degree of variability in a set of scores.

standard error The standard deviation of a theoretical sampling distribution, such as a sampling distribution of means.

*standard scores Scores expressed in terms of standard deviations from the mean, with raw scores transformed to have a mean of zero and a standard deviation of one; also called *z* scores.

statement of purpose A broad declarative statement of the overall goals of a study.

statistic An estimate of a parameter, calculated from sample data.

statistical analysis The organization and analysis of quantitative data using statistical procedures, including both descriptive and inferential statistics.

statistical conclusion validity The degree to which conclusions about relationships and differences from a statistical analysis of the data are legitimate.

statistical control The use of statistical procedures to control extraneous influences on the dependent variable.

statistical inference The process of inferring attributes about the population based on information from a sample, using laws of probability.

statistical power The ability of the research design and analysis to detect true relationships among variables.

statistical significance A term indicating that the results from an analysis of sample data are unlikely to have been caused by chance, at some specified level of probability.

statistical test An analytic tool that estimates the probability that obtained results from a sample reflect true population values.

*stepwise multiple regression A multiple regression analysis in which predictor variables are entered into the equation in steps, in the order in which the increment to *R* is greatest.

stipend A monetary payment to individuals participating in a study to serve as an incentive for participation and/or to compensate for time and expenses.

strata Subdivisions of the population according to some characteristic (e.g., males and females); singular is *stratum.*

stratified random sampling The random selection of study participants from two or more strata of the population independently.

*structural equations Equations representing the magnitude and nature of hypothesized relations among sets of variables in a theory.

structured data collection An approach to collecting information from participants, either through self-report or observations, in which the researcher determines response categories in advance.

study participant An individual who participates and provides information in a study.

subgroup effect The differential effect of the independent variable on the dependent variable for various subsets of the sample.

subject An individual who participates and provides data in a study; term used primarily in quantitative research.

substantive theory In grounded theory, a theory that is grounded in data from a single study on a specific substantive area (e.g., postpartum depression); in contrast to *formal theory.*

summated rating scale A composite scale with multiple items, each of which is scored; item scores are added together to yield a total score that distributes people along a continuum (e.g., a Likert scale).

survey research Nonexperimental research in which information regarding the activities, beliefs, preferences, and attitudes of people is gathered by direct questioning.

*survival analysis A statistical procedure used when the dependent variable represents a time interval between an initial event (e.g., onset of a disease) and an end event (e.g., death); also called *life table analysis*.

symmetric distribution A distribution of values with two halves that are mirror images of each other; a distribution that is not skewed.

systematic sampling The selection of study participants such that every *k*th (e.g., every 10th) person (or element) in a sampling frame or list is chosen.

table of random numbers See *random number table*.

tacit knowledge Information about a culture that is so deeply embedded that members do not talk about it or may not even be consciously aware of it.

target population The entire population in which the researcher is interested and to which he or she would like to generalize the results of a study.

taxonomy In an ethnographic analysis, a system of classifying and organizing terms and concepts, developed to illuminate the internal organization of a domain and the relationship among the subcategories of the domain.

template analysis style An approach to qualitative analysis in which a preliminary template or coding scheme is used to sort the narrative data.

test statistic A statistic used to test for the statistical significance of relationships between variables; the sampling distributions of test statistics are known for circumstances in which the null hypothesis is true; examples include chi-square, *F*-ratio, *t*, and Pearson's *r*.

test–retest reliability Assessment of the stability of an instrument by correlating the scores obtained on repeated administrations.

*testing threat A threat to a study's internal validity that occurs when the administration of a pretest or baseline measure of a dependent variable results in changes on the variable, apart from the effect of the independent variable.

theme A recurring regularity emerging from an analysis of qualitative data.

theoretical notes In field studies, notes detailing the researcher's interpretations of observed behaviour.

theoretical sampling In qualitative studies, the selection of sample members based on emerging findings as the study progresses to ensure adequate representation of important themes.

theory An abstract generalization that presents a systematic explanation about the relationships among phenomena.

theory triangulation The use of competing theories or hypotheses in the analysis and interpretation of data.

thick description A rich and thorough description of the research context in a qualitative study.

think aloud method A qualitative method used to collect data about cognitive processes (e.g., problem solving, decision making), involving the use of audio recordings to capture people's reflections on decisions as they are being made or problems as they are being solved.

time sampling In observational research, the selection of time periods during which observations will take place.

time series design A quasi-experimental design involving the collection of data over an extended time period, with multiple data collection points both before and after an intervention.

time triangulation The collection of data on the same phenomenon or about the same people at different points in time to enhance the validity of the findings.

topic guide A list of broad question areas to be covered in a semistructured interview or focus group interview.

transferability The extent to which findings can be transferred to other settings or groups—often used in qualitative research and analogous to generalizability in quantitative research.

treatment The experimental intervention under study; the condition being manipulated.

treatment group The group receiving the intervention being tested; the experimental group.

trend study A form of longitudinal study in which different samples from a population are studied over time with respect to some phenomenon (e.g., annual Gallup polls on abortion attitudes).

triangulation The use of multiple methods to collect and interpret data about a phenomenon so as to converge on an accurate representation of reality.

true score A hypothetical score that would be obtained if a measure were infallible.

trustworthiness The degree of confidence qualitative researchers have in their data, assessed using the criteria of credibility, transferability, dependability, and confirmability.

t-**test** A parametric statistical test for analyzing the difference between two means.

*two-tailed tests Statistical tests in which both ends of the sampling distribution are used to determine improbable values.

Type I error An error created by rejecting the null hypothesis when it is true (i.e., the researcher concludes that a relationship exists when in fact it does not—a false positive).

Type II error An error created by accepting the null hypothesis when it is false (i.e., the researcher concludes that *no* relationship exists when in fact it does—a false negative).

typical case sampling An approach to sampling in qualitative research involving the selection of participants who highlight what is typical or average.

unimodal distribution A distribution of values with one peak (high frequency).

unit of analysis The basic unit or focus of a researcher's analysis; in nursing research, the unit of analysis is typically the individual study participant.

univariate descriptive study A study that gathers information on the occurrence, frequency of occurrence, or average value of the variables of interest, one variable at a time, without focusing on interrelationships among variables.

univariate statistics Statistical procedures for analyzing a single variable for purposes of description.

unstructured interview An oral self-report in which the researcher asks a respondent questions without having a predetermined plan regarding the content or flow of information to be gathered.

unstructured observation The collection of descriptive information through direct observation that is not guided by a formal, prespecified plan for observing, enumerating, or recording the information.

validity The degree to which an instrument measures what it is intended to measure.

validity coefficient A quantitative index, usually ranging in value from .00 to 1.00, that provides an estimate of how valid an instrument is.

variability The degree to which values on a set of scores are dispersed.

variable An attribute of a person or object that varies, that is, takes on different values (e.g., body temperature, age, heart rate).

variance A measure of variability or dispersion, equal to the standard deviation squared.

vignette A brief description of an event, person, or situation about which respondents are asked to describe their reactions.

visual analog scale A scaling procedure used to measure certain clinical symptoms (e.g., pain, fatigue) by having people indicate on a straight line the intensity of the symptom.

vulnerable subjects Special groups of people whose rights in research studies need special protection because of their inability to provide meaningful informed consent or because their circumstances place them at higher-than-average risk of adverse effects; examples include young children, the mentally retarded, and unconscious patients.

weighting A correction procedure used to arrive at population values when a disproportionate sampling design has been used.

*Wilcoxon signed ranks test A nonparametric statistical test for comparing two paired groups based on the relative ranking of values between the pairs.

*Wilk's lambda An index used in discriminant function analysis to indicate the proportion of variance in the dependent variable unaccounted for by predictors; $\lambda = 1 - R^2$.

within-subjects design A research design in which a single group of subjects is compared under different conditions or at different points in time (e.g., before and after surgery).

*z score A standard score, expressed in terms of standard deviations from the mean.

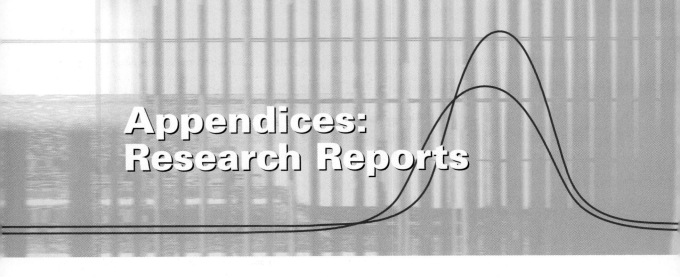

Infant, Mother, and Contextual Predictors of Mother–Very Low Birth Weight Infant Interaction at 9 Months of Age

Nancy Feeley, Laurie Gottlieb, Phyllis Zelkowitz

ABSTRACT. This prospective study examined how characteristics of infants (i.e., birth weight and perinatal illness severity), mothers (i.e., anxiety and level of education), and the social context (i.e., maternal received and perceived helpfulness of support) related to mother–very low birth weight (VLBW) infant interaction in 72 dyads. Infant, mother, and contextual factors were assessed at 3 and 9 months of age, and mothers and infants were observed in teaching interactions at 9 months. Dyads whose interaction was more sensitive and responsive included mothers who were better educated and less anxious at 3 months and reported higher perceived support at 3 months. The findings highlight the importance of maternal education and well-being in the parenting of VLBW infants. *J Dev Behav Pediatr 26:24–33, 2005.* Index terms: *very low birth weight, mother–infant interaction, maternal anxiety, maternal support, maternal education.*

Considerable evidence suggests that children born with a very low birth weight (VLBW) (<1500 g) are at greater risk of a variety of developmental difficulties including cognitive, learning, behavioral, and socioemotional problems compared with their normal birth weight (NBW) counterparts.[1–8] The quality of interaction between

Reprinted with permission from *Developmental and Behavioral Pediatrics* (2005; 26[1]: 24–33).

a mother and her infant is one particular aspect of the VLBW child's early environment that appears to have long-lasting effects on later development. Although early sensitive and responsive parent–child interaction is important for the healthy development of all children, it appears to have even stronger effects on the development of VLBW children.[9,10] An increasing number of studies provides consistent evidence that sensitive and responsive interaction between a mother and her VLBW infant in the early years of life is predictive of the child's cognitive, language, and social development outcomes in toddlerhood, the preschool years, and as late as adolescence.[11–16]

Given that sensitive and responsive interaction appears to be critical to the optimal development of VLBW children, it would be important to understand what factors are related to mother–VLBW infant interaction. Greater understanding of these factors is needed to identify mother–infant dyads at risk of having difficulty interacting sensitively and responsively and to develop effective intervention programs. Only a handful of studies has examined factors related to mother–infant interaction in VLBW dyads, and these studies have found that the infant's birth weight,[17] the severity of infant's illness in the perinatal period,[17,18] maternal psychological distress[19–21] and education,[22] and various dimensions of maternal support[23–25] were related to mother–VLBW infant interaction.

Infant Factors and Mother–Very Low Birth Weight Infant Interaction

Previous studies have examined the association between birth weight and the interactive behavior in VLBW dyads and found that these variables are related. However, the findings have been mixed and fail to paint a clear picture of how these variables are related. Lower birth weight has been associated with greater maternal stimulation, caregiving, and holding[17] as well as greater maternal verbal stimulation and duration of caregiving.[26] In contrast, others have found that lower birth weight was associated with lower maternal sensitivity, greater maternal intrusiveness, and fewer maternal affective attunements as well as less positive infant affect and greater infant negative expressions.[27] This lack of consistency of findings across studies is typical of the literature on mother–VLBW infant interaction and has been attributed to methodological issues, as studies have examined different mother and infant behaviors with different coding systems, at different ages, and in different settings and situations.[21] To summarize, birth weight appears to be related to interaction, but the direction of the relationship is not yet clear.

Although a few studies have observed no differences in the interactive behaviors of ill VLBW, less ill VLBW, and healthy NBW infants,[18] the majority of previous studies have reported differences in at least some of the interactive behaviors of ill VLBW infants compared with their healthy VLBW and NBW peers. Ill VLBW infants have been observed to be less likely to increase the complexity of their play,[28] do more passive looking and less vocalizing, and engage in less functional play than both other groups of infants.[29] Ill VLBW children have demonstrated less self-directed behavior and more inappropriate responses to maternal directives than healthy VLBW children, even after accounting for child I.Q. and maternal interactive behavior.[30] Therefore, most current evidence suggests that perinatal illness appears to adversely affect the interactive capabilities of VLBW infants.

Infant perinatal illness may also affect mothers' interactive behavior. Although some have observed that mothers of ill VLBW infants provide more care and stimulation to their infant,[26] others have found that mothers of ill infants provide less stimulation as they touched, smiled less, and looked in face less than mothers of well VLBW infants.[18] Levy-Shiff et al[31] found that greater perinatal illness severity was associated with increased holding by mothers but decreased stimulation and argued that perhaps illness severity may have a differential effect on different types of maternal behavior. In sum, previous studies suggest that infant birth weight and perinatal illness severity are related to both mother and infant interactive behaviors; however, the direction of these relationships remains for the most part unclear.

Mother Factors and Mother–Very Low Birth Weight Infant Interaction

Descriptive studies of mothers of preterm VLBW infants have revealed that mothers are anxious about many aspects of their children's health, development, care, and future.[32–35] Furthermore, mothers of VLBW infants appear to be more anxious than mothers of NBW infants in the first few weeks after birth.[36–38] Despite this evidence, only two studies have investigated how maternal anxiety affects a mother's ability to engage in sensitive and responsive interactions with her infant. Wijnroks[39] reported that mothers who recalled being highly anxious during the neonatal intensive care unit hospitalization were more intrusive, more active, and less sensitive in interactions with their infants, whereas Singer et al[20] found that high maternal concurrent anxiety was related to less maternal verbal behavior and less prompting to feed in feeding interactions. These findings suggest that both recollected anxiety and concurrent anxiety are associated with maternal interactive behavior and that anxiety may adversely affect sensitivity and responsivity in VLBW dyads.

Studies employing different methods of measuring mother–child interaction in a variety of settings with children of varying ages have consistently found that more highly educated mothers behave differently than less well educated mothers.[40] More specifically, more highly educated mothers have been found to be more sensitive and responsive with their infants.[41] Although maternal education appears to play an important role in mother–infant interaction, it may be particularly critical for the optimal parenting of children born with a VLBW. One of the strongest predictors of sensitive and responsive interaction in the Infant Health and Developmental Program, a large multisite intervention study with low birth weight infants, was maternal education.[22]

Contextual Factors and Mother–Very Low Birth Weight Infant Interaction

Previous studies of VLBW dyads have found a relationship between various dimensions of support (i.e., available support, received support, satisfaction with support) and maternal interactive behavior. Greater available support has been associated with more optimal later interactive behavior.[16,42] Although greater received support for parenting has been found to be positively related to maternal touching and holding,[24] mothers were asked to recall the support that they received several months previously; thus, these data might reflect what support was available to them rather than support that they actually received. Crnic et al[23] found that greater maternal satisfaction with support was positively associated with later maternal interactive behavior.

Most previous studies of the factors associated with mother–VLBW infant interaction share several important limitations. First, most studies have examined the relationship between a single factor and mother–infant interaction. Theorists have argued[43–45] and empirical evidence from studies with NBW children provides support for the notion[46–48] that to understand parental functioning, multiple sources of influence must be examined simultaneously. Furthermore, both theory and research point to the importance of three particular categories of factors that influence parenting behavior, namely, characteristics of the child, the parent, and the social-contextual environment in which the child and parent are situated. Thus, it is becoming increasingly apparent that to understand parenting behavior and functioning, researchers need to examine multiple infant, parent and contextual sources of influence simultaneously.[43,44,49] Nonetheless, those few studies that have examined multiple factors have included child and parent factors, neglecting to include contextual factors such as mother's support. A final limitation of most previous research is that samples have not been restricted to VLBW infants but included infants weighing as much as 2500 g at birth.

The Current Study's Purpose

The current study sought to improve on previous research by moving beyond the examination of single factors to the simultaneous examination of multiple infant, mother, and contextual factors that may be associated with interaction. We examined the extent to which a model that included six infant, mother, and contextual factors predicted mother–VLBW infant interaction. Furthermore, the relationship was examined prospectively and the sample was limited to infants weighing less than 1500 g at birth.

Two characteristics of the infant were examined in the current study, birth weight and perinatal illness severity, because these characteristics may affect both infant and maternal interactive behavior. The infant's size may affect their ability to emit social cues and respond to their interactive partner. Furthermore, VLBW infants of the same birth weight may differ markedly in their abilities as social partners due to their medical condition in the perinatal period.[50] Mothers may be fearful of stimulating or handling an infant that is tiny or ill.

Two maternal factors were considered: anxiety and education. Mothers of VLBW infants have been found to be more anxious than mothers of NBW infants. Anxious mothers may be preoccupied with their own concerns and less able to tune into their infants' needs and respond appropriately[22] and may also be more intrusive and controlling due to anxieties about their infants' behavior and development. Thus, we decided to examine the relationship of maternal anxiety to mother–infant interaction. Better educated mothers of VLBW infants may be more knowledgeable about the capabilities and developmental needs of infants and/or more likely to seek information about how to interact sensitively with a VLBW infant.

The contextual factors examined in this study were two dimensions of maternal support: received support and perceived helpfulness of received support. We sought to extend this avenue of research by simultaneously examining the relationship of two dimensions of maternal support to mother–VLBW infant interaction, i.e., received support specific to the task of parenting and the mothers' subjective evaluation of their received support. Mothers who receive support for their parenting (i.e., advice, assistance with child care) and feel that this support eases their parenting efforts may be better able to attend to their infants' needs and interact sensitively and responsively.

Thus, our major objective was to assess the relationship between this set of six infant (i.e., birth weight, perinatal illness severity), mother (i.e., anxiety and level of education), and contextual (i.e., received support and perceived helpfulness of support) factors and mother–VLBW infant interaction. We tested the hypothesis that the infant, mother, and contextual factors would explain significant and unique portions of the variance in the interactive behavior of VLBW dyads. Based on previous studies, we hypothesized that interactions would be more sensitive and responsive when the infants' birth weights were higher and perinatal illness severity was lower, when mothers were less anxious and better educated, and when mothers' received support and perceived support were higher.

METHOD

A prospective design was used to examine the relationship among the set of six infant, mother, and contextual variables and mother–very low birth weight (VLBW) infant interaction. Infant, mother, and contextual variables were assessed at 3 and 9 months of age (corrected for prematurity), and at 9 months interaction was also observed.

Participants

The participants were mothers whose infants weighed less than 1500 g at birth, were born at less than 32 weeks' gestation, and were hospitalized in one of two participating neonatal intensive care units (NICUs) in a Canadian urban center. Only mothers living with the infant's father (married or cohabiting to control for martial status) and able to read English or French were included. Mothers were excluded if their infant had a major congenital anomaly, required a surgical intervention that necessitated transfer to another hospital for more than 72 hours, or had a major motor or sensory handicap (e.g., blindness). Mothers of multiples (i.e., twins or triplets) were included, but a single infant from each multiple set was randomly selected and included in the sample.

The study received ethical approval by the institutional review boards at both sites, and 158 mothers who met the inclusion criteria were invited to participate while their infant was in the NICU. Sixty mothers refused to participate at the outset (38%), most stating they were too overwhelmed or busy. A total of 98 eligible mothers gave informed consent; however, as the study proceeded, five mothers were found to be ineligible (one infant died after enrollment, two mothers separated from their partner, one mother was unable to respond to questionnaires, and one mother's infant was found to have a severe visual deficit). At the 9-month visit, eight mothers withdrew due to lack of time. Thirteen mothers were not included in the analyses because data collection occurred too late. The final sample of 72 participants represented 47% of the potential eligible sample (n = 153).

Participants were compared with nonparticipants on selected variables. Nonparticipant mothers were younger (30.2 years vs 32.2 years, $p = .00$), their infants weighed less at birth (1019.3 g vs 1099.7 g, $p = .01$), were born earlier (27.9 weeks' gestation vs 28.6 weeks', $p = .02$), and were sicker during the NICU hospitalization (Revised Nursery Neurobiologic Score [NBRS] of 4.2 versus 3.0, $p = .00$) compared with infants of participating mothers. Selected sociodemographic characteristics of the 72 mothers and infants who participated are presented in Table 1. Sixty-nine percent (n = 50) of the women were married, and 57% (n = 41) were first-time mothers. Although 85% (n = 61) of the mothers had been born in Canada, 15% (n = 11) had been born elsewhere. At 9 months, 58% (n = 42) of mothers were not employed outside the home, and 72% (n = 52) were the infant's primary caregiver. Most of the infants were singletons; however, 18% (n = 13) were born of a set of twins or triplets. Fifty-four percent of the infants (n = 39) were boys, and 17% (n = 12) were small for gestational age (defined as weight more than 2 SDs below the mean).

TABLE 1   Characteristics of Mothers and Infants (n = 72)

VARIABLE	MEAN	SD	RANGE
Mother's age, yr	32.3	5.5	21–45
Mother's education, yr	13.8	3.0	8–24
Mother's duration of partner relationship, yr	6.7	4.2	1–21
Infant birth weight, g	1099.7	266.5	545–1525
NBRS[a]	3.0	3.0	0–12
Infant's gestational age, wk	28.6	2.6	23–32
Infant's APGAR score	4.8	3.2	0–9
Infant's duration of hospitalization, days	72.2	31.1	26–153

Variable (infant)	n	%
Oxygen in NICU[b]		
≤28 days	43	61
>28 days	27	39
Intraventricular hemorrhage		
None	57	79
Grade 1 or 2	15	21
Grade 3 or 4	0	0
Periventricular leucomalacia		
Yes	6	8
No	66	92
Hospitalized between ages 0 and 3 mo[c]		
Yes	9	13
No	60	87
Hospitalized between ages 3 and 9 mo[d]		
Yes	9	14
No	54	86

NBRS, Revised Nursery Neurobiologic Score; NICU, neonatal intensive care unit.
[a]Median of the Revised Nursery Neurobiologic Score was 2.0.
[b]n = 70; some data unavailable.
[c]n = 69; some data unavailable.
[d]n = 63; some data unavailable.

Procedure

Data collection occurred in the family home when the infant was 3 and 9 months of age (corrected age). At the first home visit, mothers completed the battery of questionnaires. At the second home visit, mothers first responded to the same questionnaires and then performed the teaching task with their infant.

Measures

Mother–Infant Interaction. Mother–infant interaction was assessed with the Nursing Child Assessment Teaching Scale (NCATS), a well-established observational measure designed to assess the teaching interactions of parents with children between birth and 3 years of age.[51] Teaching interactions may be particularly important to study with VLBW dyads because the teaching task challenges the dyad[41] and places demands on the infant's joint attention skill, a skill that is especially difficult for VLBW infants.[52]

The total NCATS teaching score consists of 73 dichotomous items, with 50 items tapping parent behaviors and 23 items assessing infant behaviors. Higher scores indicate more sensitive and responsive interaction. Evidence supports the predictive validity of this measure for both normal birth weight (NBW) and VLBW samples.[51] Internal consistency has been evaluated, and Cronbach's alpha for the total NCATS score is high (i.e., .87). The administration of the teaching task was performed according to the NCATS guidelines in that five teaching tasks suitable for infants 6 to 12 months of age were chosen from a list of possible tasks (i.e., pull a car by the string, turn book pages). Mothers were asked to indicate which of the tasks that their infant could not perform, and this task was attempted. Any other persons present were asked to leave the room, and the interaction was videotaped. The observed interactions ranged from 2 to 13 minutes in duration (mean = 5.5 minutes, SD = 2.6). The videotapes were scored at a later date by a NCATS trained rater blind to the infants' medical history. A randomly selected subset of interactions (i.e., 20%) were scored independently by a second trained rater, and the kappa coefficient was 0.72, indicating high interrater reliability.

Infant Perinatal Illness Severity. Infant perinatal illness severity was measured with the Revised Nursery Neurobiologic Score (NBRS) developed by Brazy et al.[53] The measure includes seven items that assess the presence, severity, and duration of medical events thought to be associated with the risk of later abnormal neurodevelopment including mechanical ventilation, anaerobic metabolism (i.e., blood pH levels), seizures, intraventricular hemorrhage, periventricular leukomalacia, infection, and hypoglycemia. The total NBRS score is the sum of the scores for individual items, and increasing scores are indicative of greater risk of abnormal neurodevelopment. The measure is scored after a review of the infant's NICU medical record. The predictive validity of the NBRS has been established in a series of studies that have shown that NBRSs correlate with later child neurological examination scores.[54] The records of 20% of the current sample were randomly selected and scored by both a research assistant and neonatologist. The kappa coefficient was 0.85, indicating excellent interrater reliability.

Maternal State Anxiety. The mother's generalized anxiety was measured with the state portion State-Trait Anxiety Inventory (STAI), which consists of 20-items scored on a four-point scale.[55] Raw scores were converted into standardized scores, and higher scores reflect higher anxiety levels. The STAI is a widely used measure of anxiety and has been used with mothers of VLBW infants.[56] Evidence of the construct validity of the STAI has been provided by studies that have found that STAI scores increase significantly in stressful situations and decrease significantly after relaxation training.[55] Internal consistency in the current study was assessed and Cronbach's alpha coefficients were very high (.91) for both the 3- and 9-month assessments.

Maternal Received and Perceived Helpfulness of Support. The Support in Parenting (SIP) is a self-report measure, consisting of 14-items, seven-items that assess the perceived frequency of instrumental, emotional, and informational support received from the respondent's social network and seven items that assess their subjective evaluation of the extent to which the support received helped them cope with the demands of parenting. This questionnaire was developed for the purposes of this study and is an extension and modification of the "Help I Get" questionnaire.[57] The SIP yields two scores, a received support score and a perceived helpfulness of received support score. Higher scores are indicative of greater received support and greater perceived helpfulness of support. The face validity of the measure was confirmed by a panel of clinical experts and mothers. Further evidence of validity was demonstrated as mothers' SIP received support and perceived helpfulness scores (for the spouse) correlated significantly with the Pattison et al[58] psychosocial inventory of support from the spouse ($r = .58 - .60$) and with a measure of the quality of mothers' marital relationship (Dyadic Adjustment Scale[59]) ($r = .27 - .37$). Internal consistency was high for both the received support and perceived helpfulness scores (Cronbach's alpha coefficient .79–.87 range).

RESULTS

This section is divided into two sections. In the first section, descriptive statistics and preliminary analyses are presented, as are comparisons between 3 and 9 months. The second section is concerned with an examination of the important predictors of mother–very low birth weight (VLBW) infant interaction.

Descriptive Statistics and Comparisons of Mothers at 3 and 9 Months

Table 2 provides a summary of the mean, SD, and range for each of the independent (at 3 and 9 months) and dependent variables. As mother's anxiety and received and perceived support were assessed at two points in time, paired t tests were conducted to assess whether mothers' scores differed from 3 to 9 months. No significant differences between mothers' mean scores at 3 and 9 months were found on any of these variables.

Pearson product moment correlations were used to examine the interrelations among the variables. Correlation matrixes were computed for both the 3- and 9-month data. Table 3 reports the correlations at 3 months. Lower infant birth weight was associated with greater infant perinatal illness severity. Greater maternal perceived support at 3 months was related to higher maternal education and greater maternal received support at 3 months. More sensitive and responsive interaction at 9 months was related to lower maternal anxiety at 3 months, greater maternal education, and greater perceived support at 3 months. Only one

TABLE 2	Summary of Measures for Mothers (n = 72)		
MEASURE	**MEAN**	**SD**	**RANGE**
STAI[a]			
3 mo	45.9	8.4	35–71
9 mo	46.5	8.4	35–68
Received support			
3 mo	7.8	3.6	2.3–21.0
9 mo	8.2	4.8	0.6–24.0
Perceived helpfulness			
3 mo	18.9	3.0	11.0–26.8
9 mo	19.1	2.9	12.2–27.0
NCATS total, 9 mo	50.9	5.0	37–60

STAI, State Anxiety Inventory; NCATS, Nursing Child Assessment
Teaching Scale.
[a] Standardized STAI scores are reported and used in analyses.

correlation among the variables at 9 months was significant (Table 4). Greater maternal perceived support at 9 months was associated with greater received support at 9 months. In preliminary univariate analyses, we examined whether various maternal sociodemographic characteristics were related to mother–infant interaction. Maternal age, parity, multiple birth status, duration of relationship with spouse, and numbers of hours employed outside the home at 9 months were not related to interaction. Maternal occupation status was related to mother–infant interaction. However, occupation status was highly correlated with education ($r = .74, p = .00$), a mother factor already in the model; thus, it was not added to the model. Also we examined whether various infant characteristics were related to mother–infant interaction. Infant gender, gestational age at birth, APGAR score at birth, duration of neonatal intensive care unit (NICU) hospitalization, neurological problems in the first 3 months (including intraventricular hemorrhage, periventricular leukomalacia, hypotonia, and hypertonia), intraventricular hemorrhage, and small for gestational age were not related to mother–infant interaction at 9 months.

TABLE 3	Correlations Among Study Variables at Three Months (n = 72)					
VARIABLE	**1**	**2**	**3**	**4**	**5**	**6**	**7**
Weight	—	−0.61**	−0.13	0.08	−0.20	−0.13	−0.23*
Illness		—	0.10	−0.04	0.19	0.07	0.15
Anxiety			—	−0.17	0.09	−0.09	−0.26**
Education				—	0.02	0.24**	0.38***
Received					—	0.54***	−0.09
Perceived						—	0.24**
Interaction							—

All tests of significance are two tailed.
*$p = .055$; **$p < .05$; ***$p < .01$.

TABLE 4	Correlations Among Study Variables at Nine Months (n = 72)						
VARIABLE	1	2	3	4	5	6	7
Weight	—	−0.61**a	−0.08	0.08	−0.04	−0.11	−0.23*
Illness		—	−0.07	−0.04	0.10	0.20	0.15
Anxiety			—	−0.09	−0.12	−0.14	−0.11
Education				—	0.12	0.02	0.38***a
Received					—	0.70**	0.00
Perceived						—	0.16
Interaction							—

a Reported in Table 3.
*p = .055; **p < .05; ***p < .01.

Predictors of Mother–Infant Interaction

In this study, six independent variables were hypothesized to be relevant in explaining interaction: infants' birth weight, infants' perinatal illness severity, mothers' level of education, mothers' state anxiety, mothers' received support, and mothers' perceived helpfulness of support. The dependent variable was the Nursing Child Assessment Teaching Scale (NCATS) total score. To test the hypothesis that the infant, mother, and contextual factors would explain significant and unique portions of the variance in interactive behavior, a hierarchical regression equation was computed. The variables were entered in the following order. In step 1, the infant variables were entered because these variables were considered to be temporal prior to the remaining independent variables.[60] In step 2, the mother set of variables as assessed at 3 months was entered. Finally, in step 3, the set of contextual variables as assessed at 3 months was entered. This tested the extent to which the combination of six independent variables predicted interaction 6 months later.

Table 5 displays the results of the hierarchical regression analyses. The model was significant and explained 33% of the variance in the NCATS total score. Four variables contributed significant unique variation to the prediction of the NCATS total score: mother's education, mother's anxiety at 3 months, mother's received support at 3 months, and mothers' perceived helpfulness of support at 3 months. Although the variable received support was a significant predictor within this regression analysis, an examination of the zero-order correlation between this variable and the NCATS total score revealed that the correlation was not significant and essentially equal to zero. Moreover, the absolute value of the zero-order correlation (i.e., .09) was much smaller than the part correlation (i.e., .29). This signals the presence of a suppressor variable.[61] Received support suppressed variance in perceived support that was irrelevant to the prediction of the NCATS score. Therefore, received support was not given any importance in the interpretation of the results. Dyads whose interactions were more sensitive and responsive at 9 months were characterized by mothers who were better educated and less anxious at 3 months and perceived that the support that they received at 3 months was helpful to their parenting efforts. There was a reliable increase in the prediction of the NCATS total score when adding mother and contextual variable sets.

TABLE 5	Predictors of Mother–Infant Interaction at Nine Months (n = 72)			
PREDICTOR VARIABLE	**B**	**SEB**	**β**	**△R^2**
Step 1: infant				
Birth weight	−0.00[a]	0.00	−0.22	
Severity of illness	0.02	0.25	0.01	0.05
Step 2: mother				
Education	0.60	0.17	0.37**	
State anxiety, 3 mo	−0.14	0.06	−0.23*	0.21**
Step 3: contextual				
Received support, 3 mo	−0.40	0.17	−0.29*	
Perceived helpfulness, 3 mo	0.43	0.21	0.26*	0.06*

Overall model: R^2 = 0.33, F = 5.3, p = .00, R^2 adjusted = 0.27.
[a]Birth weight is small because it was measured in grams.
*p < .05; **p < .01.

We also examined the extent to which the combination of six independent variables as assessed at 9 months predicted mother–infant interaction observed concurrently. The same approach and order of entry for the independent variables as described above were adopted. However, in this concurrent model, the 9-month State-Trait Anxiety Inventory (STAI) and Support in Parenting (SIP) data were included. This model was also significant and explained 28% of the variance in the NCATS total score. Mothers' education and mothers' perceived helpfulness of support at 9 months remained important predictors; however, maternal anxiety at 9 months was not an important predictor of interaction.

A significant proportion of the mothers in this sample (18%) were mothers of multiples. We conducted the analyses excluding mothers of twins and triplets, and the findings differed. Only maternal education was a predictor of interaction. In further analyses, we compared mothers of multiples to mothers of singletons on all key study variables as well as various maternal sociodemographic and infant health characteristics, and the only difference was that mothers of multiples were more anxious at both 3 and 9 months (t = −2.1, p = .01 and t = −2.4, p = .02, respectively).

DISCUSSION

The purpose of this study was to examine the extent to which a model of six infant, mother, and contextual factors predicted mother–very low birth weight (VLBW) infant interaction and to examine which of these factors were important predictors. We found that mothers who were more anxious early on when their infant was 3 months old had less sensitive and responsive later interactions with their infants at 9 months. This finding is consistent with studies that have found that mothers' concurrent psychological distress was related to less optimal maternal interactive behavior in feeding interactions with VLBW infants[20,21] and interactions with VLBW toddlers.[62] Our data extend this avenue of research by specifically linking state anxiety to interaction and provide evidence of a relationship between anxiety and interaction in a different situation (i.e., teaching interaction). Furthermore, our prospective data suggest that mothers' early anxiety may affect later interaction. An alternative explanation for the observed association between anxiety and interaction is that the experience of having difficult interactions with a VLBW infant may lead to high maternal anxiety. Conceivably, infants of the more anxious mothers may have been poorer interaction partners soon after birth, and this may have given rise to high maternal anxiety at 3 months as well as a continued pattern of interaction characterized by low sensitivity. However, in our previous work, we found that maternal anxiety early in the neonatal intensive care unit (NICU) hospitalization was associated with less optimal interactive behavior at 3 months.[63] Thus, it seems likely that early maternal anxiety affects interactive behavior.

Although a decrease in the mean state anxiety score of mothers might have been anticipated as the infants developed and the critical neonatal period had receded, anxiety did not decrease significantly over the 6-month interval, and this may be noteworthy. Few data exist on the anxiety of mothers of VLBW infants after discharge from the NICU. Nonetheless, the continued high maternal anxiety that we observed is consistent with the results of two studies that have examined longitudinally the psychological distress of mothers of VLBW infants.[38,64] Why might mothers' anxiety remain relatively elevated when the infants were 9 months old? Wijnroks[39] argued that mothers may relive the traumatic experiences of the early perinatal period for many months afterward. It is also possible that mothers' continued elevated anxiety state might reflect high trait anxiety. There is some evidence that the infants of anxious mothers have a significantly lower average birth weight and tend to be born prematurely.[65,66] Furthermore, an association between maternal anxiety during pregnancy (as assessed with the State-Trait Anxiety Inventory [STAI]) and increased uterine artery resistance has been reported.[67] Women with increased anxiety were more likely to have abnormal uterine artery blood flow than those with less anxiety. Maternal anxiety may affect blood flow to the fetus and hence fetal growth and explain the association between maternal anxiety and low birth weight. It may be that women high in trait anxiety may be more likely to experience high state anxiety during pregnancy and thus have reduced blood flow through the uterine artery, contributing to the premature birth of a VLBW infant. These women may also experience elevated state anxiety with premature birth and may remain highly anxious for many months after this stressful event. Continued high anxiety may adversely affect their ability to interact sensitively and responsively with their infant.

One subgroup of mothers that may be a risk of increased anxiety is mothers of twins and triplets. Exploratory analyses revealed that mothers of multiples were more anxious than mothers of singletons when the infants were both 3 and 9 months of age. Mothers of infant twins and triplets have reported worries about their abilities to adequately feed, care, and support their infants; finances; lack of time for other duties and activities; obtaining child care assistance; and dealing with the special challenges of developing a relationship with multiple infants simultaneously.[68] These numerous concerns may give rise to higher anxiety in mothers of multiples. This subgroup of mothers of VLBW infants warrant further investigation to better understand their experience and how it may affect both their parenting and the development of their children.

In this study, we chose to assess anxiety and not depression because we considered that anxiety might be more closely related to the types of interactive behaviors that have been observed in mothers of VLBW infants (i.e., overactive and intrusive). As it is well known that anxiety and depression are highly correlated and we did not assess both anxiety and depression, we cannot conclude that it is anxiety and not depression that is related to mother–infant interaction.

The findings also indicated that maternal education was an important predictor of interaction. Higher maternal education was associated with greater sensitivity and responsivity. This observation is consistent with those of previous investigations that have also found that more highly educated mothers tend to obtain higher NCATS scores[69,70] and with recent evidence that maternal education may play an important role in the parenting behavior of mothers of VLBW infants.[16] Hoff-Ginsberg and Tardif[40] noted that the influence of maternal education on parenting may be derived from internalized characteristics of mothers that differ according to level of education. Perhaps better educated mothers may acquire more knowledge about a VLBW infant's capabilities and needs, and this in turn may allow them to be more effective. Support for this explanation is provided by a study that observed an association between maternal education and knowledge of child-rearing practices among mothers of VLBW infants.[22] The influence of maternal education on parenting is also thought to be derived from factors external to the mother, associated with maternal education, that enhance the mother's ability to be sensitive and responsive.[40] Support of this explanation for the association between maternal education and sensitive and responsive parenting was found in exploratory analyses that we conducted that revealed that in our sample, better educated mothers were more likely to be married and employed in a white-collar occupation and report better marital quality and higher perceived helpfulness of support. Further study is needed to advance our understanding of how maternal education influences interaction in VLBW dyads.

We also found that mothers who reported greater perceived helpfulness of support had interactions that were more sensitive and responsive, and this association is consistent with previous studies of both VLBW[23] and normal birth weight (NBW) dyads[71] that have found that mothers' positive evaluation of their support was related to interaction. Although perceived helpfulness of support was an important predictor in this study, received support was not. This finding suggests that mothers' appraisal of their support may be more critical to the development of sensitive parenting than the amount of support received. It has been argued that the fit between what a parent needs and support received may be most important for parent functioning,[72] and our findings lend support to this viewpoint. Further research is needed to clarify what type of support, provided by whom, and when it is perceived as helpful by mothers of VLBW infants.

We found that perceived helpfulness of support at 3 months was related to interaction 6 months later. Previous studies of VLBW dyads[16,23] have also reported that support in the early months after discharge from the hospital was related to later interaction. Miller-Loncar et al[73] found that mothers' support influenced their ability to adopt a child-centered perspective, and a child-centered perspective in turn influenced mothers' interactive behavior. If a child-centered perspective mediates the association between support and interaction, this may explain how early support influences parent behavior later.

A few limitations of our study warrant consideration. We observed interactions when the infants were 9 months old, and the factors that shape interaction at this time may not be generalizable to other points in time. Also context is an important factor that shapes the actions of interactive partners[74]; thus, caution should be exercised in generalizing findings concerning home teaching interactions to interactions in other situations or settings. For example, maternal education may be particularly important in the teaching interactions that we observed but less so in other types of interactions such as feeding interactions.

Although the observation of interaction was brief, NCATS scores have been found to correlate with behavior in much longer naturalistic observations,[69] and maternal behavior appears to be moderately stable over time.[74] Thus, it is reasonable to expect that our observations may be representative of what transpires in a teaching interaction in the home. Many of the mothers whom we approached chose not to participate, stating they were too overwhelmed. Furthermore, non-participants also differed from participants in that their infants weighed less at birth, were born earlier, and were sicker in the NICU. Thus, there may have been a systematic underrepresentation of mothers who were highly anxious or mothers whose infants were in poorer medical condition while in the NICU. Finally, the size of our sample was small, and, thus, the number of variables that we could include in our model was also small. Many other infant, mother, and contextual variables may shape the interaction between mothers and VLBW infants. For example, we did not have developmental assessments on the infants, and infant development status may be an important infant factor to consider in future investigations.

This study provides evidence regarding specific psycho-social factors that contribute to shaping sensitive and responsive interaction between a mother and her VLBW infant. Greater understanding of these factors is needed to develop intervention programs to foster optimal interaction and to identify which dyads might be more likely to have difficulty developing sensitive and responsive interaction and benefit most from intervention. Anxious mothers, less well educated mothers, and mothers who perceived that the support that they receive is not helpful may be those mothers who could benefit from intervention during the NICU hospitalization that could foster more sensitive and responsive interaction.

REFERENCES

1. Anderson P, Doyle LW, Victorian Infant Collaborative Study Group. Neurobehavioral outcomes of school-age children born extremely low birth weight or very preterm in the 1990s. *JAMA*. 2003;289: 3264–3272.
2. Boardman JD, Powers DA, Padilla YC, Hummer RA. Low birth weight, social factors, and developmental outcomes among children in the United States. *Demography*. 2002;39:353–368.
3. Bhutta AT, Cleves MA, Casey PH, Cradock MM, Anand KJS. Cognitive and behavioral outcomes of school-aged children who were born preterm: a meta-analysis. *JAMA*. 2002;288:728–737.
4. Greenberg MT, Carmichael-Olson H, Crnic KA. The development and social competence of a preterm sample at age 4: prediction and transactional outcomes. In: Friedman SL, Sigman MD, eds. *The Psychological Development of Low-Birthweight Children*. Norwood, NJ: Ablex Publishing; 1992:125–155.
5. Hack M, Flannery DJ, Schluchter M, Cartar L, Borawski E, Klein N. Outcomes in young adulthood for very-low-birth-weight infants. *N Engl J Med*. 2002;346:149–157.
6. Saigal S. Long-term outcome of very low-birth-weight infants: kindergarten and beyond. *Dev Brain Dysfunct*. 1995;8:109–I18.
7. Saigal S. Follow-up of very low birthweight babies to adolescence. *Semin Neonatol*. 2000;5:107–118.
8. Weindrich D, Jennen-Steinmctz C, Laucht M, Schmidt MH. Late sequelae of low birthweight: mediators of poor school performance at 11 years. *Dev Med Child Neurol*. 2003;45:463–469.
9. Landry SH, Smith KE, Swank PR, Assel MA, Vellet S. Does early responsive parenting have a special importance for children's development or is consistency across early childhood necessary? *Dev Psychol*. 2001;37:387–403.
10. Landry SH, Smith KE, Swank PR. The importance of parenting during early childhood for school-age development. *Dev Neuropsychol*. 2003;24:559–591.
11. Beckwith L, Rodning C. Dyadic processes between mothers and preterm infants: development at ages 2 to 5 years. *Infant Ment Health J*. 1996;17:322–333.
12. Cusson RM. Factors influencing language development in preterm infants. *J Obstet Gynecol Neonatal Nurs*. 2003;32:402–409.
13. Fewell RR, Casal SG, Glick MP, Wheeden CA, Spiker D. Maternal education and maternal responsiveness as predictors of play competence in low birth weight, premature infants: a preliminary report. *J Dev Behav Pediatr*. 1996;17:100–104.

14. Landry SH, Smith KE, Swank PR. Environmental effects on language development in normal and high-risk child populations. *Semin Pediatr Neurol.* 2002;9:192–200.
15. Moore JB, Saylor C, Boyce G. Parent-child interaction and developmental outcomes in medically fragile, high-risk children. *Child Health Care.* 1998;27:97–112.
16. Smith KE, Landry SH, Swank PR. The influence of early patterns of positive parenting on children's preschool outcomes. *Early Educ Dev.* 2000;11:147–169.
17. Levy-Sniff R, Mogilner MB. Mothers' and fathers' interactions with their preterm infants during the initial period at home. *J Reprod Infant Psychol.* 1989;7:25–37.
18. Minde K, Whitelaw A, Brown J, Fitzhardinge P. Effect of neonatal complications in premature infants on early parent-infant interactions. *Dev Med Child Neurol.* 1983;25:763–777.
19. Halpem LF, McLean WE. "Hey mom, look at me!" *Infant Behav Dev.* 1997;20:515–529.
20. Singer L, Davillier M, Preuss L, et al. Feeding interactions in infants with very low birth weight and bronchopulmonary dysplasia. *J Dev Behav Pediatr.* 1996;17:69–76.
21. Singer LT, Fulton S, Davillier M, Koshy D, Salvator A, Baley J. Effects of infant risk status and maternal psychological distress on maternal-infant interactions during the first year of life. *J Dev Behav Pediatr.* 2003;24:233–241.
22. Gross T, Spiker D, Haynes CW. *Helping Low Birth Weight Babies: The Infant Health and Development Program.* Stanford, CA: Stanford University Press; 1997.
23. Crnic KA, Greenberg MT, Slough NM. Early stress and social support influences on mothers' and high-risk infants' functioning in late infancy. *Infant Ment Health J.* 1986;7:19–33.
24. Feiring C, Fox NA, Jaskir J, Lewis M. The relation between social support, infant risk status and mother-infant interaction. *Dev Psychol.* 1987;23:400–405.
25. Zarling CL, Hirsch BJ, Landry SH. Maternal social networks and mother-infant interactions in full-term and very low birthweight, preterm infants. *Child Dev.* 1988;59:178–185.
26. Beckwith L, Cohen SE. Preterm birth: hazardous obstetrical and postnatal events as related to caregiver infant behavior. *Infant Behav Dev.* 1978;1:403–411.
27. Levy AK, Coll CT, Meyer EC, et al. Mother-infant interaction in preterm infants: influences of biological and environmental risk. Paper presented at: International Conference for Infant Studies; April 18–21, 1996; Providence, RI.
28. Landry SH, Garner PW, Swank P, Baldwin CD. Effects of maternal scaffolding during joint toy play with preterm and full-term infants. *Merrill Palmer Q.* 1996;42:177–199.
29. Garner PW, Landry SH, Richardson MA. The development of joint attention skills in very-low-birth-weight infants across the first 2 years. *Infant Behav Dev.* 1991;14:489–495.
30. Landry SH, Chapieski ML, Richardson MA, Palmer J, Hall S. The social competence of children bom prematurely: effects of medical complications and parent behaviours. *Child Dev.* 1990;61:1605–1616.
31. Levy-Shiff R, Sharir H, Mogilner M. Mother-and father-preterm infant relationship in the hospital preterm nursery. *Child Dev.* 1989;60:93–102.
32. Bidder RT, Crowe EA, Gray OP. Mothers' attitudes to preterm infants. *Arch Dis Child.* 1974;49:766–770.
33. Casteel JK. Affects and cognitions of mothers and fathers of preterm infants. *Matern Child Nurs J.* 1990;19:211–220.
34. Jeffcoate JA, Humphrey ME, Lloyd JK. Disturbance in parent-child relationship following preterm delivery. *Dev Med Child Neurol.* 1979;21:344–352.
35. McCain GC. Parenting growing preterm infants. *Pediatr Nurs.* 1990;16:467–470.
36. Blanchard LW, Blalock SJ, DeVellis RF, DeVellis BM, Johnson MR. Social comparisons among mothers of premature and full-term infants. *Child Health Care.* 1999;28:329–348.
37. Gennaro S. Postpartal anxiety and depression in mothers of term and preterm infants. *Nurs Res.* 1988;37:82–85.
38. Singer L, Salvator A, Guo S, Collin M, Lilien L, Baley J. Maternal psychological distress and parenting stress after the birth of a very low-birth-weight infant. *JAMA.* 1999;281:799–805.
39. Wijnroks L. Maternal recollected anxiety and mother-infant interaction in preterm infants. *Infant Ment Health J.* 1999;20:393–409.
40. Hoff-Ginsberg E, Tardif T. *Socioeconomic Status and Parenting. Handbook of Parenting: Volume 2. Biology and Ecology of Parenting.* Mahwah, NJ: Lawrence Erlbaum; 1995:161–188.
41. Barnard KE, Hammond MA, Booth CL, Bee HL, Mitchell SK, Spieker SJ. Measurement and meaning of parent-child interaction. In: Morrison FJ, Lord C, Keating DP, eds. *Applied Developmental Psychology.* Vol. 3. San Diego: Academic Press; 1989:39–80.
42. Smith KE, Landry SH, Miller-Loncar CL, Swank PR. Characteristics that help mothers maintain their infants' focus of attention. *J Appl Dev Psychol.* 1997;18:587–601.
43. Dunst CJ, Trivette CM. Looking beyond the parent-child dyad for the determinants of maternal styles of interaction. *Infant Ment Health J.* 1986;7:69–80.
44. Lamb ME. On the familial origins of personality and social style. In: Laosa LM, Sigel IE, eds. *Families as Learning Environments for Children.* New York: Plenum Press; 1982:179–202.

45. Vondra J, Belsky J. Developmental origins of parenting: personality and relationship factors. In: Luster T, Okagaki L, eds. *Parenting: An Ecological Perspective*. Hillsdale, NJ: Lawrence Erlbaum; 1993:1–33.
46. Bogenschneider K, Small SA, Tsay J. Child, parent and contextual influences on perceived parenting competence among parents of adolescents. *J Marriage Fam*. 1997;59:345–362.
47. van Bakel HJA, Riksen-Walraven JM. Parenting and development of one-year-olds: links with parental, contextual, and child characteristics. *Child Dev*. 2002;73:256–273.
48. Woodworth S, Belsky J, Crnic KA. The determinants of fathering during the child's second and third years of life: a developmental analysis. *J Marriage Fam*. 1996;58:679–692.
49. Belsky J. The determinants of parenting: a process model. *Child Dev*. 1984;55:83–96.
50. Eckerman CO, Oehler JM. Very-low-birth-weight newborns and parents as early social partners. In: Friedman SL, Sigman MD, eds. *The Psychological Development of Low Birthweight Children*, Norwood, NJ: Ablex Publishing; 1992:91–124.
51. Sumner G, Spietz A. *NCAST Caregiver/Parent-Child Interaction Teaching Manual*. Seattle: NCAST Publications, University of Washington, School of Nursing; 1994.
52. Landry SH. Preterm infants' responses in early joint attention interactions. *Infant Behav Dev*. 1986;9:1–14.
53. Brazy JE, Goldstein RF, Oehler JM, Gustafson KE, Thompson RJ. Nursery Neurobiological Risk Score: levels of risk and relationships with nonmedical factors. *J Dev Behav Pediatr*. 1993;14:375–380.
54. Brazy JE, Eckerman CO, Oehler JM, Goldstein RF, O'Rand AM. Nursery Neurobiologic Risk Score: important factors in predicting outcome in very low birth weight infants. *J Pediatr*. 1991;118:783–792.
55. Spielberger CD, Gorsuch RL, Lushene R, Vagg PR, Jacobs GA. *State-Trait Anxiety Inventory for Adults*. Palo Alto, CA: Consulting Psychologists Press; 1983.
56. Miles MS, Funk SG, Kasper MA. The stress response of mothers and fathers of preterm infants. *Res Nurs Health*. 1992;15:261–269.
57. Pridham KF, Van Riper M. *Fathers' Help and its Relationship to Maternal Behaviour With Preterm and Term Infants Through the First Year. Third International Family Nursing Conference*. Montreal: McGill University; 1994:76.
58. Pattison EM, Llamas R, Hurd G. Social network mediation of anxiety. *Psychiatr Ann*. 1979;9:56–67.
59. Spanier G. *Manual for the Dyadic Adjustment Scale*. New York: Multi-Health Systems; 1989.
60. Cohen J, Cohen P. *Applied Multiple Regression/Correlation Analysis for the Behavioral Sciences*. 2nd ed. Hillsdale, NJ: Lawrence Erlbaum; 1983.
61. Tabachnick BG, Fidell LS. *Using Multivariate Statistics*. 3rd ed. Philadelphia: HarperCollins Publishers; 1996.
62. Assel MA, Landry SH, Swank PR, Steelman L, Miller-Loncar C, Smith KE. How do mothers' childrearing histories, stress and parenting affect children's behavioural outcomes? *Child Care Health Dev*. 2002;28:359–368.
63. Zelkowitz P, Bardin C, Papagcorgiou A. Medical and psychological factors related to parental behavior with very low birthweight infants. *Pediatr Res*. 2000;47:36A.
64. Thompson RJ, Oehler JM, Catlett AT, Johndrow DA. Maternal psychological adjustment to the birth of an infant weighing 1500 grams or less. *Infant Behav Dev*. 1993;16:471–485.
65. Hedegaard M, Henriksen TB, Secher NJ, Hatch MC, Sabroe S. Do stressful life events affect the duration of gestation and risk of preterm delivery? *Epidemiology*. 1996;7:339–345.
66. Perkin MR, Bland JM, Peacock JL, Anderson HR. The effect of anxiety and depression during pregnancy on obstetric complications. *Br J Obstet Gynaecol*. 1993;100:629–634.
67. Teixera JMA, Fisk NM, Glover V. Association between maternal anxiety in pregnancy and increased uterine artery resistance index: cohort based study. *BMJ*. 1999;318:153–157.
68. Holditch-Davis D, Roberts D, Sandelowski M. Early parental interactions with and perceptions of multiple birth infants. *J Adv Nurs*. 1999;30:200–210.
69. Tesh EM, Holditch-Davis D. HOME inventory and NCATS: relation to mother and child behaviors during naturalistic observations. *Res Nurs Health*. 1997;20:295–307.
70. Onyskiw JE, Harrison MJ, Magill-Evans J. Past childhood experiences and current parent-infant interactions. *West J Nurs Res*. 1997;19:501–518.
71. Hann DM. A systems conceptualization of the quality of mother-infant interaction. *Infant Behav Dev*. 1989;12:251–263.
72. Belsky J, Vondra J. Lessons from child abuse: the determinants of parenting. In: Cicchetti D, Carlson V, eds. *Child Maltreatment: Theory and Research on the Causes and Consequences of Child Abuse and Neglect*. New York: Cambridge University Press; 1989:153–202.
73. Miller-Loncar CL, Landry SH, Smith KE, Swank P. The role of child-centered perspectives in a model of parenting. *J Exp Child Psychol*. 1997;66:341–361.
74. Holden GW, Miller PC. Enduring and different: a meta-analysis of the similarity in parents' child-rearing. *Psychol Bull*. 1999;125:223–254.

NANCY FEELEY, Ph.D.

*Centre for Nursing Research, S.M.B.D. Jewish General Hospital and
McGill University School of Nursing, Montreal*

LAURIE GOTTLIEB, Ph.D.

McGill University School of Nursing, Montreal

PHYLLIS ZELKOWITZ, Ed.D.

*Institute for Community and Family Psychiatry, S.M.B.D. Jewish General Hospital,
Montreal, Quebec, Canada*

Received July 2004; accepted October 2004.

Address for reprints: Nancy Feeley, Ph.D., Centre for Nursing Research, Room A-811, S.M.B.D. Jewish General Hospital, 3755 Cote St. Catherine Road, Montreal, Quebec, Canada H3T 1E2; e-mail: nancy.feeley@mcgill.ca.

Acknowledgments. *This study was funded in part by grants from Fonds de la recherche en sante du Quebec, Social Sciences and Humanities Research Council of Canada, Order of Nurses of Quebec, McGill University Faculty of Graduate Studies, and Montreal Children's Hospital Foundation. We acknowledge the assistance of Carole Cormier, Raymonde Gagne, Lucy Wardell, Robin Canuel, Dr. Claudette Bardin, and Professor Rhonda Amsel.*

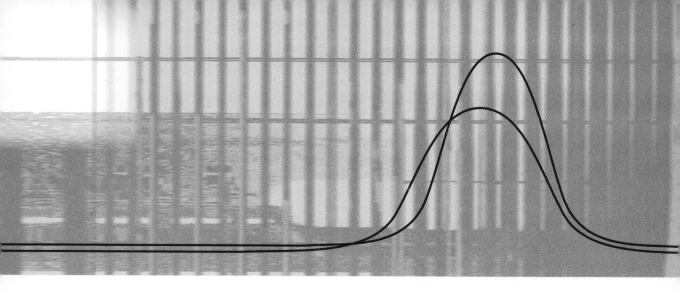

B.

Birth Trauma: In the Eye of the Beholder

Cheryl Tatano Beck

▶ **Background:** The reported prevalence of posttraumatic stress disorder after childbirth ranges from 1.5% to 6%.
▶ **Objective:** To describe the meaning of women's birth trauma experiences.
▶ **Methods:** Descriptive phenomenology was the qualitative research design used to investigate mothers' experiences of traumatic births. Women were recruited through the Internet, primarily through Trauma and Birth Stress (TABS), a charitable trust located in New Zealand. The purposive sample consisted of 40 mothers: 23 in New Zealand, 8 in the United States, 6 in Australia, and 3 in the United Kingdom. Each woman was asked to describe the experience of her traumatic birth and to send it over the Internet to the researcher. Colaizzi's method was used to analyze the 40 mothers' stories.
▶ **Results:** Four themes emerged that described the essence of women's experiences of birth trauma: To care for me: Was that too much too ask? To communicate with me: Why was this neglected? To provide safe care: You betrayed my trust and I felt powerless, and The end justifies the means: At whose expense? At what price?
▶ **Conclusions:** Birth trauma lies in the eye of the beholder. Mothers perceived that their traumatic births often were viewed as routine by clinicians.
▶ **Key Words:** birth trauma, phenomenology, PTSD, qualitative research

Reprinted with permission from *Nursing Research* 2004; 53[1]: 28–35.

In her 1878 novel *Molly Bawn*, Margaret Wolfe Hungerford, an Irish-born 19th century romance novelist, first penned the phrase "beauty is in the eye of the beholder." Beauty is not the only quality or phenomenon that lies in the eye of the beholder; birth trauma also does. What a mother perceives as birth trauma may be seen quite differently through the eyes of obstetric care providers, who may view it as a routine delivery and just another day at the hospital. The reported prevalence of posttraumatic stress disorder (PTSD) after childbirth ranges from 1.5% (Ayers & Pickering, 2001) to 5.6% (Creedy, Shochet, & Horsfall, 2000). Although there is a reported prevalence of PTSD after childbirth, little research has aimed at an understanding of this phenomenon from the women's experience. This phenomenologic study investigated the meaning of women's birth trauma experiences.

LITERATURE REVIEW

A review of the literature on birth trauma showed limited research on the trauma itself rather than its aftermath, PTSD. This literature review focused on the studies that investigated traumatic births and their risk factors as well as research on the components of physical-emotional-mental birth trauma that can lead to the development of PTSD. Birth trauma is an event occurring during the labor and delivery process that involves actual or threatened serious injury or death to the mother or her infant. The birthing woman experiences intense fear, helplessness, loss of control, and horror.

Three studies were found that discussed elements of birth trauma, although their main focus was on identifying the prevalence of diagnosed PTSD resulting from childbirth.

In the United Kingdom, women ($N = 500$) volunteered to participate in research on psychological stress related to obstetric or gynecologic procedures. Advertisement in newspapers and magazines was the method of recruitment. A small number of women ($n = 102$) in this sample described their experiences of obstetric or gynecologic procedures as "terrifying" and "still affecting them now" (Menage, 1993). These women completed the PTSD Interview questionnaire (Watson, Juba, Manifold, Kucala, & Anderson, 1991). Of the 102 women, 30 met the *Diagnostic and Statistical Manual* (DSM-III-R) criteria for a diagnosis of PTSD. These women with a diagnosis of PTSD resulting from birth trauma reported that during the procedures, they felt powerless, lacked information about the procedures, experienced physical pain, perceived unsympathetic attitudes of the healthcare providers, and lacked a clearly understood consent on their part for the procedures. As compared with the nontrauma group, the women with trauma had experienced significantly more infant death and a higher number of invasive procedures.

In a cross-sectional study of all the women who had given birth over a 1-year period in an obstetric department in Sweden, Wijma, Soderquist, and Wijma (1997) reported that 28 of 1,640 women (1.7%) met the criteria for PTSD. Factors related to the women's experience of PTSD after childbirth included a history of psychiatric counseling, a negative cognitive appraisal of the past delivery, nulliparity, and a negative contact with the delivery staff.

Creedy, Shochet, and Horsfall (2000) conducted a prospective, longitudinal study in Australia. Recruited into the study during their third trimester, the women completed various questionnaires including the State Trait Anxiety Inventory (Spielberger, Gorsuch, &

Lushene, 1983). Eligibility criteria for inclusion in the sample required that participants be older than 18 years, in the third trimester of pregnancy, at low risk for obstetric complications, and able to understand English. Telephone interviews with the women ($n = 499$) 4 to 6 weeks post-partum explored their perceptions of the labor and delivery care and the presence of trauma symptoms. The DSM-IV diagnostic criteria for acute posttraumatic stress disorder were met by 28 mothers (5.6%). These stressful birth events included extreme pain, fear of the mother for her life or that of her infant, and a perception of a real or actual lack of obstetric care. Two variables were associated significantly ($p < .0001$) with acute trauma symptoms: a high degree of obstetric intervention and dissatisfaction with the care received during labor and delivery.

The following three studies focused on traumatic births and posttraumatic stress symptoms. No formal diagnosis of PTSD was included as part of the research.

In Sweden, Ryding, Wijma, and Wijma (1998) interviewed women ($N = 53$) approximately 2 days after emergency cesarean delivery to determine whether this trauma met the stressor criterion of PTSD. Other sample criteria besides the experience of an emergency cesarean included use of the Swedish language and delivery of a live infant who had not been transferred to another hospital for special care. In this study, 29 mothers (55%) reported experiencing intense fear of death or injury to themselves or to their baby during the delivery process, which fulfilled the stressor criterion of DSM-IV. The most common fear was related to concerns that the baby would die or be injured. The mothers who feared for their own lives had experienced a painful labor. The findings showed that 8% of the women were angry because they felt that the delivery staff had treated them very badly. These mothers felt violated and helpless during the care provided by the delivery staff.

Czarnocka and Slade (2000) assessed the prevalence and potential predictors of posttraumatic stress symptoms with a sample of women ($N = 264$) in the United Kingdom. Eligibility criteria specified women who (a) were older than 18 years, (b) had delivered a healthy infant, (c) spoke English, and (d) had no immediate plans of moving out of the area. At 6 weeks postpartum, the mothers completed the Post-Traumatic Stress Disorder Questionnaire (PTSD-Q) and Interview (Watson et al., 1991). In this assessment, 3% of the sample ($n = 8$) reported symptoms on the PTSD-Q indicating clinically significant levels of the three posttraumatic stress dimensions: intrusions, avoidance, and hyperarousal. Regression analysis showed the following significant predictors of posttraumatic stress symptoms related to childbirth: low levels of perceived support from labor and delivery staff and partner and low perceived control during labor.

One study conducted in the United States investigated the prevalence and predictors of psychological trauma experienced by women during childbirth (Soet, Brack, & Dilorio, 2003). Women were recruited from childbirth education classes. In late pregnancy, the women ($N = 103$) completed questionnaires measuring such concepts as locus of control and social support. Approximately 4 weeks after delivery, a follow-up interview was conducted by telephone. The mother's experience of birth trauma was measured using the Traumatic Event Scale (TES) (Wijma et al., 1997). In these interviews, 35 women (34%) reported traumatic births. Significant predictors of birth trauma included cesarean delivery, medical intervention, long painful labor, feelings of powerlessness, inadequate information, negative interaction with medical personnel, and differences between expectations and the actual event of childbirth.

The literature review found only one qualitative study that had investigated traumatic births. Women who perceived having traumatic deliveries were recruited by health visitors when they brought their infant for the 8-month well baby checkup. Allen (1998) interviewed women ($N = 20$) in the United Kingdom 10 months after their delivery who perceived that they had experienced distressing labor. Grounded theory analysis showed that the core category related to a traumatic birth experience was the mothers' feelings of not being in control of events or of their own behavior. Causal factors leading to the perception of a traumatic birth were the belief that the baby would be harmed, past experiences in labor, and pain during labor. The mothers tried to gain control by seeking reassurance and knowledge provided by staff and partners.

Seng (2002) acknowledged the complexities of conducting research on PTSD and childbearing. A conceptual framework for research was developed to study the effects of past and current abuse and posttraumatic stress on childbearing women. Seng's framework emphasized PTSD as a potential mediator in the relation between trauma and adverse childbearing outcomes. By both behavioral and neuroendocrine pathways PTSD can be a possible mechanism for adverse maternal and infant outcomes using Seng's conceptual framework, studies can be designed where treatment for PTSD and decreasing high life event stress can potentially decrease association between PTSD and negative childbearing outcomes.

The literature review found a limited number of studies on birth trauma. These quantitative studies focused on identifying predictors of PTSD that related to childbirth. None of the studies investigated the long-term effects of birth trauma for women. Current PTSD knowledge does not address the meaning of a traumatic birth for women. The purpose of the current phenomenologic study was to investigate the following research question: What is the essential structure of women's experiences of birth trauma?

METHODS

Research Design

Descriptive phenomenology was the qualitative research design chosen for the study of mothers' experiences of traumatic births. Husserl's (1970) descriptive (eidetic) phenomenology was the philosophical underpinning for this study. In phenomenology, the nature of a phenomenon (i.e., what makes something what it is without which it could not be what it is) is investigated (Husserl, 1962). Phenomena as they are experienced consciously are described without theories about causes and as free as possible from unexamined preconceptions and presuppositions (Spiegelberg, 1975). One assumption of descriptive phenomenology is that for any human experience there are distinct essential structures that make up that phenomenon regardless of the particular person who experiences it. These essential structures are discovered by studying the particulars encountered in the lived experience.

An understanding of these essential structures requires phenomenologic reduction (Husserl, 1960), in which researchers attempt to put aside temporarily any presuppositions they may hold about the phenomena they are studying, allowing phenomena to come directly into view without distortion by the researchers' preconceptions. "Bracketing" is the term used by Husserl (1960) to describe this process of peeling away the layers of interpretation so the phenomena can be seen as they are. Bracketing does not eliminate perspective, but brings the experience into clearer focus.

Procedure

After approval had been obtained from the university's institutional review board, women were recruited via the Internet primarily through Trauma and Birth Stress (TABS), a charitable trust located in New Zealand. Trauma and Birth Stress was founded by five mothers who had experienced birth trauma. This self-help organization supports women who have experienced birth trauma and educates about birth trauma and the resulting PTSD.

Members of TABS were informed of the study by a packet sent to each of them by regular postal mail from the chairperson of TABS. Two letters were included in the packet. The first letter was written by the chairperson as an introduction to the study. The researcher wrote the second letter, explaining her role and describing the research program. An announcement recruiting women also was placed in the TABS newsletter. Women interested in participating had two options: e-mail or regular postal mail. In addition to recruitment through TABS, a few mothers learned of the study from the researcher's university Web site. Finally, two women from Australia joined the study after hearing a joint presentation on PTSD after childbirth by the chairperson of TABS, a psychiatrist, and the researcher.

A purposive sample was used to gain perspectives from the participants who had experienced the phenomenon investigated in the study. The sample criteria required that the mother had experienced birth trauma, was willing to articulate her experience, and could read and write English. Ability to use the Internet was not a sample criterion. The mothers who chose the Internet as the means of participation e-mailed the researcher concerning their interest. The researcher then sent the interested women two attachments: an informed consent form and directions for participating in the study. After reading both documents, the women had the opportunity of e-mailing the researcher with any further questions about the study. They electronically signed the informed consent form and returned it to the researcher by attachment. The mothers who chose to participate in the study by regular postal mail contacted the chairperson of TABS, who then sent them the informed consent form. Each mother was asked to describe her experience of traumatic birth in as much detail as she could remember and wished to share.

Of the 40 mothers, 38 participated in the study through the Internet. They sent their birth trauma stories as attachments to the researcher. The remaining two women wrote their experiences of birth trauma and sent them by regular postal mail to the researcher. After the researcher read each mother's birth trauma story, she e-mailed the woman if she had any questions or needed clarification concerning what had been written. Two participants also sent the researcher boxes of journals they had written chronicling their traumatic birth experiences and the PTSD that followed. Data collection extended over an 18-month period.

Data Analysis

The study used Colaizzi's (1978) method of data analysis, which consists of the following seven steps:

1. Read all the participants' descriptions of the phenomenon under study.
2. Extract significant statements that pertain directly to the phenomenon.

3. Formulate meanings for these significant statements.
4. Categorize the formulated meanings into clusters of themes.
5. Integrate the findings into an exhaustive description of the phenomenon being studied.
6. Validate the exhaustive description by returning to some of the participants to ask them how it compares with their experiences.
7. Incorporate any changes offered by the participants into the final description of the essence of the phenomenon.

A portion of the audit trail for the data analysis can be found in Table 1, which includes selected examples of significant statements and corresponding formulated meanings. With regard to the clustering of the formulated meanings around the four themes, the largest number of formulated meanings clustered around themes 1 and 2, followed by themes 3 and 4.

Colaizzi's (1978) process for thematic analysis was used. Once the formulated meanings were organized into clusters of themes, these clusters were referred back to the

TABLE 1	Selected Examples of Significant Statements and Their Formulated Meanings for Two Themes	
THEME NO.	**SIGNIFICANT STATEMENTS**	**FORMULATED MEANINGS**
1. To care for me: Was that too much to ask?	When you returned to my labor room and I was vomiting and shaking and no longer handling the contractions, you never reassured me or explained what was happening.	The woman felt uninformed and lacked reassurance about her labor process.
	Lying indecently and asking why the curtain behind me was open and could they close it. I felt exposed to the outside world!	The mother felt stripped of her dignity as her privacy was not respected.
2. To communicate with me: Why was this neglected?	While waiting for a scan for retained placenta fragments, I read my chart and learned for the first time my congenitally deformed baby was born alive. I thought he had been born dead and that they had brought him back to life. I went into a real inner panic and made me think, "what else don't I know or haven't they told me."	The mother panicked and became distrustful of her health care providers once she learned that information about her baby had been withheld from her.
	The midwife never told me or my support people where she was going, what she was doing, how long she would be, or what to do if I needed help.	During labor the woman felt abandoned by her primary clinician.

women's original birth trauma stories for their validation. At this stage of thematic analysis, the researcher must not be tempted to ignore data or themes that do not fit (Colaizzi).

The four themes were validated by nine mothers who had participated in the study. This group of mothers, who met with the researcher while she was in New Zealand, felt that none of the results needed to be changed. In addition, four mothers who had participated in the study and one father reviewed this article before it was submitted for publication. All agreed that the results captured the essence of their birth trauma experiences. The rationale for not including all the participants for validation of the results was that once some of the women had written their story, they did not want to revisit it again.

RESULTS

Sample

The purposive sample consisted of 40 mothers who perceived that they had experienced birth trauma. The length of time since their traumatic deliveries ranged from 5 weeks to 14 years. The mothers lived in New Zealand ($n = 23$), the United States ($n = 8$), Australia ($n = 6$), and the United Kingdom ($n = 3$). According to the diagnoses, 32 of the women (80%) had PTSD attributable to birth trauma, whereas 8 women (20%) had experienced PTSD symptoms, but had not yet gone for mental healthcare after delivery. The mean age of the sample at the time the women participated in the study was 34 years (range, 25–44 years). Of the 40 women, 34 were married, 3 were divorced, and 3 were single. Of the 15 women who shared their education level, 1 had graduated from medical school, 4 had completed graduate school, 8 had graduated from college, 1 had a partial college education, and 1 had graduated from high school. Sixteen of the women were primiparas, whereas 24 were multiparas. Eighteen of the women (45%) had undergone cesarean deliveries, whereas 22 (55%) had delivered vaginally. Almost an equal number of birth traumas in this sample had occurred during cesarean and vaginal deliveries. Labor had been induced for 17 of the mothers. Two mothers delivered twins and one mother had triplets. Three mothers in the sample were bipolar, and one had experienced prenatal depression with this most recent pregnancy.

Themes

The study results clearly show that birth trauma is in the eye of the beholder. The birth traumas identified by the women in the sample are presented in Table 2. The concept of birth trauma involves traumatic experiences that may occur during any phase of childbearing. During any phase, the trauma may be classified as a negative outcome including a stillbirth, an obstetric complication (e.g., an emergency cesarean), or psychological distress (fear of an epidural).

THEME 1. TO CARE FOR ME: WAS THAT TOO MUCH TO ASK?

I am amazed that 3 1/2 hours in the labor and delivery room could cause such utter destruction in my life. It truly was like being the victim of a violent crime or rape.

TABLE 2	List of Birth Traumas	
▶ Stillbirth/infant death		▶ Forceps/vacuum extraction/skull fracture
▶ Emergency cesarean delivery/fetal distress		▶ Severe toxemia
▶ Cardiac arrest		▶ Premature birth
▶ Inadequate medical care		▶ Separation from infant in NICU
▶ Fear of epidural		▶ Prolonged, painful labor
▶ Congenital anomalies		▶ Rapid delivery
▶ Inadequate pain relief		▶ Degrading experience
▶ Postpartum hemorrhage/manual removal of placenta		

What could have happened to this woman and others to turn the delivery process into a rape scene? Perceived lack of a caring approach during such a vulnerable time was one of the core components in this scenario for a traumatic birth. The mothers reported that feeling abandoned and alone, stripped of their dignity, lack of interest in them as unique persons, and lack of support and reassurance all contributed to their birth trauma. One mother said she "felt betrayed by a system that is supposedly there to care for me."

The women who participated in this study reported that their expectations for their labor and delivery care were shattered. One mother painfully stated:

> The labor care has hurt deep in my soul and I have no words to describe the hurt. I was treated like a nothing, just someone to get data from. The nurse took my pulse, temperature, blood pressure, and weight without talking to me as a person. She then asked about teeth, colds and smoking without acknowledging me as a person. She left me, tears rolling down my face.

A multipara who had an induced labor said:

> I felt like just a vessel into which you poured hormones hoping for the quick release of another baby.

The adjectives used by the mothers in this study to describe the care they had received during the delivery process included "mechanical," "arrogant," "cold," "technical," and "lack of empathy." For example, within 24 hours of giving birth, one mother had to say goodbye forever to her beloved newborn daughter. As her baby was dying in the neonatal intensive care unit (NICU), her husband took lots of photos until the film ran out. She and her husband asked for more film and ignored the disapproving looks of the staff members. They wondered:

> Was this too much to ask for—for us it was our only opportunity to do this before our daughter died.

The mothers reported that being stripped of their dignity also played a part in birth trauma. As one young Puerto Rican mother recounted:

> They had me in all kinds of positions (including all fours) to hear the heartbeat with a stethoscope, and about 20 students came in the room without my permission. All I heard them saying was that I was now 7½ dilated. By the way, while I was on all fours, I was trying to cover my bottom by holding the gown, and a nurse took my hands from the gown. So, I felt raped, and my dignity was taken from me.

During the delivery process, some women were shaken to the core by feeling abandoned and alone, as illustrated by the following quote:

> I had a major bleed and started shaking involuntarily all over. Even my jaw shook and I couldn't stop. I heard the specialist say he was having trouble stopping the bleeding. I was very frightened, and then it hit me. I might not make it! I can still recall the sick dread of real fear. I needed urgent reassurance, but none was offered.

THEME 2. TO COMMUNICATE WITH ME: WHY WAS THIS NEGLECTED?

At times, the mothers perceived that the labor and delivery staff failed to communicate with their patients. During a traumatic birth, women often felt invisible. Clinicians spoke to each other as if the woman were not present. One woman who was having her first baby recalled:

> After an hour trying to deliver the baby with a vacuum extractor, the obstetrician said it was too late for an emergency cesarean. The baby was truly stuck. By now the doctors are acting like I'm not there. The attending physician was saying, "We may have lost this bloody baby." The hospital staff discussed my baby's possible death in front of me and argued in front of me just as if I weren't there.

The following segment of a mother's story dramatically illustrates how someone merely communicating with her and explaining what was happening could have prevented her birth trauma:

> The doctor turned on this machine that sounded like a swimming pool pump. He proceeded and hurriedly showed me the piece that was to be inserted into me. It was chrome metal and extremely large in circumference. Next thing he begins to pull on this hose, which was the extension of the suction. He gritted his teeth and pulled. I felt sick. On the end of this machine was our baby's head. He used every ounce of his male strength to pull the baby out. I was horrified, I started to imagine, and any minute now a head will come out, ripped off of its body. I was really in shock. He had his foot up on the bed, using it as leverage to pull. All of a sudden, the loud sucking machine made an even louder noise, and it broke suction. The doctor fell back and nearly landed on his bum. Blood came spurting out of me, all over him. That was it for me. I thought he'd ripped the head off. He then swore and said hurriedly, "Get the forceps." I can still remember the feeling of him ripping the baby out of me. It was the most awful unnatural devastating feeling ever. Well, finally out came this baby. I was, by this stage, still stuck in my own private horror movie, visualizing my baby being born dead with half of its head missing. The pediatrician was standing beside the doctor, and I assumed that he would take the dead baby away. But, much to my horror and surprise, the doctor pulled out this blood red baby and threw it onto my tummy. I screamed, "Get him off of me!" I cried my eyes out!

Clinicians also at times failed to communicate among themselves, which influenced the women's perceptions of their deliveries as traumatic. For example, labor was induced for one woman who had experienced a previous serious vasovagal reaction before pregnancy and it came time for her to receive an epidural. She was terrified because the midwife did not tell the anesthetist about her history. As this mother shared,

> I remember my husband trying to tell the anesthetist that I was fearful of a vasovagal attack. The midwife should have been doing that. My husband kept saying, "My wife, my wife." He could not remember what to say. I was terrified for my life. My soul was in agony because the medical people did not know the situation. I was terrified to the core of my being. I called out, "I'm scared, I'm scared." Not scared of the needle, scared for my life.

THEME 3. TO PROVIDE SAFE CARE: YOU BETRAYED MY TRUST AND I FELT POWERLESS

Women began their labors confident that the delivery staff would provide safe care. The women entrusted their lives and that of their unborn baby into the hands of these clinicians. At times, women perceived that they received unsafe care, which ignited terror in them as they feared for their own safety and that of their infants, but felt powerless to rectify the dangerous situation. As one mother vehemently recounted:

> I remember believing that the labor and delivery team would know what was right and would be there should things go wrong. That was my first mistake. They didn't and they weren't! I strongly believe my PTSD was caused by feelings of powerlessness and loss of control of what people did to my body.

One brief scenario vividly illustrates this third theme. Shortly before becoming pregnant the second time, one mother had surgery to repair a hiatal hernia. During this pregnancy, gestational diabetes developed, and at 28 weeks a scan detected a mass in the brain of her fetus. Her desired birth plan was to have a cesarean delivery to save her baby the distress of a vaginal birth. The doctor "pressured" her into a trial of labor because her first delivery had been so straightforward and rapid. The doctor assured her that if she got into any difficulties she could "easily convert to cesarean." As this mother explained,

> I went into the delivery room assured that my baby and I would be in safe hands. I got into difficulties at 9 p.m. with severe abdominal pain and felt something was terribly wrong. I was in what I describe as "white pain," a terrible ripping pain. I told the staff something was wrong and I begged for a cesarean. I was refused without an examination. An epidural was administered without an examination. I was pushing for hours to no avail, flat on my back, numb from the waist down and feeling that my vague pushes were killing my unborn daughter. I started to die inside. The whole of my genital area was swollen to resemble a baboon. My daughter was posterior, brow presenting, and I continued in second stage labor actively pushing for over 6 hours. My daughter was distressed and her heartbeat kept disappearing. An episiotomy was cut without so much as eye contact with me. My daughter was born flat, resuscitated with Apgars of 2 and 6, and taken to the NICU. After being stitched up, I went to see my baby, and I didn't recognize her, felt no bond, nothing. She wasn't my baby; my baby had died. In my mind, my efforts to give birth had killed her. After delivery I was incontinent. The familiar stomach pain returned. My hiatus hernia repair had now failed. I later had repair surgery to reattach a part of my labia majora. I had an anal sphincter repair and my pelvic floor was refashioned at the same time. I'm waiting for a repeat hiatus hernia repair, and I am still going to physiotherapy to improve the incontinence. During labor, I had expected pain, and I had expected a powerful experience. I expected that, if necessary, medical staff would intervene to keep us safe. Why didn't anyone use their professional judgment? That was what I expected from them. I have posttraumatic stress disorder.

THEME 4. THE END JUSTIFIES THE MEANS: AT WHOSE EXPENSE? AT WHAT PRICE?

Mothers believed that the bottom line in considering a delivery a successful and fulfilling experience was the outcome of the baby. If the baby was born alive with good Apgar scores, that was what mattered to the labor and delivery staff and even to the mother's family and friends. The safe arrival of a live, healthy infant symbolized the achievement of clinical efficiency and of professional and fiscal goals. Mothers perceived that their traumatic deliveries were glossed over and pushed into the background as the healthy newborn took center stage. Why put a damper on this celebration by focusing on the mother's traumatic experience giving birth!

One woman had been hospitalized with chronic sciatica 20 years earlier when she was 18 years old. She received an epidural steroid injection for treatment. As the woman recalled,

> The needle hit a nerve in my back and created a frightful situation where I could not move and had such a horrible sensation I vowed on the spot never ever to have another epidural.

Submitting to her most dreaded epidural and saying goodbye to her dreams of a vaginal delivery, this woman experienced an out-of-body experience as she lay on the delivery table hemorrhaging. She wrote,

> I would have done anything to have this baby and did everything, even stuff I didn't want to. All I get told when dealing with the residual emotional effects is, "You should be happy with the outcome."

After an hour of pushing, one primipara was offered forceps. The epidural was topped up, but not given enough time to work properly, nor was it checked. The mother felt the cut, the forceps going in, and her body tearing as the doctor pulled the baby out. She screamed loud and long. She shared that she

> was congratulated for how "quickly and easily" the baby came out and that he scored a perfect 10! The worst thing was that nobody acknowledged that I had a bad time. Everyone was so pleased it had gone so well! I felt as if I had been raped!

Women, who perceived that they had experienced traumatic births viewed the site of their labor and delivery as a battlefield. While engaged in battle, their protective layers were stripped away, leaving them exposed to the onslaught of birth trauma. Stripped from these women were their individuality, dignity, control, communication, caring, trust, and support and reassurance.

DISCUSSION

The birth traumas experienced by the mothers in this study have been identified previously such as emergency cesarean deliveries (Ballard, Stanley, & Brockington, 1995; Soet et al., 2003), long, painful labors with inadequate pain relief (Ballard et al., 1995; Fones, 1996; Soet et al., 2003), epidurals (Ballard et al., 1995; Fones, 1996), forceps deliveries (Fones, 1996), fetal or newborn deaths (Ballard et al., 1995; Turton, Hughes, Evans, & Fainman, 2001), premature infants and infants in the NICU (DeMier, Hynan, Harris, & Manniello, 1996; Holditch-Davis, Bartlett, Blickman, & Miles, 2003), degrading experiences (Menage, 1993), and perceptions of unsafe care during childbirth (Creedy, et al., 2000). Creedy et al. (2000) reported that the perception of unsafe care had a significant additive effect on birth trauma symptoms for women who also had a high level of obstetric intervention during their labor and delivery.

Parts of the four themes that describe the essence of a traumatic birth have been reported in previous studies, but nowhere has the totality of the experience been reported. Aspects of theme 1 (To care for me: Was that too much to ask?) have been mentioned by Ballard et al. (1995), Menage (1993), and Wijma et al. (1997). Theme 2 (To communicate with me: Why was this neglected?) appears in the research of Ballard et al. (1995), Creedy et al. (2000), Menage (1993), and Soet et al. (2003). The mothers' feelings of powerlessness and loss of control (theme 3) have been echoed previously by Allen (1998), Czarnocka and Slade (2000), Menage (1993), and Soet et al. (2003). Maes, Delmeire, Mylle, and Altramura (2001) reported that loss of control is a significant component of the traumatic event for many mothers who experience PTSD. Theme 4 (The end justifies the means: At whose expense? At what price?) has not been specifically addressed in any previous research. Whereas some of the mothers in this study felt as if they had been raped, the clinicians appeared to the women as oblivious to their plight. The mothers perceived that the clinicians focused only on the successful outcomes of clinical efficiency and live healthy infants.

In reviewing this manuscript before it was submitted for publication, two mothers made a special point to emphasize the importance of this fourth theme. The one mother wrote:

> For me the most telling statement remains, "The end justifies the means: At whose expense? At what price?" For me, this sums up my situation and many others I know of.

The other mother said:

> This I believe is the actual contributing factor toward PTSD occurring. As no one is comfortable enough in themselves to be honest with the mother and the partner too I might add. So let's just breathe a sigh of relief and focus on the fact that the baby arrived.

Besides providing safe care, what is it that clinicians can do to help prevent traumatic births? At a woman's admission to labor and delivery, it is important that clinicians take a careful history from her regarding any particular fears she may have about giving birth, such as needle phobia. If a woman has had previous deliveries, this admission history should include questions on whether previous deliveries were perceived as traumatic. Identification of any possible contributing factors to birth trauma can alert clinicians so that special care can be taken regarding these factors.

During labor and delivery, clinicians should strive to enhance a woman's sense of control by offering her options when possible. Many events during the delivery process are, however, out of the control of both the obstetric care providers and the mothers. Obstetric care providers need to discuss with the women the means of delivery, and not just the outcome. When hopes for the best laid birth plans are dashed, women's unmet expectations regarding their anticipated birth process need to be addressed by clinicians. Mothers' perceptions of birth trauma can be based not only on the event, but also on their unmet expectations regarding the event.

Church and Scanlan (2002) alert clinicians to have a proactive role in preventing PTSD after childbirth by vigilantly watching mothers during the postpartum period for recognition of early trauma-related symptoms: a dazed appearance, withdrawal, or temporary amnesia. Knowing that birth trauma lies in the eye of the beholder, they should treat every woman as though she were a survivor of a previous traumatic experience (Crompton, 2003).

REFERENCES

Allen, S. (1998). A qualitative analysis of the process, mediating variables, and impact of traumatic childbirth. *Journal of Reproductive and Infant Psychology, 16,* 107–131.

Ayers, S., & Pickering, A. (2001). Do women get posttraumatic stress disorder as a result of childbirth? A prospective study of incidence. *Birth, 28,* 111–118.

Ballard, C. G., Stanley, A. K., & Brockington, I. F. (1995). Post-traumatic stress disorder (PTSD) after childbirth. *British Journal of Psychiatry, 166*, 525–528.

Church, S., & Scanlan, M. (2002). Posttraumatic stress disorder after childbirth: Do midwives play a preventative role? *The Practicing Midwife, 5*, 10–13.

Colaizzi, P. F. (1978). Psychological research as the phenomenologist views it. In R. Valle & M. King (Eds.), *Existential phenomenological alternatives for psychology* (pp. 48–71). New York: Oxford University Press.

Creedy, D. K., Shochet, I. M., & Horsfall, J. (2000). Childbirth and the development of acute trauma symptoms: Incidence and contributing factors. *Birth, 27*, 104–111.

Crompton, J. (2003). Posttraumatic stress disorder and childbirth. *Childbirth Educators New Zealand Education Effects*, summer, 25–31.

Czarnocka, J., & Slade, P. (2000). Prevalence and predictors of posttraumatic stress symptoms following childbirth. *British Journal of Clinical Psychology, 39*, 35–51.

DeMier, R. L., Hynan, M. T., Harris, H. B., & Manniello, R. L. (1996). Perinatal stressors as predictors of symptoms of posttraumatic stress in mothers of infants at high risk. *Journal of Perinatology, 16*, 276–280.

Fones, C. (1996). Posttraumatic stress disorder occurring after painful childbirth. *Journal of Nervous and Mental Disease, 184*, 195–196.

Holditch-Davis, D., Bartlett, T. R., Blickman, A. L., & Miles, M. S. (2003). Posttraumatic stress symptoms in mothers of premature infants. *Journal of Obstetric, Gynecologic, and Neonatal Nursing, 32*, 161–171.

Hungerford, M. W. (1878). *Molly Bawn*, London: Smith, Elder and Company.

Husserl, E. (1960). *Cartesian meditations* (Trans. D. Cairns). The Hague: Martineus Nijhoff.

Husserl, E. (1962). *Ideas: General introduction to pure phenomenology.* New York: MacMillan.

Husserl, E. (1970). *The crisis of European sciences and transcendental phenomenology* (Trans. D. Carr). Evanston, IL: Northwestern University Press.

Maes, M., Delmeire, I., Mylle, J., & Altramura, C. (2001). Risk and preventive factors of posttraumatic stress disorder (PTSD). *Journal of Affective Disorders, 63*, 113–121.

Menage, J. (1993). Posttraumatic stress disorder in women who have undergone obstetric or gynecological procedures. *Journal of Reproduction and Infant Psychology, 11*, 221–228.

Ryding, E. L., Wijma, K., & Wijma, B. (1998). Experiences of emergency Cesarean section: A phenomenological study of 53 women. *Birth, 25*, 246–251.

Seng, J. S. (2002). A conceptual framework for research on lifetime violence, posttraumatic stress, and childbearing. *Journal of Midwifery and Women's Health, 47*, 337–346.

Soet, J. E., Brack, G. A., & Dilorio, C. (2003). Prevalence and predictors of women's experience of psychological trauma during childbirth. *Birth, 30*, 36–46.

Spielberger, C., Gorsuch, R., & Lushene, R. (1983). *Manual for the state-trait anxiety inventory.* Palo Alto, CA: Consulting Psychological Press.

Spiegelberg, H. (1975). *Doing phenomenology: Essays on and in phenomenology.* The Hague: Martinus Nijhoff.

Turton, P., Hughes, P., Evans, C. D., & Fainman, D. (2001). Incidence, correlates, and predictors of posttraumatic stress disorder in the pregnancy after stillbirth. *British Journal of Psychiatry, 178*, 556–560.

Watson, C. G., Juba, M. P., Manifold, V., Kucala, T., & Anderson, E. D. (1991). The PTSD interview: Rationale, description, reliability, and concurrent validity of a DSM-III-based technique. *Journal of Clinical Psychology, 47*, 179–189.

Wijma, K., Soderquist, J., & Wijma, B. (1997) Posttraumatic stress disorder after childbirth: A cross-sectional study. *Journal of Anxiety Disorders, 11*, 587–597.

Cheryl Tatano Beck, DNSc, CNM, FAAN, is Professor of Nursing, University of Connecticut School of Nursing, Storrs.

Accepted for publication September 18, 2003.

The author thanks Sue Watson, the Chairperson of Trauma and Birth Stress (TABS), a charitable trust in New Zealand, for her unwavering support and enthusiastic assistance with this research project. Without her help, this research study would never have come to fruition. To all the courageous women who shared their most personal and powerful stories of birth trauma, the author is forever indebted.

Corresponding author: Cheryl Tatano Beck, DNSc, CNM, FAAN, University of Connecticut, School of Nursing, 231 Glen-brook Road, Storrs, CT 06269-2026 (e-mail: Cheryl.beck@uconn.edu).

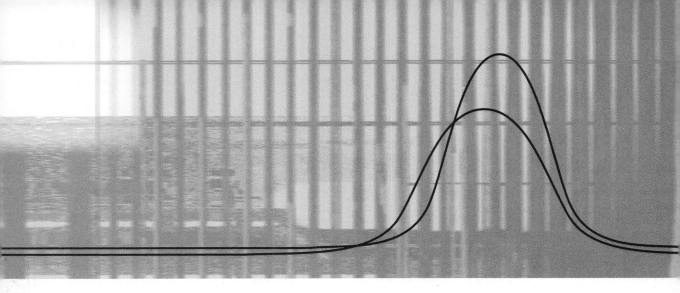

C.

Postoperative Arm Massage: A Support for Women With Lymph Node Dissection

Cheryl Forchuk, Pat Baruth, Monique Prendergast, Ronald Holliday, Ruth Bareham, Susan Brimner, Valerie Schulz, Yee Ching Lilian Chan, Nadine Yammine

- ▶ **Purpose/objective:** To evaluate the usefulness of arm massage from a significant other following lymph node dissection surgery.
- ▶ **Design:** Randomized clinical trial with a pretest-posttest design. Data were collected prior to surgery, within 24 hours post surgery, within 10 to 14 days post surgery, and 4 months post surgery.
- ▶ **Sample:** 59 women, aged 21 to 78 undergoing lymph node dissection surgery and who had a significant other with them during the postoperative period.
- ▶ **Methods:** Subjects were randomly assigned to intervention and control groups. Subjects' significant others in the intervention group were first taught, then performed arm massage as a postoperative support measure.
- ▶ **Research main variables:** Variables included postoperative pain, family strengths and stressors, range of motion, and health related costs.
- ▶ **Findings:** Participants reported a reduction in pain in the immediate postoperative period and better shoulder function.
- ▶ **Conclusion:** Arm massage decreased pain and discomfort related to surgery, and promoted a sense of closeness and support amongst subjects and their significant other.
- ▶ **Implication for nursing practice:** Postoperative massage therapy for women with lymph node dissection provided therapeutic benefits for patients and their significant other. Nurses can offer effective alternative interventions along with standard procedures in promoting optimal health.
- ▶ **Key Words:** Arm massage; Lymph node dissection; Pain reduction

Reprinted with permission from *Cancer Nursing* (2004; 27[1]: 25–33).

Women diagnosed with breast cancer frequently undergo lymph node surgery to assist in the staging of the disease. The pain and discomfort from this surgery can create an additional burden at this point in their journey. In addition to the immediate postsurgical pain, women may experience longer-term sequelae, such as reduced range of motion (ROM) and function in the affected arm, and/or lymphedema.[1–4] The purpose of this investigation was to examine the usefulness of arm massage by a significant other in the immediate postoperative period.

CURRENT KNOWLEDGE

Breast cancer is a serious disease with an estimated lifetime risk of around 1 in 9 for every woman in Canada and the United States. Breast cancer is the most common cancer to affect women (excluding nonmelanoma skin cancer).[5,6] Although the mortality rate from breast cancer has been consistently decreasing, the rate of detection of breast cancer has steadily risen; this pattern is occurring due to the screening programs and improved treatment methods.[5] For those women diagnosed with the disease, current management includes some type of breast surgery and/or adjuvant therapy. Surgical options include a partial mastectomy/lumpectomy with axillary node dissection, or modified radical mastectomy with axillary node dissection. Emotionally, both surgeries can be devastating for women and their significant others. Following surgery, women work through the turmoil of the cancer diagnosis, as well as disturbances to body image, pain, and altered sensation, including numbness/tingling to the underside of the affected arm.[2–4]

Lymph Node Dissection

During lymph node dissection surgery, the woman's arm is draped and abducted as needed throughout the procedure. The positioning of the arm during surgery can cause pain from muscle cramping and stiffness in the immediate postoperative period. Discomfort may lead to a reluctance or difficulty in moving the arm. Further complications may include reduced range of motion and fluid accumulation.[1,2,4,7] In studies investigating weakness, stiffness, pain, and ROM restriction of the arm following breast surgery, pain and loss of sensation were reported by greater than 50% of patients.[1,2,8–10]

Massage

Massage has been used for breast cancer patients who develop lymphedema. Lymphedema or swelling of the affected arm is a potential complication related specifically to lymph node removal. Lymphedema is a complication found in about 12% of all women who have undergone breast surgery and lymph dissection[2] and can constitute a handicap for patients and impede their daily functional abilities[1,2,10,11]; massage therapy or manual lymph drainage may be recommended.[9,12,13] Physiotherapists generally accept the notion of gentle massage, or effleurage strokes. Self-administered retrograde massage and backward massage strokes have been routinely prescribed to patients and have been included in a multidisciplinary treatment approach for lymphedema.[9]

Nurses, physical therapists, and massage therapists commonly practice a technique using hand strokes from the distal portion of the limb to the proximal in a circular pattern[14]; this helps to redirect fluid from one area of the body to another. Furthermore, effleurage, light manual rubbing,[12] a classical type of massage, retrograde self-massage, and gentle, rhythmic stroking may result in a mild pressure gradient, assisting in removing edema from the affected limb; these techniques may be administered by a properly trained therapist, nurse, or by the patient's significant other following adequate instructions and proper demonstrations.[15]

Massage therapy has been well documented in the literature as an effective treatment intervention for lymphedema secondary to breast surgery.[9,12,14,16,17] However, the concept of massage therapy as a preventative measure to the development of lymphedema has not been described in the literature.

Pain

Massage therapy has also been used frequently as nonpharmacological alternative to reduce pain.[12,18,19] Bredin[20] determined that massage therapy reduced numbness and pain of the affected arm. Weinrich and Weinrich[21] found that massage decreased the intensity of pain in male cancer patients. Gibson[22] and Joachim[23] concluded that massage assisted in providing better control over pain.

Range of Motion

Le Vu et al[1] concluded that massage therapy improved the range of motion in the shoulder of the affected arm. Patients that were subjected to circular massage and mobilization of their arm experienced a 15% improvement in shoulder extension and an 18% improvement in abducting their affected shoulder. Consequently, Le Vu et al[1] recommend initiation of massage therapy and mobilization of the affected limb on the first day postoperatively.

HYPOTHESES

It was hypothesized that individuals receiving arm massage from a significant other following lymph node dissection surgery would have greater immediate comfort and fewer functional constraints compared to women receiving the standard postoperative treatment. Functional constraints were defined as constrains that affect women's ability to use their arm and shoulder in activities of daily living.

Subhypotheses

Specific subhypotheses considered in addressing immediate comfort examined differences between individuals receiving arm massage from a significant other following lymph node dissection surgery and control groups, receiving standard postoperative treatment, in relation to

1. reduction of pain; and
2. perceived control and comfort of significant other.

Subhypotheses associated with fewer functional constraints in individuals receiving arm massage from a significant other following lymph node dissection surgery at 2 weeks and 4 months considered

1. swelling;
2. range of motion;
3. shoulder function; and
4. costs.

DESIGN

The design was a randomized clinical trial with measures taken (1) prior to surgery, (2) within 24 hours post surgery, (3) within 10 to 14 days post surgery, and (4) four months post surgery.

Sampling

Sampling was initially completed with 14 individuals in order to pilot the procedure, test the instruments and determine the power required for a final sample. Based on a power of .80 and $P < .05$, a minimum of 25 participants per group would be required. There were 30 participants per group recruited to allow for dropouts. Only one person dropped out (due to death). There were no refusals to participate.

Inclusion Criteria

Inclusion criteria were

1. 18 years of age or older;
2. diagnosed with breast cancer, and scheduled for lymph node dissection;
3. planning on having significant other (spouse, family, or friend) present in post surgical period (at least 1 hour immediately after leaving post anesthesia care unit);
4. both woman with breast cancer and significant other consent to participate and able to make informed consent by understanding the nature of participation; and
5. proficient in English to the degree necessary to participate in interviews.

Exclusion Criteria

The following would exclude potential subjects from participation in the study:

1. Diagnosed with an organic brain disease; and
2. Preexisting disorder affecting functional ability of affected arm or lymphatic system.

Demographics

Demographic data were collected, including age, marital status, and educational level. Other descriptive data included length of time since diagnosis of breast cancer, type of surgery, and relationship to significant other.

Procedure

Significant others were given a demonstration of the massage techniques on participants, to show them a variety of techniques and positions of comfort (see Appendix). They were instructed to ask their significant other if they would like a massage to help ease the discomfort postoperatively. Likewise, patients were asked to request the massage as often as they felt that they needed it, to help with pain relief. Although 10 minutes was offered as a suggested length of massage, there were no set parameters with respect to length of time or number of massages; massage was meant to be used as needed, as would be pain analgesia. Additionally, a written demonstration sheet outlining the massage techniques in different patient positions were distributed to significant others (Appendix). Participants were then asked to demonstrate their massage technique to ensure proper administration of the intervention. One registered nurse, prepared at the masters level, performed all the teaching and demonstrations in order to avoid variance from multiple teachers.

Measures

The timing and frequency of data collection measures are summarized in Table 1.

Postoperative Pain and Pain Control

Postoperative pain was measured using the numeric rating scale (NRS). Subjects were asked to rate their pain at its most, least, and average each day, on a scale from 0 to 10 (10 being worst pain). They were also asked to rate from 0 to 10 the amount of pain control they experienced from their medication. Intervention group participants were also asked to rate the pain control they experienced from their massage. NRS is a simple and valid method of measuring pain[24] and has been used by other researchers to measure cancer pain intensity.[24,25] Jensen, Turner, and Romano[26] concluded in their study that the 0–10 NRS provided adequate sensitivity to measure pain effectively in most patients. Participants in the study were adults (Mean age = 42 years) diagnosed with chronic pain ($N = 124$); 60% of patients were female; the primary area of pain included low back, head, leg, neck, and shoulder/arm.[26] Paice and Cohen[25] stated that NRS is an uncomplicated and an easy to

TABLE 1	Timing and Frequency of Data Collection				
MEASURES	**PREOPERATION**	**24 H**	**10–14 D**	**4 Mo**	**DAILY RECORD**
Demographics form	x				
Pain numeric rating scale					x
Family stress	x	x	x	x	
Shoulder function	x		x	x	
Range of motion	x		x	x	
Girth of limb (swelling)	x	x	x	x	
Health related costs	x		x	x	
Frequency of massages					x
Feedback on massage				x	

understand rating tool; the majority of subjects in their study preferred using the NRS and experienced no evident difficulties in understanding the tool.

Frequency of Massage

Frequency of massages was recorded on a Post Operative Arm Massage Record developed by the investigators. The record involved a checklist format that subjects could complete each evening.

Family Stress and Strengths

The Family Stressor Inventory was used to measure the family's level of stress and strengths.[27] This instrument contains subscales for both general family stress and issue-specific family stress as well as family strengths. The inventory generates both qualitative and quantitative information regarding family health.[28] Hanson[28] further added that the inventory is simple to administer and interpret; it concentrates both on the individuals and the family unit; and combines both the strengths and stressors of a family. For this study, the inventory's internal consistency and measure through Cronbach alpha was found to be .90.

Shoulder Function

Shoulder function was measured using the disability section of the Shoulder Pain and Disability Index (SPADI). [29] The SPADI is a subjective shoulder function status measure that has been shown to be responsive to clinical change.[29] It uses a visual analogue scale and has a reliable Cronbach alpha of .9321 and test-retest reliability intraclass correlation (ICC) of 0.655.[30]

Range of Motion

Shoulder ROM was quantified using a procedure outlined by Norkin and White.[31] Boone, Azen, and Lin[20] reported that intertester reliability was lower than intratester reliability for weekly measurements of active ROM of lower and upper extremities. Riddle, Rothstein, and Lamb[21] made repeated-passive range of motion (PROM) measures of shoulder flexion, extension, abduction, horizontal abduction, and external and internal rotation in 2 groups of 50 subjects; intratester intraclass correlation coefficients for all motions ranged from 0.87 to 0.99. The ICC for the intertester reliability of horizontal abduction and external rotation measures ranged from 0.84 to 0.90.[21] These values indicate that ROM measurement should be conducted ideally by one trained individual throughout the study to ensure a standardized approach to measurement.

Swelling

Volume of the limb was calculated based on measuring the circumference of the limb at 4-in intervals.[22] An adapted formula for the volume of a cylinder is used to determine the volume of the arm from the wrist to the axilla.[23] A comparison between surface measurements and water displacement volumetry for the quantification of leg edema was completed in 1981 by Einar Stranden and a correlation coefficient of 0.98 was obtained.[22]

Costs/Utilization of Health Care Services

Health-related costs were determined using a modified Health and Social Services Utilization Form,[32] an instrument designed to assess direct and indirect costs of health and social services in Ontario. Subjects were asked to report the frequency of such things as physician visits, visits to emergency rooms, and subsidization of expenses such as transportation and homemaker services. At data collection points 10 to 14 days and 4 months, subjects were questioned regarding the health and social services they had used in the previous month, as well as related costs, including the number of hospitalizations since surgery. To calculate annual utilization the monthly rates are extended to 12 months.[32] Browne et al[32] validated a portion of the form by having 141 patients' reports on laboratory tests compared to clinical records. Observed agreement ranged from 0.72 to 0.99. When this was adjusted for chance agreement the Kappa statistic was 0.48 to 0.89.

ANALYSIS

Descriptive statistics were completed for all variables. *T*-tests were carried out comparing responses of women in the control group to women in the intervention group for the following measures: pain control, family strengths and stressors, shoulder function, ROM, and girth measurement. The stated measures tested hypotheses related to comparing the intervention group to the control group. The Statistical Package for Social Sciences was used in the data analysis.

RESULTS

Sample Characteristics

The study included 59 women diagnosed with breast cancer. Thirty were in the intervention group and 29 were in the control group. Slightly more than half ($n = 33$, 55%) of the women had a lumpectomy/partial mastectomy with axillary node dissection, 13 (21.7%) had a total mastectomy and axillary node dissection, 10 (16.7%) had a modified radical mastectomy and axillary node dissection, 3 (5%) had axillary node dissection alone, and 1 (1.7%) reported other. Their ages ranged from 21 to 78 with a mean of 56.19. The majority were married or had a common law partner (88.1%). Three women had an education level of primary school or less, 12 had some secondary, 15 had completed secondary, 13 had a community college diploma, and 14 had a university degree. The majority of women ($n = 48$, 80%) reported previous experience with massage therapy.

The majority of significant others were spouses ($n = 49$, 83.1%), 4 (6.8%) were parents, 2 (3.4%) were other relatives, 1 (1.7%) was a friend, and 3 (5.1%) were reported as "other." Significant others' educational level included 9 individuals with university degrees (15.3%) and 18 who had completed secondary school (30.5%). Eight (14.8%) of the significant others had previous experience with massage therapy.

Postoperative Pain Control and Pain Control

Pain was recorded on a daily record, provided to subjects at the time of enrollment. Subjects were asked to complete this record each day, as long as they had pain. Pain records were then collected at 2 weeks postsurgery or could be mailed in to the researchers.

Pain control in the immediate postoperative period for both the intervention and control group is described in Table 2. On the first day postoperation, women in the intervention group reported significantly greater [$t(40) = 2.31$, $P < .05$] pain control than reported by the control group. On the second day postoperation, women in the intervention group reported significantly lower [$t(36) = 2.38$, $P < .05$] pain *when pain was at its least* than reported by the control group. On the third day postoperation, women in the intervention group reported significantly lower [$t(36) = 2.68$, $P < .05$] pain *when pain was at its least* than reported by the control group. Past the third day postoperation, there were no significant differences in terms of pain control between the two groups.

Frequency of Massage

The average number of massages varied over the first 3 days post-operatively (see Table 2). The number of massages peaked on Day 4, with an average of 2.69, and a range of 0 to 10. One of the participants in the intervention group never received massage. After Day 4 women reported progressively less use of massage.

Family Stress and Strengths

Overall, there were some differences between the groups' ratings of family strengths and stressors. During the preoperative interview, women in the control group ($M = 4.28$,

TABLE 2	Postoperative Pain Control in the Intervention and Control Group		
	DAY 1	DAY 2	DAY 3
Intervention group			
Average number of massages			
Mean	1.72	2.28	2.44
Range	0–5	0–6	0–8
SD	1.41	1.45	2.13
Pain control from massage			
Mean (%)	39.5	57.06	54.44
Range (%)	0–100	0–100	0–100
SD	39.19	39.5	37.31
Pain control from medication			
Mean (%)	83.18	88	87.81
Range (%)	0–100	50–100	60–100
SD	28.64	14.62	13.29
Control group			
Pain control from medication			
Mean SD (%)	84.74	84.38	80.31
Range (%)	50–100	50–100	50–100
SD	16.45	13.02	12.44

SD = 0.75) rated the overall physical health of their families significantly higher [$t(46.73)$ = 2.07, $P < .05$] than women in the intervention group ($M = 4.23$, SD = 0.91). At the second follow-up visit, 10 to 14 days post surgery, women in the control group ($M = 4.68$, SD = 0.67) rated overall family functioning significantly higher [$t(43.65)$ = 2.06, $P < 0.05$] than women in the intervention group ($M = 4.24$, SD = 0.88). At the third follow up, 4 months after surgery, women in the intervention group ($M = 4.57$, SD = 0.60) rated fostering family table time and conversation significantly higher ($t(37.48) = 2.78$, $P < 0.05$) than women in the control group ($M = 3.91$, SD = 0.95).

Shoulder Function

At the initial measurement prior to surgery, there were no significant differences between the groups on the SPADI disability scale. At the second follow-up visit, women in the intervention group reported significantly less difficulty than the women in the control group with the following tasks:

1. washing their back;
2. putting on an undershirt or a pullover;
3. placing an object on a high shelf; and
4. removing something from their back pocket (see Table 3).

By the third follow-up there were no significant differences between the intervention and control groups on the disability scale.

Range of Motion

ROM measurement was not performed at the first follow-up, 24 hours post surgery. There were no statistical differences in ROM between the intervention and control groups at the second and third follow-up visits.

Swelling

At the second follow-up, women in the intervention group had significantly higher (20 cm) proximal girth measurements than women in the control group (see Table 4). Similarly,

TABLE 3 **Significant Shoulder Function Differences Between the Intervention and Control Group**

TASK	INTERVENTION GROUP		CONTROL GROUP		
	Mean	SD	Mean	SD	T value ($P < .05$)
Washing their back	2.86	2.98	4.89	3.48	53
Putting on an undershirt or pullover	2.2	3	4.04	3.36	52
Placing an object on a high shelf	3.03	3.4	5	3.56	52
Removing something from their back pocket	1.23	2.32	2.94	3.04	49

TABLE 4	Girth Measurements for Intervention and Control Groups at Follow-up 2		
	INTERVENTION GROUP	CONTROL GROUP	t, P values
Proximal girth measurements			
Mean	16.95 cm	16.20 cm	$t(53) = 2.02, P < .05$
SD	1.49	1.15	
Ulnar styloid measurements			
Mean	26.20 cm	2.38	$t(52) = 2.07, P < .05$
SD	25.27 cm	2.37	

women in the intervention group had significantly higher base of ulnar styloid measurements than women in the control group. These differences remained significant during the third follow-up. The difference seemed to be based on a single outlier. When the outliers from follow-up 2 (30.5 cm for 20 cm proximal girth measurement and 20 cm for ulnar styloid measurement) were removed the differences between the intervention and the control group became nonsignificant [proximal girth measurements: $t(52) = 1.80, P = .078$; ulnar styloid measurements $t(51) = 1.81, P = .077$]. Similarly, when the outliers from follow-up 3 (22.20 cm for 20 cm proximal girth measurement and 38.50 cm for the ulnar styloid) were removed from the analysis, the difference between the control and the intervention became nonsignificant [proximal girth measurements: $t(48) = 1.91, P = .062$; ulnar styloid measurements: $t(48) = 1.98; P = .053$].

Costs/Utilization of Health Care Services

There were no significant differences between the groups in terms of costs related to health care utilization. In general, patients in both groups had 1 to 2 appointments with their surgeons after surgery. They were also seen by their family physicians once and some had more consultations with nurses ($t = 0.996, P = .324$). Since patients in both groups had similar diagnoses, the type and quantity of postoperative tests done in hospital and out of hospital were similar ($t = 1.655, P = 1.104$).

In addition to the specific medication prescribed by their physicians, painkillers and vitamins were the common medication taken by patients of both groups ($t = .716, P = .477$). Thus, the costs related to health care utilization for both groups are similar. On the other hand, the insignificant difference ($t = 1.423, P = .161$) amongst groups in social costs (eg, loss of income of patients and significant others) may be partially attributed to the large amount of missing data (almost half) for this section of the questionnaire. Missing data was attributable to discomfort of participants in disclosing financial information.

Feedback From Intervention Group

Participants in the intervention group reported a sense of closeness and support they have felt with their partners while receiving the massage. Subjects described how the massage was something "lighthearted" to do in a stressful time. Another report stated that the massage was more effective in dealing with pain in the postoperative period than medication and that an added factor was that there are no "side effects" to deal with in massage. Several other descriptors included "relaxing," "enjoyable," and "fostering intimacy." Negative feedback received was related to the massage ending too soon. Participants felt that 10-minute massages, as it was suggested by the study, were not long enough.

LIMITATIONS

This study demonstrates some encouraging trends regarding massage as a therapeutic intervention for women following surgery for breast cancer. However, one of the prerequisites to participate in the study was the availability of a significant other; therefore, women with no significant other are not represented in this study. An additional limitation of this study was related to incomplete data sets. In particular, women tended to stop filling out the pain measurement instrument after the first week postoperatively and felt uncomfortable about disclosing financial information. Furthermore, more than one research assistant completed measurement of ROM and girth width, which could have contributed to the insignificant difference in ROM and girth width between the intervention and the control group. The sample size of 59 may not have been sufficient to determine differences.

DISCUSSION

The average number of received massages varied amongst the women; massage was performed when women felt they needed it, with no prescribed time and duration. Nonetheless, the number of received massages consistently increased to reach a peak on the fourth postoperative day, with an average of 2.69 massages, and a range of 0 to 10. Benefits of massage in the immediate postoperative period was evident with a significant improvement of shoulder function in the intervention group. Although there were no significant differences between the groups in their ROM, women in the intervention group experience significant improvement of their shoulder function as identified on the SPADI scale (see Table 3). Essentially, the questions on the SPADI scale tested the women's range of motion in carrying out daily activities. LeVu[1] concluded similar findings in their study. After determining the positive effects of massage on ROM, LeVu[1] recommended the initiation of massage on the first postoperative day.

Moreover, the use of massage was accompanied by some pain relief. Both women in the intervention and the control group experienced similar ranges of pain relief from medication. However, women in the intervention group endured less pain (39.5% less pain on the first postoperative day, 56.07% on second postoperative day, and 54.44% on third postoperative day) after receiving arm massage from a significant other. It appears that the positive effects of massage are transient, but do help during the initial stages of recovery in terms of pain management and return to normal function. These results concur with the findings of Bredin[33] who concluded that massage following breast mastectomy reduced pain and discomfort associated with the affected side. Additionally, Ferrell-Torry and Glick[34] declared that following 15 minutes of massage for cancer patients, their perception of pain decreased significantly.

In addition to the physiological benefits of postoperative arm massage by a significant other, women experienced a range or emotional and mental benefits. Women reported being comfortable and relaxed during massage. Bredin[33] determined that massage assisted her subject in relaxing and generated a "great" feeling. Women and their significant other felt that massage promoted a sense of closeness and support during a stressful time. Arm massage promoted the involvement of a significant other in the treatment. Bredin[33] described the touch of a massage as a method of communication that expresses the other person's willingness to tolerate and accept the woman after her disfiguring surgery.

IMPLICATIONS FOR NURSING PRACTICE

The majority of studies completed by both physiotherapy and nursing describe chronic management of lymphedema and ongoing range of motion difficulties. The notion of health prevention and recommendations for the need to study alternate prevention strategies has been suggested. An opportunity to explore the effects of massage therapy in the early postoperative period following breast related surgery exists. The National Cancer Institute (NCI) of Canada suggests a list of exercises appropriate for the immediate, early, and late postoperative period following mastectomies.[16] While much of the NCI teaching focuses on preventative strategies, the notion of gentle massage therapy is excluded; the effect of the addition of massage to the usual exercise program is another area of interest. Furthermore, teaching the significant other the simple massage technique may provide a tangible helping role that traditionally has not existed.

CONCLUSION

Breast cancer and mastectomy inflict an extensive range of problems that women and their families are forced to endure. Often after surgery, the women's daily living activities are affected by the complications. Simple activities such as mobilizing the arm and putting on clothes can become very difficult. Massage therapy, in this study, helped minimize some of these restrictions.

Teaching significant others to perform a simple massage on the affected arm after lymph node surgery has several benefits. Women in the intervention group expressed great satisfaction and beneficence from massage. Arm massage decreased pain and discomfort and improved their shoulder function in the immediate period after surgery. Additionally, massage was a way that significant others could demonstrate support. Many women found the massage relaxing and fostering a sense of closeness at a difficult juncture.

REFERENCES

1. Le Vu B, Dumortier A, Guillaume MV, Mouriesse H, Barreau-Pouhaer L. Efficacité du massage et de la mobilisation du member supérieur après treatement chirurgical du cancer du sein. *Bull Cancer*. 1997;84: 957–961.
2. Voogd AC, Ververs JMMA, Vingerhoets AJJM, Roumen RMH, Coebergh JWW, Crommelin MA. Lymphoedema and reduced shoulder function as indicators of quality of life axillary lymph node dissection for invasive breast cancer. *Br J Surg Soc*. 2003;90:76–81.
3. Kuehn T, Klauss W, Darsow M, et al. Long-term morbidity following axillary dissection in breast cancer patients-clinical assessment, significance for life quality and the impact of demographic, oncologic and therapeutic factors. *Breast Cancer Res Treat*. 2000;64:275–286.

4. Erickson VS, Pearson ML, Ganz PA, Adams J, Kahn KL. Arm edema in breast cancer patients. *J Natl Cancer Inst*. 2001;93(2):96–111.

5. National Cancer Institute of Canada. *Canadian Cancer Statistics 2000*: Toronto, Canada: National Cancer Institute of Canada; 2000.

6. National Alliance of Breast Cancer Organization. NABCO: fact sheets about breast cancer in the USA 2002. New York. Available at: www.nabco.org/index.php/7/rl-sections/1/39. Accessed June 21, 2002.

7. Brennan M, DePompolo R, Garden F. Focused review: postmastectomy lymphedema. *Arch Phys Med Rehabil*. 1996;77:S74–S80.

8. Maunsell E, Brisson J, Deschenes L. Arm problems and psychological distress after surgery for breast cancer. *Can J Surg*, 1993:36:315–320.

9. Bass SS, Cox CE, Salud CJ, et al. The effects of postinjection massage on the sensitivity of lymphatic mapping in breast cancer. *Am Coll Surg*. 2001;192(1):9–16.

10. Brennan MJ, Miller LT. Overview of treatment options and review of the current role and use of compression garments, intermittent pumps, and exercise in the management of lymphedema. *Am Cancer Soc*. 1998;83(12):2821–2827.

11. Schijven MP, Vingerhoets AJJM, Rutten HJT, et al. Comparison of morbidity between axillary lymph node dissection and sentinel node biopsy. *Eur J Surg Oncol*. 2003;29:341–350.

12. Billhult A, Dahlberg K. A meaningful relief from suffering. *Cancer Nurs*. 2001;24(3):180–184.

13. Williams AF, Vadgama A, Franks PJ, Mortimer PS. A randomized controlled crossover study of manual lymphatic drainage therapy in women with breast cancer-related lymphoedema. *Eur J Cancer Care*. 2002;11: 254–261.

14. Humble CA. Lymphedema: incidence, pathophysiology, management, and nursing care. *Oncol Nurs Forum*. 1955;22:1503–1509.

15. Brennan M, Miller L. Overview of treatment options and review of the current role and use of compression garments, intermittent pumps, and exercise in the management of lymphedema. *Cancer Suppl*. 1998;83:2821–2827.

16. Granda C. Nursing management of patients with lymphedema associated with breast cancer therapy. *Cancer Nurs*. 1994;17:229–235.

17. Kirshbaum M. Using massage in the relief of lymphedema. *Prof Nurse*. 1996;11(4):230–232.

18. Dicken SC, Lerncr R, Klose G, Cosimi AB. Effective treatment of lymphedema of the extremities. *Am Med Assoc*. 1998;133:452–458.

19. Gillham L. Lymphoedema and physiotherapists: control not cure. *Physiotherapy*. 1994;80:835–843.

20. Boone DC, Azen S, Lin CM. Reliability of goniometric measurements. *Phys Ther*. 1978;58:1355–1360.

21. Riddle DL, Rothstein JM, Lamb RL. Goniometric reliability in a clinical setting. *Phys Ther*. 1987;67: 668–673.

22. Stranden E, Oslo J. A comparison between surface measurements and water displacement volumetry for the quantification of lymphedema. *City Hosp*. 1981;31:153–155.

23. Farncombe M, Daniels G, Cross L. Lymphedema: the seemingly forgotten complication. *J Pain Symptom Manage*. 1994;9(4):269–276.

24. Kremer E, Atkinson JH, Ingelzi RJ. Measurement of pain: patient preference does not confound pain measurement. *Pain*. 1981;10:241–248.

25. Paice JA, Cohen FL. Validity of a verbally administered numeric rating scale to measure cancer pain intensity. *Cancer Nurs*. 1997;20(2):88–97.

26. Jensen MP, Turner JA, Romano JM. What is the maximum number of levels needed in pain intensity measurement? *Pain*. 1994;58:387–392.

27. Mischke KB, Hanson SM. *Pocket Guide to family Assessment and Intervention*. St Louis: Mosby; 1991.

28. Hanson SMH. Family assessment and intervention. In: Hanson SMH, Boyd ST, ed. *Family Health Care Nursing: Theory, Practice, and Research*. Philadelphia: FA Davis Co; 1996:147–172.

29. Williams JW Jr, Holleman DR Jr, Simel DL. Measuring shoulder function with the shoulder pain and disability index. *J Rheumatol*. 1995;22:727–732.

30. Roach KE, Budiman-Mak E, Songsiridej N, Lertratanak Y. Development of a Shoulder Pain and Disability Index. *Arthritis Care Res*. 1991;4(4):143–149.

31. Norkin CC, White DJ. *Measurement of Joint Motion: A Guide to Goniometry*. Philadelphia: FA Davis Co; 1985.

32. Browne G, Arpin K, Corey P, Fitch M, Gafni A. Individual correlates of health services utilization and the cost of poor adjustment to chronic illness. *Med Care*. 1990;28(1):43–58.

33. Bredin M. Mastectomy, body image and therapeutic massage: a qualitative study of women's experience. *J Adv Nurs*. 1999;29:1113–1120.

34. Ferrell-Torry A, Glick OJ. The use of therapeutic massage as a nursing intervention to modify anxiety and the perception of cancer pain. *Cancer Nurs*. 1993;16(2):93–101.

APPENDIX: INSTRUCTIONS FOR MASSAGE

Positioning

It is important that the patient is comfortable and her arm is fully supported. She can lay on her side with her arm supported on 1 or 2 pillows.

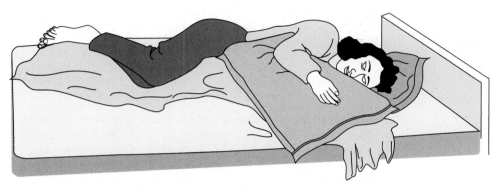

Or she can lay on her back with her arm on 1 or 2 pillows.

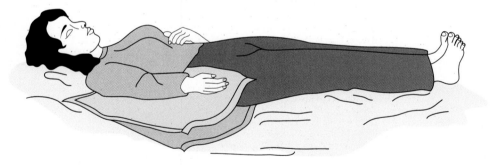

Her clothing should be loose so that her arm and shoulder are free. A sleeveless night gown or loose T-shirt would be okay. You should not use any creams, lotions, or powders.

Technique

The first stroke uses light pressure under your palm. Start at her hand and gently glide your hand over her shoulder. Keeping your fingertips in contact with her skin, follow the same path down to her hand. Repeat the stroke again in a smooth rhythm. The pressure may be increased gradually as is comfortable.

Another stroke is done with only your fingertips. Starting at her hand, glide your fingertips over her shoulder. Return, following the same path. Repeat the stroke again in a smooth rhythm.

The third stroke is called *kneading* and is done in circles. You can use your whole hand or just your fingertips. Use gentle pressure in the upward circle and less on the way down. This stroke is good for the shoulder or neck muscles.

You can use these strokes on her arm, shoulder, or neck. Do not massage the underarm area. If she is uncomfortable, try changing your position or the amount of pressure you are using.

Cheryl Forchuk, RN, PhD; Pat Baruth, RN, MScN; Monique Prendergast, BScPT; Ronald Holliday, MD, FRCS, FACS; Ruth Bareham; Susan Brimner, RMT, CLDT; Valerie Schulz, MD, FRCPC (Anaesth), MPH; Yee Ching Lilian Chan, PhD; Nadine Yammine, RN, BScN, BSc, MScN (candidate)

From the University of Western Ontario (Dr Forchuk), Lawson Health Research Institute (London Health Sciences Centre) (Drs Forchuk and Holliday, Ms Baruth and Prendergast), London, Ontario, Canada; Department of Family Medicine, London Regional Cancer Centre/London Health Sciences Centre, University of Western Ontario, London, Ontario, Canada (Dr Schulz); Michael G. DeGroote School of Business, McMaster University, Hamilton, Ontario, Canada (Dr Chan); and the Faculty of Health Sciences, School of Nursing, University of Western Ontario, London, Ontario, Canada (Ms Yammine). Ms Bareham is a Breast Cancer Survivor and Ms Brimmer is in Private Practice.

We thank the Canadian Breast Cancer Research Initiative and the National Cancer Institute of Canada for the funding to conduct this study, and the London Health Sciences Centre Research Inc for the funds for the pilot work.

Corresponding author: Cheryl Forchuk, RN, PhD, Lawson Health Research Institute, 375 South St, Rm C201 NR, London, Ontario, Canada N6A 4G5 (e-mail: cforchuk@uwo.ca).

Accepted for publication October 16, 2003.

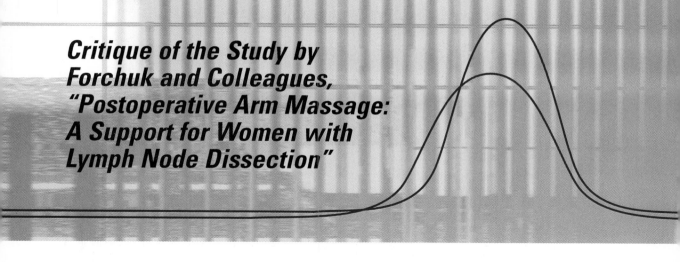

Critique of the Study by Forchuk and Colleagues, "Postoperative Arm Massage: A Support for Women with Lymph Node Dissection"

OVERALL SUMMARY

Overall, this was a good study that used a strong (experimental) research design to test a promising intervention that could easily be adopted by nurses to promote better patient outcomes among women with lymph node dissection. The small sample size, however, undermined study validity in a number of ways, including its internal validity (the experimental and control group were not equivalent at the outset, which is more likely to happen with a small sample), external validity, and, especially, statistical conclusion validity. The absence of statistical controls for preexisting group differences in the analysis and the erratic pattern of findings make interpretation of the results difficult—especially in the absence of a guiding conceptual framework. The study is best construed as a good pilot study of an intervention of great relevance to nursing that merits additional refinement and testing.

TITLE

The title of this report indicates the independent variable (postoperative arm massage) and the population of interest (women with lymph node dissection), but it does not communicate that the study was a test of an intervention, nor that the intervention involved a significant other. (In fact, the title could be for a nonempirical review paper.) Also, the title does not indicate what the outcome variables were—perhaps because there were so many of them. Nevertheless, a more informative title might have been something like the following: "The Effect of Postoperative Arm Massage by a Significant Other on Pain and Functional Constraints in Women with Lymph Node Dissection."

ABSTRACT

The abstract was, in general, excellent, summarizing all major features of the study in a succinct but thorough fashion. There was, however, one problem with the abstract. The claim that the arm massage "*promoted* [emphasis added] a sense of closeness and support amongst subjects and their significant other" is not supported by the data. Information about the subjects' emotional responses was gathered qualitatively from women in the experimental group only—that is, the emotional and mental benefits were not evaluated as part of the experimental design, and therefore language implying a causal connection is not appropriate. It would have been better to say that the intervention "was perceived to be helpful in promoting closeness and support by the women and their significant other."

INTRODUCTION

The introduction to this study was well organized. There were several sections, including an introductory paragraph that provided a statement of the problem and purpose statement, a section on "Current Knowledge," and a section labelled "Hypotheses."

Problem Statement

The first paragraph set the stage for the rest of the report by articulating the problem: women who undergo lymph node surgery experience postsurgical pain and other consequences. The purpose of the study ("to examine the usefulness of arm massage by significant other in the immediate postoperative period") was then presented at the end of the first paragraph. This was a convenient placement for the statement of purpose, so that readers could readily find it—although a bit more could have been said here about what the researchers meant by "usefulness." Nevertheless, the researchers targeted a problem of considerable clinical significance to nursing.

Literature Review

The literature was reviewed in a section labelled "Current Knowledge." The review was organized into four subsections that provided background information on the following: lymph node dissection, massage, pain, and range of motion. The section on lymph node dissection summarized research on the consequences and complications of lymph node dissection, providing support for the researchers' statement of the problem. The next section summarized research on the effectiveness of massage as a treatment for lymphedema; the researchers noted the absence of studies on the use of massage as a *preventive* measure, thereby providing a rationale for conducting this study. The last two sections described research on massage in relation to two key outcomes, pain and range of motion.

Overall, the literature review was quite brief, but it was well written, organized, and up-to-date, with many studies published after the year 2000 cited (its thoroughness could not be determined without undertaking our own review, of course). One concern is that the researchers again overstated the confidence that can be placed in findings from nonexperimental studies. The review indicated that "Bredin determined that massage therapy reduced numbness and pain of the affected arm," but Bredin's study was not experimental (primarily qualitative), and so it should not have been the basis for drawing conclusions about the effectiveness of massage as an intervention. Yet another issue is that the literature review provided little information about the confidence we can place on the findings from earlier studies (i.e., the review did not comment on the *quality* of existing evidence).

Another concern is that the review did not describe any literature relating to the effect of massage on psychosocial variables such as family stress, which was one of the outcome variables. Indeed, the researchers did not offer a rationale for including this outcome in their study. Evidence tying massage interventions to the use of health care services and to costs—two other outcomes of interest in this study—also was not summarized, and we do not know if this is because there *is* no existing literature on these topics, or if the review neglected to cover these topics.

One final issue is that it would have been useful for the researchers to conclude their literature review section with a brief summary statement that laid out what is known or not known and why their study would contribute to knowledge.

Hypotheses

In addition to providing a purpose statement in the first paragraph, the researchers devoted one section of the introduction to a statement of their hypotheses. Their overall hypothesis was well stated: "individuals receiving arm massage from a significant other would have greater immediate comfort and fewer functional constraints compared to women receiving the standard postoperative treatment."

The researchers also presented subhypotheses, which are elaborations of the main hypothesis. For example, they indicated that "greater immediate comfort" would be tested as the effect of the intervention on "reduction of pain" and "perceived control and comfort of the significant other." It is not clear, however, what was meant by "comfort of the significant other." Both pain and pain control were outcomes that were measured and described in the subsection called "Measures," but "comfort of the significant other" does not appear to have been measured and tested in this study—unless this "comfort" variable was operationalized as "family stress and strengths." This needs clarification.

One other point is that the subhypotheses elaborating on the effect of the intervention on functional constraints listed "cost" as one of the outcomes to be considered. It could be argued that this is not really a subset of the hypothesis on functional constraints, and could have been elevated to a higher status in their hypothesis hierarchy.

Framework

One final issue concerning the introduction to the report is that Forchuk and her colleagues did not include any discussion of the conceptual or theoretical underpinnings of their study. It would have been useful for the researchers to discuss what it is about the intervention that might be expected to result in "greater immediate comfort" and "fewer functional constraints." Did the researchers envision the massage as having its expected effects primarily as a physiologic response? (This is suggested but not elaborated on with the statement in the subsection labelled "Massage": "this helps to redirect fluid from one area of the body to another"). Or did they conceptualize the massage as having beneficial effects primarily through an emotional/psychological mechanism? An emotional mechanism must have been partly envisioned, given that the researchers examined the effects of the intervention on a psychological variable, family stress and strengths.

This concern about the study's conceptual framework is not merely about the absence of an intellectual context—there are methodologic implications. The intervention can be thought of as having multiple components, the effects of which are hard to disentangle. Is the key ingredient in the intervention the presence and concern of the significant other? Is *touch* the key ingredient? Or is it the actual massage? This is the very common "black box" problem that many evaluations of interventions face. If the researchers had given more thought to what the underlying causal mechanism might be, they might have designed a somewhat different study (e.g., with multiple comparison groups, as discussed later in this critique).

The study's conceptual framework should also influence the researchers' choice of outcome variables, but in this study, the underlying rationale for the choice of outcomes is not always clear. For example, the rationale for concluding that the intervention might affect family stress was not articulated. Indeed, it might be wondered if a measure of marital relationships or marital satisfaction would have been a better choice, inasmuch as the great majority of significant others were husbands.

METHOD

The method section was very nicely organized, with numerous subheadings so that readers could easily locate specific elements of the design and methods.

Research Design

Forchuk and her colleagues chose a very strong design to test the effectiveness of the arm massage by a significant other—a pretest–posttest experimental design that involved random assignment of study participants to an experimental (E) group or a control (C) group. The research design is one that has the potential for strong internal validity—that is, for permitting inferences about whether the intervention caused beneficial outcomes. Unfortunately, as it turns out, the E and C groups were not perfectly equivalent at the outset, which makes it difficult to rule out selection biases. More will be said about this issue later in this review.

Data were collected before surgery and then at three later points within 24 hours after surgery, 10 to 14 days after surgery, and 4 months later. This design was intended to capture immediate outcomes of the intervention as well as longer-term outcomes. Although it is commendable that the researchers followed-up on women after they left the hospital, it would have been useful for the researchers to explain why the 4-month point was chosen. Again, had the researchers developed a coherent conceptual framework, there likely would have been a cogent rationale for the scheduling of data collection.

As we noted previously, even though the intervention was nicely described, there is some ambiguity about what components could be responsible for driving any observed effects. As strong as the research design is, it would have been even stronger if there had been additional comparison groups. For example, if the researchers wanted to know if the significant other was key to the intervention's success, then a third group could have been assigned to receive the massage from a member of the health care staff. Or if the researchers wanted to disentangle the effect of the massage from support from a significant other, a third group of patients could be assigned to simply being touched or given moral support by the significant other in a structured fashion—without the massage. These are issues that future researchers should attend to in designing replications.

The Intervention

The researchers provided a good description of the intervention in a section labelled "Procedure," supplemented by an appendix that provided detail about the massage. The intervention involved teaching and demonstrations by a single masters-prepared nurse, to "avoid variance from multiple teachers." There was, unfortunately, considerable variance in the treatment from the point of view of the patients: frequency and duration of massages varied from dyad to dyad—there was no consistent "dose" of treatment. In fact, one woman received no massage at all. Moreover, there was no attempt to check on the massage technique the significant others used once the training was completed, so women probably were receiving massages of varying efficacy. The effect that this variability had on the study results is difficult to determine—the researchers did not examine "dose" (frequency or duration of massage) or quality of massage in relation to outcomes, perhaps because the small sample size likely would have led to ambiguous findings. The lack of control that the researchers had over the actual massage probably reduced the power of the analysis (i.e., undermined statistical conclusion validity). On the other hand, the lack of control probably *enhanced* external validity: In the real world, nurses instructing significant others on the benefits and techniques of an arm massage would not be able to mandate a specified number or quality of massages.

Another concern with the report is that the counterfactual was not described at all. The only allusion to the control group was in the statement of the hypotheses, which indicated that the control group received "standard postoperative treatment." We do not know what such treatment entailed; in evaluating the study, it is especially important to know whether standard treatment involved encouraging or discouraging the presence, support, or participation of significant others.

Study Sample

The sample for the study included 59 subjects, 30 of whom received the intervention. Commendably, the researchers conducted a pilot study that enabled them to refine the study and calculate an effect size for a power analysis to estimate sample size needs. This analysis suggested that a sample of 50 would be adequate to achieve standard statistical criteria. However, the report did not actually provide information about the effect size, nor did it indicate *which* outcome variable was used in the power analysis. The choice undoubtedly influenced their conclusions about the adequacy of such a small sample. That is, if another outcome variable had been used, the effect size might have been smaller, and this would have suggested a larger sample. The findings of this study suggest that a larger sample would have been desirable.

The report did a nice job of summarizing the inclusion and exclusion criteria for the study, and also of describing sample characteristics, which makes it easy for readers to understand groups to which the findings could be generalized.

Validity Issues

Overall, Forchuk and her colleagues used some strong methods in designing their study, but nevertheless the design resulted in some problems. In terms of internal validity, the experimental design they chose should have resulted in few threats to the study's internal validity. Unfortunately, however, there is some evidence that randomization was not totally successful in equalizing the two groups, which means that the threat of selection cannot be ruled out. Regrettably, we do not know as much as we should about selection biases because the researchers did not provide information about the demographic comparability of the E and C groups. But we do know the groups were different in terms of family characteristics because the C group members had higher preintervention ratings for overall physical health of their families than the E group (mentioned in the "Results" subsection on "Family Stress and Strengths"). In all likelihood, the two groups were different initially in other respects as well.

The small sample size (which the researchers acknowledged as a study limitation) probably played a role in undermining the study's internal validity. It is more difficult to equalize groups with a small number of subjects because one or two "outliers" (atypical subjects) can skew the averages; with a large sample, atypical values tend to cancel each other out. Indeed, the researchers themselves admitted that they may have had a problem with outliers. In the subsection on "Swelling" in the "Results" section, they noted that an outlier may have distorted the averages.

The small sample size limited the generalizability of the findings as well. The positive results are suggestive, but it would be imprudent to conclude with confidence that these positive effects would be observed in different settings and with different people, given that only 30 women received the intervention. On the positive side, however, the description of the sample does suggest diversity in terms of the women's age and educational background, which would enhance the generalizability of the findings.

Statistical conclusion validity is also affected by small sample sizes. Several E and C group differences were not statistically significant, and we cannot determine whether this reflects insufficient statistical power (e.g., a Type II error) or the lack of effectiveness of the intervention for some outcomes. Statistical conclusion validity could also have been undermined by the variability of the treatment (different "doses" for different women); it would also have been affected by the control group treatment—although this cannot be determined because there is no information on what that treatment was. For example, if the "standard treatment" involved any encouragement to significant others to spend time with, touch, support, or otherwise participate in the women's recovery, this would mean the two groups were exposed to conditions that were not distinctive in some respects.

One final validity issue concerns blinding, which the report does not mention as having occurred. The participants and significant others could not be blinded—the E group members were aware of getting the treatment, and the C group members were aware of *not* getting it. The report did not mention what the study participants were told about the study, but perhaps the C group members (and E group members for that matter) altered their behaviour based on their expectations about the study, regardless of the intervention itself. Significant others in the C group, for example, may have been more vigilant and solicitous of the patients than they otherwise would have been. The report did not mention whether the research assistants responsible for measuring girth width (swelling) and range of motion were blinded to the patients' group assignments, as would ideally be the case. In the absence of an explicit assurance, we must conservatively conclude that blinding did not occur. (Because the differences between the groups on these measures were not statistically significant, there is less of a concern of bias than would be true if an intervention effect had been found because expectations would tend to bias observers in the direction of the hypotheses.)

Measures

The section on "Measures" included many laudable features, as well as some shortcomings. Of particular note, the section lacked information about data collection procedures. For example, the report did not indicate who collected the data, how self-report instruments were administered (orally or in writing), and where follow-up data were collected (i.e., in the participants' homes, in clinics, and so on).

Most of the outcome measures that the researchers selected appear to have been thoughtful choices that were adequately described in the report. Table 1, which outlined the timing and frequency of administering the various measures, provided an excellent summary. Most of the measures seemed to be an appropriate measure of the outcome variables in which the researchers were interested, and for most, the researchers provided some information about the measure's quality. For example, the measure for shoulder function was a scale with adequate internal consistency and test–retest reliability. The report did not provide evidence relating to the validity of the measures, but for the most part, their measures had high face validity, such as the measures of pain and range of motion.

It appears that the range-of-motion measurements were collected by multiple research assistants, which the authors themselves described as a study limitation. However, the problem is not so much that there were multiple data collectors as that there is no information about the reliability of these measurements. The researchers should have described how these data collectors were trained, and also should have required high interrater reliability during training before allowing them to collect the data.

Although the measures used in this study generally seemed appropriate, there was no discussion of why a measure of family stress and strengths (the Family Stressor Inventory) was included. This outcome was not mentioned in the hypotheses, nor was there a discussion of how it might be affected by the intervention. One further thought is that the researchers did not collect any information from the significant others, who were the true recipients of the researchers' teaching intervention. The researchers could have measured a number of outcomes with the significant others (e.g., their well-being, their sense of efficacy, their feeling of closeness to the patient) and could also have obtained valuable information from those in the E group about their experiences (e.g., Was the training clear? Did it motivate them to perform the massage? What improvements to the intervention could be made? Why did they perform the number of massages they did?).

The researchers apparently *did* collect qualitative data from the women in the E group regarding their perceptions of the treatment, that is, for the results described in the subsection "Feedback From the Intervention Group." However, there is no information in the report about how or when these data were collected, how many women were questioned, what exactly was asked, or how it was recorded and analyzed.

Ethical Aspects

The authors did not provide much information (which does not mean that there were ethical transgressions). No mention was made of having the study approved by a Research Ethics Board, for example. The only information in the report was a notation in the "Inclusion Criteria" subsection that both the women and their significant other had to consent to participate and be able to make informed consent. There is no indication in the report that the subjects were harmed, deceived, or mistreated in any way.

RESULTS

The results section addressed each of the study hypotheses, and also included an analysis of the qualitative feedback regarding reactions to the intervention from women in the treatment group. It would have been useful to learn more about how these data were gathered, as just noted, but the information was valuable and offered some suggestions about how the intervention might be improved (e.g., longer massages).

The statistical analyses focused on group differences on the outcome variables, that is, whether the E and C groups differed significantly in terms of pain, perceptions of pain control, swelling, range of motion, shoulder function, family stress and strengths, use of health care services, and health care costs. It also would have been possible to present statistical information about changes over time for most of these outcomes (e.g., how family stress changed from baseline to 4 months after surgery), but the researchers chose to focus on tests of their hypotheses.

One notable absence in the "Results" section, as previously mentioned, was a table summarizing E and C group characteristics at the outset. The text provides a description of the overall sample, but it is important for readers to understand whether the two groups were similar with respect to demographic characteristics and baseline measures of the outcomes—that is, whether randomization was successful in equating the groups with regard to key attributes.

The researchers used *t*-tests to compare group means on the outcomes. This statistical test is technically appropriate for comparing group means, but it is not the most powerful or suitable procedure—especially when there is evidence that the groups were not perfectly equivalent at the outset. It is not clear why the researchers chose not to use analysis of covariance, using baseline measures of the outcome variable as the covariate. This analytic strategy would have added precision and strengthened the internal validity of the study because it would have statistically adjusted for any initial group differences. ANCOVA might have even changed some of the conclusions, but this is impossible to speculate about because the researchers did not share much descriptive information—for example, what the range-of-motion scores for the two groups were at baseline and at the two follow-up points when this variable was measured.

The findings indicated that the women in the E group reported greater pain control and less pain than women in the C group in the first few days after surgery. There were also favourable and significant group differences with regard to shoulder function 10 to 14 days after surgery. Thus, even with a small sample size and the absence of statistical controls, there were significant and encouraging group differences in the predicted direction for these outcomes. However, contrary to prediction, there appeared to be significantly more swelling in the E than in the C group (Table 4). The authors attribute this group difference to the effect of a single outlier, meaning that one woman in the E group had extremely high measurements. When the outlier was removed from the analysis, the group difference was no longer significant (although it just missed significance, and would have been significant with a larger sample). The legitimacy of removing the outlier is not clear, but the researchers should have also used statistical controls (ANCOVA) for this analysis, in particular. With or without the outlier, the hypothesis regarding swelling being lower in the E group was not supported. The findings with regard to family stress and strengths were erratic, sometimes favouring the E group and sometimes favouring the C group. With regard to health care costs and utilization, there were no significant group differences, although one difference relating to social costs approached significance. Overall, given some of the design and analytic problems already mentioned, the pattern of findings is not easily interpreted, but some of the positive results are nevertheless of considerable interest.

DISCUSSION

Forchuk and her colleagues began their discussion with a review of some of the study's limitations. They made note of the biggest problem (small sample size), but failed to note other important ones (lack of blinding, selection bias). The researchers also noted that the study's generalizability was limited by the fact that only women who had a significant other could be included in the study.

The discussion and interpretation of the findings focused exclusively on the positive results. Similarly, the implications for nursing practice were developed with the positive findings in mind. A more balanced analysis of the study, factoring in the study limitations and the nonsignificant or contrary results, would have been desirable. On the other hand, it would appear that there is value in the researchers' assertion that "teaching the significant other the simple massage technique may provide a tangible helping role that has traditionally has not existed." The authors would have done well to urge replications and extensions of the study so that the evidence regarding the effectiveness of a massage for women with lymph node dissection could be strengthened.

GLOBAL ISSUES

This report was well written and well organized but would have benefited from the inclusion of some additional details. The results section had a nice mixture of text and tables, but the tables could have been organized somewhat better and had more information. For example, a table with E and C differences for all major outcomes (including baseline and follow-up means and standard deviations) would have been useful. A particularly regrettable presentational lapse is the absence of sufficient information for computing effect sizes, which would be needed to include this study in a meta-analysis. One last issue is that there appear to be some errors in the tables (which could be the fault of the publisher and not the authors). For example, the pain scores were described as ratings from 0 to 10, and yet the means in Table 2 were double-digit numbers, for example, 83.18 for the experimental group on Day 1. Moreover, the row label indicates "Mean (%)," so it is not clear what information is being provided—means or percentages.

RESPONSE FROM CHERYL FORCHUK

Thanks for the critique. Overall the comments are accurate with regard to what is in the report.

It is mentioned that we did not specify which outcome measure was used for the sample size calculation—in fact, all outcome measures were used, and the results reflected the largest sample size required by any measure (in this case costs).

The research assistants were blinded until the last data collection period. They then opened an envelope (after all other measures were collected) so that they would know whether or not to ask the additional questions about feedback related to the intervention.

Ethics approval was through both the university and hospital.

All these points were of course in earlier drafts (including much more on the data collection procedure, etc.) and had to be removed to meet the page limitations. I think your critique will be useful to students—but they also need to know about page limitations of journals.

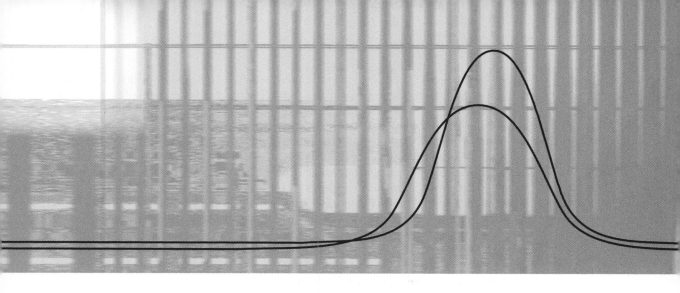

D.

Redefining Parental Identity: Caregiving and Schizophrenia

P. Jane Milliken, Herbert C. Northcott

When parents try to assume responsibility for an ill adult-child with schizophrenia, the law, mental health practitioners, and often the ill person reject their right to do so. Consequently, these parents regard themselves as disenfranchised, i.e., lacking the rights required to care properly for their loved ones. Redefining Parental Identity, a grounded theory of caregiving and schizophrenia, traces changes in a parent's identity and caregiving during the erratic course of the child's mental illness. Participants were a purposive sample of 29 parent caregivers from 19 families in British Columbia, Canada, caring for 20 adult children. This understanding of their experience will be helpful to parents of people with schizophrenia, professional practitioners, and those involved in mental health care reform.

S chizophrenia causes disability in the form of impaired social functioning that lasts for a protracted period, often the rest of the individual's life. Community care for the mentally ill has proven effective where there is appropriate discharge planning, coordinated case management, and the necessary social supports, both formal and informal, for patients and their families (Stein & Test, 1980: Reynolds & Hoult, 1984). Unfortunately, reports of patients' "falling through the cracks" of the mental health care system (Isaac & Armat, 1990; Torrey, 1995, 1997) remain prevalent. The consequences of this include homelessness or inadequate housing (Mechanic & Rochefort, 1990; Torrey, 1988), poverty (Lurigio & Lewis, 1989), victimization, and/or criminalization of the mentally ill (French, 1987), as well as a "revolving door" cycle of hospital admission-discharge-readmission

Reprinted with permission from *Qualitative Health Research* (2003: 13[1]: 100–113) © 2003 Sage Publications.

(Geller, 1992). In the process of deinstitutionalization, a significant amount of care has been transferred from professionals to inadequately prepared lay people—frequently the ill person's family. Consequently, with schizophrenia having its onset in adolescence or young adulthood, the burden of providing consistent care generally falls by default to the individual's parents.

Studies of family care for mentally ill persons are, for the most part, either descriptive or focused on identifying the tasks required to provide technical aspects of care (see, for example, Hatfield & Lefley, 1987; Thornton & Seeman, 1991; Torrey, 1995). Theoretical models of caregiving generally follow the stress paradigm (Biegel, Sales, & Schulz, 1991; Maurin & Boyd, 1990) and emphasize both ongoing family disruption (Terkelsen, 1987) and the endless duration of caregiving (Howard, 1994). Many researchers have measured caregiver burden (Pickett, Cook, & Solomon, 1995; Wright, 1994) or the degree of expressed emotion in the family as a risk factor for the sufferer's relapse (Brooker, 1990; Hogarty, 1985).[1]

Research employing interpretive methodologies is less common. Tuck, du-Mont, Evans, and Shupe (1997) outline the phenomenological transformations in family life and the grief suffered by parents when an adult-child has schizophrenia. They note that these parents must reformulate what it means to be a parent to their changed relative. The present study revealed parents undergoing this reformulation sporadically in response to the erratic course of their adult-child's illness. Chesla (1991) identified a typology of four approaches to parental caregiving for schizophrenia: engaged care, conflicted care, managed care, and distanced care. We agree with Chesla's conclusion that conventional research into caregiver burden misses the distinctions among these groups of parents; however, we suggest that by grouping parents' caring practices in this way, we can describe a particular family only at a given point in time. Over the course of the illness, parents are likely to vary their caring practices in response to the adult-child's illness trajectory and the involvement of mental health professionals. Consequently, we saw the need for a grounded theory study to explain the subjective and emotional experience of parental caregiving in schizophrenia. As an exploratory method, grounded theory, with its emphasis on social interaction, is "the method of choice when we want to learn how people manage their lives in the context of existing or potential health challenges" (Schreiber & Stern, 2001, p. xvii).

Due to the unforeseen but often tragic consequences of deinstitutionalization, health care professionals and policy makers need a more thorough understanding of caregiving for people with serious mental illnesses. Knowledge of the consequences of caring for a mentally ill family member is essential in planning for better psychosocial rehabilitation services. To this end, the Canadian Alliance for Research on Schizophrenia called for psychosocial research "to evaluate the concrete and complex interactions of specific families in order to identify positive attributes which could, in turn, predict improved outcome" (1994, p. 14). This study directly addresses these points, to help us understand the challenges of schizophrenia for families and to inform mental health researchers with interests in grief, caregiver burden, and quality of life.

METHOD

Following university research ethics approval, we recruited participants through the newsletters of the British Columbia Schizophrenia Society and the Caregivers Association of British Columbia. Others were recruited through snowballing or, in one case, after the study was mentioned on a local radio program. We interviewed 29 parents from 19 middle- or working-class families, many of whom were retired (mean age = 62)—both parents in 10 families, the mother in 6 families, and the father in the remaining 3.

In total, the interviewed parents had 6 daughters and 14 sons afflicted with schizophrenia, two of whom had died in the 5 years prior to the study. Of the remaining 18, daughters averaged almost 30 years of age (range = 21–38), having been diagnosed on average at just over age 20, whereas the sons averaged 32 years (range = 23–42) and were diagnosed about 6 months earlier on average than the daughters (mean = 19.6). None of these young adults had ever been married and none were employed at the time of the interview. Most had lived with their parents for extended periods during their illness, but only four did so at the time of the study. The rest were about equally divided between group homes and semi-independent or independent apartments. In total, these parents had been caregiving for schizophrenia for an average of 11.5 years (range = 0.5–23 years) after their child's diagnosis; however, many of these children were also ill for a lengthy period before being diagnosed.

If roughly one third of people with schizophrenia recover, one third have a variable disease course, and one third remain chronically ill (Walsh, 1985), this group is more chronic than average. Nevertheless, this study examines a wide variation in parental experience. The grounded theory of redefining parental identity that emerged from this study illustrates their diverse caregiving experiences and should help us understand caregiving by other parents in similar circumstances.

In-depth, audiotaped interviews of approximately 1.5 to 2 hours were held in a private setting chosen by each participant. This was generally the parents' home. Couples, except for one, were interviewed separately. We guaranteed confidentiality and anonymity, and informed participants of their right to withdraw at any point. Near the end of the project, several participants had follow-up interviews, which were aimed at theoretical elaboration, saturation of incomplete categories, and verification of the theory. The final tally was 32 interviews, for a total of 53 hours. The interviews were transcribed verbatim to preserve the richness of the data.

Initially, we asked participants broad, open-ended questions to elicit both the positive and negative consequences of caring for a family member with schizophrenia. In keeping with the constant comparative method of grounded theory, data collection and analysis proceeded concurrently. We coded transcripts phrase by phrase and collapsed similar codes into increasingly broad categories. Over time, the interview questions changed as analytic categories became saturated or participants introduced new categories that generated new hypotheses to be explored during further data collection. As the theory developed, we validated the emerging concepts against the stories of new interviewees and in follow-up interviews with selected respondents, using theoretical sampling. Data collection ended when the interviews produced no new categories and the analysis revealed the basic social problem experienced by these parents and the ways in which they work through it.

A GROUNDED THEORY OF REDEFINING PARENTAL IDENTITY

In general, a grounded theory serves to explain the process through which a social problem common to the participant group is resolved. The basic social problem identified in this study is that parents believe they have the right and responsibility to care for, protect, and make decisions for children whom they do not see as capable of caring for and protecting themselves or making appropriate decisions in their own best interests. However, when a child is deemed an adult, this belief is not sanctioned by society, which denies parents that right. In response, parents whose adult-children suffer from schizophrenia engage in the basic social process (BSP) of redefining their parental identity and thus adapting their caregiving.

The socially prescribed change in parental caregiving for teens and young adults is toward freedom from management and direction. Parents are expected to socialize their children toward independence, and as this happens, parents anticipate that their own responsibilities will decrease accordingly. Ultimately, parents expect to be emancipated from active parenting.

After a child is diagnosed with schizophrenia, the parents' identity shifts. Initially, they find themselves disenfranchised from the role they expected to fulfill; then, they find new ways to exert their rights and responsibilities, thus establishing a new parental role. We have identified four parental identities, and the transitions between them, that constitute seven stages of a BSP called Redefining Parental Identity. The stages, parent of a teen or young adult, becoming marginalized, the disenfranchised parent, embracing the collective, the reenfranchised parent, evaluating my life, and the emancipated parent, are summarized in the following sections of this article.

Parent of a Teen or Young Adult

Adolescence, characterized by young people's testing the limits of their independence, can be challenging for both parents and teenagers. Parents need to find a comfortable balance between granting freedom and providing supervision, with a gradual increase in freedom and a corresponding decrease in supervision, until the child achieves independent adult status. Accordingly, parents expect that the adolescent period will be time limited and that eventually they will be able to invest more time and effort on their personal interests and adult relationships. This anticipation of freedom from the constraints of parenting is rooted in the promise of their children's aspirations and remembrance of their children's early achievements, behavior, and personality. Thus, parents of teens and young adults can be described as *anticipating liberty*[2] *while tolerating adolescent challenges*. Participants in this study described their children's early development as normal, with positive traits outweighing negative qualities and lacking any indication of impending mental illness. None of these parents was overly surprised when grades began to slip and/or behavior deteriorated during adolescence, and only two of the parents suspected antisocial attributes as signaling mental-health problems. Eventually, however, all of these parents found that they could no longer view their son's or daughter's conduct as normal teenage behavior.

Becoming Marginalized

This initial status passage,[3] or transition, for these parents involves *becoming alarmed* and *assuming responsibility* for the child, but also *encountering barriers*. Parents in all but four of these families[4] reached a crisis point when the child's personality, behavior, and relationships with family and friends became so disruptive, bizarre, or dangerous that the changes could no longer be disregarded. Their children became excessively angry, depressed, anxious, isolated, or preoccupied, and family relationships suffered. Insomnia and street drug use were common, as was an attraction to nonmainstream religious groups and a propensity to disappear abruptly, often to live on the streets. When contacted by the child for money or by the police or social workers, parents willingly rescued their children and brought them home, often at considerable expense.

Rising concern compelled the parents to assert more control and assume responsibility for helping and protecting their child. Reluctantly, parents admitted to suspicions of mental illness and consulted a doctor or mental health professional, often taking the young person involuntarily to the hospital, sometimes with the help of the police. Still, a diagnosis and treatment were not always obtained. Some of the young people, fearing hospitalization, were able to cover up their symptoms long enough to fool the authorities. For example, the police released one daughter, who immediately disappeared again and was returned much later by an elderly couple who found her wandering on the beach. At home, after being revived from the cold, she

> became completely hysterical, throwing herself on the floor, hiding from monsters, and just totally disorganized, [with] paranoid delusions. She was again convinced that Michael the archangel was after her and was going to gouge out her eyes. She thought that I had murdered her brother and chopped him up and buried him in the backyard, that I had murdered Teresa[5] [her mother] and replaced her with an android. I went downstairs... and phoned the police again. They came with two cars, four officers, and an ambulance. They took her to the hospital. This time they realized that she was ill and she was admitted. (Bruce)

Once the diagnosis of schizophrenia was made, parents found that their influence on their children's care was severely limited. These "children" had reached the age of majority or were otherwise deemed to be responsible for their own decisions. Parents learned that even when a psychotic person loses the right to self-determination, professional caregivers, rather than parents, have the authority to direct care. Although parents believe they know their child better than anyone else, psychiatrists and other professionals seldom consulted or even listened to them. Yet, paradoxically, the young person was often discharged to the parents' home and care. The majority of these parents discovered that their ability to take responsibility for their child was effectively blocked by the law, by mental health professionals, and often by their own child. When these parents realized that they had no formally recognized right to assume that responsibility, they had, indeed, become marginalized and, consequently, they assumed a new parental identity. They now saw themselves as disenfranchised.

The Disenfranchised Parent

Parents felt obliged to safeguard their loved one's health and welfare and to ensure that professional help was obtained early to avoid another crisis. Nevertheless, they continually met obstructions whenever they tried to intercede on their child's behalf. At this stage, they described a miserable existence composed of *maintaining vigilance, grieving alone,* and *grasping at straws.* One father observed,

> The only thing that keeps her alive during those periods is our resourcefulness. You know, our vigilance. So even though she is an intelligent 26-year-old woman, it is still as though you have a 2-year-old you're worried is going to run out in front of a car, because she does do things like that. (Bruce)

Life revolved around constant surveillance, watching carefully for signs that the hallucinations, delusions, and bizarre behavior that characterize schizophrenia were returning or worsening. Watching a loved one deteriorate and feeling powerless to intervene is painful for parents, who see a young person becoming increasingly socially withdrawn, emotionally deprived, and lacking in motivation. A mother whose son committed suicide after a decade of illness said,

> As he got sicker and sicker his personal hygiene went down the drain. He frequently smelled bad the last few years of his life because I guess he just didn't have energy to shower. One of the people that came to his memorial service was the barber. The barber was a big deal in our life because when we could get him to agree to go to the barber, quite often he went to the barber's home so he wouldn't have to meet other people, and this man was very understanding. (Sue)

Parents watched over their child's psychiatric treatment, trying to ensure compliance with medication and keeping track of developing side effects. In an underfunded system, many parents become, by default, their child's case manager. Although a few were able to establish communication with practitioners, most either lacked access to health care providers or perceived that practitioners did not respect their opinions. Gwen knew the pattern of her son's illness well. When he stopped taking his medication, fired his psychiatrist, and switched to a psychologist, she tried to avert a relapse:

> I had phoned his counselor who actually had an MA in psychology, and I said to him, "You know, Colin was definitely becoming ill again, heading for a breakdown, I don't know if you realize this because he is very clever at concealing it." And he said, "Oh well, what makes you think he is?" And I said, "Well, one of the things is that he is reading the Bible constantly and this has always been one of the early symptoms." So he said in a very sarcastic voice, "Oh, I see. Because your son is reading the Bible, you think he should be on medication?" (Gwen)

A parent's vigilance is also motivated by fear: fear of schizophrenia, fear for the ill child's safety and future, and sometimes fear of his or her violent behavior. Parents feared that they would be unable to cope or that they might provoke a relapse, that their child would never recover, and that another child or grandchild would also become ill. The unpredictability of schizophrenia was particularly difficult, as one mother's story illustrates:

> I've realized that it's not so much the things that happen, though a lot of really painful disturbing instances have happened, but they are quite short, the instances in themselves. It's the fear in between. It's the remembering and the anticipation and the wondering if you can cope with it. It's like waiting for the other shoe to fall all the time. If you could just get that under control, you would be stronger to deal with the instance and you would recover from them more quickly because you wouldn't be anticipating the next one. (Maggie)

Initially, most parents learn about schizophrenia from the media, where violent behavior is often emphasized. In these families, violence was relatively infrequent and seldom reached the severity found in the press. Still, several of these parents were attacked by their offspring—one mother fatally. More commonly, violent acts were directed at property or themselves. Eight of these young people had attempted suicide—one successfully.

Furthermore, especially when they stopped taking medication, the ill persons' lifestyle made them vulnerable to victimization. Many of these young people ran away from home, took illegal drugs, and lived on the streets for months at a time. Three of these young people were beaten up in major cities far from home. Several had money and belongings stolen. Parents worried about their child contracting sexually transmitted diseases. Even those living semi-independently or in apartments were easy targets for burglary.

Not surprisingly, these parents reported high levels of stress, born out of feelings of frustration, powerlessness, and poor self-esteem:

> Elaine and I watched the powerlessness that we sensed, that grew in over the 2-year period. You know how sometimes you have a gut feeling you are in a losing situation? That's how I felt the entire time. Every time we'd lose something. (Fred)

Extra expenses, such as supplementing their child's limited social assistance, airline tickets to bring a runaway home, replacing damaged belongings, and moving expenses following eviction, add financial strain. Frequent crises, coupled with their determination not to give up and to try to normalize life for the rest of their family, only add to the pressure.

From the diagnosis of their child's schizophrenia onward, these parents experienced emotions that are associated with grief, as described below:

> What I grieve every day is [her lack of a] functional life. I grieve that every day, for Anne. Every day. Anne is never out of my thoughts and I say, "How could that happen?" How could that happen to others too? Not just Anne, but how could the illness be so cruel? Cruel, right in the bloom days, that's when it flares up. Anne will never see those years again. (Teresa)

Disenfranchised in their caregiving, their grief is also disenfranchised (Doka, 1989). This child is not dead but instead has become like a stranger.[6] Although parents grieve for the child that they once had, our society provides only rituals to help ease grief following physical death. In addition, totally preoccupied with caring for their ill child, many parents become socially quite isolated. Consequently, although they grieve for the person their child once was and for the life that they hoped their adult-child would have, they have little opportunity to communicate or share their grief with others. They grieve alone.

At this point, parents will grasp at any straw, looking for answers and, especially, for a cure. They desperately seek out second opinions, new and experimental treatments, and more knowledge about schizophrenia. Whether these parents learned anything about schizophrenia from their child's psychiatrist was a matter of luck. Some had doctors who were helpful and forthright in giving them information and describing the possibilities in terms of prognosis. Others—like Gwen and Irwin, who were told only to prepare for a "bumpy ride"—were given the diagnosis and nothing else. Information gleaned from various sources was often conflicting or overly technical. Instead, these parents needed practical advice from others in similar circumstances. Reaching out for that kind of help signaled a redefinition of parental identity beyond being disenfranchised.

Embracing the Collective

Requiring practical information about caring for someone with schizophrenia and an opportunity to communicate with people who understand their plight leads many parents to a support group. In British Columbia, the B.C. Schizophrenia Society usually provides this service. By *connecting with others,* they quickly learn that they no longer face mental illness alone. They find empathic people with whom they can speak honestly. In addition, they learn useful ways to approach people, either personal acquaintances or mental health service providers, who are less understanding. The Schizophrenia Society also offers a library of books and videotapes, organized educational programs, and monthly meetings with knowledgeable guest speakers. As a bonus, they make new friends.

> If you want to get on top of the disease, you have to get access to that information, and experience, and counseling, and support. And the monthly meetings for some people are tremendous. Right off the bat they can unburden themselves and people will just understand and they will say, "Well, when you do so and so", "If you try such and such" or "This piece of information will tell you how to access that". And that's when the support starts to roll out. [long pause] That's the one piece of advice that just stands a mile high in my view. [You need to] talk to people that have been there. (Michael)

In time, these new friends become their primary reference group, which leads parents to *redefining their child*. Having been blocked so often in their attempts to help their own ill child and to influence his or her care, these parents began working for the betterment of all those who suffer from this devastating illness. They realized that helping everyone with schizophrenia in turn benefits their own child. Thus, they appear to have expanded the scope of their parenting and to have symbolically redefined their "child" as the community of people affected by schizophrenia, both patients and other families. Once they have fully embraced the collective, they have entered the next identity, the Reenfranchised Parent.

The Reenfranchised Parent

The identity of Reenfranchised Parent allows these parents to regain their parental rights and responsibilities by *taking on the "system"* through doing volunteer work, advocating for the mentally ill, and providing public education about schizophrenia. These parents develop and apply their personal skills and efforts toward mental health care reform, improving community services, raising public awareness about schizophrenia, and trying to reduce the stigma against mental illness. For example, they advocate for low-cost housing that supports varying degrees of independence; culturally appropriate care for ethnic minorities; family services, including respite care; and the promotion of research. Because of their efforts, parents (and other family members) are increasingly being included in treatment planning:

> When I spoke to the staff at [the psychiatric hospital], I said that finally family members are being included in a discussion and a treatment plan and, I said, it's a little bit like women getting the vote, that it was something they had to fight for, and it should have been a natural process. And so I say the whole question of including family in the treatment and discussion isn't something that should have been fought for. It should have been there from day one. (Willow)[7]

Although parents approach their volunteering and advocacy with enthusiasm, change is not easily won and the difficulties inherent in taking on an entrenched bureaucracy soon become apparent. *Being disillusioned* with the system centers around three broadly defined problem areas. First, parents observe limited funding for mental health services in comparison to the technologically exciting fields of health care. They also perceive poor accountability in the mental health system when policy makers, program directors, and individual therapists make promises that they fail to deliver. Finally, they observe the political maneuvering involved in health care reform and become discouraged when changes in mental health programming appear to be based on either political pressure or economic restraints rather than clear scientific evidence of efficacy. As Teresa wryly noted, politicians can afford to ignore the mentally ill because few psychiatric patients vote.

On a positive note, parents no longer have to grieve alone; instead, they are *mourning together.* The work that they do is valued and shared by others in the Schizophrenia Society and represents an acceptable public expression of their loss, at last allowing them to accept their situation and come to terms with their grief. According to Michael, acceptance means that you might still experience sadness and discouragement, but you never return to really deep despair.

With time, often many years, the ill son or daughter improves somewhat, and perhaps benefits from supportive housing and community services. The parents are older. Although their volunteer activity was satisfying, they become tired. Many have developed their own health problems, some of which might be stress related. Confronting their aging, they begin to reassess how they wish to spend their remaining years.

Evaluating My Life

At this time, parents engage in two evaluative processes: *acknowledging realities* and *identifying their personal needs.* Realistic expectations for their child's future evolve from their recognition of the ill person's social functioning and the acceptance of the chronic nature of schizophrenia. In essence, the parents adopt the stranger but continue to hope for a better future; however, these more limited hopes center on their child's achieving contentment and what Margaret referred to as "reasonable times of happiness." After years of being preoccupied by their child's illness, they can begin to focus more on themselves or on other long-ignored interests and move toward the status of the Emancipated Parent.

The Emancipated Parent

How parents periodically reconstruct their parental identity can be interpreted as a journey toward the ideal type of the Emancipated Parent, when parents expect to maintain a relationship with their children but withdraw from direct control and decision-making. They anticipate eventually enjoying the successes of their self-sufficient offspring, content in a significant amount of well-earned mutual independence. When a child is ill, the parents' journey toward emancipation is delayed, and their position depends on the location of the child on his or her individual illness trajectory (Strauss, 1975). Although the lives of all of the parents who participated in this study and their ill children improved, mutual independence was an unattainable goal. Once a child's diagnosis is confirmed, the specter of schizophrenia never completely disappears. Evelyn stated it in this way:

> I guess for every person, you bring the baby home from the hospital and you teach them to be independent and you look forward to the wedding day when they are totally off your hands, and yet if you have a child who is affected with an illness, a chronic illness like schizophrenia, the pattern is going to be slightly different. In a sense, you are never totally the emancipated parent.

For these parents, the end point was a hybrid identity combining (in various degrees) the Reenfranchised Parent and movement toward Emancipation. Indeed, parental emancipation can be a relative thing for all parents, and complete independence is a myth that occurs only in what Willow called the "airy fairy TV family." Perhaps no parent ever truly gets there, whether the children are healthy or not. Still, for parents of children with schizophrenia, emancipation remains more elusive than it is for many others.

DISCUSSION AND CONCLUSION

Although the above overview describes Redefining Parental Identity as a linear process, it seldom (if ever) is. The self-identities of these parents respond to the fluctuating course of the child's schizophrenia illness trajectory. With each relapse, parents tend to regress toward disenfranchisement; with improvement, they once again move forward.

Although the terms *caring* and *caregiving* are often used interchangeably in the caregiving literature, some authors draw a distinction that is important for this grounded theory. For example, Fisher and Tronto (1990) define four interconnected components of caring: caring about, taking care of, caregiving, and care-receiving. *Caring about* involves paying attention to a person's needs. *Taking care* of implies assuming responsibility for those needs, whereas caregiving is "the hands-on work of maintenance and repair" (p. 40). *Care-receiving* is the child's response to *caregiving* and is influenced by the extent to which the caregiver and receiver agree about what is required.

For these families, the connections among the four components of caring were disrupted, and conflicts arose among parents, the ill adult-child, and other caregivers. Parents cared about their loved one and tried to take care of and provide caregiving to the adult-child. Unfortunately, they frequently lacked basic resources, including time, knowledge, and the necessary skills. More fundamentally, they lacked legal and societal permission to do so. Thus, the vital "taking care of" link between parents' caring about and their caregiving was disrupted. Their lack of authority blocked the connection between their moral and legal responsibilities for caring.

Fisher and Tronto (1990) state, "One of the most pervasive contradictions involved in taking care of concerns the asymmetry between responsibility and power" (p. 43). They contend that bureaucratic requirements for a division of labor, a hierarchy of power and authority, and the standardization of routines and policies cause contradictions and poor integration among the phases of caring. Such features are characteristic of the mental health system. In Fisher and Tronto's estimation, resolving these conflicts requires us to consider caring to be a contextual process. The immediate context of schizophrenia is the family within which it occurs and, to address the contradictions that exist among the components of caring, care for people with schizophrenia must incorporate the needs of their families.

Instead, the tendency has been to disregard and silence families. Feminists explain that oppression hinges on the silencing of women and other marginalized groups by those with power (Belenky, Clinchy, Goldberger, & Tarule, 1986; Gilligan, 1993). A parallel can be drawn to the experience of these parents whose voices are silenced when professional caregivers decline to consult, inform, or even listen to them in regard to their child's illness, treatment, and prognosis. As a result, these parents are similar to other oppressed and marginalized groups. At the same time, like women more generally in our society, they are expected to care for their ill children. Even if not overtly asked to do so, they are driven to assume that responsibility when no one else takes a perpetual interest in the child's well-being.

The concept of disenfranchisement of rights is important in conceptualization and measurement of caregiver burden. Statistical models of caregiver burden should incorporate a measure of powerlessness or, alternatively, mastery—something that few researchers besides Noh and his associates have done (Noh & Avison, 1988; Noh & Turner, 1987). Similarly, the suggestion by Reinhard (1991) to include grief in any study of caregiver burden is supported here. Finally, caregiving for someone with schizophrenia lasts for a protracted period, often decades. Most studies of caregiver burden provide us with a snapshot understanding of subjective and objective burden measured once, usually relatively soon after the patient has left the hospital. Only Pai and Kapur (1982) measured burden over time and then for only 6 months. If burden and mastery are assessed later in the proves, when a caregiving parent has reached the stage of The Reenfranchised Parent, mastery will likely have increased and burden will have decreased. Thus, there is a need for long-term studies of caregiving to track the changes in burden over time.

One means of testing and refining a grounded theory is to investigate how well the theory can be extended to other groups with similar experiences. Changes in parental identity might help explain caregiving for parents' adult children who are disabled by other mental illnesses like bipolar illness, by catastrophic accidents causing quadriplegia or brain injury, or by drug or alcohol addiction. The theory may also extend to sibling caregivers, who must redefine their identity as brothers and sisters. As well, the applicability of the model to parent caregivers from diverse cultural backgrounds should be assessed.

In addition to the above implications for research, the study highlights a number of issues for mental health care reform. Professional caregivers must recognize the contribution that families make to the patient's therapy but also accept professional responsibility to provide care for family caregivers. Respect, compassion, and education for family members, including practical advice about how to interact and communicate with a psychotic person, should be included in the treatment plan, not left for family members to obtain on an ad hoc basis. Case management and assertive community treatment are the cornerstones of a safe and comprehensive community program rather than the responsibility of parents. Care must come to the ill person and his or her family, not the other way around. To accomplish this, community programs must be staffed sufficiently well to ensure that caseloads are manageable.

Finally, in-patient treatment should be readily available whenever a mentally ill person is psychotic, to ensure that parents are not forced to try to manage a son or daughter who has been turned away from the emergency department. Parents told me that policy makers must address how the legal system defines "danger to oneself and others" and institute a more liberal application of commitment to psychiatric care. Refusal of treatment combined with an inability to provide an appropriate level of self-care should be considered as dangerous to self. Although such measures might be perceived by some as patriarchal and an infringement of patients' rights, they are necessary to achieve more humane treatment of the mentally ill and vital for countering the disenfranchisement of caregiving parents. With mental health care improvements that more fully incorporate the needs of families, parents who might never become emancipated from caregiving would at least be less disenfranchised.

NOTES

1. Milliken (2001) describes selected characteristics of this caregiving experience that are particularly difficult for mothers.

2. Within each state of this BSP are secondary social processes that define the parent's activities in that stage. Throughout this article, italics are used to identify these subprocesses.

3. The final phase of the constant comparative method is to link a new grounded theory with the relevant literature. In doing so, we discovered that Redefining Parental Identity is an empirical example of the formal grounded theory of status passage (Glaser & Strauss, 1971). According to Glaser and Strauss, status passage involves a change from one social status to another with "a loss or gain of privilege, influence or power, and a changed identity and sense of self, as well as changed behavior" (p. 2).

4. Four of the ill adolescents accessed medical help before their parents recognized the need, one of them following a suicide attempt. One young woman was successful in hiding her delusions and hallucinations from her family until her psychiatrist admitted her to the hospital. In the other three cases, the parents were preoccupied with additional family problems. For example, the father in one family was terminally ill.

5. Pseudonyms have been used to ensure anonymity of participants and their family members.

6. All parents talked of how their son or daughter had changed since becoming ill and about how difficult it was to know how to react to or talk to this new person. Seven parents used the term "stranger" or said that someone else had taken over their child's body. Other authors have also used the same term when referring to how a family member with schizophrenia has changed (Hatfield, 1978, p. 358; Tuck, du-Mont, Evans, & Shupe, 1997, p. 118).

7. To emphasize Willow's point, we originally called this identity Parental Suffrage, to underscore the parents' own suffering, their tolerance of others, and their engagement in a cooperative and political process aimed at obtaining better understanding and treatment of people affected by schizophrenia. Ultimately, enhancing these collective rights introduces opportunities for parents to reclaim some individual rights and responsibilities with regard to their adult offspring.

REFERENCES

Belenky, M.F., Clinchy, M.F., Goldberger, N.R., & Tarule, J.M. (1986). *Women's ways of knowing*. New York: Basic Books.

Biegel, D.E., Sales, E., & Schulz, R. (1991). *Family caregiving in chronic illness: Alzheimer's disease, cancer, heart disease, mental illness, and stroke*. Newbury Park, CA: Sage.

Brooker, C. (1990). Expressed emotion and psychosocial intervention: A review. *International Journal of Nursing Studies, 27*(3), 267–276.

Canadian Alliance for Research on Schizophrenia. (1994). A national strategy for research on schizophrenia. *Journal of Psychiatry and Neuroscience, 19*(5, Suppl. 1), 3–49.

Chesla, C.A. (1991). Parents' caring practices with schizophrenic offspring. *Qualitative Health Research, 1,* 416–468.

Doka, K.J. (1989). Disenfranchised grief. In K.J. Doka (Ed.), *Disenfranchised grief: Recognizing hidden sorrow* (pp. 3–11). Lexington, MA: Lexington Books.

Fisher, B. & Tronto, J. (1990). Toward a feminist theory of caring. In E.K. Abel & M.K. Nelson (Eds.). *Circles of care: Work and identity in women's lives* (pp. 35–62). Albany: State University of New York Press.

French, L. (1987). Victimization of the mentally ill: An unintended consequence of de-institutionalization. *Social Work, 32*, 502–505.

Geller, J.L. (1992). A historical perspective on the role of state hospitals viewed from the era of the "revolving door". *American Journal of Psychiatry, 149*(11), 1526–1532.

Gilligan, C. (1993). *In a different voice: Psychological theory and women's development*. Cambridge, MA: Harvard University Press.

Glaser, B.G., & Strauss, A.L. (1971). *Status passage*. Chicago: Aldine.

Hatfield, A.B. (1978). Psychological costs of schizophrenia to the family. *Social Work, 23*, 355–359.

Hatfield, A.B., & Lefley, H.P. (Eds.). (1987). *Families of the mentally ill: Coping and adaptation.* New York: Guilford.

Hogarty, G.E. (1985). Expressed emotion and schizophrenic relapse: Implications from the Pittsburgh study. In M. Alpert (Ed.), *Controversies in schizophrenia* (pp. 354–365). New York: Guilford.

Howard, P.B. (1994). Lifelong maternal caregiving for children with schizophrenia. *Archives of Psychiatric Nursing, 8*(2), 107–114.

Isaac, R.J., & Armat, V.C. (1990). *Madness in the streets: How psychiatry and the law abandoned the mentally ill.* New York: Free Press.

Lurigio, A.J., & Lewis, D.A. (1989). Worlds that fail: A longitudinal study of urban mental patients. *Journal of Social Issues, 45*(3), 79–90.

Maurin, J.T., & Boyd, C.B. (1990). Burden of mental illness on the family: A critical review. *Archives of Psychiatric Nursing, 4*(2), 99–107.

Mechanic, D., & Rochefort, D.A. (1990). Deinstitutionalization: An appraisal of reform. *Annual Review of Sociology, 16*, 301–327.

Milliken, P.J. (2001). Disenfranchised mothers: Caring for an adult child with schizophrenia. *Health Care for Women International, 22*(1–2), 149–166.

Noh, S., & Avison, W.R. (1988). Spouses of discharged psychiatric patients: Factors associated with their experience of burden. *Journal of Marriage and the Family, 50*, 377–389.

Noh, S., & Turner, R.J. (1987). Living with psychiatric patients: Implications for the mental health of family members. *Social Science & Medicine, 25*(3), 263–271.

Pai, S., & Kapur, R.L. (1982). Impact of treatment intervention on the relationship between dimensions of clinical psychopathology, social dysfunction and burden on the family of psychiatric patients. *Psychological Medicine, 12*, 651–658.

Pickett, S.A., Cook, J.S., & Solomon, M.L. (1995). Dealing with daughters' difficulties: Caregiving burden experienced by parents of female offspring with severe mental illness. *Research in Community and Mental Health, 8*, 125–153.

Reinhard, S.C. (1991). Living with mental illness: Effects of professional contacts and personal control on caregiver burden (Doctoral dissertation, Rutgers University, 1991). Dissertation Abstracts International, 50/07, 2717.

Reynolds, I., & Hoult, J.E. (1984). The relatives of the mentally ill: A comparative trial of community-oriented and hospital-oriented psychiatric care. *Journal of Nervous and Mental Disease, 172*(8), 480–489.

Schreiber, R.S., & Stern, P.N. (2001). *Using grounded theory in nursing.* New York: Springer.

Stein, L.I., & Test, M.A. (1980). Alternative to mental hospital treatment: I. Conceptual model, treatment program, and clinical evaluation. *Archives of General Psychiatry, 37*, 392–397.

Strauss, A. (1975). *Chronic illness and the quality of life.* St. Louis: C.V., Mosby.

Terkelsen, K.G. (1987). The meaning of mental illness to the family. In A.B. Hatfield & H.P. Lefley (Eds.). *Families of the mentally ill: Coping and adaptation* (pp. 128–150). New York: Guilford.

Thornton, J.F. & Seeman, M.V. (1991). *Schizophrenia simplified.* Toronto, Canada: Hogrefe & Huber.

Torrey, E.F. (1988). *Nowhere to go.* New York: Harper and Row.

Torrey, E.F. (1995). *Surviving schizophrenia* (3rd ed.). New York: HarperCollins.

Torrey, E.F. (1997). *Out of the shadows: Confronting America's mental health crisis.* New York: John Wiley.

Tuck, I., du-Mont, P., Evans, G., & Shupe, J. (1997). The experience of caring for an adult child with schizophrenia. *Archives of Psychiatric Nursing, 11*(3), 118–125.

Walsh, M. (1985). *Schizophrenia: Straight talk for family and friends.* New York: William Morrow.

Wright, E.R. (1994). Caring for those who "can't": Gender, network structure, and the burden of caring for people with mental illness. (Doctoral Dissertation, Indiana University, 1994). Dissertation Abstracts International, 55/02, 380.

P. Jane Milliken, R.N., Ph.D., is an assistant professor in the School of Nursing, University of Victoria, British Columbia, Canada.

Herbert C. Northcott, Ph.D., is a professor in the Department of Sociology, University of Alberta, Edmonton, Canada.

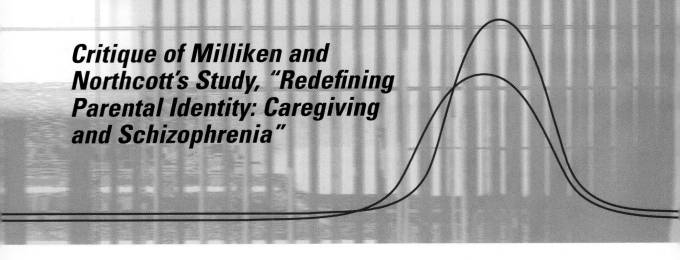

Critique of Milliken and Northcott's Study, "Redefining Parental Identity: Caregiving and Schizophrenia"

OVERALL SUMMARY

Overall, Milliken and Northcott conducted an interesting and important grounded theory study. The description of the results was filled with thick, rich slices of data on the seven stages of redefining parental identity that the researchers discovered through their research. The study has implications for nurses practicing in nursing home settings, as well as for public policy makers and advocates in mental health care. The researchers could have enhanced their report somewhat, however, by providing more detail about their methodologic decisions and the theoretical underpinnings of grounded theory (i.e., about symbolic interaction). They also provided only limited information about their efforts to enhance the rigour of their study.

TITLE

The title identified the name of the researchers' grounded theory: "Redefining Parental Identity." Their use of a gerund ("redefining") helped to alert prospective readers that this was a grounded theory study. The title could have been improved, however, by alluding to the fact that the focus was on parents caring for *adult* schizophrenic children. Here's one possibility: "Redefining Parental Identity: Caregiving to Adult Children With Schizophrenia."

ABSTRACT

The abstract succinctly and clearly summarized some of the main features of the study. Milliken and Northcott described the research problem, the study purpose, the specific qualitative research design that was used, the study participants, and the study significance. The authors could have provided a bit more information, however—the abstract was about 120 words, although 150 words are permitted by the journal. For example, the abstract could have provided more information about the method of data collection (in-depth interviews) and more specifics about the findings, such as that they discovered a seven-stage process of *redefining parental identity* that involved four parental identities with transitions between them. Also, in stating the study's clinical significance, the authors would have been prudent to offer more tentative conclusions, given the scale of the research. That is, it would have been more appropriate to state, "This understanding *might* be helpful..." rather than "... will be helpful."

INTRODUCTION

The introduction of Milliken and Northcott's report set the stage for the research by identifying the problem, articulating the phenomenon of interest, reviewing some of the literature, stating the purpose of the research, and indicating the study's significance.

Problem Statement

The introduction made it clear that the phenomenon of interest was parents' caregiving of an adult child with schizophrenia. The authors articulated the problem in the very first paragraph: with deinstitutionalization of the mentally ill, the burden of care is often transferred by default to families, who may be inadequately prepared for their role. This is a problem that is certainly relevant for nurses, as well as for other health care professionals and for those involved in mental health care reform.

Literature Review

In the first two paragraphs, Milliken and Northcott cited some relevant literature on family caregiving for mentally ill persons in general. In the third paragraph, the authors described two relevant qualitative studies of parental caregiving of children with schizophrenia. There are, however, additional studies that the researchers could have cited that might have provided a somewhat stronger context for their study. For example, Pejlert (2001) conducted a phenomenological study of the experiences of parents caring for an adult child with a severe mental illness (Pejlert, A. [2001]. Being a parent of an adult son or daughter with a severe mental illness receiving professional care: Parents' narratives. *Health and Social Care in the Community, 9,* 194–204). Another possible reference is a phenomenological study by Australian nurses on caring for a family member with chronic mental illness (Jeon, Y. H., & Madjar, I. [1998]. Caring for a family member with chronic mental illness. *Qualitative Health Research, 8,* 694–706). It is not particularly unusual, however, for qualitative studies to have literature reviews that are not comprehensive.

One other comment about Milliken and Northcott's literature review is that they used language that overstates the confidence that can be placed in research findings, for example, "Community care for the mentally ill *has proven effective* [emphasis added] when there is appropriate discharge planning...." The phrase *"has been found to be effective"* would have been better.

Study Purpose and Rationale

The report did not explicitly state any research questions. Milliken and Northcott did, however, state the purpose of the study, which was "to explain the subjective and emotional experiences of parental caregiving in schizophrenia." They also indicated that the broader goal was "to help us understand the challenges of schizophrenia for families."

In the concluding paragraph of the introduction, Milliken and Northcott provided an excellent rationale for undertaking this research. They stated that the Canadian Alliance for Research on Schizophrenia specifically asserted the need for research on the "complex interactions of specific families in order to identify positive attributes" that could affect improved mental health outcomes. They noted that their study directly addressed this need.

Framework

Milliken and Northcott noted that there have been some in-depth studies of parental experiences in caring for children with mental illness, but pointed out that there is little information about processes *over time*—over the whole trajectory of the child's illness. The congruence between the research problem and the paradigm and methods used was excellent. Milliken and Northcott chose a naturalistic paradigm for their study so that the voices of the parents could shed light on the phenomenon of interest. The authors chose grounded theory as their approach. This was a good match for the aim of the study, which was to "explain the subjective and emotional experiences of parental caregiving in schizophrenia." The authors chose this method because of its emphasis on social interaction and its ability to help them learn how the parents of schizophrenic adult children manage their lives.

One shortcoming of the introduction, in our opinion, is that Milliken and Northcott did not address the theoretical basis underlying grounded theory, that is, symbolic interaction. The introduction section of the report would have been strengthened by describing symbolic interaction and its ties to grounded theory and by referencing some primary sources for the readers.

METHOD

The method section of the report was brief but described the overall approach, sampling, data collection and analysis, and ethical concerns.

Approach

The methods Milliken and Northcott used to collect and analyze their data were congruent with the research tradition, grounded theory. The authors stated they used constant comparison, which is the appropriate method in a grounded theory study. The researchers should have, however, referenced the primary source for this approach, and should also have identified *which* grounded theory method was followed, such as Glaser and Strauss, 1967. (In the introduction, the authors cited a secondary source for the grounded theory method, i.e., Schreiber and Stern, 2001.)

Milliken and Northcott indicated that their design decisions unfolded during the course of data collection, and such an emergent design is proper in a grounded theory study. As one example, the researchers noted that, "over time, the interview questions changed" as their analysis progressed. They also made decisions to reinterview some participants "aimed at theoretical elaboration, saturation of incomplete categories, and verification of a theory."

Research Sample

Initially, the researchers sampled by convenience, through the assistance of two organizations: the British Columbia Schizophrenia Society and the Caregivers Association of British Columbia. The researchers were fortunate to have the cooperation of these two agencies, which were able to put them in touch with a number of families. (The eligibility criteria for the study were not, however, provided in the report.) The researchers also used snowballing; that is, they asked participants if they knew of other families who might be appropriate for and interested in the study. Again, this was an excellent source: the findings themselves revealed that the family members made contact with others in similar circumstances ("connecting with others" was part of the parents' process of redefining their identity). It appears that Milliken and Northcott did not use theoretical sampling in their initial recruitment of study participants. However, they reported that theoretical sampling (the respected sampling approach in grounded theory studies) was used to select participants for their follow-up interviews, which was commendable. Specific examples of their theoretical sampling would have proved helpful.

The researchers used the principle of saturation in their sampling decisions: they indicated that "data collection ended when the interviews produced no new categories and the analysis revealed the basic social problem experienced." The researchers were able to recruit an adequate sample for a grounded theory study (29 parents from 19 families), and achieved a sample with considerable diversity in terms of socioeconomic status, age and gender of their children, their children's living arrangements, and length of time caring for their children with schizophrenia. Commendably, the authors pointed out that their sample included families experiencing more chronic mental illness than is typical in schizophrenia, but that they were able to recruit families with "wide variation in parental experience." The sample's demographic characteristics—including characteristics of the parents and those of their children—were adequately described.

Data Collection

The researchers' actual data collection procedures were not explained in detail, and a bit more information might have been helpful to readers. For example, the report did not state who conducted the interviews. Did one or both authors do the interviewing—or were the interviews conducted by a research assistant? Also, the researchers did not indicate the length of time they spent data collecting, although they did mention that they conducted

32 interviews in total (3 were second interviews) and that they analyzed 53 hours of interviews. Their in-depth interviews were about 1½ to 2 hours, which are sufficiently long to obtain rich detail, and were conducted in a private setting. Parents, except for one couple, were interviewed separately (there was no information on why the exception occurred). Interviews were audiotaped and then transcribed verbatim, which helped to preserve the richness and accuracy of the data.

Milliken and Northcott's interviewing technique was appropriate for a grounded theory study. They started interviews at the beginning of the study using broad, open-ended questions regarding caring for an adult child with schizophrenia. As the grounded theory developed, the interview questions changed. Questions then focused on saturating categories and on exploring new categories introduced by the participants. Toward the end of data collection, several participants (but how many?) were involved in follow-up interviews to help with saturation of incomplete categories. Some specific examples of the initial questions and the more focused and follow-up questions would have been helpful.

The researchers relied exclusively on self-reports as their source of data. Use of participant observation in addition to these interviews could have strengthened the study design. It might not have been possible to observe the parents in interaction with their children, but there might have been other opportunities for observation—for example, parents interacting with health care providers, or parents attending a support group meeting.

Rigour

Regarding enhancement of rigour, Milliken and Northcott did not have a separate section in their report on this topic, as is the case in an increasing number of qualitative reports, nor did they explain their efforts to ensure the trustworthiness of their data analysis in much detail. The methods they used to enhance the trustworthiness of their data included audiotaping and transcribing the interviews and collecting data until saturation was achieved. Member checking was also used ("we validated the emerging concepts . . . in follow-up interviews with selected respondents"). But many other methods could have been used (and perhaps they were, but the report did not state this). For example, there is no mention of investigator triangulation—did the analysis involve efforts to corroborate the coding and interpretation of the analysts? There is also no indication of peer debriefing, nor of efforts to search for disconfirming evidence. The issue of reflexivity also was not reported; no mention was made of keeping a journal, memos, or field notes. No specific examples of their audit trail for collapsing similar codes into more abstract categories were provided for readers. Specific illustrations of their decision-making process would have strengthened the report.

Ethics

With regard to the ethical aspects of this study, the authors did not specifically indicate that the participants signed an informed consent, but they did state that "we guaranteed confidentiality and anonymity, and informed participants of their right to withdraw at any point." The study received approval from the university Research Ethics Board.

RESULTS

Milliken and Northcott described their process of data management and data analysis in general terms. For example, "we coded transcripts phrase by phrase and collapsed similar codes into increasingly broad categories." No specific data were presented to illustrate the steps taken for analysis. Apparently missing from their data analysis was theoretical coding, which is an essential component of the constant comparative method. The report did not offer insights into how the categories were related to each other.

Milliken and Northcott could have strengthened their results section considerably by including a figure depicting the seven stages of their substantive theory on redefining parental identity. A figure would have communicated clearly the four different parental identities and the transitions between them. Without a figure, it is difficult for readers to develop an overview of the processes that the parents experienced.

Nevertheless, Milliken and Northcott's analysis appears to have yielded insightful findings on parental caregiving and schizophrenia. The authors allowed the basic social problem to emerge from the data. The basic problem was that parents believed they had a right and obligation to care for and protect their adult children; however, inasmuch as their children were adults, society and health care providers did not sanction this. Milliken and Northcott then identified the basic social process of redefining parental identity. They reported four parental identities, and the transitions between them led to seven stages of redefining parental identity. Milliken and Northcott did an excellent job summarizing their substantive theory. The excerpts they chose from the participants' interviews were powerful.

DISCUSSION

The major findings of this grounded theory of redefining parental identity were discussed in the concluding section of the report. Milliken and Northcott began by pointing out, to their credit, that the process they outlined in the report is seldom as linear as described. They astutely observed that the children's trajectory of illness brought with it relapses, parental regression to a prior identity, and then forward progress once again.

A major portion of the Discussion focused on their findings in relation to the theoretical writings of Fisher and Tronto (1990), who described four interconnected components of caring. This discussion provided an insightful further interpretation of what these parents experienced in caring for their adult children. However, it would have been useful if the researchers had also linked their findings to prior studies, especially studies of the experiences of parents of adult children with a mental illness. As it is, we cannot easily ascertain whether the findings are congruent with earlier research.

Milliken and Northcott did discuss an important feature of their study, namely that it offered a glimpse into the issue of caregiver burden over an extended time span. They commented on the limitations of efforts to capture a snapshot of caregiver burden, usually soon after a patient leaves formal care, and noted the need for longitudinal studies of how caregiver burden evolves over time.

The authors did not, unfortunately, describe the limitations of their study, nor did they address the issue of the transferability of the findings. They did, however, discuss the implications for clinical practice and issues for mental health care reform. And, as noted, they also made suggestions for future research. One such suggestion focused on testing and refining the grounded theory to examine how well it can extend to other groups with similar experiences, such as bipolar illness.

GLOBAL ISSUES

Milliken and Northcott's report was well written and well organized. The description of the method section could have been more detailed, however, with specific examples for illustration, but the description of the findings was rich and vivid. The process of redefining parental identity was filled with meaningful evidence for nursing practice.

RESPONSE FROM JANE MILLIKEN

I am in complete agreement with the critique. A number of your comments and suggestions for strengthening the article were actually met in the research but stemmed from having to reduce a 320-page dissertation down to article length. I was quite surprised, in fact, when you mentioned that interviews were the only source of data, given that I had also engaged in, admittedly limited but still significant, participant observation at monthly meetings of the BC schizophrenia society and also had a number of short documents and poems that parents had written. On checking the article, however, I was amazed to find that I had neglected to mention those.

Index

Page numbers in bold indicate glossary entries.

C